THE NATURE DOCTOR

A MANUAL OF TRADITIONAL AND COMPLEMENTARY MEDICINE

❋ THE ❋ NATURE DOCTOR

DR H.C.A.VOGEL

A MANUAL OF TRADITIONAL AND COMPLEMENTARY MEDICINE

FOREWORD BY **JAN DE VRIES**

Instant
Improvement
Inc.

The Nature Doctor is not intended as medical advice. Its intent is solely informational and educational. Please consult a health professional should the need for one be indicated.

THE NATURE DOCTOR

Published by arrangement with Dr. H.C.A. Vogel
Copyright © Verlag A. Vogel, Teufen (AR) Switzerland 1952, 1991
ALL RIGHTS RESERVED

German title: *Der kleine Doktor*
New English edition prepared by Harry Selbert
Drawings by Verlag A. Vogel

Library of Congress Cataloging-in-Publication Data

Vogel, H. C. A., 1902-
    [Kleine Doktor. English]
    The nature doctor : a manual of traditional and complementary medicine / H.C.A. Vogel ; foreword by Jan de Vries.
        p.   cm.
    Translation of: Der kleine Doktor.
    Includes index.
    1. Herbs—Therapeutic use   I. Title.
    RM666.H33V64   1991
    615'.321—dc20   91-25186
                                                                        CIP
ISBN 0-941683-27-3 (Hardcover)

Fourth Hardcover Printing, 1994

Printed in the United States of America

Published by Instant Improvement, Inc., 210 East 86th Street New York, New York 10028, with the permission of Keats Publishing, Inc., New Canaan, CT.

Contents

Foreword   xvii
Preface   xix
A Doctor in Your House   xxiv

Part One

Treatments to Try Out   1
Burns and Scalds   1
Cuts, Scratches and Grazes   1
Inflammation of the Eyes   2
Colds   2
Catarrh   2
Hoarseness   3
Chilblains and Cold Feet   3
Tired Feet and Legs   4
Haemorrhages and Haemophilia   5
Abdominal Disorders   5
Heartburn   5
Digestive Upsets and Cramps   6
Constipation   6
Diarrhoea   7
Slimming   8
Headaches   9
Facial Neuralgia   9
Your Iron – a Help for Aches and Pains   9
Urine Retention   10
Combatting the Accumulation of Uric Acid   10
Limewood Charcoal Powder   10
Curing Rheumatic and Arthritic Ailments without Medication   11
Corn (Maize) and Millet Porridge   11
Itching and Burning of the Skin   12
Eczema and Other Skin Eruptions   12
Boils   13

Whitlows (Paronychia)   13
Swelling and Bruises   13
Insect Stings and Bites   14
Insect Stings in the Mouth and Throat   15
False Sea Onion (*Ornithogalum caudatum*)   15
Convulsions   16
Excessive Libido   16
Conclusion of Part One   16

Part Two

Fever – an Alarm Bell   19
Cooperating with Nature   22
Pain – an Alarm Bell   23
The Correct Thing to Do   24
Heed the Warning   25
Advice for Expectant and Nursing Mothers   26
Dealing with Calcium and Silica Deficiencies   29
Dangerous Influences during Pregnancy   30
Mastitis (Inflammation of the Breast)   32
Infertility – the Pros and Cons of Hormone Treatment   33
Two Solutions to Consider   33
Other Important Observations   34
Infant Care   35
Baths   35
Skin Care   37
Remedies   37
Infant Nutrition   39
Mother's Milk   39
Solid Food   41
Infants' Complaints   42
Cradle Cap (Crusta lactea)   42
Infantile Eczema   44
Children's Diseases   46
Measles   48
Mumps   50
Whooping Cough   50
Coeliac Disease   51
Poliomyelitis   53
Influenza   54
Virus Influenza   55
Checklist for the Treatment of Influenza   56
The Brain   57

What Can Damage the Brain?   59
Taking Precautions   60
The Pituitary Gland (Hypophysis)   60
The Master Gland   60
Care of the Small Wonder Gland   61
Headaches – their Causes and Treatment   62
The Tongue   63
The Sensation of Taste   63
Other Capabilities of the Tongue   64
The Tongue Can Be a Blessing   65
Taking Care of the Eyes   66
The Lacrimal Glands   68
Simple Remedies for Eye Problems   69
Infectious Suppuration of the Eyes and Mouth   69
The Nose   70
The Functions of the Nose   71
Treatment for Nasal Problems   72
Inflammation of the Ear (Otitis)   73
Middle Ear Infections   74
Sinus Infections   75
Sore Throats   76
The Treatment of Sore Throats   77
Hay Fever   78
Leucorrhoea and What to Do about It   79
Colds   81
During a Change of Season   81
Vitamin and Calcium Deficiencies   83
Foods that Build Up Resistance to Colds   84
Other Remedies to Build Up Resistance   84
Guarding against the Consequences of Infectious Diseases   85
The Remarkable Laws of Immunity   86
Laws We Should All Take Note Of   86
Why Natural Antibiotics Are Necessary   88
Building Up Resistance   88
Various Antibiotics in Practice   88
Natural Antiobiotics   89
Improving the Value of Raw Food   92
**Looking after your Health – the Best Prevention against
   Respiratory Diseases**   92
Various Causes   92
Adequate Nutrition   94
Skin Care and Other Precautions   95

The Importance of Joy and Correct Breathing	95
Asthma	96
Nervous Asthma	96
Bronchial Asthma	96
Cardiac Asthma	98
Important Factors in the Treatment of Pulmonary Diseases	99
Calcium	100
How to Overcome Calcium Deficiency	101
The Lesser Known Benefits of Calcium	104
Our Blood – a Mysterious Fluid	105
The Lymphatic System – the White Bloodstream	107
Functions of the Lymphatic System	107
How to Keep the Lymph Healthy	100
Tuberculosis and Cancer	110
Lymphoadenoma	111
Looking After our Capillary System	111
Our All-Important Circulation	112
The Marvellous Design of the Circulatory System	113
The Important Function of the Arteries	114
Narrowing and Hardening of the Arteries	115
Arteriosclerosis, Coronary Thrombosis and Heart Attacks	117
Embolism and Thrombosis	119
Preventative Treatment	119
Calcification and Calcium Preparations	120
Older People and Calcium	122
Diets for Hypertension, Arteriosclerosis and Other Signs of Old Age	124
A Recommended Diet	125
Normalising the Blood Pressure through a Wholegrain Rice Diet	128
What Can You Expect to Achieve?	129
Low Blood Pressure (Hypotension)	129
What Relief is Available?	130
Other Remedies and Treatments	131
Varicose Veins	132
Sclerosing	133
Surgery	134
Natural Regeneration	135
Phlebitis (Inflammation of the Veins)	137
Leg Ulcers	137
Circulatory Disorders	138
Chilblains	138

Gangrene	139
Haemorrhoids	140
The Treatment of Haemorrhoids	140
The Heart – an Indefatigable Organ	141
The Heart's Matchless Activity	141
Complications Deserving Attention	142
Interesting Help for the Heart	143
Lycopus europaeus – **a Remedy for Palpitations**	144
Modern Heart Poisons	145
Stress – Pace and Haste	145
Smoking	146
Only One Heart!	147
Beware of Heart Attacks	148
Finding a Happy Medium	149
Recommended Changes	150
Athlete's Heart	150
Angina Pectoris	151
An Old Country Remedy	153
The Woody Partitions inside the Walnut	153
Sick without a Sickness	154
Hyperthyroidism	155
Neurodystonia (Autonomic Nervous Disorders)	155
Visible and Invisible Goitre	156
Causes and Cures	157
Post-Operative Treatment of Goitre	158
Goitre and Iodised Salt	158
Iodine	160
Where Iodine Can Be Found	161
The Effects of Iodine Deficiency	161
Menstrual Problems	162
Menopausal Problems	163
The Kidneys	164
Noteworthy Characteristics of the Kidney Structure	164
Harmful Influences	165
How to Detect Kidney Disorders	166
Kidney Colic	167
The Urinary Bladder	170
Inflammation of the Bladder (Cystitis)	170
Bed-wetting (Enuresis)	171
Prostate Trouble	173
Inflammation of the Testicles (Orchitis)	174
Skin Disorders	175

Eczema and Other Skin Eruptions 175
When a Tendency to Eczema Runs in the Family 177
Psoriasis 179
Nettle Rash (Urticaria) 181
Simple Remedies for Neuritis 182
What Is an Allergy? 183
What Can Be Done about Allergies? 184
A Fast Cure for Shingles (*Herpes zoster*) 184
Spasms and Cramps 185
Our 'Nasty' Sympathetic Nervous System 186
Prevention Is Better than Cure 187
Insomnia 187
Some Reliable and Inexpensive Remedies for Insomnia 189
Epilepsy – New Views concerning its Treatment 191
Reasoning on the Evidence 192
Tragic Hereditary Factors 193
Basic Qualifications for Starting a Family 194
The Treatment of Psychosomatic Illnesses and Mental Disorders 195
The Meaning of the Word 'Soul' 195
The Interaction of Mind and Body 196
Natural Treatment 196
From my Own Experience 197
New Approaches to these Problems 197
Nursing Patients with Mental Problems 198
Weight Control (Overweight and Underweight) 201
Guidelines for Slimming without Danger 203
The Stomach 206
Hunger and Appetite 206
Stomach Disorders 207
Gastric Acid 208
Gastric Ulcers 210
Poisoning of the Stomach and Intestines 212
Causes 212
Successful Treatment 213
Special Guidelines 214
Appendicitis 215
Non-Surgical Treatment 216
Diarrhoea 217
Is Constant Diarrhoea Harmful? 217
Effective Treatment 218
Chronic Constipation 219

The Dangers of Leaving Constipation Untreated   219
Natural Remedies   220
Do Starchy Foods Cause Constipation?   223
Two Soups to Open the Bowels   224
Dysbacteria   225
Intestinal Parasites   226
Threadworms and Roundworms   227
Tapeworms   230
Dangers of the Tropics   232
Hidden Dangers – Parasites and Micro-organisms   233
Tropical Diseases   234
Precautionary Measures   237
The Liver and Gallbladder   239
Causes and Symptoms of Liver Disorders   239
Liver Disorders and Nutrition   243
Treating Infectious Diseases of the Liver and Gallbladder   249
Oil Cure for Gallstones   250
Jaundice   252
The Pancreas   253
Proper Care of the Pancreas   255
A Diet for Diabetics   256
Multiple Sclerosis   258
The Real Cause   258
The Symptoms   258
Various Approaches to Treatment   259
Arthritis and Gout   262
Can Tomatoes Cause Cancer and Arthritis?   264
Rheumatoid Arthritis   265
The Living Cell   272
Cell Metabolism   273
Sick Cells   273
The Degenerated Cell   273
The Spectre of Cancer   276
A Question Still Unanswered   277
Is Cancer a Localised Disease or One Affecting the Whole
   System?   278
Is Cancer Communicable?   280
Susceptibility to Cancer Despite a Healthy Life-Style   281
Birthmarks and Cancer   282
Smoker's Cancer   284
Deadly Dangers in the Water   286
Beware of Carcinogenic Substances   287

Seven Basic Rules for the Prevention of Cancer   288
Remedies for Cancer   292
Bacteria and Viruses   293
Bacteria   293
Viruses   294
AIDS – Worse than Cancer   297
Our Teeth   299
Healthy Teeth and their Defence Action   299
Dead Teeth   301
Care of the Teeth   303
Periodontal Disease (Periodontitis)   308
Beautiful Hair – a Natural Adornment   309
The Structure of the Hair   309
Hair Colour   310
Care of the Hair   311
The Skin   313
The Functions of the Skin   313
Sensible Skin Care   319
Impetigo   324
Biological Treatment   324
Reliable Remedies for Fungal Infections (Mycosis)   325
Diseases of the Nails   325
The Feet – our Faithful Servants   326
The Structure of the Feet and the Need for Proper Care 327
Care of the Feet   327
Dealing with Excessive Foot Sweat   330
High Heels or None at All?   331
Walking Barefoot   332
Periostitis   334
Strained Ligaments and Sinews, Sprained Ankles   335
Back Problems   336
Hernias (Ruptures)   337
Preventative Measures   337

A Selection of Medicinal Herbs   338
How a Good Herbal Remedy Is Developed   338
How Herbal Remedies Can Be Used   341
Alpine Plants and Lowland Plants – Which Are of Greater
   Value?   344
Angelica (*Angelica archangelica*)   347
Bear's Garlic/Ramsons (*Allium ursinum*)   349
Butterbur (*Petasites officinalis [hybridus]*)   350

Comfrey (*Symphytum officinale*) 355
Maidenhair Tree (*Ginkgo biloba*) 359
Horsetail/Shave Grass (*Equisetum arvense*) 362
Lady's Mantle (*Alchemilla vulgaris*) 364
Lily of the Valley (*Convallaria majalis*) 365
Mistletoe (*Viscum album*) 366
Mugwort (*Artemisia vulgaris*) 367
Nettles (*Urtica dioica, Urtica urens*) 368
Oats (*Avena sativa*) 370
Papaya (*Carica papaya*) 372
Pimpernel Root (*Pimpinella saxifraga*) 374
Purple Coneflower (*Echinacea purpurea* and *angustifolia*) 376
Sea Onion or Squill (*Scilla, Urginea maritima*) 380

Wild Fruits and Berries 382
Barberry (*Berberis vulgaris*) 382
Hawthorn (*Crataegus oxyacantha*) 383
Juniper Berries (*Fructus juniperi*) 384
Rose Hips (*Rosa canina*) 385
Rowan Berries (*Fructus sorbi*) 387
Sea Buckthorn (*Hippophae rhamnoides*) 387

*A Brief Guide to Selected Homoeopathic
   Remedies* 390
Aconitum napellus (Aconite, Monkshood) 390
Atropa belladonna (Belladonna, Deadly Nightshade) 391
Coccus cacti (Cochineal) 393
Guaiacum officinale (Guaiac, Resin of *Lignum vitae*) 393
Kalium iodatum (Potassium iodide) 394
Lachesis 394
Daphne mezereum (Daphne, Spurge Laurel) 395
Sepia officinalis (Sepia) 396
Tarentula cubensis 396
Urtica dioica, Urtica urens (Stinging Nettle) 397

Four Biochemical Remedies 398
Calcarea fluorica (Calcium Fluoride) 398
Natrum muriaticum (Cooking or Table Salt, Sodium
   Chloride) 399
Natrum sulphuricum (Glauber's Salt, Sodium Sulphate) 400
Terra Silicea purificata (Silica) 401

Seasonings   404

Culinary Herbs Are Medicines   404
Garlic (*Allium sativum*)   409
Garlic Milk   410
Onion (*Allium cepa*)   411
Shallot (*Allium ascalonicum*)   412
Cress   412
Horseradish (*Armoracia rusticana*)   413
Black or Spanish Radish (*Raphanus sativus*)   415
Salt as a Medicine   415

Various Diets and Treatments   417

Serious Vitamin Deficiency in the Spring   417
Internal Cleansing in the Spring   419
Programmes to Purify the Blood   422
Kelp and 'Spring Fever' or Fatigue   424
Water and its Therapeutic Effects   424
The Therapeutic Value of the Sea   427
Alternating Hot and Cold Water Therapies   429
Steam Baths at Home   430
Sitz Baths and their Medicinal Value   430
The Schlenz Method (Baths of Increasing Temperature)   433
Kuhne's Cold Water Treatment   436
Revulsion by Means of Stimulation (Irritation) Therapies   438
The Medicinal Value of Clay   439
Herb Poultices   441
The Potato as a Remedy   444
Papain – its Origin and Uses   445
The Therapeutic Effects of Milk   448
The Curative Effects of Wheat Germ Oil   451
Honey – its Specific Therapeutic Effects   454
The Medicinal Value of Honey   455
The Wonder Jelly for Queen Bees – Royal Jelly   456
Pollen   458
The Curative Properties of Chicken and Chicken Fat   460
Red Slug Syrup (*Arion rufus*)   461

Questions of Nutrition   463

Natural Wholefood   463
Helpful Diets for the Sick   475
Fasting   480
Fattening-Up Diets   483

How Much Food Do We Need?   483
Vitamins   484
Overcoming Protein Deficiency   492
Eating Vegetables and Fruit at the Same Meal   493
Fruit and Vegetable Juices – their Effects on You   495
Difficulties in Adjusting to a Raw Food Diet   500
Berries   502
Be Careful with Stone Fruit   505
Fruit Sprayed with Pesticides   508
Rhubarb   509
Sugar   509
The Value of Canned and Bottled Fruit   514
Our Daily Bread   516
Whole Wheat and Other Cereals   519
Wheat Germ   521
Buckwheat (*Fagopyrum esculentum*)   523
What You Should Know about Potatoes   525
Oils and Fats   527
The Importance of Oil Seeds and Fruits   532
Almonds   535
Walnuts   535
Milk and Dairy Farming   536
Yogurt   540
Coffee   542
Sauerkraut (Fermented White Cabbage)   545
The Art of Cooking Depends upon Proper Seasoning   547
Cooking Salt   550
Yeast and Yeast Extract   551

Miscellaneous Topics   553
Impoverished Earth, Rich Sea   553
No Life without Iodine   554
Poisons that Are Difficult to Eliminate   557
Look Out – Metallic Salts Are Hazardous   562
Copper Cookware   566
Are Synthetic Fibres Detrimental to Health?   567
Animals and Insects as Carriers of Disease   569
Climatic Influences   571
The Sun Means Life and Death   572
Intense Heat and its Dangers   575
Breathing Means Life   577
Fresh Air   582

Oxygen as a Healing Factor   583
The Effects of Smoking   584
Stress – a Disease of Modern Times   587
Housing Problems and Sickness   589
Taking Health into Consideration when Building a House   590
Questions of Health and the Protection of Nature   593
Television and Health   596
The Need to Relax   599
Tiredness – a Natural Symptom   601
What Is Exhaustion?   605
Natural Sleep   606
What Do Dreams Tell Us about Ourselves?   612
The Symptoms of Old Age   615
Gratitude – a Remedy   617
The Therapeutic Power of Music   619
The Therapeutic Power of Peace and Quiet   621
Happiness Means Health   624
Recommendations for Breakfast   632
Recommendations for Lunch (Midday Meal)   634
Recommendations for Supper (Evening Meal)   635
Important Basic Rules for the Healthy and the Sick   635
Fasting – a Means to Combat the Damage Caused by
    Civilisation   637
Emptying the Bowels – Indispensable for Juice Diets   641
Health Benefits from Taking Vegetable Juices with a Specific
    Purpose   643
A. Vogel's Rheumatism Cure   651
Are Nitrates Poisonous?   653
The 'Nature Doctor' Takes his Leave   654
A Special Note   655
Index   659

Foreword

In my mind I often relive my first meeting with Dr Vogel. It was not a lengthy meeting, yet it was to determine my future in more ways than one. During that fateful meeting I immediately realised how exceptional a person Dr Vogel was in his chosen field. It was with fascination that I listened to what this talented man had to say and I was delighted when the possibility arose for me to be trained by him.

It is now almost thirty-five years since that first meeting; in the meantime I have worked for him and worked with him, both of which I still consider a privilege. I have been able to observe him in his work with patients and have listened to him conduct lectures for thousands of people. Over the years, his tremendous knowledge has confirmed my impression of his exceptional qualities.

In those early days of our acquaintance Dr Vogel inspired in me the fervent wish to follow in his footsteps and I subsequently did everything possible to be trained to become like him, that is, to be able to help those who are suffering.

Over and over again he has surprised me by being such an excellent tutor. One only needs to read the first section of this book, one of the many Dr Vogel has written. He generously shares his ideas with the reader and in so doing passes on invaluable advice on a wide range of health problems.

I consider it a privilege to have been asked to write a foreword to this book, not only because of my admiration for Dr Vogel, but also because I have been able to turn to his books for guidance on countless occasions in order to help the thousands of people whom I have attended to at my own clinics.

In this new edition he has sought to advise the reader on new methods that are of specific relevance to today's environmental and ecological conditions.

I carefully adhere to Dr Vogel's philosophies which he has taught me over the years and I know that one of his main aims is to instruct his patients and the general public alike in the many natural ways in which suffering and pain can be relieved. As he often points the way to the simple methods available to us in nature, I have no doubt that this book will find a place in many households as a useful source of valuable information and sensible advice on treatment without side effects.

I once joined Dr Vogel on a walk through the Jura mountains, accompanied by a group of medical students. The educational value of this exercise was most impressive as he pointed out the many roots, herbs, leaves, berries and flowers along our path and explained to us their medicinal value. Dr Vogel's great knowledge and the secrets he revealed to us added greatly to the enjoyment of this walk. An even bigger revelation awaited us when we arrived at our destination. Although our guide was considerably older than any of us, Dr Vogel was the only one among us who was not totally exhausted. Surely this alone must stand as clear proof of the value of his philosophies!

Jan de Vries
Auchenkyle
Southwoods
Troon
Scotland

Preface

A Lifetime Devoted to Serving my Fellowman

It was in 1952 when I decided to publish the results of thirty years of experience in naturopathy, the treatment of disease by natural means and remedies. With the very first edition of *The Nature Doctor* (*Der Kleine Doktor*, in my native language) I hoped to stimulate a greater awareness of traditional natural medicine, to help the sick and aid the healthy to prevent illness and disease, withholding nothing that could be of benefit to my fellow man. Would I succeed?

The answer speaks volumes: since those small beginnings not only has the number of items and pages steadily grown in the course of more than fifty editions, but over 1½ million families around the globe have bought the book in one of the twelve languages in which it is published and with it have acquired a 'resident doctor' right in their own homes. That *The Nature Doctor* has proved an invaluable source of advice in days of sickness and of good health, making all my literary efforts most worthwhile, is seen in the gratifying number of letters still pouring in from appreciative readers.

So why publish another edition for the English-speaking public? I would like to reply by giving two related reasons. First, the constant changes in conditions and circumstances of our modern world call for adaptation in order to keep abreast with new developments. And second, there is my own personal involvement, my entire life being devoted to serving my fellow man, a kind of mission, if you will, urging me to enlighten, encourage and help towards a healthier body and mind.

As regards the latter, I am happy to see the worldwide fast-growing interest in natural medicine, phytotherapy (the use of plant medicines), homoeopathy, biochemical treatment, aromatherapy and other forms of alternative medicine. At the same time the modern way of life has given rise to new diseases, or an increase in the incidence of once lesser-known ailments, like viral diseases, chronic post-virus fatigue syndrome, candida albicans, stress, depressions, and AIDS, to mention but a few. Hence the need for up-to-date information, which prompted me to take on the arduous task of preparing a new edition of *The Nature Doctor*, including information on the most recent results of research, a chapter on viruses and bacteria, and details of some newly developed natural remedies.

But good health involves more than taking remedies. If we want to live healthy, happy and joyful lives, we must endeavour to re-establish the proper relationship between ourselves – the whole body and mind – and nature. There is no other way to lead a happy and satisfied life. If we violate nature, its harmony is destroyed, for we are part of nature. In the same way, all medical research is a waste of time if these holistic interrelationships are not taken into consideration.

I have always shown deep respect for nature and relied on it exclusively. Nature has been my most influential teacher and cherished university. It has been my endeavour to observe nature, to listen to it, in order to learn how to treat it and how we can use it beneficially.

I was born in October 1902 in Aesch near Basel, Switzerland. From my earliest childhood I remember that nature with its endless variety of plants and animals has always impressed and fascinated me. My thirst for knowledge, my curiosity, urged me to roam the fields, meadows and woods. My father and my grandmother in particular introduced me to the beauties of the colourful and often mysterious Creation around us. I used to wonder about things like ants, beetles, frogs and lizards until I began to understand more about them and acquire a deep sense of respect for every living creature. I esteem life as sacred. For this reason none of the body care products I have developed over the years are tested on animals, a practice that I am deeply opposed to.

My love of nature was behind my drive to explore and investigate, and led me to travel around the globe. The 1950s and 1960s were devoted to field research among native tribes in Africa, North and South America, Australia and Tasmania. I lived among them, sharing their work, their joys, their sadnesses. I was not motivated by a spirit of sheer adventure; I was keenly interested in their life-style, their diet and environment, their mind and body, and the connections and interrelations between these factors.

My fondest memories concern the Sioux Indians in South Dakota, where I spent some time. I was touched and thrilled to discover that we had a common understanding and loving respect for nature in spite of our different cultural and religious backgrounds. Nature is sacred to the American Indians and must not be destroyed. They understand that it can be used beneficially in many ways without having to violate it. Chief Black Eagle, with whom I was united in a bond of friendship, put it this way: 'I take a plant, put it in the earth, propagate it; nothing is destroyed, but I use it for myself in a natural way.'

I feel deeply indebted to the Sioux Indians for their knowledge of exceptional herbs which they shared with me. An outstanding example is *Echinacea*, the purple coneflower. I watched Indian women chew *Echinacea* leaves and apply the pulp to wounds and injuries. It was even effective in combatting the poison from venemous snakes, and particularly in cases of high temperatures and badly healing skin eruptions. Later I experimented with this plant and experienced its successful effects on my own body. I took some coneflower seed back to Europe with me, acclimatised the plant in cultivation, and developed a remedy from the flowers, leaves and roots that is now an accepted part of efficacious treatment with plant extracts.

As a nutritionist I discovered among such primitive peoples the real cause of the ever-increasing cases of 'diseases of civilisation' despite the astronomical amounts of money being spent on health and medical care. It is excess protein in the diet. Most of us eat two or three times more protein than is needed, in the form of meat, eggs, cheese and fish. Of course, protein is necessary in our diet, but too much of it triggers protein-storage diseases. Protein foods also produce excess acid, and the constant state of hyper-acidity in the body is one of the causes of cancer because protein is used in cell formation and also promotes cell proliferation, as in tumours, but also as in rheumatism, gout and arthritis. I found that these diseases are virtually unknown among people who still live close to nature.

I myself have been a vegetarian for seventy years. My diet consists of nothing but natural, unadulterated, excess-alkaline food, with a high proportion of raw foods, just as is the custom among primitive peoples, who follow such a diet unconsciously. They still live in harmony with nature, the exact opposite of the modern fast-food culture. *The Nature Doctor* advises on this subject more specifically in the course of this book. Primitive peoples have no knowledge of civilisational or mental diseases. The Congo pygmies, for example, dance for joy every day, even though it rains almost daily and they hardly ever see the sun shine through the thick forest canopy.

Finding the balance between nature, body and mind has been my endeavour and philosophy, a holistic approach. I formulated my concept – which has since been proved thousands of times over – to tackle the cause of an illness or disease, and to work in harmony with nature, never against it. Ignorance and unreasonableness regarding our body's requirements contribute up to 80 per cent to our falling ill. Today's orthodox medical opinion in the main still holds to the fundamentally wrong view that it is the illness or disease itself, the symptom, that has to be treated and if possible combatted or suppressed by strong drugs. *The Nature Doctor* is designed to help us regain our basic confidence in nature, which has been pushed aside and ignored as a result of technical and scientific progress. But thousands of years of empirical medicine, proven in practice, cannot simply be brushed aside without inviting trouble.

In my long life I have collected bit by bit and expanded the traditional and empirical knowledge of European folk medicine. My activities in the interests of sick as well as healthy people began in Teufen in the Appenzellerland. This is where I established a clinic based on naturopathy, gathered medicinal plants at the foot of the Swiss Alps and first prepared extracts from fresh plants. I discovered early on that these tinctures were more effective than those made from dried plants. Driven by my love of the Creator, nature and my fellow human beings, I have communicated my knowledge freely in innumerable lectures on all continents, and since 1929 I have reported my experiences and observations as a nature practitioner and researcher in my monthly periodical called *Gesundheits-Nachrichten* (A. Vogel's Health News). Some items which first appeared in this magazine have been included in *The Nature Doctor*, others have been published in my other books, *The Liver, the Regulator of Your Health, Health Guide Through Southern Countries, Subtropics, Tropics, and Desert Zones* (a guide for holidaymakers and those living in those regions), *Nature – Your Guide to Healthy Living*, and the most recent title, *Cancer – Fate or Disease of Civilisation?*

There is not one single home remedy, piece of advice, herbal or homoeopathic remedy mentioned in *The Nature Doctor* that has not been tried and tested by myself and thousands of patients. The reader can follow the recommendations with full confidence in nature and the body's inherent defence mechanism, or immune system.

To find your way about, look at the table of contents at the beginning, and to locate a specific subject, illness or remedy, check the comprehensive subject index at the back. In many instances you will find remedies drawn from nature's bountiful medicine chest, and natural treatments that need no outsider to help in their application. Of course, there are also cases when the advice of a qualified practitioner is indicated.

I am now in my eighty-eighth year and feel the proof of my philosophy confirmed in my own life. I still enjoy working every day; I am still chairman of the board of directors of the Bioforce Company, manufacturers of natural remedies, health foods and body care products, a company I established in 1963 to cope with the great demand for natural remedies and which now operates worldwide.

I still enjoy attending meetings and conferences, and meet regularly with doctors, scientists and researchers specialising in the field of natural plant medicine (phytotherapy). On these occasions I am often amazed to find that their latest knowledge usually confirms and vindicates what I have been propagating over seven decades in my books and lectures and have experienced with innumerable patients as a nature doctor – that man is a unit of body and mind, a marvel of nature that is subject to nature's laws.

If we seek and hope to achieve a real cure, whether in the case of a single patient or of the whole human race, that is, the survival of our natural environment, we cannot expect to achieve success unless we subject ourselves in everything to nature's balanced laws. For I am firmly convinced that despite the great achievements and advancements of modern medical science we ourselves – even with the most sophisticated medical equipment – cannot do the healing. Only nature can heal and cure. We can help and support nature and its laws that make a cure possible.

And it is with this in mind that I beg the reader to consider and apply the information contained in this latest edition of *The Nature Doctor*. Good health to you!

Dr. H. C. Alfred Vogel

A Doctor in Your House

What is the purpose of having a copy of *The Nature Doctor* in your house? Well, its simple but important task is to make you aware of the many natural remedies that are readily available in your home and immediate surroundings. When a sudden emergency arises or if you suffer from some persistent ailment, simply pick up *The Nature Doctor*, locate the appropriate entry and see what help is at your disposal to alleviate the pain or overcome the problem.

Of course, I don't know whether you live in a pretty little village or a small town. I have no idea whether you have to be content with living in the built-up area of a large city or whether you have chosen to live on a farm close to nature in the quiet countryside far away from other houses, villages or towns. You may have chosen to settle in a country where distance means nothing. You may even be a forester whose home may be a solitary house among the trees, or live high up in the mountains.

Whoever you are and no matter where you live, it will be to your advantage to consult *The Nature Doctor* in your hour of need, at least until you can call your family doctor who may be able to give you further assistance. Often, however, in an emergency the immediate help offered by *The Nature Doctor* may be sufficient to overcome your problem, because the right remedy given at the right time usually has successful results.

Perhaps you think that you and your family are assured of enjoying good health and that no misfortune could ever befall you. It often happens that day after day you go about your business and various tasks without anything happening to disturb the rhythm of your life. But suddenly something goes wrong – an accident occurs, be it ever so slight, an illness strikes, a cold or a bout of flu – and the daily routine is upset. At such times you will be glad of the immediate help provided by *The Nature Doctor*.

So what do you have in your house or nearby that will give you quick and reliable help? The size of your figurative medicine chest will depend largely on where you live and what can be found in and near your home. It may be that some of the remedies you need can be found in the kitchen, the larder or the cellar. You may even have some things stored in the attic that could be most useful to you. And if you have a garden, there are many plants that can come to your assistance. Better still, if you live in the country you will find an even more abundant supply of help in the fields, woods and meadows. If, however, you live in a town, you will simply have to keep your eyes open when out walking, because you can still find many plants that will be useful in times of need.

Should you run out of the usual remedies you keep in your house, our many little plant friends can act as preventative measures as well as remedies for less serious complaints. The number of medicinal plants found hidden in the woods, sprouting in fields and meadows, growing along river banks and streams is so great that *The Nature Doctor* would be more than twice its present size if it attempted to describe all the wonderful help nature's garden has to offer.

To begin with, *The Nature Doctor* will acquaint you with some of the remedies to be found right among your everyday supplies. You will be astonished to learn that many food items can have a medicinal use, for instance flour, sugar, water, oil, salt, eggs, soft white cheese ('quark'), potatoes, carrots, cabbage, radishes, onions, garlic, horseradish and parsley – to name but a few.

Welcome *The Nature Doctor* into your home and read it carefully. It will reveal many of the remedies that have been in your home all the time without your knowing it.

At first glance, the volume and diversity of suggestions and advice may appear confusing, but a careful examination of the comprehensive index at the back of the book will help you to quickly find the information you are seeking.

The simple examples found in Part One of the book will no doubt whet your appetite and encourage you to consult the more detailed sections that follow.

Part One

Treatments to Try Out

'Can I really trust your simple natural remedies?' you may ask at first. 'Will they encourage me to consult you whenever I am in need?'

'Of course,' the 'Nature Doctor' replies, 'try them and see for yourself!'

Burns and Scalds

Burns from flame or fire and scalds from boiling liquids call for quick action. Immerse the affected part of the body immediately in *cold water*. Where this cannot easily be done, apply a cold compress. Cover the burn with gauze, or with a clean cloth if a large area is affected, until medical help can be obtained. To avoid infection, do not puncture any blisters. In cases of third-degree burns, immediate medical attention should be sought if complications are to be prevented. *St John's wort oil* has also proved to be an effective remedy for burns and scalds.

Cuts, Scratches and Grazes

Superficial scratches and small wounds which prove difficult to heal can be dealt with quite simply. Use *concentrated whey (Molkosan)*, which is one of nature's best cleansing agents. Then dust the wound with *biological calcium powder* (for example *Urticalcin*) and, for two nights running, apply *soft white cheese* (quark). Should these items not be available, soak some *wheat grain* (which needs to be minced afterwards) or *bran* in fresh milk. Then cover the wound with the resulting mash and you will find that this also acts as a thorough cleanser. Once again dust the wound with biological calcium powder and after two days of treatment apply pulped *cabbage leaves*, preferably using Savoy cabbage for the best results. Cabbage leaf poultices have proved more effective than many modern remedies. If the wound is stubborn, causing swelling or

1

discoloration, and if everything else seems to have failed, you must not lose patience but continue the treatment with cabbage leaf poultices for weeks or even months. Alleviation will be experienced even in serious cases and a complete cure is often possible.

Inflammation of the Eyes
Lengthy exposure to the reflection of the sun on water or snow can make the eyes sore. Do you know what to do when you or someone in your family are affected in this way and perhaps the eyes begin to burn during the night? The remedy is quite simple. All you need to do is take the white of an *egg*, beat it lightly, spread it on a cloth, and bandage the eyes with it. The burning sensation will subside and the patient will be able to sleep. It is more than probable that the inflammation will have diminished, if not disappeared, by the morning. If no egg is available, *soft white cheese* (quark) or even a piece of *raw meat* (veal, beef or chicken) will achieve similar results. These well-proven remedies can be used whenever you need them, including cases of snow-blindness caused by the intense reflection of sunlight from snow and ice.

Colds
A 'streaming cold' is best treated with *onions (Allium cepa)*. Dip a slice of freshly cut onion into a glass of hot water. Remove the onion after only one or two seconds, allow the water to cool and sip this throughout the day. This is also an excellent remedy for spring colds. If, in addition, you place half an onion on your bedside table, you will inhale its odour while sleeping, thus reducing the tendency to catarrh and alleviating your cold. An *onion poultice* applied to the neck during the night is equally effective. Another way to help rid yourself of a cold is by sniffing up *salt water, lemon juice,* or a natural *calcium powder* (for example Urticalcin).

Catarrh
Perhaps you are prone to frequent colds and suffer from catarrh. If you have a *pine, larch* or any other pinaceous tree in your garden, take some of the *buds* which can always be found in various stages of growth on these trees. By chewing these buds slowly and thoroughly throughout the day, replacing them with fresh ones from time to time, the catarrh will be eliminated within a few days. So, when you go skiing or out for a walk, watch out for pine trees and take the opportunity to avail yourself of this

simple but effective remedy. Before retiring at night, dampen a cloth with *oil* (cooking or salad oil), wrap it around the neck and cover with a *woollen scarf* to keep it warm. This will help to clear up any irritating cough.

Hoarseness

The berries of the *mountain ash*, also known as *rowan*, are a good remedy for hoarseness. There may be a tree in your garden, or in a neighbour's, or you may remember seeing one on country walks. At the same time, you can look out for the *pimpernel*. To combat hoarseness, chew either rowan berries or pimpernel root, fresh or dried. Keep chewing these for as long as possible and let the insalivated juice run down the throat. This simple treatment makes hoarseness disappear in no time at all. Of course, you do not need to use both remedies together; either one on its own will no doubt help you. When you have lost your voice, rowan berries and pimpernel root are two of the best cures available.

Chilblains and Cold Feet

Have you ever wondered what causes these two unpleasant complaints? It is unlikely that you would be troubled with them if you saw to it that your vascular system, particularly the veins, were kept free from congestion. But if you do suffer, *hot and cold foot baths* can help. Begin by immersing your feet in hot water for several minutes, then place them in cold water and keep them there for the equivalent number of seconds; in other words, if you soak your feet for two or three minutes in hot water, leave them for only two or three seconds in the cold water. This procedure may be repeated 6–8 times at a session. Finish off with cold water, rub your feet vigorously with a towel and then apply a little oil (preferably *St John's wort oil*), if you like. This treatment will soon bring the circulation back to normal.

A much older but less known method of improving the circulation is that of *walking barefoot in the snow*. If your house or apartment has a veranda which becomes covered with snow in winter, you have the ideal location for this. Incidentally, this is a similar treatment to *treading cold water*, a form of hydrotherapy connected with the Kneipp method (see page 334). To start with, practise snow-walking for ten seconds, then thirty seconds, gradually building up to 2–3 minutes. However, a word of caution is called for here. Take care not to do this to the point where you start to feel chilled. After completing the exercise, and without drying your feet, go back inside to your warm bed. Do this every morning for several days in a row. If you have no balcony or veranda and have to leave your house to do your snow-walking, wear warm slippers to go outside, remove them quickly and start stamping around in the snow, preferably fresh snow. If at all possible, dry your feet vigorously with a towel before replacing your slippers to go back inside. Again, this treatment should be repeated for several days and you will be surprised to see how the chilblains disappear.

In order to prevent a return of the problem the following winter, *soak your feet* (for at least twenty minutes) regularly during the summer months in water to which *wild thyme* or *hay flowers* (*hayseed*) have been added. It is also helpful to go barefoot whenever possible so as to toughen up your feet.

You can also rub your feet with *lemon juice*. Let them dry naturally and then apply oil, *olive oil* being the best. In other areas, especially in the north, it is customary to use *paraffin* instead of lemon, although the smell is not as pleasant.

If you live near a place where cheese is made you may be able to obtain *whey*, which can be added to a foot bath. Sour whey is to be preferred to sweet for this purpose because of its more powerful action. These foot baths, although recommended for the summer period, can also be taken in winter as an alternative to the hot and cold baths or snow-walking. The water for the foot bath should be kept at blood temperature (37 °C/98.6 °F) by adding hot water whenever necessary; you can also, of course, add a decoction of herbs. The feet should be immersed for about thirty minutes and then rubbed with lemon. Finally, apply a poultice of pulped *cabbage leaves* and leave this on overnight. This treatment will not only do wonders for your chilblains, but will also be helpful when you suffer from skin eruptions.

Tired Feet and Legs

Should you be troubled with tired feet and legs, finding them even slightly swollen at the end of the day, bathe them in *potato or vegetable water*. Then wrap them immediately in a *cloth* that has been *covered with hot salt*. Do this every evening for a few days and the tiredness in your feet will disappear. If you have some *hay flowers* or other *herbs* handy, prepare an infusion and add salt, preferably sea salt, which is more effective than common salt. This salty herbal foot bath will also help you get rid of the tiredness, as well as relieving hot, burning feet. Swollen feet, especially ankles, can be a sign of heart trouble, but *The Nature Doctor* will deal with this later (see pages 138–9).

Haemorrhages and Haemophilia
If you know someone who frequently suffers from heavy nose bleeds, or who is a 'bleeder', any advice will be welcome. What can you do if the bleeding will not stop because the normal clotting ability is impaired? This can be a serious problem unless you know that applying a piece of *fresh raw chicken* is the only natural remedy to stop the bleeding if it is caused by haemophilia. However, if it is only a temporary disturbance it can be effectively dealt with by means of a herb called *tormentil*. *The Nature Doctor* will inform you fully a little later on.

Abdominal Disorders
Girls and women frequently suffer from venous congestions in the abdomen. *Water treatment* brings great relief, and it is recommended that a long *sitz bath* (hip bath) be taken once or twice a week to combat these disorders. For expectant mothers, this kind of treatment will also make confinement easier, thus benefiting the baby. Later on, it will help prevent difficulties arising during the menopause. The body responds to such regular care, and will give you far less trouble at these critical times than it would do otherwise.

Heartburn
A number of simple remedies exist for heartburn, a symptom of indigestion experienced as a burning sensation which may rise into the chest, even causing regurgitation of acid from the stomach into the gullet and mouth. All you need do first is to grate a *potato* as finely as possible, then put this in a cheesecloth and press out the juice. Dilute with warm water, one part juice to two or three parts water. Drink this juice every morning before breakfast, before lunch and at night before retiring. For the best results, prepare fresh each time.

If you still feel some discomfort, take a teaspoon of *wood ash* mixed in a little warm water after eating. This may produce the desired result. Just pour warm water over the ashes and drink them down. If you have no wood ash, common *charcoal*, preferably from limewood, can be crushed and mixed with a little water, porridge or other *cereal*. The charcoal is easier to swallow when prepared in this way and will serve to neutralise the stomach acid.

5

If you do not find the idea of taking wood ash as described above appealing, pour hot water over them and brew in the same way you would make a pot of tea, straining through a fine sieve or cheesecloth. This liquid will also neutralise the gastric acid. *Clay* (white or yellow) dissolved in a little water is equally effective.

In the absence of any of these remedies, sipping *fresh milk* will give temporary relief. Uncooked *oatflakes*, eaten dry and well masticated, are known to serve the same purpose and should be preferred to the more harmful bicarbonate of soda. If, however, you want to normalise the secretion of the gastric juices permanently, you will have to *modify your diet*: keep off spicy food, abstain from white sugar and white flour products, and use less salt. Drinking tea made from *centaury* and *Centaurium extract* has also proved helpful.

If none of these remedies produces the desired effect, it may be that the heartburn is caused by dysfunction of the gallbladder or by intestinal worms. In these cases, the appropriate treatments would be required. Both of these complaints are dealt with in Part Two of this book.

Digestive Upsets and Cramps
Eating too much, or food that causes the pancreas to go on strike, can result in abdominal cramps. A *hot shower* will help dispel the cramps if you remain under it for 10–15 minutes until the stomach area becomes bright red. If you have no shower you can achieve the same result by applying *hot moist compresses*. Follow up by applying a *poultice of chopped raw onion* or *pulped cabbage* on the stomach. The fermentation will cease, the cramps will subside, and you will be back to your usual self. Be sure to *chew your food thoroughly*, allowing it to become well mixed with saliva. If these simple suggestions do not help you must see your doctor, for there is a possibility of a perforation of the stomach, the presence of gallstones, or perhaps an inflammation of the appendix.

Constipation
Soaked *prunes*, taken first thing in the morning and last thing at night, will often remedy the problem of constipation. Young *stinging nettles* boiled in milk have also been found helpful. After removing the nettles, drink this milk every morning on rising. This simple remedy is equally effective in cases of migraine headaches accompanied by bilious vomiting. Stinging nettles eaten raw, as a salad, are also a wonderful remedy, being good for the blood.

The simplest remedy for constipation is to drink a glass of hot water first thing in the morning. But if this does not do the trick, eat a few slices of *fig paste*, which you can make yourself in the following way. Take 100 g (3½ oz) of figs, 100 g (3½ oz) of raisins, 20 g (0.7 oz) of senna pods (preferably powdered) and 20–50 g (0.7–1.75 oz) of ground linseed. Mix all the ingredients together, grind into a paste and shape this into rolls. Cut off slices as you need them.

There is also a special *soup* for sluggish bowels which you eat in the morning with a little *crispbread* or *wholegrain bread*. To make it, cook together freshly ground whole wheat, a small chopped onion and a crushed clove of garlic. When it is ready, add some chopped parsley and a spoonful of olive oil. This simple breakfast has cured many of their constipation. For more stubborn cases, however, ground *linseed* or *psyllium seed* should be added.

In Part Two, where constipation is dealt with in greater detail, a recipe for herb soup to relieve especially stubborn cases is given (see page 224).

Sometimes just a *change in diet* will provide the answer. Avoid anything that may have a constipating effect if your bowels are already sluggish. Sudden constipation, followed by diarrhoea, could indicate a tumour in the colon and medical attention should therefore be sought.

It may be that the constipation has psychological causes or is due to a weak nervous state, exhaustion or some mental anxiety. If so, it is essential to restore the *psychological balance* to ensure sufficient *sleep* and *relaxation*. Plenty of *exercise* should be taken, particularly if the sufferer has a sedentary occupation.

Diarrhoea

If your children, especially babies, have diarrhoea, give them finely grated *apples*. As an extra help, follow up with *oatmeal porridge*. Older children can take the *oatflakes* raw. They should chew them thoroughly, insalivating well, and preferably not be given anything else to eat for a few hours. For very stubborn cases of diarrhoea there is a simple plant that helps almost without exception. This herb, called *tormentil*, has already been recommended for haemorrhages.

Put bad cases of diarrhoea on a 'tea day'. What does this mean? Depending on the gravity of the case and the child's age, nothing but herb teas are given for 6–12, or even up to 24 hours. The following herbs are recommended: *Silvery lady's mantle (Alchemilla*

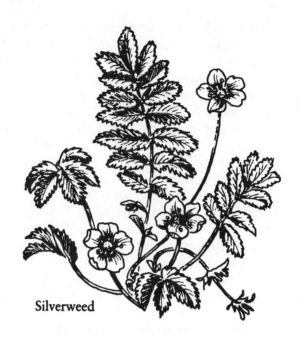

Silverweed

alpina), *bilberry leaves, sage, Iceland moss, silverweed (Potentilla anserina*), and *tormentil*. Furthermore, it is advisable to take activated *charcoal (Biocarbosan* contains charcoal and charcoaled coffee) to absorb the toxins present in the system. *White clay* has a similar effect. Food may be directly responsible for poisons entering the intestinal tract or the toxins can originate inside through putrefaction and excessive fermentation in the bowels, causing diarrhoea. Whatever the case may be, use activated charcoal to combat such upsets.

Slimming
Do you want to lose weight? If so, beware of harmful reducing methods. For example, do not eat five or six lemons a day for the sake of a shapely waist, because this could do irreparable damage to your liver. Follow a *sensible diet*, avoiding all starchy foods. If you must have meat, choose a little veal. Eat plenty of salads, seeing to it that you have a good variety at each meal. You may include steamed vegetables such as leeks, fennel, chicory, celery or celeriac, salsify and carrots. Fruit can be eaten in the mornings and evenings.

From time to time you will find it beneficial to have a *'juice day*', drinking nothing but juice, for example carrot juice. In the autumn, you may like to have a day when you only drink freshly pressed grape juice.

However, be very careful that your slimming does not harm your health. *Sitz baths* (hip baths) with sea salt and herbs that stimulate circulation are most beneficial for people who are overweight. In the kitchen, too, use only *sea salt (Herbamare)* for seasoning as the trace elements it contains will stimulate the internal metabolism and will help to dispose of superfluous fat. If you take *seaweed (kelp)* at the same time, your slimming diet will be even more successful. More detailed advice on the subject of weight control is given in Part Two of this book (see pages 201–7).

Headaches
Recurring headaches of any sort can be relieved by applying *onion* or *horseradish poultices* to the nape of the neck, the calves of the legs or soles of the feet. In this way headaches caused by an inflammation may be alleviated or even eliminated. However, since headaches may be brought on for various reasons, it is essential to discover the cause and treat it. Any treatment that only kills the pain can be dangerous. *Petadolor* is an excellent herbal remedy for headaches.

Facial Neuralgia
Excruciating spasmodic pain in the face originates in the nerves. The best and most effective remedy for this is a *hot shower* directed against the face, or, failing that, *hot water compresses*. These should be reapplied frequently so that they are as hot as you can bear them. Stubborn cases will need a *hot herbal compress*. It is sometimes necessary to continue this treatment for up to half an hour before the pain subsides and you begin to feel better. In cases where an abcess, sinusitits or glaucoma is the cause of the pain, these simple applications will not remedy the problem.

Your Iron – a Help for Aches and Pains
It is astonishing to realise the things you can do with an ordinary domestic iron. Neuralgic and rheumatic aches and pains resulting from a chill can be alleviated by rubbing the affected parts with *St John's wort oil*. Or, if you would rather, soak a cloth in the oil and cover with this. Then cover the oiled skin or cloth with a dry cloth and gently iron over with an iron at its lowest setting, for example 'synthetic fibres'. This procedure is quite easy to do. The

heat from the iron will thin the oil, making absorption easier. The effect of this simple treatment is so good that the pain is eased almost immediately. Take care, however, not to have the iron too hot, as you do not want to burn the skin.

Urine Retention
Elderly men who suddenly find themselves unable to pass water during the night will greatly benefit from a *herbal steam bath*. Make an *infusion of camomile or any other herb*, then add this to boiling water in a largish container. Place a narrow board over the container so that the patient can sit above the rising steam. Wrap a blanket or bath towel around the patient to retain the steam. This treatment will stimulate the flow of urine, bringing great relief, and the doctor will not have to be called out in the middle of the night to perform a catheterisation, a most unpleasant procedure. Should the retention of urine be caused by the prostate, further advice can be found under the entry on 'Prostate Trouble' (see pages 173–4).

Combatting the Accumulation of Uric Acid
This is often a long drawn-out battle. If simple remedies such as *parsley tea* are not enough to ease your painful limbs and joints, take a *herbal bath* using any herbs you have available. When you check your stock of herbs in the spring, planning to gather fresh ones, use what you have left in your baths, or make an infusion of cut grass and add this to the bath. Make sure the water is around blood heat (37 °C/98.6 °F); remain completely submerged, with only your nose visible, for 10, 15 or 20 minutes, even as long as half an hour. Have someone turn on the hot water so that the temperature can slowly rise to 38 °C (100 °F), and if you can stand it, to 39 °C (102 °F), following the *Schlenz method* (see pages 433–6). While submerged, have someone brush you vigorously with a stiff brush. If you take this bath once a week, you will be rid of your aches and pains.

To reinforce the treatment place a *poultice of pulped cabbage leaves* on the aching areas and drink plenty of raw *vegetable juices*. Be sure to eat enough alkaline foods and avoid offal, such as liver, kidneys and sweetbread, as well as alcohol.

Limewood Charcoal Powder
Those who suffer from gastric acidity, problems with the stomach and intestinal mucous membranes, or the consequences of protrac-

ted jaundice, should definitely take charcoal powder, preferably from limewood. You can make it yourself by grinding pieces of limewood charcoal. Take this powder in a little milk and, although milk on its own is not always suitable for patients with liver trouble or protracted jaundice, in combination with limewood charcoal powder it is very effective.

Curing Rheumatic and Arthritic Ailments without Medication
Begin your treatment in the morning by drinking half a glass of raw *potato juice* on an empty stomach; if you like, dilute it with a little warm water. All meals should consist of natural, organically grown foods. Detailed information on 'Natural Wholefood' is found in another section of this book (see pages 463–74).

An hour before lunch eat two or three *juniper berries;* chew them thoroughly, insalivating well, and swallow. After lunch swallow 2–4 whole *mustard seeds.* To quench your thirst during the day drink the water in which *potatoes* have been boiled.

Painful areas and arthritic deformities should be treated with different *poultices;* on the first day use pulped cabbage leaves; on the second day clay and on the third day, soft white cheese (quark).

Let me also remind you of a very old but effective treatment for sciatic and rheumatic pains, the *formic acid therapy.* Once every two weeks place the painful limb, say your leg or arm, in an anthill and leave it there long enough for the ants to inject their acid. Then, wipe them off with a brush or cloth and let the formic acid do its work. This is a simple, absolutely natural injection that does not cost you a penny.

Anyone who persists in the use of these simple methods of treatment, and in eating natural foods, will not only alleviate serious cases but cure them, even where the doctor has given up hope. However, if the patient suffers from a slipped disc or other disc trouble, it will be necessary to consult a good chiropractor.

Corn (Maize) and Millet Porridge
An excellent poultice for rheumatic and some arthritic pains can be made with corn (maize) or millet porridge. If you want to increase the circulation, producing hyperaemia, these poultices are most suitable since they remain hot for quite a while.

Prepare the porridge in the usual way, but without adding anything, and apply as hot as you can bear it.

Itching and Burning of the Skin

This condition, wherever it may be experienced, is always exceedingly troublesome. When applied externally, *potatoes* often give relief. Peel a raw potato and cut a slice, or grate it finely, and rub on the affected part, even on the face. But this treatment alone may not be sufficient. Quite often the kidneys are to blame for the condition and you will have to observe the treatment indicated in the section on kidneys at the same time (see pages 175–83). It may also be possible that the itching is a symptom of some liver disorder. In this case it will be necessary to consider the advice given under the heading 'Liver Disorders and Nutrition,' (see pages 243–9); the recommended diet for liver patients will be particularly useful. What is more, diabetes and intestinal worms may also cause itchy skin, as can the popular remedy *arnica*, if the patient is sensitive.

Eczema and Other Skin Eruptions

When treating eczema and other skin eruptions, it is essential to make sure that the kidneys, liver and intestines are working properly. Bathing the affected area in warm *whey*, preferably sour whey (*Molkosan*), is excellent. If you can spend your holidays in the country near a dairy where you can obtain whey, you may be able to do this regularly during your stay. Using bran to bathe the eruptions is also effective. Since eczema is sometimes difficult to cure and may require a great deal of time, you should not forget that the cause may not be internal but external. Some people are allergic to certain substances and plants, for example arnica. Your skin may be allergic to terpenes, in which case you would have to keep away from plants that contain them, such as conifers, and of course floor polishes and other products made with turpentine. Even camomile can provoke eczema, and so can *Rhus toxicodendron* (poison ivy), and the primula has been known to cause urticaria. So your eczema may well have one of these external causes. As soon as the right one is identified and the necessary measures taken, the eczema will disappear.

Children may break out in a rash when they overindulge in fruit. Strawberries can cause urticaria. In every case it is good to treat and stimulate the kidneys.

Skin rashes can also have their origin in poisoning or in a vitamin deficiency. It is therefore good to avoid eating, for example, sulphurised dried fruit, and fresh fruit or vegetables that have been sprayed with chemicals. Organically grown *spinach* and young

12

stinging nettles, preferably prepared as salad and dressed with *lemon juice* or *Molkosan*, will eradicate the deficiency and cure the rash in no time at all. Drinking tea made from *wild pansy* (heartsease) will reinforce the healing process.

Boils
Whenever you notice a hot, red swelling under the skin, or if you already have one or more boils, you can help to bring them to a head in the following way. Boil some ground *linseed*, or better still, *fenugreek seed* in water. Apply the resulting hot mash and this will soften the spot and draw the pus to the surface, enabling you to discharge it. If you have neither linseed nor fenugreek available, use hot mashed *potatoes* for a similar result. The wound can then be cleansed with highly diluted *Molkosan*. Then sprinkle with *lactose* (milk sugar), or better still, biological *calcium powder (Urticalcin) and apply pulped cabbage leaves.* You will be pleased to see how quickly this simple treatment works. As an additional support for the healing process, take *yeast extract* or *dried yeast* as a dietary supplement. Finally, do not forget to have your urine tested for sugar whenever you have boils.

Whitlows (Paronychia)
A whitlow is a painful, pus-producing infection of tissues around the nails of a finger or sometimes a toe. It appears quite unexpectedly and its discomfort impels you to take immediate steps to get rid of it. Soak the affected finger or toe in *hot water* (37–38 °C/98–100 °F) two or three times a day, for an hour each time, and be sure to keep the water warm. This treatment can effect a cure relatively quickly, but if not, ask a doctor to lance the finger in order to drain off the pus and prevent stiffening. It is also useful to know that not only hot water but also soft soap can be of help. Just spread the soap on the finger, bandage it and leave on overnight.

Swelling and Bruises
Any simple swelling or bruise responds well to treatment with *cabbage leaf poultices*. If these prove to be too strong, alternate with a *clay pack*. Mix the clay with an infusion of *horsetail* or any *other herb* for a better effect. Alternating the poultices from one day to the next is beneficial because clay reduces the swelling and cabbage leaves contain healing properties and also draw out toxins. This double action ensures a rapid cure.

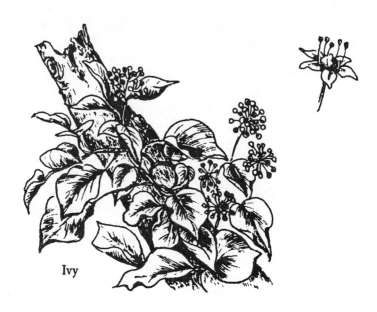

Ivy

Insect Stings and Bites

What a shock it is when you are stung by a bee or a wasp!
Immediately, you try to pull out the sting and suck out the poison
that has been injected, because you do not know how the body
will react. The pain is best alleviated by means of *ivy*. Perhaps you
have an ivy vine climbing up the garden wall or a tree, but if not
you should easily be able to find some in a nearby forest or wood.
Take a few leaves and some bark, crush them between your fingers
and rub onto the sting. Of course, it would be better if you already
had some *ivy tincture* in the house. This is quite easy to prepare.
Gather ivy leaves and cut off some of the green bark, then pass
them all through a mincer. Pour alcohol over the mash and let it
stand for a week or so. When ready, press through a sieve, filter
and bottle. A few drops of this tincture rubbed lightly on a sting
will quickly relieve the pain. Also effective are compresses made
with *salt water* to which a few drops of ivy tincture have been
added. Any of these treatments will prevent extensive swelling and
will neutralise the poison.

Fern (bracken) is an excellent remedy for bites from gnats and
similar insects. In tropical regions fern is the next best thing to
mosquito nets for protection. Stuff pillows and mattresses with
fern and you will not only be protected against all kinds of unwel-

come insects, even bed bugs, but will also have a means of relief from rheumatism. Fortunately, education has brought about great changes in matters of hygiene and such unpleasant invaders affect us much less nowadays than in the past, except perhaps in some old farmhouses. Nevertheless, it is helpful to know that rubbing fern on an insect bite helps to avoid any unpleasant consequences.

Insect Stings in the Mouth and Throat

It is unpleasant to be stung anywhere, most of all in the mouth or throat. This can happen if you fail to notice a wasp or bee on your bread and honey or in fruit. The very moment that the insect is pressed against the palate it will sting you, and this can lead to serious problems. What can you do? Dab the sting or gargle with *whey* or *whey concentrate (Molkosan)*. If these are not available, use concentrated *salt water* instead to reduce the swelling and prevent choking. You can help yourself in this way until a doctor arrives. Gargle repeatedly with a solution of salt water – two tablespoons of salt to 100 ml (¼ pint) of water. After a while the poison will begin to disperse and will also be partially drawn out by the salt water. After gargling, a *clay pack* or *cabbage leaf poultice* applied to the neck will be of further help in reducing the poison's effect. As a good antidote, take *clay* and, if possible, biological *calcium tablets (Urticalcin)* as well.

If you add a few drops of *ivy tincture* to the salt water the effect will be better still. The preparation of ivy tincture is described in the previous entry.

In the case of hornet stings it is imperative to see your doctor immediately or go to an ear, nose and throat hospital, because there is a greater danger of choking (oedema of the glottis).

False Sea Onion (*Ornithogalum caudatum*)

This onion is related to the lilaceous plant known as starflower. Its crushed leaves when used as a poultice are an effective remedy for a number of ailments; for example, wrap around the neck to alleviate headaches and sore throats; for rheumatism apply to the painful areas. They are also efficacious in cases of blood poisoning, suppurations and serious insect stings. Where splinters or thorns are buried in the skin and difficult to extract, the crushed leaves will draw them to the surface, thus averting the need for more unpleasant treatment.

Convulsions

If your children have ever had the frightening experience of convulsions – and the problem is not uncommon – you will know that there is very little that can be done to help. Yet there is a herbal remedy that is hardly known, *chickweed*, its botanical name being *Stellaria media*. This simple weed can be found in the fields almost the whole year round, giving you ample opportunity to gather it. It is the best possible remedy for children's convulsions. An infusion of chickweed has to be taken only a few times, whether made from fresh or dried weeds, and the unpleasant symptoms of these convulsions will disappear, often never to return. At the same time, chickweed strengthens the heart and it is this that makes it especially important when treating children. Chickweed is seldom mentioned in books on herbalism because its medicinal uses are very limited. Nevertheless, it deserves full recognition since its effect in curing convulsions is absolutely astounding. What a blessing it will be if the distressed parents can find it in the garden in their hour of need!

Excessive Libido

The excessive need for, or preoccupation with, sexual activity can be quite a problem but it is possible to do something about it. Drink an infusion of *wormwood* one day and of *hops* the next, continuing to do this regularly over a period of time.

Vegetables cooked with *soda* are also helpful; this method is used in prisons and certain other institutions as a preventative measure. However, this treatment is detrimental to health if resorted to for any length of time, although the degree of harm inflicted will depend upon the individual's susceptibility.

Instead, therefore, it would be better to restrict one's diet to food that is sexually less stimulating, and include plenty of *lemon juice*. Be sure to avoid eating eggs, oysters and celery.

Take *cold showers* and *Kuhne treatments* (see pages 436–8) for a calming effect.

Conclusion of Part One

At the beginning of this section the 'Nature Doctor' asked you to try out some of his simple natural remedies. How did you get on? Have you been encouraged to consult the rest of the book in which he presents more detailed information and reveals more of nature's secrets to benefit you even further? You will not be disappointed if you do.

In the second part of *The Nature Doctor* you will find a wide range of remedies and treatments for many different ailments, as well as additional advice for some of those already discussed. Given the great number of problems that arise in life, and not wanting to hold up publication, he did not cover everything, although he touched briefly on certain subjects. The 'Nature Doctor' wants all those who gladly accept nature's ways to benefit from his extensive knowledge and practical experience gained over the years.

His advice is in harmony with nature. It will increase your skill in caring for the sick and introduce you to a great variety of remedies.

All that's offered, examine more,
Then keep and use the best.
Of friends' advice you must make sure,
Man's brain oft fails the test.

All the things that in harmony are
With the laws of the One above,
Do only good, won't harm or mar,
Give a blessing – the way of love.

Plants' vital forces are on tap,
Natural, complete – just take.
Unadulterated, pure, fresh sap,
It's for one's own health's sake.

If, in time, progress you make,
Happy with the Maker's ways,
And pure foods you only take,
Success will bless your days.

First published in *Neues Leben* (May 1929).

Part Two

Fever – an Alarm Bell

If only everyone realised that a fever is nature's alarm bell, and actually a defence against harmful invaders, we would allow nature to take its course and give it our full support. Instead, in our mistaken fear and ignorance, we all too often run for things like aspirin and quinine to bring down a temperature the moment it rises above normal. We should stop to ask ourselves whether we know better than the natural processes that work within us. Why do we always want to reduce a fever? Why are we not grateful for it? Why do we not listen to the advice of those who know and understand its value?

Even in ancient times it was recognised that a fever has healing powers. One physician of that time said, 'Give me the power to induce a fever and I will show you the way to cure all disease.' Although his statement may be somewhat exaggerated, nevertheless, it is intrinsically true. Exceptions, of course, are the high temperature experienced in cases of suspected tuberculosis, Graves' disease, paratyphoid fever, endocarditis, and iron deficiency anaemia. It is generally known that a low body temperature can have a serious outcome because the physician's skill will not be enough to save the patient if complications set in and his body is unable to generate more heat. We would do well, therefore, to listen to the teachings of the physicians of antiquity and regard a fever as the healing agent it is. We should be constantly aware that a fever is our ally in the fight against disease, unless it is a fever induced by drugs, that is, by allopathic medicines.

What happens, though, if the body temperature keeps on rising and the patient is faced with an untimely demise? Did we not learn in school that we are in mortal danger when our temperature reaches 40.5 °C (105 °F)? So, should we let it rise and run the risk of dying as a result?

19

This will not happen if we simply use our gift of observation. Indeed, we do not have to go far to find an example that will illustrate the effectiveness of fever. We all know that for a stove to work well it must be properly ventilated. If it is, we can increase the heat as much as we like without damaging the stove. But if it is not, the coals will smoulder, with serious consequences to the stove. The grate may be damaged by the intense heat if the air flow from beneath it is allowed to become blocked. However, if the stove is properly cleaned out and the air can circulate freely, you will avoid the need to replace a damaged grate.

When applied to the human body, the principle behind this illustration will help us to know what to do. In fact, we will understand that a fever is, in a manner of speaking, nothing but an accelerated burning-up process. Therefore, we must see to it that the excretory organs are kept open, just as a fire needs good air circulation. The metabolic waste products must not be allowed to accumulate in the body but must leave it, in the same way as the 'ashes' must be cleared from the grate. Good bowel function is absolutely necessary for this, as is the adequate working of the kidneys and the skin. Give due consideration to these three factors and a fever will have hardly any damaging consequences.

When a feverish condition exists, the natural therapy method requires that first of all the bowels be thoroughly cleansed. An *enema* made from an infusion of herbs can be given, or a *natural laxative* taken. If the oral laxative proves ineffective, introduce it into the rectum.

A diuretic will help to stimulate the kidneys. One of the best remedies is *goldenrod (Solidago)*, but if this is not readily available use *horsetail (shave grass)*. An infusion of *parsley, onions* or *juniper berries* may also be effective. Should none of these be available, make an infusion of *rose hips* which, although relatively mild in its effect, is still better than nothing.

Once the kidneys are working properly, elimination through the skin must also be stimulated. *Hot compresses* are always indicated for the treatment of a feverish condition. If you are uncertain as to the correct procedure, ask for a practical demonstration at a home-nursing class or obtain some written instructions. To go about it the wrong way can do more harm than good. However, a compress for the chest or buttocks should not be too difficult to handle; just take care that there are no spaces between the skin and the compress. If the patient is well wrapped, he will soon begin to perspire. If he then complains of being too hot, you can always

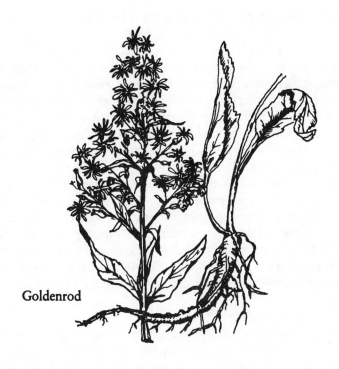

Goldenrod

apply *cold compresses to his calves* or put *socks soaked in vinegar* on his feet. It will not be long before the patient begins to feel more comfortable and so able to sleep. You now see how simple the natural solution is. There is really no need to give way to fear and make use of harmful pills and potions.

While nature's ways are quite simple, we tend to seek a far more complicated solution to our troubles. A prescription written in Latin, which most of us do not understand, seems to inspire more confidence than nature's easy way. We want a quick reaction, faster than natural treatment can give. Of course, we never admit that the sometimes dire consequences of such proceedings actually prove this method of treatment to be wrong. The simple and natural procedure which everyone is able to understand without any difficulty and apply in his own home, is considered to be backward and unorthodox.

Nutrition is another factor that merits our attention while a fever lasts. Normally the patient is not hungry and does not want to take anything. This is nature's way of indicating that feeding would not only be useless but actually harmful, since the digestive

21

system is almost inactive. Encouraging a fever patient to eat will not help him at all. Often, however, in these situations we want to spoil the patient with something special. We want to show him how much we care by preparing a juicy steak, fried eggs with cheese and other attractive combinations. However, it must be pointed out that a fever patient should not receive any protein or other food that is difficult to digest, only fruit juices being indicated. Should none be available, give him a little kidney tea or some water. If you wish, these may be sweetened with cane sugar. Alternatively, just use plain water with a natural product added (Molkosan or a herbal remedy). However, the best liquids are still fruit juices, and the fever patient will enjoy these more than anything else. Squeeze some grapes or oranges; the fresh juice will provide nutritive salts and vitamins. Let him sip the cool juice slowly and he will feel truly refreshed. It is not often that a patient cannot tolerate fruit juices, but if this is the case, a good nonalcoholic wine can be given. Diluted Molkosan is equally beneficial.

Cooperating with Nature
If the fever is assisted as described above, rather than suppressed, the temperature will not continue to rise, but will decrease slowly. This is nature's way, so do not try to make it come down faster. When the temperature rises it remains high until everything that has to be eliminated has been burned up; only then will it begin to drop. This is the natural process. Anything done in haste in reality only suppresses and does not eliminate, as we might be led to believe. At best, a sort of armistice will be achieved, but never the removal of the actual cause of the problem. Everything not eliminated through perspiration, the urine and the stools remains in the body, and these toxic residues can cause a relapse at any time.

You may have a temperature and the wonderful little tablets you take to get rid of it actually relieve your very bad sore throat. However, what you have done has not eliminated the toxins and the trouble may suddenly surface somewhere else in the body and in a different way. Pericarditis or rheumatic fever, perhaps even pneumonia, may attack you. We are all too familiar with the story of how a new drug can cure a disease with amazing speed, yet bring unpleasant side effects with it. Surely even orthodox medicine must begin to conclude from experience that 'wonder' drugs do not get to the root of the disease and that nature can neither be circumvented nor overpowered with impunity. The wild animal is often wiser than civilised man when it comes to knowing what nature requires for healing and recuperation.

In future, therefore, refuse to be guided by misguided views and dulled instincts. If we follow nature's lead, it can only be for our good. If, on the contrary, we ignore its direction, we are the ones who will suffer. We should always consider fever as nature's alarm bell, and need not fear it. If we cooperate with nature instead of resisting, it will be to our mutual benefit.

Pain – an Alarm Bell

Just as fever is nature's alarm bell, so does pain act as a warning of disruption in the harmonious workings of the body. But what can you do about sudden pain? Do you feel grateful for the warning that something somewhere in the body has to be put right? Will you try and find out what is causing the pain in order to treat it correctly? Oh no, for this is too time-consuming and we are not inclined to endure pain any longer than we have to. As soon as it arises we want to expel it. Of course, there are many proprietary drugs available for killing pain, which means you would have to be crazy if you continued to suffer longer than necessary!

How short-sighted this attitude is! Consider how differently we react when it comes to repairing, say, our car or some other machine. What motor mechanic believes that the fault has been rectified if he simply plugs his ears so that he cannot hear the rattling? Will he not rather be a credit to his trade by trying to get to the bottom of the problem and repair it before a wheel comes off or some other serious trouble develops? That is what we do with a machine, but the human body, which is much more delicate, we treat superficially, even though pain – that alarm bell – may be warning us that there might be something seriously wrong. In no way should pain ever be ignored or bypassed, which is what you are doing if you simply take a painkiller.

It is interesting to note that nature is always ready to make amends for our mistakes; so if we are conscious of them and willing to learn from them we will avoid making the same ones again. How strange, therefore, that we can be so thoughtless and, for instance, fail to draw the right conclusion when an analgesic no longer gives the relief that it used to. Instead of admitting to ourselves that the analgesic effect did not mean that the cause of the pain had been cured and that we were acting contrary to nature, we foolishly take ever stronger drugs in order to suppress the pain at all costs.

The Correct Thing to Do

The conscientious doctor will most certainly do his best to find out the cause of the pain. For example, if the patient complains about pain in the region of the liver, the doctor will not simply prescribe a painkiller, but will check for symptoms of a liver disorder. He will ask whether fats disagree with the patient, what is the colour of the stool, in short, he will do all that is necessary to get to the root of the trouble. Having diagnosed the cause, he can then prescribe the appropriate remedy. At the same time, he will indicate the right kind of *diet*, including a course of *carrot juice*. *Radishes* will be permitted only in very small quantities as a remedy, since large amounts can do considerable harm to the liver. This is how the doctor will inform his patient about the best way he can help himself to improve his health.

The same doctor will proceed in a similar way if a patient complains about pain in the kidneys. He will ask whether the skin over the area feels tight, as if being contracted. He will also want to know the colour of the urine and the quantity expelled daily. If the answers lead him to suspect a kidney disorder, he will then analyse the urine in order to obtain more specific information. He may discover albumen, red and white blood corpuscles, perhaps some cylindrical or epithelial cells from the bladder, the renal pelvis or the kidneys themselves, as well as bacteria. Even if only traces of these are present in the urine, he will advise the patient to take the precautions of adopting a *low-salt diet* and wearing *warm clothing* to avoid catching colds and chills. Recommended *herbal teas* would be *horsetail, birch leaves* and *Rhizoma graminis* (couch grass root), as well as *parsley*. In addition, the doctor will advise the use of *warm compresses* to ease the painful area.

The above examples show what the doctor must do to discover the cause of pain, in order to prescribe the appropriate medication and treatment. There is no other way. Merely alleviating pain, the symptom, will be of no service to the body. People who habitually swallow analgesics little realise that their constant headaches may well be due to persistent constipation. Who would think that the toxins remaining in the bowels could be the cause of such headaches? Would it not be more appropriate to take steps to improve the bowel function instead of resorting to a constant succession of pills and powders? First for constipation, next, for a headache, and then for constipation again! And if, some twenty-five years later, cancer of the bowels is diagnosed, the patient will not be able to understand it, especially where there is no history of cancer in his family.

Heed the Warning

Some doctors fail to diagnose and treat the root cause of a patient's chronic constipation and merely prescribe a laxative. So it is not surprising that in time the patient will suffer serious consequences. It would be much better if the doctor were to consider the patient as a whole, that is, regarding his body as a unit and realising that what affects one organ will also influence others.

The same principle applies to abdominal pains experienced by many women. Often, leucorrhoea and menstrual cramps are neglected and their cause, restricted circulation, remains untreated.

Of course, there are some people who instinctively know what to do in such circumstances, whereas others have no idea whatsoever. It is the latter group who need guidance and advice.

Sitz baths (hip baths) relax the abdomen and relieve congestions. It is helpful if infusions of *herbs* such as hay flowers, camomile or juniper leaves are added to the water. The temperature of the bath should not rise above 37 °C (98.6 °F), so as not to make the blood rush to the head. Since the patient should remain in the bath for half an hour, she should maintain the required temperature by adding hot water. These hip baths will do much to relieve the cramps, and if they are continued over a period of time even the leucorrhoea may be cured. It stands to reason that every woman should give the best possible care to her abdomen, rather than letting congestions, irritations and inflammations linger and so endanger the vital organs it contains. Even the smallest upsets can, in time, develop into bigger and more serious ones. So do not neglect these early signs of trouble if you want to avoid ending up on the operating table. Rather than suffer such unpleasant consequences of neglect, it is simpler to take good care of yourself.

When it comes to the care of plants we use much more common sense than is often exercised towards our body. If a tree in your garden produces a shoot that you can see will grow in the wrong direction, you are not likely to wait until it is a branch as thick as your arm before sawing it off. Rather, you will remove it immediately – yes, 'nip it in the bud'. Because you know that 'big oaks from little acorns grow'. The same principle applies to pain. It should never be merely palliated but rather accepted for what it is, nature's early warning system. Therefore, it is essential to treat

25

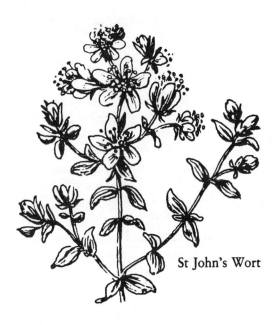

St John's Wort

the cause of the pain before it can develop into something more serious.

Advice for Expectant and Nursing Mothers

During pregnancy and even afterwards, the mother's happiness is often marred by such troubles as phlebitis (inflammation of the veins), thrombosis and embolism.

A few words of advice on how to help and perhaps even avoid these problems will undoubtedly be welcomed by all mothers. There are certain herbs which, when combined, work wonders for the veins. In cases of phlebitis, varicose veins and thrombosis this blend is so effective that we are happy to name the herbs for the benefit of expectant and nursing mothers. They are:

−*St John's wort (Hypericum perforatum)*,
− *Yarrow (Achillea millefolium)*, and
−*Arnica root (Arnica montana)*.

Tea made with these herbs is an excellent remedy for the afore-mentioned troubles. It would be even better to use the juices derived from the fresh plants, that is, the fresh herb extracts, since they are stronger.

All expectant mothers should make a note of this simple medication, because it has brought fast relief to hundreds of women – particularly nursing mothers – who suffered from varicose veins and ulcerated legs.

The therapeutic action of each of the herbs is as follows. The fresh plant extract made from St John's wort flowers and buds is an effective wound-healing remedy, as is St John's wort oil. It is an excellent remedy for severe pain in cases of injury to the nerves, concussion and injuries to the spinal cord; where the nerves are badly affected; for post-operative pains and for neuralgias, especially headaches resulting from mental strain and overexertion.

Yarrow, or millefolium, fresh plant extract is primarily indicated as a remedy for varicosis, haemorrhoids, varicose veins, venous obstructions in the abdomen and in the legs, also when there is a rush of blood to the head, frequent and excessive nosebleeding, and haemorrhaging of the bladder.

Arnica is another good remedy for the treatment of the veins, mainly in cases of stagnation of blood in veins and injuries to the soft tissue; it also relieves the symptoms of aching, heavy and tired legs and ankles. Moreover, arnica has an extraordinary effect in helping to restore the mother's organs after childbirth. Varicose veins, which are often a feature of pregnancy, can be combatted by means of this plant. It is also an excellent and reliable remedy for high blood pressure, even after a stroke, heart trouble or any similar disturbance caused by restriction of the veins. Arnica has proved its worth in the treatment of ulcerated legs, but for this purpose the extract made from the root, not the flowers, is indicated. The flowers and the tincture obtained from them are only for external use.

Pulsatilla (pasqueflower or wind flower) is another remedy for circulatory disorders. It belongs to the family that includes the buttercup and *must not* be taken as a tea because of its strong, almost poisonous effect. For this reason it should be used only in homoeopathic potency. There are no restrictions on the three herbs described above, which are quite safe.

An excellent tonic for the veins is *Aesculaforce*, a fresh herb preparation made from horse chestnut, sweet clover (also called melilot), witch hazel and arnica. The medicinal value of horse chestnut for the venous circulation has been clinically proved. Witch hazel is also prized for venous problems, and can be used internally and externally. Sweet clover strengthens the capillaries and improves the venous return, and since arnica stimulates the

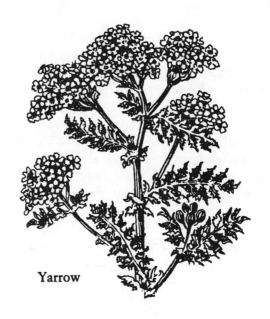

Yarrow

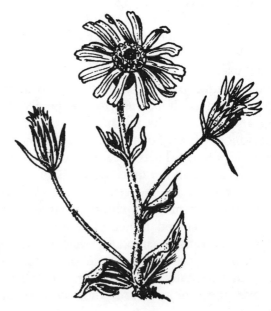

Arnica

circulation, it is an ideal choice to complement the other fresh herbs.

For morning sickness during pregnancy there are three simple remedies. *Nux vomica 4x* usually disperses the unpleasant nausea from the first day. In some exceptional cases, if this should prove ineffective, try *Ipecacuanha 3x* or homoeopathic *Apomorphinum 4x*. For why should the mother-to-be endure the discomfort of morning sickness for weeks on end, which could mar the joyful anticipation of the coming event, when harmless homoeopathic remedies can make things so much easier?

For a trouble-free pregnancy and confinement it is further advisable to take the calcium preparation *Urticalcin*, in addition to the fresh herbs already indicated, together with a natural vitamin supplement, such as *Multi-Vitamin Capsules* or *Bio-C-Lozenges*.

Dealing with Calcium and Silica Deficiencies

It can happen that some time after the baby is born a mother develops signs of trouble with the glands and the lungs, possibly even tuberculosis. In such cases the disease has usually been latent, or the susceptibility to it was already present. Great demands are made on the body during pregnancy, which could cause an inherent weakness to manifest itself. It is generally known that the growing foetus requires large amounts of calcium in its development, so if the mother does not take care to provide her body with the necessary calcium – which she could well do – nature will not allow the unborn baby to suffer. As the foetus cannot look after itself, the calcium it is lacking will be automatically drawn from the mother's body, from her bones, teeth and tissues. Of course, this will make her own body deficient. The old saying that 'each child costs a mother a tooth', meaning that the demand for calcium is very great during pregnancy, is all too true. It is therefore important to eat plenty of *calcium-rich foods* during pregnancy, especially raw foods and, if possible, in a form that is easily absorbed. Finely grated raw carrots, cabbage salad, raw sauerkraut and other foods rich in calcium should be eaten daily. Good *calcium preparations* should also be taken, but not the more commonly sold lactic acid calcium. It is better to use preparations that contain plant calcium. Calcium obtained from nettles, for example, and other plants is much more readily assimilated.

In addition, it will be necessary to take *silica*. Plants containing silica, such as horsetail, hemp nettle (*Galeopsis*) and various others, are ideally suited for this purpose. You can either prepare infusions or use the fresh plant extracts. *Vitamin D* is also essential, for if it is lacking, calcium will not be fully assimilated and utilised by the body. Oranges, cod-liver oil, various emulsions containing cod-liver oil, and all natural products and nutriments containing vitamin D are indicated for this purpose. *Vitaforce* is a very good and balanced formula incorporating some of these substances.

Another important factor to consider is the efficiency of the kidneys and the skin. If these excretory organs are in any way obstructed, accumulations of uric acid and other metabolic waste matter will cause metabolic disorders and may prevent the assimilation of calcium.

Special attention must be given to the way you eat, that is, you should eat slowly, chewing the food thoroughly so that it becomes well mixed with saliva.

Returning to calcium for a moment, it has been observed that lack of calcium causes disturbances in the glands with internal secretions; the lymph glands can also be impaired. This can lead to flatulence, internal fermentation and putrefaction in the bowels, thus poisoning the system.

If all these factors are considered and care is taken to avoid the problems described, you will have a fairly good chance of escaping illness. It is, of course, impossible to evade every infection, but a bloodstream supplied with the necessary calcium and silica can deal with them much more easily. So, if your teeth are bad, if you are susceptible to colds, sore throats or other infectious diseases, or if you suffer from swollen glands, then you would do well to take the advice given. Why not put into practice the wisdom of the old proverb, 'Prevention is better than cure'? There is no more appropriate time to get into the habit of recognising suspicious symptoms and taking the required steps to counteract them.

Dangerous Influences during Pregnancy
Nothing gives greater happiness to a woman than giving birth to a healthy baby. No young person can fully understand the meaning of parental bliss until parenthood is realised. But how great is the distress when a sickly child is born, or worse, a deformed child, perhaps with twisted limbs, hands or feet missing, or any other of those terrible deformities which, unfortunately, can occur. How terrible must be a mother's feeling of guilt when she has to admit to herself that she might bear some or all of the blame for this calamity. Scientific research has shown that the first four to eight weeks, even the first three months of pregnancy, are the most

crucial as far as harmful influences on the developing life in the womb are concerned. Some suggestions are given below on what a mother-to-be can do to best prevent abnormalities in the developing baby.

NUTRITION AND EXERCISE
Anyone who appreciates the importance of proper nutrition will readily understand that the food of the mother-to-be should be as natural and free from additives as possible. As regards quantity, she need not eat more than she was used to before she became pregnant.

A pregnant woman should make sure to inhale plenty of oxygen to guarantee the best conditions for the child's development. This is best achieved by undertaking activities outdoors in the fresh air, for example by taking walks through forests, woods and fields. On the other hand, busy roads and streets with a lot of traffic polluting the air should be avoided.

ALCOHOL, NICOTINE AND RADIATION
It should be sufficiently well known today that alcohol in the body at the moment of conception may already have frightful consequences. It is therefore utterly irresponsible to beget and bear children while indulging in alcohol. Unfortunately, this often happens after parties where heavy drinking has taken place, even though such thoughtlessness may lead to a tragedy. Every mother-to-be should understand the risk and dangers of alcohol and make it her duty to abstain from it throughout her pregnancy.

It is equally irresponsible of women to smoke during pregnancy and while nursing. Research has shown that only a few hours after smoking, nicotine is already present in the mother's milk. Who, then, can guarantee that during pregnancy the poison will not reach the placenta – and the unborn baby – just as quickly?

If at all possible, X-rays, radium therapy and any other type of radiation used in modern therapies should be avoided. Unfortunately, it is impossible to escape the radiation that contaminates the air as a result of nuclear explosion drifts, since it is not in our power to do anything about it.

CHEMICAL MEDICINES
Every pregnant woman should firmly refuse to take chemical medicines for headaches or similar complaints; nor should she take sleep-inducing drugs. Most of us will remember the shocking news

about thalidomide and the tragedy it caused to possibly thousands of mothers who gave birth to deformed babies. This example alone should warn and convince any pregnant woman of the great danger of taking chemical medicines during pregnancy and while still nursing. Then it was thalidomide, tomorrow it will perhaps be a sulphonamide, and later it may be yet another product that will trigger the damage. Thus, it is better to use chemicals to clean your windows and floors and put them to other technical uses, but do not take them as medicines.

Pregnant women should take note and value their maternal duties more highly than the desire to use chemical medicines to obtain quick relief from headaches, indisposition or insomnia. On the other hand, there are plenty of harmless remedies made from plants that will help to alleviate such temporary problems. So why expose yourself to danger and reap irreversible consequences? Experience continues to confirm that natural remedies can truly aid a person without producing harmful after effects. Nevertheless, because of the unnatural conditions and unhealthy views to which we are subjected in this day and age, many people still seem to find it more expedient to rely on palliatives rather than trying to cure their ailments in a natural way. The results of their mistaken thinking should be evidence enough that the apparent detour required to adopt more natural means of healing is definitely worthwhile.

Mastitis (Inflammation of the Breast)
An inflammation which has been improperly treated, or not treated at all, frequently leaves nodules, or knots of cells, in the breast. This may possibly lead to breast cancer in later years. Gynaecologists are always on the alert when having to examine the breasts of patients, because breast cancer is very often detected. The breast being susceptible in this regard, it should be given more than the usual care and attention.

Inflammation of the breast can develop from a simple bruise. More frequently, however, an inflammation appears after delivery, during the period of lactation or at the time of weaning. It is imperative to treat an inflammation immediately, since lumps may form that lead to cysts. In cases where an abscess forms, it is best to let it come to a head and break open by itself. Of course, it may also be opened surgically. In either case scars will remain as the scar tissue will have lost its elasticity.

TREATMENT AND PRECAUTIONS
An inflammation of the breast is treated externally as well as internally. For internal treatment *Echinaforce* has proved to be extremely valuable. The use of *arnica tincture* and Echinaforce are indicated for external application. Rub them gently on the affected part, alternating between the two remedies. If the area is sensitive, the regular application of *warm compresses* with *mallow* or *sanicle* infusions will achieve faster results. For an even better healing effect, add to the infusion 5–10 drops of Echinaforce and arnica tincture.

Women who are breast-feeding and would like to reduce their milk supply may do so by rubbing the breasts with *lovage tincture* and taking an *infusion of lovage*, this herb being excellent for the purpose. In cases of miscarriage or stillbirth the milk will need to be removed with a breast pump until the remedies have decreased the flow. To prevent milk fever and inflammation of the breasts, every effort should be made to stop the production of milk by natural means. We recommend oiling the breasts regularly and, especially, rubbing the nipples with *St John's wort oil* or *Bioforce Cream* once or twice a week. This provides the additional benefit of preventing the skin from cracking.

Infertility – the Pros and Cons of Hormone Treatment

Women who would love to have children but remain childless often do everything in their power to fulfil their natural desire. This is understandable, since an unfulfilled yearning for children may lead to severe mental and emotional suffering. There are, of course, some women who have little or no desire at all for a child. Although they do not suffer by not having children, they do miss out on the joys of motherhood and the many natural pleasures which children bring to the home.

Two Solutions to Consider

The inability to have children is often connected with a hormone deficiency. In such cases there are two possibilities that can be pursued. First, the body may be stimulated in such a way that its own production of hormones is improved. On the one hand, this can be achieved through *hydrotheraphy*, by means of *sitz baths* (hip baths), alternating *hot and cold baths*, the *Kuhne treatment* and similar methods. On the other hand, stimulation of the circulatory system will boost the supply of blood to the abdomen, which in turn will step up the production of hormones and may eventually lead to pregnancy.

For stimulating the circulation remedies such as *Aesculaforce, Aesculus hippocastanum* and *Urticalcin* can be of great benefit, especially when supplemented by *wheat germ* or *wheat germ oil* (capsules). Although outdoor exercise and deep-breathing in the open air are necessary for the natural regeneration of the body, sporting activities should not be overdone. Rather, one's whole way of life should be normal and balanced. This is the natural and safe course of action to take first of all.

Some, however, immediately resort to the alternative course to overcome infertility since it may possibly assure quicker results, that of hormone treatment, especially treatment with gonadotropins. There are, however, certain risks involved. The degree of sensitivity of the female body varies greatly from one individual to the next and it is not easy for a doctor to find the right dose. Most people will be aware of the unpredictable results that an overdose of hormones can have. It is possible that a number of eggs become ready to be fertilised, resulting in twins, triplets or an even greater number of children. This would certainly be too much of a good thing, even for the woman who may have suffered previously on account of her childlessness. It is therefore preferable to try out the first solution, stimulating the hormone-producing glands in a natural way. Only if these efforts fail should one contemplate hormone treatment as a last resort.

Other Important Observations
In this context it is appropriate to take a closer look at the opposite method, the curbing of normal hormone production in the female body. Gynaecologists have observed that the inhibitory effect lasts only as long as the agent, for example the contraceptive pill, is taken. If a woman stops taking the 'pill', her body may react in such a drastic way that the end result will be multiple births. When they consider the risks of having triplets or quintuplets, some women may begin to realise the drawbacks of hormonal contraception and have second thoughts about taking the 'pill'.

Furthermore, some doctors have found that the taking of hormone preparations like contraceptive pills can increase the risk of developing cancer. This underlines the warning to women not to commit gross offences against nature, because of the unpleasant repercussions and detrimental side effects that may result.

Infant Care
Experience being a good teacher, no doubt many of our parents'
methods in caring for their children were very good. Some of their
ways, however, were quite wrong, since they were based on old
customs that do not meet the demands of modern hygiene. Just
think of the almost superstitious fear of water which led them to
believe that bathing, especially if frequent, was bad for the health.
There are still some older people who have never sat in a bath tub
and, what is more, who actually boast about it! When you read that
in days gone by children were carefully protected from exposure to
light, air, sun and water, so that they would not catch cold, you
may smile for knowing better, thinking it was a story from the
ancient past. But not so; it was the custom in our parents' or
grandparents' time. Again, it was also feared that children would
develop crooked limbs unless they were so tightly wrapped that
they were rendered practically immobile. Even today in some parts
of Italy we find evidence of babies so bandaged up that they look
like mummies. It is, therefore, not surprising that infant mortality
was once much greater than it is today.

Baths
Frequent baths are absolutely essential for a baby, not only for
hygienic reasons but also because of their importance in maintaining proper skin activity. Bathing removes congestions and stimulates the functions of internal organs and the endocrine glands. We
must not forget that the baby had been in the warm, even temperature of the mother's womb for nine months, protected from the
discomforts of the outside world and hidden under the mother's
heart. The newborn baby is suddenly introduced into a much
cooler environment to which its little body has to adapt. For this
reason the baby's first baths should never be hotter than blood
temperature, that is, not more than 37 °C (98·6°F). In summer the
water may even be a little cooler, especially if the water has been
warmed by the sun. The lively splashing and joyful shouts bear
witness to the pleasures babies derive from their baths. This can
also be seen in their frequent protests at being taken out of the
bath when they evidently think they should be allowed to stay
longer.
    Any medicinal additions to a baby's bath should be chosen with
the greatest care, since they can do much harm. It is impossible to
stop babies from sucking their wet fingers and swallowing some
of the bath water. Therefore, additions like pine essence or cubes

35

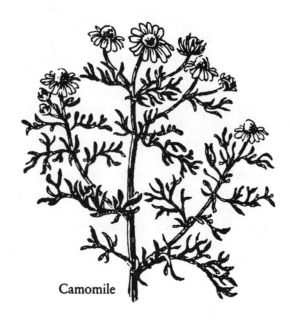

Camomile

containing the green iridescent colouring *Natrium fluorescentum* should be avoided. The same warning applies to acrid herbs like celandine and cranesbill which, although of great benefit for eczematous skin troubles and rashes, if used at all, should be added in only the smallest quantities. Babies have very sensitive skin and even seemingly harmless herbal additions to their bath water can cause quite unexpected reactions. The bath herbs listed below, however, are recommended for baby care. In all cases, only weak infusions should be used, since light stimulation is to be preferred for babies.

— *Horsetail* contains organic silica and exerts a beneficial influence upon the skin.
— *Lemon balm* is indicated for nervous babies who need soothing.
— *Lady's mantle* will give elasticity and tone to the tissues when they are spongy and flabby. (In cases of a tendency to hernia, this herb will help to strengthen the tissues.)
— *Camomile* is good for indigestion, stomach aches and minor metabolic disturbances.
— *Marigold* is useful when the skin is sensitive and affected by

rashes and impurities. (The flowers may be used as well as the leaves.)
- *Wild thyme*, also called Mother of Thyme, has proved its worth as an excellent bath herb and is especially valuable for babies who catch colds easily. Parents who themselves have weak lungs should give their babies this herbal bath from time to time.
- *Ribwort* should not be underestimated as a help in cases of a weak bladder; however, such a tendency does not become apparent in babies until they are toilet trained.

Skin Care
For cleansing the skin it is best to use a mild, super-fatted soap, 'baby soap'. Remember, the daily use of soap is not absolutely necessary. After bathing the baby a good skin oil should then be applied, but one that does not contain strong essential oils. One of the best is *St John's wort oil* with a tiny amount of mandarine, orange or lemon oil added (*Bioforce Body Oil*).

It is enough to oil the baby's whole body twice a week. The legs may be oiled every day, using St John's wort oil. Oiling is always better than powdering, as powder blocks the pores, absorbs the urine and encourages the growth of bacteria. Experience has shown that oiling is the better way and that it also prevents sores. If redness or soreness should appear, rub the skin lightly with a good woolfat cream, either genuine *lanolin* or *Bioforce Cream*, which also contains St John's wort oil.

Remedies
Household remedies and other medicines should be chosen with the greatest care. Babies react quickly to even the smallest dose and can tolerate only very light stimulants without suffering ill effects. This is especially true of teas (herbal infusions) and great care must be taken because an apparently harmless herbal tea can trigger serious upsets.

Homoeopathic remedies are ideal for the treatment of children. In fact, babies should only be given such remedies and it is lamentable that paediatricians do not prescribe them more frequently. Many allopathic drugs do more harm than good even for adults, so how much less would a young child be able to cope with their adverse effects? The amazing results achieved by homoeopathy should convince many doubters; they cannot be explained away as being 'imaginary' or 'psychological' effects, as some opponents try to do, for it can hardly be expected that babies and young children imagine these things.

It should be stressed again that infusions of herbs (teas) for small children should be very weak indeed, barely coloured. The herbs listed below have been found to be effective.

– *Fennel* (or *anise* if no fennel is available) belongs to the most common group of household remedies. Fennel, anise, caraway and dill are the so-called 'warming teas'. Whenever there is anything wrong with your baby's digestion, a weak fennel infusion will be of great benefit and will help the mother to remedy a temporary indisposition.

– *Yarrow*, given as a very weak infusion, is good for diarrhoea and loss of appetite. If this fails to stop the discharge, add a small pinch of *tormentil* and give teaspoonfuls of this weak infusion throughout the day.

– *Goldenrod* is a reliable remedy when the kidneys are out of order. The fresh plant extract from this herb, either as *Solidago* or as an ingredient in *Nephrosolid*, is one of the best and most effective medicines for the kidneys and the bladder. If you cannot obtain any goldenrod, a weak *rose hip* or *horsetail* infusion can be used instead.

– *Whey concentrate* (*Molkosan*) is a good antiseptic for minor injuries. This is a natural lactic acid product which can be used in the same way as iodine, although it is certainly less harmful than iodine.

– *Hypericum* can also be used as an antiseptic, and dabbed on externally. Dr Joseph Schier and other well-known paediatricians have recommended this simple remedy made from St John's wort even for the prevention of tetanus.

Calcium deficiency shows itself in various ways and can still be found quite frequently among small children. It prevents them from developing properly and makes them prone to catching frequent colds. If the mother wants an inexpensive, natural and good calcium preparation, she can make one up herself by doing the following. Pick some young fresh *nettles*, which can be found in most places, maybe right by the house or in the garden. Next, take some *egg shells*, which are on hand in practically every kitchen. People who live by the sea might like to use *oyster shells* instead. Crush the shells together with the fresh nettles and leave to dry in the air. Once pulverised, a light green powder will result. The child should take half a teaspoon of this 2–3 times daily. After a few months the teeth will improve and, in time, will become noticeably stronger. The bones will benefit also, and the susceptibility to colds and catarrh will diminish. If preparing this powder is too much of a bother, simply use *Urticalcin*, a ready-made calcium product containing stinging nettles.

If, in addition, the child has a deficiency of vitamin D, then you have the basic cause of rickets. Although serious cases of rickets, resulting in underdeveloped or deformed bones, are now extremely rare, less severe forms of rickets are still seen even today. It may seem strange, but children suffering from this mild form of rickets are usually very lively, react to everything quickly and their facial expression is almost too intelligent for their age. They tend to be precocious and always remind me of an apple that has grown ripe too soon. On closer examination the apple proves to be worm-eaten, and that is actually why it has ripened prematurely.

Such children who lack both calcium and vitamin D need help and can be helped. Homoeopathic or biochemical calcium triturations are excellent for this purpose, for example *Calcarea phos. 6x, Calcarea fluor. 12x* (for the teeth) and *Silica 12x*. The calcium preparation *Urticalcin* contains several calcium salts in various potencies, as triturations, as well as *Urtica* (as a vitamin D carrier), and is therefore also an efficacious remedy. *Orange juice* and *cod-liver oil* are rich in vitamin D and are highly recommended. Furthermore, *carrot juice* or the concentrate *Biocarottin*, which is made from fresh carrot juice, is another natural remedy for overcoming calcium deficiency.

Infant Nutrition

Mother's Milk
Mother's milk is the only natural and perfect food for a young baby. Nothing is more important for the infant's well-being and health in later life. This has been proved time and again by statistics on infant mortality which show that bottle-fed babies have a far greater death rate than those who have been breast-fed. In fact, the most crucial time for the baby is its first few days of life, when circumstances may decide whether it will live or die.

Even in animals we can see how nature does not tolerate any interference without serious consequences. Any farmer or country person knows how difficult it is to raise young animals, for example lambs, without their mother's milk, however strong they may seem at birth. Even the best lambs sometimes die if they are given cow's milk, or even if they are fed sheep's milk obtained from a ewe other than its own mother. Nothing is better for the newborn animal and its healthy development than its own mother's milk. A calf must have cow's milk, a lamb must have sheep's milk, and babies must have human milk. It alone is physiologically and biologically right in its composition to give the new human body what it needs for proper growth, for the development of the bone structure, nervous system and all the organs and tissues.

Breast milk, especially the very first secretion called colostrum, contains enzyme-like substances, nutritive salts and vitamins, some of which are known to us but others unknown; these cannot be found in any other food in the same quality and proportions. Moreover, breast milk is the source of immunising agents and alexins that protect the baby from diseases. Herein lies one of the greatest secrets of why very young breast-fed babies are immune to certain infections.

The argument that suckling a baby damages a mother's health and beauty can be refuted as unfounded because there is sufficient evidence to the contrary. A mother who is reasonably healthy actually benefits from breast-feeding, since during the time of nursing, under normal circumstances, the glands with internal and external secretions will function more efficiently and abundantly. The absorption of food and its vitamins is at its best at this time. The womb returns to normal much more easily in nursing mothers than in those who renounce their natural privilege and bottle-feed their offspring. Also, there is no doubt that a lasting psychological rapport and harmony are established between the mother and her breast-fed baby. In this way both mother and child profit by this natural relationship, as is always evident when we refrain from interfering with the Creator's natural laws.

For normal development and effective resistance to disease in the years to come, the foundation laid by breast-feeding is of the greatest importance to the baby. Experience and medical statistics prove that breast-fed babies recover from children's diseases much more easily and with fewer complications than bottle-fed children of a similar constitution.

Young mothers are sometimes unhappy and nervous when the flow of milk does not appear on the very first day. But it should be remembered that this would be quite unnatural as the baby should not receive any food during the first twenty-four hours of life. At the beginning, the breasts produce only the highly nutritious colostrum; the actual milk does not appear before the third, and sometimes on the fourth to the sixth, day. So, young mothers, do not despair when things do not immediately turn out in the way you may have expected. Later, if your milk supply is not enough to satisfy the baby, a few drops of *Urtica* every day, or a few tablets of calcium complex with *Urtica* (*Urticalcin*) will help the flow. Further useful information may be found in the section on cradle cap (*Crusta lactea*) on page 42.

Solid Food

Mothers often complain that their babies become constipated when they are fed brown rice gruel. It may well be that babies are more sensitive and that rice is more constipating than barley gruel, but because of its nutritional value it should not, on any account, be left out of the child's diet. The constipation can always be counteracted by natural means. Ground *linseed* is very good for the bowel action and should be added to the brown rice gruel. The amount to be used depends upon the child's reaction, but half a teaspoonful will usually be adequate. In this way the child will not be deprived of the goodness of brown rice.

Whole rye also makes a nutritious gruel. It may not be quite so creamy but it is certainly valuable, especially during teething. Rye contains not only calcium but also calcium fluoride, which is essential for the development of tooth enamel.

The best programme is to feed the baby alternatively rice, rye, barley, oat, perhaps even millet and buckwheat gruels, together with various juices, either carrot or fruit. Care must be taken, however, not to mix vegetable juices with fruit juices. In fact, it would be wise to avoid using more than one kind of fruit juice per meal, since sensitive babies may have difficulty in digesting the mixture. It would be better to mix one fruit juice with *almond cream*. This may be available already prepared from health food stores or can be made by grinding some almonds very finely and crushing them with a pestle and mortar; then mix with water in a blender. Mix the almond cream with the fruit juice in a blender and you will have the best food not only for your baby but even for older children and adults. Babies with cradle cap (see below) should definitely be put on *almond milk*, and if you want to clear up the condition, *Violaforce* and *calcium* must be added to their diet.

Infants' Complaints

Cradle Cap (Crusta Lactea)

Cradle cap in babies gives the parents a lot of trouble. Though many think that it is due to external factors, such as infections, this is not so. It is simply an abnormal oversensitivity, a so-called trophic allergy, possibly also a symptom of deficiency. If you deal with the causes the condition will soon disappear. On the other hand, the baby may have been born with the weakness of oversensitivity. Initially, treat the underlying cause: good digestion is important, so if anything goes wrong in this respect, the bowels should be normalised with the aid of *brown rice gruel, buttermilk* and other natural means.

In the case of breast-fed babies, the cause of cradle cap may be in the mother's diet. Unfortunately, few mothers pay much attention to the fact that anything they ingest, especially medicines, finds its way into their milk and is passed on to their babies. For example, a mother may be constipated and take a laxative. Then her breast-fed baby suddenly has a bout of diarrhoea. The baby is treated with all manner of things, without success, until bottle-feeding is resorted to and the diarrhoea finally stops. What a pity, though, since the infant is deprived of the best food for it – breast milk. With a little knowledge and forethought the upset would never have occurred in the first place.

While she is breast-feeding, a mother should not take any laxatives that contain aloe and other strong substances. Instead, linseed preparations, such as *Linoforce, psyllium seed* and similar remedies are harmless and can be used to regulate the bowels. Other medicines are also known to enter into the composition of milk when the mother has taken them. Among the most common of these are Luminal and many other barbiturates which are used to make up various sedatives and sleeping pills, as well as bromide, morphia and mercury preparations, quinine, salicylic acid and many remedies for rheumatism, iodide of potassium, alcohol and nicotine.

If a baby is indirectly fed such drugs we must not be surprised to see its health adversely affected. So, if your baby has cradle cap, think about the drugs you might be taking. If you have the unpleasant habit of smoking, you should certainly give it up while you are breast-feeding. Think of your child. Would you want your baby's health upset because your irresponsibility means it has to try and cope with poisonous nicotine?

Even during pregnancy nicotine has an adverse effect on the

unborn child. You can prove this to yourself by means of a simple experiment. Place a stethoscope on the mother's abdomen and count the child's heartbeats. Then let the mother smoke just one cigarette and then count the beats again. You will note that they have increased by eight per minute! Once the mother and her partner have convinced themselves of this overstimulation, they will be in no doubt that the mother should give up smoking at once.

Certain foods can affect the mother's milk in the same way as drugs. I have often seen a child's cradle cap disappear within a few days if the mother avoids eating egg white. It is, therefore, especially important to adopt a healthy diet while breast-feeding, as set out in another section of this book (see pages 39–41). Nursing mothers should remember that they are eating for both themselves *and* the baby.

Try to breast-feed your baby for as long as possible. But if, in spite of changing your own diet, the child's condition remains unaltered, then replace a meal by giving a bottle of *almond milk* or *buttermilk*. Babies suffering from cradle cap respond well to this less fatty food. *Violaforce*, the fresh plant extract made from wild pansy, can be added to buttermilk to enhance its curative effect.

If the ailing child is already weaned, instead of cow's milk give the child almond milk only. However, this requires accurate weight control. Some babies cannot assimilate vegetable protein and will lose weight. In such cases, if a protein supplement in the form of soy flour does not produce the necessary weight gain, animal protein, in this case milk, will have to be resorted to once more. Frequently, goat's milk or sheep's milk is better tolerated than cow's milk. Older children suffering from very stubborn cases of cradle cap should be given wheat germ. In all cases, nothing but natural remedies should be employed, never chemical preparations.

Sometimes the natural treatment brings very quick relief, but there are other cases that require more time and patience. As an example, one worried mother wrote to me asking for advice on how to cure her little daughter's cradle cap. She also sent a sample of the child's urine, an analysis of which revealed the existence of a liver problem. Almond milk and diluted carrot juice, to be given as a bottle-feed, were recommended, as well as a biological calcium preparation to rectify the girl's calcium deficiency. Mild stimulation of the kidneys was also necessary, for which a very weak *kidney tea* with a little *Solidago* (goldenrod) was prescribed. In addition,

Violaforce was prescribed; this is the best remedy for cradle cap and the one that especially guarantees a successful result. For external treatment it was recommended that the mother use *St John's wort oil* and then dust with *Urticalcin* powder. Bran baths are excellent for this too.

A year later the mother sent us the following brief note: 'Last year you helped us cure our little girl's cradle cap. Thank you ever so much.'

Another letter we received from a nurse reads:

'At the moment I am looking after two children. The boy, now 15 months old, had cradle cap last year. You sent me a calcium complex (Urticalcin), *Viola tricolor* and whey concentrate. Thanks to your excellent remedies the condition cleared up within a fortnight.'

In this particular case, diluted *whey concentrate (Molkosan)* was used to dab on the rash. Excellent results have also been achieved by dabbing on *Echinaforce*, a fresh plant preparation made from *Echinacea*. Water and soap are quite unsuitable for cradle cap and must be avoided. Instead, use oil, preferably St John's wort oil, to cleanse the baby's skin. It is indeed good to know that cradle cap can be successfully treated with these natural remedies, sparing the children permanent harm.

Infantile Eczema
Children's dermatitis or infantile eczema is a distressing condition, since it is not only a strain on the child, but also on the parents, due to the constant extra care and attention the child has to receive.

In 1964, at the Convention of the German Society for Child Therapy held in Munich, Dr Holt, an American paediatrician at New York University, presented the viewpoint that the 'tar therapy' was still the best method for the treatment of infantile eczema and that using tar extract of 5 per cent was also more economical than treating with steroid ointments. Also of considerable interest was Dr Holt's concession that infantile eczema is much easier to suppress than it is to cure.

With the help of the 'tar therapy' it is relatively easy to reduce the severity of the condition from degree IV to degree I, but Dr Holt admitted that this therapy is not enough to effect a complete cure. What was not mentioned was the fact that once the tar therapy is discontinued the little patient will quickly experience a worsening of the condition. Neither was there any mention that tar, with its eleven hydrocarbons, including napthalene, has been recognised as a carcinogenic – cancer-producing – substance.

RECOMMENDED TREATMENT

Unfortunately, no other paediatrician present at the convention could offer a better therapy, although several do exist, for example a *milk- and protein-free diet* and treatment with milk enzymes, that is, with *whey*. Not one of those present explained that treating infantile eczema with whey concentrate (Molkosan) can result in unexpected cures. It is indeed unfortunate that this treatment is so little known and appreciated by the medical profession, especially considering that it has been in use for many years. Centuries ago it had already been noticed that eczema began to heal when the patient was bathed in fresh, or even better, sour whey. If *Violaforce*, a fresh plant preparation made from the wild pansy, is applied at the same time, the cure is even more striking.

Since children with eczema also tend to suffer from calcium deficiency, taking *Urticalcin* will prove helpful. This calcium preparation in powder form, if applied externally, will prevent harmful bacteria from from entering through the pores of the skin. Instead of steroid ointments, use a lanolin cream such as *Bioforce Cream*. In the end, the doctor will be delighted with his little patient's progress.

Obviously, the child's diet is another important factor. Since milk proteins are to be left out completely, the inclusion of vegetable protein is vital. In this regard soy protein or almond protein, as provided in almond cream, have proved of great value. Special attention should also be paid to providing a salt-free diet. The speakers at the paediatric convention in Munich, however, made no mention of these factors whatsoever.

The subject of nutrition brought to light an interesting discovery. The doctors reported that infantile eczema was fairly prevalent among the affluent families of Nigeria, who live according to European standards, whereas among the natives who have held on to their traditional way of life it was rare or unknown. On the basis of this finding it can be concluded that the incorrect nutrition and living habits associated with our civilisation are contributory factors to the incidence of infantile eczema.

The statement, or rather claim, that infantile eczema is an allergy does not have much support. The search for an allergen or a specific antibody will probably have little success. So why not take advantage of a natural therapy that has proved to be simple and

45

harmless in treating infantile eczema and which, in the end, does not offer just temporary relief but in many cases results in a complete cure?

Children's Diseases

Admittedly, many children's diseases can be beneficial insofar as the accompanying fever disposes of pathological material within the body that might otherwise cause more serious health problems in later life. This does not mean, however, that we should directly expose children to diseases. They will break out soon enough anyway, so the older and stronger a child is the more easily it will overcome them.

If a child's illness is correctly treated, that is to say, in a natural way and supported in the course it takes, it will be welcome as a cleansing process of the system. The fever burns up and destroys all kinds of toxins which have remained in the baby's system from the embryonic stage of development. Observant physicians agree that those who have never had any of the children's diseases accompanied by fever succumb more readily to all sorts of other diseases, even malignant ones, later on in life. This observation proves the wonderful healing power of fever.

The majority of children who do not recover easily from a children's disease owe this failure to inappropriate treatment. The worst thing that can happen to a child is the suppression of normal disease symptoms – fever and rashes – by means of chemical medicines. Remember, a fever is the internal defence reaction of the body; it burns up or destroys poisons entering from outside and those that have accumulated in the body. Rashes are often a natural way of conducting these toxins out of the system and on to the skin or through the pores. Neither the temperature itself nor its external reaction must be suppressed, because all too often the suppression results in severe damage to the heart, the nervous system or the lungs.

Chemical medicines are most harmful. Granted, it may seem convenient just to dissolve a few tablets in a glass of water, drink the solution, and see the fever obediently oblige and subside. The illness seems to fade away so harmlessly without ever reaching its climax. However, it is usually disregarded that the toxins will not have been eliminated from the body and are therefore still able to wreak damage somewhere, for example by provoking carditis, rheumatic fever, etc.

'But you can't allow the temperature to rise to a dangerous level without doing anything about it,' an overzealous nurse may object. Of course not. There is, however, a great difference between suppressing a fever and doing everything possible to encourage this internal fire. Let us always support the 'fire' and see to it that all the 'flues' are open so that it does not merely smoulder in the stove, the body, but that it really burns at full blast. All burnable wastes will then be eliminated faster, and the system will be cleansed and soon return to normal. Feverish children respond very well to the simple remedy *Ferrum phosphoricum 12x*; the tried and proven *Aconitum 4x* also helps to eliminate the toxins through the skin. If you do not yet know what course an infectious disease will take, try alternating *Aconitum 4x* and *Belladonna 4x*.

Of first importance is that the bowels are functioning properly. To achieve this, it will probably be necessary to give a small *enema*. Use an infusion of *camomile* or *horsetail*. The second important thing to watch with an infectious disease is the function of the kidneys; *horsetail tea* will be of help here, or better still, *Nephrosolid*. Thirdly, the pores of the skin must be opened to excrete toxins. To be successful, you have to follow the advice of water therapists such as Kneipp, Priessnitz and others. For effective stimulation of the skin there is nothing better than *water compresses*. Whether these should be cold or warm depends on each individual case. You can hardly go wrong with warm water compresses, but cold ones require training and skill, for you must understand when and how to use them. However, to allay any undue fear I would like to add that a body with a high temperature is not likely to chill easily and a cold pack, as a rule, will produce even greater external heat, thus reducing the internal heat.

To sum up then, we should not lose sight of the basic principle, which is never to work against nature but to direct all our efforts towards supporting the body's natural defence mechanism.

Children and adults fall victim to infectious diseases more easily if their nutrition is unhealthy and deficient. Existing deficiencies, even only slight vitamin deficiencies, encourage susceptibility to infectious diseases.

Many parents become afraid when their children have a rapidly rising temperature. But you should not forget that fevers really serve a very good purpose, because they quickly burn up the toxins in the body. Remember, too, that a child's little heart is much stronger than you might think; in fact, it can endure much more strain than that of an adult, at least in proportion to its size.

Measles

Even though in many lands this is a harmless infectious disease of childhood, in areas where it has only recently become known, for example among some American Indian tribes, the affected children often die. The causative agent is a virus, one of the submicroscopic entities that have been discovered only in more recent times. These viruses are even smaller than bacteria and cannot be seen under a normal microscope simply by colouring as can bacteria; only with the aid of modern electronic microscopes have scientists been able to study them. Even so, measles has always been considered an infectious disease because of the course the illness takes and the fact that children catch it so easily.

Most parents are familiar with the rash of pink-brownish blotches, accompanied by a high temperature. And yet, you might be uncertain as to the nature of the child's illness in its early stages, unless you check the inner cheeks in the region of the molars. In a case of measles these areas are red, and a day or two before the rash breaks out red spots with tiny white spots in the middle of them, 2–3 mm in diameter, (so-called Koplik's spots), will appear.

The disease has an incubation period of about fourteen days and it is therefore not surprising that within another ten or twelve days the next case will break out, either in your family or your neighbour's.

The first symptoms of measles can vary, but might include a head cold, nose bleeding, bronchial catarrh and conjunctivitis (with sensitivity to light, burning of the eyes and lacrimation).

Soon the child's temperature will rise to perhaps 39 °C (102 °F). It will then drop, but on the fourth day may rise again as high as 40 °C (104 °F). It usually goes down again as soon as the rash appears, but if it remains high for more than 3–4 days after its first outbreak, complications are likely to set in and more specific treatment must be given. You should immediately give the child *Lachesis 10x* to prevent the development of sepsis and apply *flannels* wrung out in a hot *infusion of herbs* (for example wild thyme) repeatedly to the affected areas. This will draw out the internal toxins through the skin. Even when the disease takes its normal course, it is advisable to apply these hot packs to bring the rash out properly. During the fever, give the child nothing but fruit juices, particularly orange and grape juice or carrot juice, the latter also being very good for the liver. If you have no juices available, give the child a mild herbal tea sweetened with honey. In addition, like all infectious diseases, a case of measles demands careful oral hygiene. For infants and smaller children, wrap a clean cloth around your finger tip, dip it in diluted whey concentrate and rub the gums, the inner cheeks and the tongue (which always become furred with measles). For older children use a soft toothbrush to disinfect the mouth.

The following remedies should be given:

— *Aconitum 4x*: 5 drops every half an hour. When perspiration has been induced and the temperature falls, it may be given less frequently.
— *Ferr. phos. 6x* (for babies use *12x*): 1 tablet every hour.
— *Belladonna 4x*: 5 drops every hour. Use when the blood rushes to the head, or with croup, conjunctivitis and ear complications.
— *Antimonium sulph. 4x* or *6x*: initially 1 tablet every 2 hours; after about three days, 2 tablets three times daily. This should be given by itself, without additional medication, when the fever has subsided. It will be sufficient to complete the cure if no complications occur.
— *Nephrosolid*: add to the fruit juice, 5 drops each time. This fresh plant preparation will help to eliminate toxins through the kidneys.
— *Cuprum acet. 4x* and *Antimonium sulph. 4x*. These should be given alternately when a hacking or whooping cough seems to be coming on.
— *Coccus cacti 4x* and especially *Thydroca* are most effective for whooping cough, if given at once when the first symptoms appear after the measles. Whooping cough can often be arrested with these remedies, without any side effects.

Children with a weak constitution who have inherited a disposition for tuberculosis and suffer from swollen glands should be treated with the following prophylactic medicines:

— *Calc phos. 4x* alternated with *6x*: 2 tablets, three times daily.
— *Urticalcin*. This is even more effective and, if given for several months, can work wonders.
— *Ars. iod. 4x*. This is indicated for thin children who grow fast. It should be taken over a period of several months in alternation with Urticalcin.
— *Kali phos. 6x*. This should be given when the lungs and bronchials are affected.
— *Sulph. 4x*. This is indicated when, in spite of packs, the rash is slow in breaking out and very mild.

When the disease has subsided the child should not be allowed outside in the cold air right away. Especially in winter, the child should be kept in bed for another week or in a warm but well-ventilated room. Such care is particularly essential for delicate children who could otherwise suffer from complications.

Mumps

This is another frequent but usually harmless childhood disease. The commonest site of trouble is in the parotid glands, but in the case of boys, the testicles and epididymis may also be affected. Serious complications can ensue when the disease is contracted by an adult male and the essential tissue of the testicles is destroyed, resulting in sterility.

An internal remedy for mumps is *Mercurius solubilis 10x*; 2–3 drops or one tablet should be taken every 2–3 hours. *Aconitum 4x* and *Belladonna 4x* should be taken in alternation every half hour (also 2–3 drops). Compresses with *whey concentrate (Molkosan)* applied to the calves are very helpful, but only when the feet are kept warm. *Hip baths (sitz baths)*, the temperature of which should be gradually increased from 36 °C to 44 °C (97 °F to 110 °F), are also excellent; after the bath the patient should be wrapped in warm blankets. If the child's bowels are not working properly, *Arabic plant essence (Arabiaforce)* is very good, but in more stubborn cases it may be necessary to give an enema. To ease the pain, apply warm compresses to the affected areas, adding a few drops of *arnica* or *calendula* (marigold) *extract* to the water. Make sure to let the child gargle with a weak solution of Molkosan. Another remedy which has proved itself over and over again is hot *St John's wort oil*. Saturate a cloth with the hot oil, or better still, mix potter's clay with St. John's wort oil, then apply to the inflamed area and cover with a very hot water bottle. This will soothe and heal. To complete the cure, give one tablet of *Silicea 12x* (silica) three times a day.

Whooping Cough

Some people still consider whooping cough to be a minor ailment, giving little thought to the distressing, hacking cough. It is, however, very important to give special attention to whooping cough, since it can cause serious complications if it is not treated properly, and may lead to permanent damage. There are a number of herbal and homoeopathic remedies for whooping cough and parents should not fail to make use of these natural treatments. Although no specific medicine exists that arrests and cures the illness completely in a given time, these remedies can reduce the intensity and duration of the attacks. First, the toxins of the pathogenic organisms have to be eliminated, as in all infectious diseases. It is also useful to do something about the patient's physical weakness so as not to encourage other infections. Whooping cough is usually followed by another illness, which is why it is important to build up the patient's general state of health as a prevention. In milder cases, the spasms will disappear after a few days.

Sometimes it will be necessary to give the child a *biological calcium preparation* and at the same time encourage the elimination of metabolic toxins through the kidneys. *Thydroca*, a fresh herb preparation containing *Drosera, Thymus, Coccus cacti, Hedera helix*, and others, is excellent for whooping cough. The homoeopathic remedies *Ipecacuanha 3x* and *Coccus cacti 3x* have also proved to be effective. As soon as the coughing attacks have stopped, the child can gradually stop taking the remedies. In their place *Santasapina* pine bud syrup can be given, as it is beneficial to continue with some medication for a little while after the cure seems to be complete.

Chest compresses are a must in cases of whooping cough. They can be either simple compresses made with a hay flower infusion or, in more severe cases, onion compresses. A horseradish poultice is stronger in its effect and a mustard poultice even more so. A correctly applied mustard poultice or a mustard bath (made using mustard powder) has saved the life of many a child who had already turned blue from a severe case of bronchiolitis (inflammation and gradual blockage of the tiniest air tubes in the lungs) and who was frantically gasping for air. But care must be taken that the skin is not exposed to the active ingredients of the mustard for too long at a time. An intense reddening of the skin is desirable, but blisters should never be allowed to form. If cases of whooping cough are treated as described above, children can be protected from serious complications.

Coeliac Disease

Since this disease causes much worry and requires great care, many parents will be relieved to learn how to go about treating it. The treatment required is similar to that used for enteritis and diarrhoea in infants and young children.

The principal remedy is *Tormentavena*; 2–5 drops are to be given 3–5 times daily, although the exact dose will depend upon the age and sensitivity of the little patient. Start by giving a low dose and gradually increase it until the stool has regained its normal consistency. *Warm hip baths* or *warm abdominal packs* prepared with camomile or horsetail infusions, given frequently, will serve as a complementary treatment.

The diet should contain plenty of *brown rice gruel,* never the polished white kind. Add a little raw carrot juice or *Biocarottin,* made with concentrated raw carrot juice; just ½ or ¼ of a teaspoonful will do. While the illness persists, for children and adults, only gluten-free cereals are indicated, rice being ideal for this purpose. White flour products and white semolina are to be strictly avoided. On the other hand, potatoes boiled in their skins and mashed, skins and all, and mixed with a little raw carrot juice are quite in order. Other vegetables, with the exception of leeks, should not be given until the child is well again.

As regards fruits, finely grated raw apples mixed with mashed bananas are permissible. Bilberries, or blueberries, can also be served. When the acute stage of the disease has passed, a little grapefruit juice may be given. *Bambu Coffee Substitute* is beneficial, but only when it is taken in small quantities.

The quantity of food eaten should be kept very low. When the digestion has become somewhat normalised (noticeable in the consistency and colour of the stools) the amount of food can gradually be stepped up. Remember, however, too much food is worse than too little. Should any food item appear to upset the patient's digestion, leave it out of the diet; the choice and combination of foods depends on the individual sensitivity of the patient. Once the stool appears normal again, the remedies can gradually be dispensed with and you may slowly try introducing other foods again. If a relapse occurs, you will have to return once more to the stricter diet. Almond milk has proved to be of great help in cases of relapse.

If these suggestions are faithfully carried out and you take the child's individual sensitivity into account, patience and perseverance will lead to a complete cure. It should be remembered, however, that due to deficient digestion, which is caused by inadequate motility of the intestine, the ingested food will be only partly assimilated and particularly the absorption of minerals will be insufficient. No wonder, then, that children who suffer from coeliac disease are very prone to fractures of the bones because of their considerable calcium deficiency. However, the susceptibility to these complications can be reduced with a preparation of biological calcium such as *Urticalcin*. At the same time, this will help to curb the tendency to spasms which, in coeliac disease, are also attributable to calcium deficiency.

Poliomyelitis

Poliomyelitis is a sinister disease, yet on the whole quite brief. The polio virus is highly infectious and its virulent toxins, if concentrated, are able to attack and destroy the nerve cells, leading to paralysis. The illness itself ordinarily lasts only about 2–3 weeks. The paralysis that follows is actually the disease's aftermath. It is therefore most important to treat the disease thoroughly and with the minimum of delay. Judging by the letters I keep receiving, it is once more necessary to remind lay people as well as professionals of the fundamental rules regarding the treatment of polio.

Some time ago, a man from central Switzerland told me that his son, a strong and healthy boy, was hospitalised for tests and observation because it was thought he might have polio. Day after day passed without the doctor in charge attempting any treatment, until the first signs of paralysis appeared in the lungs. The boy was then placed in an iron lung, but he died within a few weeks, despite having been so strong and healthy. Let me add that this incident occurred many years ago and would be most unlikely to happen with the modern approach to the disease.

Famous physiotherapists, with Sister Kenny in the forefront, have proved that a life can be saved if treatment is given without delay. It is the delay that enables the virus to destroy the nerve cells. Therefore, as soon as the first symptoms become apparent it is of the utmost importance that the patient be made to *sweat*. Use a steam cabinet, a steam bath, a sauna, a tub bath of gradually increasing temperature (Schlenz bath), or quite simply hot packs; whatever you choose the important thing is to produce copious perspiration – fast. By these means much harm can be avoided and paralysis may well be averted. If Sister Kenny's treatment had been given, the boy mentioned previously might not have lost his life.

However conservative a doctor may be, he should not close his eyes to the good results obtained by new methods of treating polio. The very first symptoms should galvanise us into action. They may suggest flu, with excessive tiredness, headaches, aching limbs, vomiting, lack of appetite, etc. Whether polio is diagnosed right away or not is of little importance. These symptoms are sufficient to warrant immediate treatment, the first of which is the above-mentioned inducement of perspiration. The effect will be beneficial even if it is happily discovered later that it was the flu and not polio.

It is advisable to back up the treatment by means of natural remedies, such as *Gelsemium 6x* and *Urticalcin*, calcium always being valuable in such cases. *Nux vomica 4x* is helpful in counteracting nausea. All these remedies contribute to improvement. As for the diet, fruit juices are indicated so as not to overburden the digestive organs. What is more, never lose sight of the necessity to rid the body of toxins, not only through heavy sweating, but also through the bowels and kidneys. Since this treatment has proved to be reliable and effective in practice, it should be tried first.

Polio epidemics occur periodically and regionally, although less so today than formerly. Hot and sultry weather seems to encourage the development of the virus, for the incidence of the disease is greater in summer than in winter. In tropical countries it continues all year round. Research specialists have found that a number of people, particularly children, although immune to the disease themselves, nevertheless are carriers of the polio virus. Among primitive peoples very few cases of polio are found and this would lead to the conclusion that the advantages and disadvantages of our civilisation are responsible for our predisposition to this disease and undermine our resistance to it. Our food and life-style, living in overheated houses, and so forth, no doubt play their part in our susceptibility.

So how can we protect ourselves from this dreadful affliction? In the same way that we should protect ourselves from all infectious diseases. The main requirement is a natural way of life. Healthy exercise is also important – and we should not become 'soft'. Plenty of fresh air, light and sunshine should be our 'companions' whenever possible. Since it is now thought with reasonable certainty that the polio virus attacks by way of the nose and mouth, do not neglect to paint your children's throats with *Molkosan* when a threat of polio occurs in your locality. By doing so we can thus protect our children from infectious diseases and build up their resistance. However, should the infection have already taken place, remember the keynote to successful treatment: detoxify and eliminate – profuse sweating and elimination through the bowels and kidneys. This will help to avert the worst.

Influenza

Fortunately, not every bout of influenza is as serious as the dreadful viral influenza that killed more people in 1918–19 than the First

World War itself. Usually it is quite a harmless illness, but since so many people do not really know what to do when infectious diseases strike, the following suggestions may be helpful. The recommendations made for influenza should be followed in cases of other flu-like and infectious diseases too.

First of all, the bowels must be cleaned out by means of a natural *plant laxative*. As long as the temperature remains above normal the patient should not eat. To quench his thirst and assist elimination, give *fruit juices*, orange, grapefruit and grape juices being the most suitable. Should the liver be affected, raw *carrot juice* should be used instead of fruit juice. Under no circumstances should the fever be reduced with chemical medicines. It is a kind of defence measure, assisting the body by burning up and destroying the viral and other toxins responsible for the illness. The elimination of metabolic waste products through the kidneys is absolutely essential, and for this purpose give a kidney tea with *Solidago* (goldenrod) or *Nephrosolid*. Moreover, we can assist the fever and induce sweating by the use of *compresses*. If the patient should still find it difficult to start perspiring, let him drink hot *elder flower tea* with lemon juice.

When the normal body temperature has stabilised, first serve *raw fruit* and other *raw foods*, followed by *light meals*, keeping to a vegetarian diet, and as soon as good health has been restored, the patient can return to his usual diet, which should, however, be a natural one.

Following these suggestions, an attack of influenza can be quickly overcome and will not mean the usual long prostration. What is more, the patient will not experience the lingering tiredness and other common after effects of flu.

Virus Influenza
Although the epidemics that have hit Europe again and again for some decades no longer kill as many victims as at first, we must nevertheless regard influenza as a serious disease, especially when we consider its possible after effects. For example, it can cause pneumonia, or an acute deterioration of a chronic liver condition; it may also affect the kidneys, pancreas and abdominal organs. It is also possible for the myocardium to suffer and eczema to break out. Rheumatism can result from an improperly or incompletely treated bout of flu. All these after effects can possibly be prevented if treatment is given until the cure is complete.

Checklist for the Treatment of Influenza
At the onset of a flu virus we should carefully consider four main aspects for successful treatment.

1. In the first place we must make use of a *physical therapy* through which we can assist the body to *excrete bacterial toxins.* At the same time, we must watch the condition of the heart during sweating cures. With this in mind, we can then proceed to induce sweating through the application of compresses, wet packs or a steam bath.

In addition to the compresses, it is also beneficial to apply *cold compresses to the calves.* The patient will then be more comfortable and able to sleep.

If the illness is affecting the heart, give the heart tonic *Cardiaforce,* or *fruit juice* sweetened with *honey.* Or simply serve *herbal tea* or just water sweetened with honey. Pure *grape sugar* (condensed grape juice) also has an immediate effect in strengthening weak heart muscles.

The body should be frequently washed with an infusion of *thyme* or *juniper needles,* even if the patient may perspire only moderately.

For a severe bout of flu, the patient should take *Podophyllum 4x, Chelidonium 4x* (celandine) and *Taraxacum* (dandelion), since these remedies are good for the liver. And as already stated, the patient should drink raw carrot juice for the liver, and apply *cabbage leaf poultices* to the liver region during the night.

If it happens to be a head or nerve flu, *Avena sativa* and *Acid. phos. 4x,* in addition to a *biological calcium preparation,* are indicated; in severe cases also *Fiebrisan* and *Echinaforce.* The simultaneous application of crushed cabbage leaves on the nape of the neck has an excellent effect.

Oral hygiene must be observed in all infectious diseases, including influenza. The patient must clean his teeth regularly and remove any coating on the tongue with a toothbrush. Gargling with *Molkosan* backs up the healing process greatly.

Patients with common influenza will benefit from *Influaforce,* a homoeopathic flu remedy (see below).

All infectious diseases make the lungs work overtime in order to burn up toxins, so the sick room should be aired frequently. Provided that the patient is well covered, a pleasantly cool room is better than an overheated one.

2. Secondly, we must employ a selection of *herbal medicines,*

such as *Nephrosolid* and *Boldocynara*, for these remedies promote increased excretion through the kidneys and liver. By taking Echinaforce we can prevent irritation and inflammation. At the beginning of the illness, the flu drops Influaforce are helpful. These drops contain *Baptisia* (wild indigo), *Lachesis 10x*, Echinaforce, *Bryonia 3x* (bryony), *Aconitum 3x* and *Solidago*, and have always proved effective in minimising the virulence of the infection.

3. *Diet* is very important for a flu patient. While fever is present, neither protein nor fat should be eaten. Going on a liquid juice diet for one or two days has proved to be very beneficial. Grapefruit juice, diluted bilberry (blueberry) juice, also blackcurrant juice alternated with diluted beetroot juice will be received as a blessing by the patient. The intake of liquids should be greater than under normal circumstances.

4. After the illness has passed, we must direct our attention to the follow-up treatment, being mindful that the period of convalescence should not be short. Even though the acute symptoms have subsided, we should still apply *physiotherapy*. Also, continue taking *diuretic* or *excretory medicines* even if the fever has subsided. This will eliminate all of the accumulated toxins so that no damage elsewhere in the body is possible.

Every bout of flu should receive follow-up treatment. In fact, with any infectious disease it is advisable to continue the treatment conscientiously until the patient has fully recovered. This is the only way to prevent after effects, which can be much more unpleasant than you think. If you become impatient, just remember that you remain prone to contracting a new infection until all vestiges of the last one have been eliminated during convalescence.

The Brain
The brain is a marvellous organ and a great gift from the Creator. We would be lost without it; we could not plan, carry out or complete anything. So we have every reason to be grateful for it every day of our life. If a person voluntarily abstains from food or is made to go hungry, and as a result loses a great deal of weight, the weight loss in the spinal cord and in the brain is hardly noticeable. The fact that everything else is affected first shows the importance of the brain as the control centre of most other processes in the body.

A good illustration of the human brain is that of the walnut. The hard shell can be compared to the cranium. The two-lobed seed resembles the cerebrum, and the skin, which peels off easily in freshly picked nuts, may be likened to the meninges. At the back of the head, between the spinal cord and the brain, lies the cerebellum, which is approximately the size of an orange.

The functions of the brain, as far as they have been discovered, are amazing. Picture, if you will, the control room of a large power plant or a modern ocean liner, or the instrument panels of a jet plane. All the numerous instruments and switches elicit our amazement and admiration. These control centres are, in a manner of speaking, the brain of, for example, the ship or plane. Everything that takes place, every change in direction, every response to the changeable elements, every command, comes from that control centre, the brain. The energy needed to make everything function is supplied by generators which produce energy, or power. When the power supply is insufficient or fails completely, it can be put down to problems in the central control because it is either malfunctioning or is out of action. This can happen even though engines and equipment have been designed and built in spectacular ways.

What can we learn from the above illustration? Energy is supplied to the brain via the bloodstream. If the blood carries all the necessary nutrients, nutritive salts and vitamins so that every brain cell receives the food it needs, then everything will function properly. Not every one of the many millions of cells has its own function. The brain is divided into work groups, called centres, and more than twenty of these centres have so far been recognised.

How an entire centre can be put out of order is seen in the case of a stroke. The attack usually occurs in the inner capsule and not the outer part of the brain or the cerebral cortex. If a blood vessel on the right side of the inner capsule ruptures, the blood supply to the outer parts of the brain is disrupted and the consequences appear on the left side of the body. This inversion is due to the fact that the cerebral hemisphere controls the opposite side of the body. Whatever we sense on the right side is registered on the left side and vice versa. If the body is able to repair the damage, the paralysis will pass and the ability to speak, which was lost, will return. If the speech centre remains disturbed, while the centre governing the connecting ideas continues to function, then the person will find himself in the embarrassing situation of thinking correctly but expressing himself in a muddled way. However, this will not happen if he writes down his thoughts instead of trying to express them verbally.

What Can Damage the Brain?

If the blood pressure is either too high or too low it will adversely affect the functioning of the brain. Dizzy spells or fainting, for example, may result from too much pressure or lack of blood flow, due to low blood pressure.

Even though this single most important control centre, the brain, is well protected by the cranium, accidents and concussions can do much damage. Just think of the many falls and bumps experienced while skiing or engaging in other types of sports. On such occasions, the head – and thus the brain – often suffers severe blows or concussion without any visible sign of injury. However, if the fall is bad enough to cause a tear in the meninges, the cerebrospinal fluid will leak out and the brain, which had previously been cushioned by this fluid, will now be more like a dead weight, resulting in pressure being exerted on the various brain centres. The person will feel nauseous, the metabolic centre will be affected, and vomiting and possibly diarrhoea will occur. The patient must lie still and rest so that the tear can heal and the brain may once again enjoy the cushioning and protecting effect of the cerebrospinal fluid surrounding it.

Alcohol and drugs can influence the brain to the extent that several centres are slowed down while others accelerate. Hence the person may lose his inhibitions and temporarily act and feel differently to how he would under normal circumstances. Permanent damage, that is, softening of the brain and paralysis, may occur when vitality decreases as a result of poisoning with metals such as arsenic and mercury. These and other poisons impair and block certain processes of the brain and the central nervous system, as is known to happen in advanced cases of syphilis. The metallic toxins may remain inactive in the body for years, only to strike the victim in later life, with tragic consequences.

Meningitis is another disease which can have grave consequences, yet it is possible to prevent it by striving to keep the circulation in good condition. If, however, one falls victim to it from contact with an infected person, every effort should be made to cure the disease without delay. One of the most effective remedies for this is *Echinaforce*. If meningitis is not treated properly it can lead to partial paralysis and other permanent damage. This should be reason enough not to take it lightly but to give it the best care and attention. The patient should be kept in a darkened room and away from all noise, since he will be very sensitive to light and disturbances. Remember, meningitis is always dangerous, not only because it can bring lasting damage to the body, but also because it might lead to death.

Taking Precautions

During the productive years of youth an active person often neglects to think about the fact that the central nervous system and brain must still serve their purpose during the autumn of life. If we wish to be sprightly and in good spirits, feeling well physically and mentally during our old age, we must see to it that the engine in the control room, the brain, is given more attention than is usual in today's world.

How many of us regularly curtail the brain's wonderful source of energy and recharging by not getting enough rest and sleep! The body may be able to take one or two exceptions, but a continuous lack of sleep will undermine the health, lead to fatigue and will gradually diminish one's efficiency and productivity. Let us therefore, first and foremost, make sure to enjoy a healthy amount of sleep, going to bed early. We should also make an effort to eat wholefoods for adequate nutrition, get enough exercise for refreshing relaxation during our free time, and avoid the poisons threatening us in so many ways.

Taking these precautions will not only contribute to our overall state of health but will render an incomparable service to our brain.

The Pituitary Gland (Hypophysis)

The pituitary, 12 by 8 mm in size (like a bean), serves our body in a similar way to that of an inconspicuous general who commands a large army, or the person in the control tower who directs and manoeuvres huge jet planes entering and leaving an international airport. This gland weighs only a few grams and was at one time regarded as a vestigial organ. But when the news of its importance began to spread through the scientific world, and it was even discovered that the anterior and posterior lobes each produce completely different hormones, the amazement was great indeed. Such a small gland, yet one with so many vital functions!

The Master Gland

The pituitary gland governs the activity of the thyroid, the suprarenal gland and the sex glands. It is known as the master gland, having the leading position among the endocrine glands. Its direct link with the central nervous system in the area of very important centres at the base of the brain, the hypothalamus, has been the subject of much research, since it appears that the pituitary gland influences all the vital processes either directly or indirectly. It also appears that, together with the thymus gland, the pituitary determines growth. Since the entire development of the sex glands and sex organs is controlled by the pituitary, a hermaphrodite condition may be attributed to impaired development or disturbed functioning of this gland. A pregnancy could never run its normal course without the cooperation of the pituitary. Diabetics have to blame their ailment not only on a failure of the islets of Langerhans – located in the pancreas – to produce sufficient insulin, but also on a functional disorder in the anterior lobe of the pituitary as a contributory factor. No matter how much bile the liver produces, the process of breaking down fat will suffer if the pituitary fails to manufacture the necessary hormones. A change in the blood pressure, too much or too little elimination of water, even the start of labour pains, are all connected with the function of the posterior lobe of the pituitary and its secretion of hormones.

Until recently, science had not succeeded in fully understanding the complex hormone structure of this interesting little gland. And this is the reason why it has not yet been possible to produce its hormones synthetically. It is always a risk to prescribe medicine that has a direct effect on the pituitary, except in small homoeopathic doses. Such medicines can have a very detrimental effect on the patient if he is sensitive to drugs.

Care of the Small Wonder Gland

As a control centre of paramount importance, the pituitary should receive extra care and attention. Because of its important functions, it is well protected in an inaccessible bony hollow at the base of the skull. The only way to care for it is by looking after one's general health. Thus, it is worthwhile supplying the body with wholesome food, sufficient sleep, exercise and oxygen by deep breathing. Even though we already know a great deal about this small gland, many of its secrets have yet to be discovered.

The instrument panel of a jet plane is a complete mystery to the layperson. A radio receiver small enough to fit in a watch casing is also a marvel of technology. But what is contained in the bean-sized gland – much of which we are still not aware of – surpasses everything the human mind has created a thousand times. Appreciating the intricate design and functions of our body, we should always show deep respect for it and avoid subjecting it thought-

61

lessly to stresses and strains that affect our health. The biblical psalmist expressed this most aptly when he wrote: 'I shall laud you [God] because in a fear-inspiring way I am wonderfully made. Your works are wonderful, as my soul is very well aware.'

Headaches – their Causes and Treatments

Headaches should never be dispelled with analgesics. Rather, you should try and discover the cause and then treat it by natural means.

Many headaches are caused by intestinal disturbances. Putrefactive processes develop gases which enter the liver through the portal vein and, from there, find their way into the bloodstream. Headaches frequently result because the nerve and brain cells are affected by the poisons circulating in the blood. Abdominal troubles and diseases can also trigger headaches. Overwork tends to erode one's nervous energy and this condition, too, may start a headache. Other problems that may cause headaches include a ruptured disc (slipped disc) resulting from strain. This cause can be successfully treated by a chiropractor. High or low blood pressure, diseases of the blood and nephritis can all trigger headaches.

Let me point out that a headache *per se* is never an illness, only a symptom pointing to an illness that is causing it. It is for this reason that taking analgesics and chemical drugs to deaden the pain is completely inappropriate. The correct thing to do is to find and then treat the underlying cause. On the other hand, you can do something about a headache by providing the nerve cells with certain biochemical salts which will lessen and often cure the pain (see 'Four Biochemical Remedies', pages 398–402). There are also homoeopathic remedies, for example *Sanguinaria canadensis* (bloodroot), which are especially good for headaches.

Headaches can also be caused by insufficient blood supply to the brain. In this case we recommend both *Petadolor* and *Ginkgo biloba*, also known as maidenhair tree. The leaves of this tree contain active properties that can do wonders for the cerebral blood supply.

Physical therapy should not be forgotten either. Relief is often obtained from *warm showers* directed on the nape of the neck and the spine, as well as massaging with *Toxeucal Massage Oil*. If the headaches stem from an upset digestive system, warm showers directed on the stomach are the answer to alleviating the pain.

Onion, horseradish or cabbage leaf *poultices* can be applied to the back of the neck in order to combat headaches successfully.

Whatever you do, natural treatments and remedies will prove more effective than chemical drugs, which merely dull the pain. It is of fundamental importance to find the cause of the headache and to treat it accordingly.

The Tongue
Just as with any one of the other organs, the tongue is a marvellous work of Creation. The singular design, structure and arrangement of this muscular organ gives it a flexibility that no other organ in the body possesses. The tongue's shape can change from flat to broad, from thin to thick, by manipulating its muscle fibres which respond to command as does a circus horse to its trainer. Yet the most interesting feature in the structure of the tongue is its surface, which, when greatly magnified, looks rather like a lunar landscape. Every elevation and every little crater-like cavity is equipped with minute receptors of taste sensations that enable us to taste and enjoy our food and drink. The mucous glands in the taste cavities see to it that there is always a small amount of local mucus or fluid present, for chemicals taken into the mouth have to be dissolved for us to taste them.

The Sensation of Taste
Nerve cells which register the sensation of taste and transmit it to the brain are arranged in a bulb-like manner. The nerve ends may be compared to the roots, while the layers of the bulb represent the reaction controls, with built-in amplifiers. To complete the illustration, in the place of the bulb's top, there are very fine hair-like nerves that register the taste sensation.

These nerve bulbs are called taste buds, because scientists compared them to the literal buds. An adult has about 3,000 of them. But did you know that we humans probably have fewer sensations of taste when eating our food than, for example, antelopes, which have about fifteen times as many taste buds as a human? If we had as many as these animals it would be much easier for us to differentiate between healthy nourishing food and that which is harmful. Thus animals are more capable than humans in distinguishing what is good for them and what is not.

Simple experiments will tell you that there are different taste zones on the tongue. If the tip of the tongue is dipped in honey water, the sensation of sweetness is immediately apparent. A little further back on the periphery of the tongue the taste of salt is registered and even further back, also on the periphery, sourness is sensed, while zones registering bitterness are found across the posterior section. The central part of the tongue is a neutral area, as it does not register any sensation of taste.

It is noteworthy that the tongue is more accurate and reliable as a test organ than many chemical reactions. For this reason a wine merchant, or a tea, coffee or olive oil processing firm will pay more attention to their experienced 'tasters' than to the analysts in a chemical laboratory.

Imagine what life would be like without the 3,000 taste buds on our tongues. What would encourage us to eat and drink if there were no pleasure in it? If you have ever had to force yourself to eat without feeling hungry you can well understand the difference. We would also lose our incentive to prepare delicious meals for our families if there were no smile of approval and enjoyment on the faces of the happy eaters. Despite its small size, the tongue is endowed with many important functions, providing much satisfaction and pleasure.

Other Capabilities of the Tongue

Even though we know something about the anatomical structure and the functions of the tongue, we have by no means exhausted the full extent of its operations and capabilities. We know, of course, that we owe the gift of oral communication to the tongue. But that is not all. The tongue is at the same time the 'voice' of the heart, the figurative seat of the ability to feel, think and make decisions. This little organ thus may be a source of blessing or curse for ourselves and others.

From the Bible we learn that horses and ships are easier to manoeuvre and control than the tongue. Though small in size, the tongue can, metaphorically speaking, ignite a 'fire' so devastating that it destroys a forest.

How sad is its influence when spreading evil gossip and, by doing so, slandering friends and dear companions. Envy and hatred, too, make use of this nimble little instrument of the soul when sending out its poisonous arrows to do harm to successful fellowmen. As slick as oil, the tongue obeys the voice of temptation, for the chosen victim cannot escape its treacherous influence. Many a tongue cannot distinguish between 'yes' and 'no', so that its contradictions, hypocrisy and lies play a part in destroying the innocent. A disappointed person may pour out the bitterness of his heart through the tongue and infect or poison others. What dreadful words may be uttered through this inconspicuous little organ in the mouth of the mentally deranged! The confused state of mind and inner conflict of such a person often seems to surface by means of the tongue. It is hard for a healthy, normal person to understand or face such an outburst.

The Tongue Can Be a Blessing

Has the tongue been given the power to speak only in order to create unhappiness? Certainly not. The apostle Paul reminded his fellow workers to consider everything lovable and well spoken of, for the contrary use of the tongue is the root of nothing but grief and vexation. Loving, heart-warming words, words of instruction and upbuilding admonition, comfort and encouragement should pass over the lips, so that this little organ of speech may truly become a blessing. But this can only be if the heart is properly conditioned, if it has the desire to be a friend to friends, to lend a helping hand to someone in need or distress, and to overcome even hostile attitudes with goodness. In this way the tongue will become a dispenser of kindness and benevolence.

What enhances and endears springtime to us? Is it not the lovely songs of birds? Their little throats fill the air with songs of gratitude, of sheer joy and devotion. We too have been endowed with the ability to sing and can, like the birds, give vent to our joyful exuberance in harmonious song.

But the tongue must learn something else: during times of distress it must keep silent, for its indiscriminate use may cause the betrayal of a friend and brother. The tongue must know how to thwart an enemy's fatal intentions and break the power of evil. Even a foolish man will be regarded as wise if he knows when to 'hold his tongue'. This did not escape the notice of King Solomon, as recorded in the Book of Proverbs. It may be why a popular proverb says, 'Speech is silver but silence is golden.' Indeed, for many, keeping silent takes greater willpower than talking.

Is it not strange that such a little organ as the tongue serves such diverse purposes? It makes food and drink appealing to us, it warns us against indulging in spoiled or even poisonous food. In fact, if we do not force our palate to take in unnatural things, if we do not expect it to call good what is really harmful, then it will reward us with its healthy power of evaluation. It is similar with the other function for which this small organ was made, the power to express feelings. The tongue can prove to be an extremely beneficial organ, but it can also turn out to be detrimental. Whether we use it as a positive or negative outlet for our emotions depends on the state of our hearts. That is why Solomon wisely advised us, 'More than all else that is to be guarded, safeguard your heart, for out of it are the sources of life.' And out of the heart's abundance the mouth speaks.

Taking Care of the Eyes

This section is not meant to deal in detail with the complex mechanism we call the eye. Instead, all it sets out to do is give some clear and helpful hints on how to preserve and protect your eyesight, and highlight the basic principles of nature involved.

Let us begin by repeating the fact that excessive brain work causes eyestrain. The more natural and free from stress is the way we live our daily lives the better it will be for our eyes. It might be added that the poor nourishment derived from today's denatured foods also contributes to the development of eye problems.

However, many of us will admit that it is not all that easy to change these things, or we may have already made some changes and want to achieve still more. How can this be done?

The answer is quite simple. Years ago, when we were not so eager to work overtime by artificial light and went to bed early, there were fewer people with painful, weak and tired eyes. So why not try a most extraordinary remedy? Why not turn the clock back and live for four weeks without electric light? How can you do this? Well, quite simply by doing without the convenience of modern lighting. You refrain from using this miracle of modern technology; you simply do not switch on the electric light. Your painful, burning, overtired eyes, which can no longer do their work efficiently, will respond to this care and rapidly recover. But in order to be well armed against the force of habit, you must plan your day carefully so that when it gets dark, you will not be tempted to turn on the light despite all your good intentions.

Years ago, the evenings were used to relax and recuperate and to prepare oneself for the rest that was to end the day. Try to do this for four weeks. It will help you to see and experience why our Creator has given us the different lights, the bright light of the sun by day and the gentle soothing moonlight by night. Just try to work hard in the soft moonlight. You will gladly desist. Why? Because if you let its magic spell work on you like an age-old lullaby, you will soon drop off and enjoy a deep, restful sleep. Truly, if you make full use of the night for rest, you will wake cheerfully with the first gleam of daylight, without feeling drowsy, or still tired and sluggish. You will not feel morose and only partially rested, turning over on the other side to sleep on into the day. What you had intended doing by artificial light, you can do more cheerfully and with much less effort in the full light of the early morning. You will be amazed at what this compliance to nature's laws can do for you; it will renew your energies and benefit your eyesight at the same time.

The unnatural strain of artificial light, which we impose on our eyes year after year, will no longer bother us if we adapt our daily routine to the coming and going of daylight. This is the natural order of things established by God and the more we set ourselves against it, the more our eyes will tire and suffer. Indeed, if things go on much longer as they do, one day it will be hard to imagine a person without spectacles. We hardly ever stop to think about the detrimental consequences of our unnatural life-style, do we? Immersed as we are in an atmosphere of artificiality, we have lost touch with nature, we are out of tune and can no longer learn and follow its natural rhythm. How would plants fare if day and night they had to live in the light, without a chance to regenerate themselves in darkness? Their cells would tire out and suffer damage and their natural functions would be impaired. Why, then, should not man, the crown of Creation, conform to the harmony of the natural laws? Why should he not use and enjoy to the full the priceless, wondrous exhilaration of the early morning hours, rather than miss out on them, lying in bed asleep while outside the sun is shining gloriously, and do during the night what was not done in the morning hours? Why should anyone create restless nights for himself, only because they did not sleep soundly during the hours before midnight, building up strength for the next day's work? If we could only reorganise our schedule of activities our eyes would indeed benefit greatly. When light fades, let us put aside our work, and when daylight comes once more, take it up again, strengthened and refreshed. Not only our eyes, but our whole body will benefit from this natural way of life.

Spring and summer encourage us especially to give this routine a try. In winter it seems more normal to wake up with the daylight but, unfortunately, at that time of the year we are also more tempted to continue our working day far into the night. In spring, then, let us start to put our good resolution into practice. Let us give our eyes the natural daylight in the earliest hours of the morning, and in the evening, let us give them a rest rather than work under artificial light. They will then recover and become strong.

The Lacrimal Glands

Is it not a marvellous thing that the lacrimal glands, or tear ducts, serve as a safety valve to reduce the internal pressure when we are under emotional stress? How unbearable it would be, even for a little girl, if she could not cry when her doll dropped on the floor and broke, or some equally frustrating thing happened. The pain seems only half as bad when salty tears roll down the cheeks like pearls. In fact, this ingenious arrangement operates much better with women than with men.

In addition to the secretion of tears when crying, the lacrimal glands, which are located just within the upper outside part of the eye socket, embedded in a little pocket, have yet another function: the tears must keep the conjunctiva and the cornea moist in order to prevent their drying out. Furthermore, bacteria, dust and other foreign particles are washed away by the tears.

Inflammation of the tear ducts themselves is rare, but that of the nasolacrimal duct and the lacrimal sac is more frequent. If this inflammation is not given immediate attention with herbal packs of *camomile* and *eyebright*, the attacking bacteria may cause a chronic condition or even the formation of abscesses. Flushing of the eyes with *warm milk* or *mallow leaf water*, to which a few drops of *Echinaforce* has been added, is a rapid cure for simple inflammations. For those who work or live in a dusty environment it is highly recommended to cleanse the area of the eyes with the lids closed by wiping them with a cotton pad soaked in Echinaforce. Do this every evening. It prevents dirt, dust and bacteria from entering the eye itself. If the lacrimal duct is blocked you must see a doctor to have it punctured. At the same time, it is important to use Echinaforce as mentioned above and to bathe the eyes with warm milk or herbal tea. If the eyes tend to be encrusted in the morning upon awakening, it is a sign of a metabolic disorder which must be treated immediately.

It is also wise to refrain from straining the eyes when there is insufficient illumination to read by. The eyes need plenty of rest, and to be closed during the night, because they work hard during our waking hours. They are indeed very precious to us, but many people forget that and do not give them the care they deserve as the indispensable gift they are. No one will deny that the eyes are instruments that we cannot do without, physically or mentally.

Blindness constitutes an extremely heavy loss. Amongst all the other wonders of Creation, the eyes are a miracle and the lacrimal glands, despite their negligible size and apparent unimportance, are a convincing symbol of a carefully thought out design to smooth the necessary but involuntary processes of our daily existence.

Simple Remedies for Eye Problems
It is a proven fact that a *carrot juice diet* has a favourable effect on the eyes on account of the provitamin A carrots contain. Anything that stimulates the circulation and the supply of blood to the eyes helps to improve their efficiency, and this is where carrot juice is most beneficial. If raw carrots are not available, use condensed carrot juice (*Biocarottin*) instead. As supporting remedies in the treatment take *Aesculaforce* and a calcium complex (*Urticalcin*), as well as *goldenrod* for the kidneys. The requirement of silica can be met by taking *Galeopsis* (hemp nettle).

Since liver disorders, constipation and overtiredness can also be the causes of eye troubles, make sure that both the liver and the bowels are functioning properly. The liver is best restored to good working order by a *liver diet* (see page 247) and by taking *Chelidonium 4x* and *Podophyllum 4x* or *Boldocynara* liver drops. Very often constipation will disappear at the same time, but if this should not be the case, use a natural remedy for it. Above all, avoid denatured foods. Instead, eat a natural diet that is low in protein and salt. If you are feeling overworked, make sure to get to sleep at least two hours before midnight and take oat extract in the form of *Avenaforce*, and *Eleutherococcus*, a remedy made from the taiga root, since both are known for their value as general tonics for the nerves and body.

Consider each case carefully and, in accordance with the diagnosed problem, choose the right remedies and treatment.

In the case of a blocked tear duct, observe the general advice already given and for external treatment apply packs made with *clay* and a *horsetail* infusion. For conjunctivitis make up an eye bath from *eyebright* and *marigold tea*.

Infectious Suppuration of the Eyes and Mouth
Infectious eye and mouth suppuration (discharging of pus or festering) can be cured in a short time if you follow the nature treatment described in the following letter I received from a mother.

'Our little boy is much better now. The pus in his eyes and

mouth stopped within about five days after we began to use your remedies. The child looked pitiful, but now he is romping around happily again. Our treatment was as follows: before meals we gave him *Solidago* (goldenrod) and a *cod-liver oil* preparation, as well as an easily assimilated calcium preparation (*Urticalcin*). After meals he took *Hepar sulph. 4x* and *Lachesis 12x*. The eyes were bathed twice daily with diluted *Aesculaforce*. Twice a day we put an *onion poultice* on his neck. Improvement of his condition was soon noticeable. We put *St John's wort oil* on his sore lips and dusted them with Urticalcin powder. During the day we gave him *fruit juice* and *horsetail tea* to drink. Several times we prepared *white clay packs* made with horsetail tea, mixed with a few drops of St John's wort oil, and applied these to his eyes. We are indeed thankful and happy that this dangerous infection has now gone, but we continue to give the child *Solidago*, cod-liver oil preparation and the easily assimilated calcium.'

As a rule, such infections are simple enough to deal with if the body is given the right kind of help, for nature cures if we support it in its performance. It is better to take no action than to give the wrong treatment. The usual attempts to suppress the symptoms in order to destroy the germs with drugs actually undermine the body's natural powers of resistance. The same foolishness is shown by those who treat plant diseases and pests. They expect to get rid of them by spraying the plants with poisonous chemicals, but succeed only in weakening or killing the plants' own natural defence mechanism. So they are forced to increase and intensify their spray programmes. Similarly, some doctors have to prescribe more and stronger drugs because the body's natural healing powers have been weakened or even destroyed. But we must remember that man is not the healer – it is nature that really performs the cure. All we ourselves can do is support the wonderful, natural self-healing powers of the body. Let us hope that this basic truth becomes once again more widely recognised and appreciated.

The Nose
Our three respiratory organs comprise the nose, the windpipe (trachea) and the lungs. Each of these three organs has a very special and important function and only a working correlation between them assures a harmless exchange of gases.

Instead of bones, the nose has cartilage plates to give it firmness. Bones would be too brittle and the danger of them breaking too great, especially if we should fall on our nose, or a ball or some other hard object hit it. Those participating in sports such as boxing or skiing would soon have nothing but an unshapely and unsightly nose if the cartilage walls were less resilient and more vulnerable. The extent to which the beauty of the face depends on the shape of the nose becomes evident after a serious accident when the nose is crushed or badly deformed. Fortunately today, a mishap of this sort can, as a rule, be easily corrected by plastic surgery.

The Functions of the Nose
The proper functioning of the nose is very important to good health. For one thing, perhaps not everyone is aware of the fact that the nose is actually an air-conditioning organ, warming the air we inhale if it is cold outside. If the air is tropically hot, a cooling system is activated to make the climate more bearable. Furthermore, the nose regulates the intake of air that is either too dry or too humid.

What a marvellous design! Not even the smallest detail is missing in all these divine provisions and it is indeed astonishing to hear people deny the existence of an omnipotent Creator, despite the many visible testimonies of divine wisdom and creative power. God alone is capable of creating something out of nothing, for only He has control over the laws he set in motion in the first place. These laws cannot come into existence by themselves, neither is their smooth operation and application left to blind chance and whim. So let us now see to what extent a small organ like the nose may serve as proof of God's creatorship.

First of all, the nose is designed in such a way that the mucous membranes keep dust and bacteria from entering the body, provided, of course, that we breathe in and out through the nose and that it is not blocked. It is true that we can also breathe through the mouth rather than the nose, but this will make us lose the benefit of the built-in screening device, exposing us to a higher risk of catching colds and infections. Mouth-breathing poses a definite threat to the throat, the bronchial passages and the lungs.

It is interesting to note that the nostrils react to pleasant and unpleasant odours by a simple dilation or contraction of the walls, thus increasing or decreasing the flow of air. Strangely enough, the nose walls (conchae) also react to cold feet. When the feet are cold the walls contract, become cold and dry and cause the glands to stop functioning, so that dust and bacteria are no longer filtered out. It is easy to see why a cold will almost inevitably result, followed by catarrh or a runny nose. You can now understand why it is important to avoid getting cold feet and inhaling bacteria by breathing through the mouth. If the mucous membranes are functioning properly they are able to destroy all cold germs entering through the nose. It is therefore a necessary requirement for good health to cultivate the habit of breathing through the nose at all times.

Treatment for Nasal Problems

If you suffer frequently from head colds it is advisable to sniff up calcium powder (*Urticalcin*) from time to time, in the way people used to take snuff years ago. When the air is cold it is also beneficial to lubricate the nasal passages regularly with a good lanolin cream. A reliable choice for this purpose is *Bioforce Cream*; it may even prevent a head cold from developing if applied early enough. When you walk too fast or run, you do not usually breathe through the nose. Hence you should try to slow down, at least enough to allow you to continue breathing through the nose. This will also be of benefit to the heart, since there will be less of a strain placed on it.

Nasal polyps may restrict the proper intake of air through the nose. Even though these growths are benign, their presence can be a source of great discomfort. The only effective cure for them is *Teucrium marum verum* (cat thyme). But should they not yield to this treatment, surgery would be indicated.

Even more bothersome than polyps is ozaena, a disease of the mucous membranes of the nose, giving off a foul-smelling discharge or odour. Relief is obtained by sniffing up or drawing in a solution containing *sea salt*, followed by sniffing up *Urticalcin* powder. For internal treatment, *Kali iod. 4x* and *Mercurius 4x* have proved very helpful.

Rhinitis (inflammation of the mucous membranes of the nose) can also be very annoying, especially in the spring with its changeable weather pattern. As for all other kinds of inflammation and infection, *Echinaforce* taken internally is a reliable remedy for rhinitis. For a more speedy cure you could also try soaking a cotton bud in Echinaforce and painting the nostrils with it. If sores or scales should develop on the inner walls of the nose, apply Bioforce Cream for an immediate healing effect.

A 'runny nose' can be stopped with relative ease. Cut a slice of fresh *onion* and dip it briefly into a glass of hot water. It is enough to dip the slice in just once, and then drink the water in small sips. This treatment will soon cure your sniffles.

Nasal catarrh or a cold, accompanied by a pus-like sticky discharge, may be cured in its acute stage by sipping a glass of hot water to which have been added five drops of *iodine tincture*. A person allergic to iodine, especially in cases of exophthalmic goitre, may obtain the same quick result by using five drops of *camphor tincture* instead of the iodine. Again, I would like to emphasise that Echinaforce taken internally and used externally will bring sure relief.

Sinusitis can cause a great deal of pain, since the infection spreads right into the sinuses and impairs our thinking processes as well. How grateful we can be for remedies such as *Cinnabaris 4x* and *Hepar sulph. 4x* and the speedy relief they are able to give. With their help, the rapidly forming pus can be drained and the patient will be free from the unpleasant infection in a relatively short time. It is important to bring about fast relief in order to prevent it from becoming chronic, since it may reach a stage where it will stubbornly resist any treatment.

Inflammation of the Ear (Otitis)
An earache should never be taken lightly as serious illness can result from it. First of all, apply a *poultice* to the neck; even if it is only onions the effect will be beneficial. Do not use chemist's ear drops; rather, go on a *fruit diet* and avoid all highly seasoned and heavy foods for a few weeks. See your doctor for *syringing*, which may be done with infusions of ribwort, camomile, marigold or lemon balm.

If a throbbing sensation is felt deep down in the ear, or if the pain is severe on one side, particularly in the right ear, and gets worse at night, *Calcarea carbonica 6x (Calcium carbonicum Hahnemann)* will help to soothe it. The patient should receive competent treatment at this stage, because inflammation of the middle ear (*Otitis media*) can develop, and this is more serious than many people think. If the pus, instead of breaking through the eardrum and draining from the ear canal, actually perforates the thin bone wall discharging into the cranial cavity, it may spread to the mastoid air cells and reach the covering of the brain and the brain itself – resulting in a critical condition.

Improperly treated infection of the middle ear can result in meningitis. Serious problems of the ear and the middle ear are often created by incompletely treated or suppressed infectious diseases such as scarlet fever, measles, whooping cough, diphtheria, influenza and tonsillitis, because they scatter their viruses and toxins throughout the body. Hence, if a relapse is to be avoided, elimination of the toxins is of the utmost importance. Improper treatment can affect the auditory nerves and cause loss of hearing; these nerves may degenerate or atrophy altogether and lead to complete deafness.

Pulsatilla, Belladonna, sulphur and *Mercurius solubilis*, in homoeopathic potencies, are the best remedies indicated for treating inflammations of the ear. At the first sign of suppuration *Hepar sulph. 12x* is very effective, and if there is a danger of septic infection, *Lachesis 12x* can still save the situation. In cases of prolonged discharge, *Silicea 12x* taken in alternation with *Causticum* (freshly burnt lime according to Hahnemann) will help. Should there be a tendency to a relapse, recourse to an occasional dose of the constitution-building remedy *Baryum carbonicum 10x* is indicated.

Anyone prone to ear problems should take the fresh plant extract of ribwort over a longer period of time. Known by its botanical name *Plantago lanceolata*, ribwort is one of the best remedies for the ears and will also sharpen the auditory senses. *Ginkgo biloba* is excellent for the same purpose and therefore recommended for people who are hard of hearing or suffer from tinnitus (ringing or buzzing in the ear).

Middle Ear Infections
Middle ear infections are frequently not given enough attention. If a child complains of earache and has perhaps a slight runny discharge which turns to pus, we put the child in a warm bed and think our duty is done. Unfortunately, however, the correct treatment is overlooked. The reason why so many people are hard of hearing and in some cases are deaf in one ear is because an inflammation of the middle ear in childhood had been neglected. Ear infections can also affect the brain, and the eyes may suffer if the infection becomes chronic. Neighbouring organs, as well as those in different parts of the body, can also be harmed. It is therefore imperative that no time is lost in treating the ear when the first symptoms of this serious condition appear, and that treatment is continued until the patient is cured.

For a chronic middle ear infection with pus the following directions will help give the patient relief. Place an *onion poultice* behind the affected ear, but if relief is not forthcoming, change to a *mustard poultice*. If even this does not produce the desired result, you will have to resort to the *Baunscheidt method* (see page 439). It is always important that the inflammation, especially in chronic cases, is drawn away from the head by some form of stimulation therapy, so that the focus of infection is drawn from the inside to the surface. Inflammation in the ears, eyes and nose can be diverted to the neck or shoulders. Internal remedies are *Belladonna 4x*, five drops every two hours, and *Ferrum phos. 6x*, two tablets also every two hours. The patient takes one of these remedies every hour, say *Belladonna* first, an hour later *Ferr. phos.*, then back to *Belladonna* again. For as long as the ear continues to discharge and suppurate, *Hepar sulph. 4x* is effective. When there is no more pus, *Silicea 12x* is indicated to stabilise the improvement. Follow up with one drop of *St John's wort oil* and one drop of *Plantago* (ribwort juice) once daily into the ear. When the ear infection is accompanied by nasal catarrh and pharyngitis, which is most likely due to the germs spreading, use *Cinnabaris 4x* and *Plantago*. You can also put five drops of *Plantago* on cotton wool and place this in the ear, replacing it every day.

This treatment will heal even a chronic inflammation so that the hearing will return to normal. On the other hand, if the described treatment is not strictly followed, the patient's sense of hearing will be endangered. The auditory nerve together with the intricate structures of the inner ear can be permanently damaged by bacterial toxins; the infection can actually cause erosion of the ossicles of the middle ear. When this happens, no treatment will restore the hearing apparatus. So never lose time in starting an intensive natural treatment as soon as problems with the ear begin to manifest themselves. Take into account the patient's general state of health and adopt a natural diet. This will help nature to heal and regenerate.

Sinus Infections

If you know how a sinus infection can come about, you will be able to see that, using natural remedies and treatment, it is quite simple to deal with the cause of this problem. For the most part, such an infection originates in the nose, especially after a head cold, sore throat, influenza, scarlet fever etc. It can also result from pus-forming bacteria in abscesses on the gums. When this happens, secretions are blocked, the circulation becomes restricted, the normal functions can no longer be sustained and the body must find another way out. The leucocytes and lymphocytes now appear on the scene to avert serious danger. The body has several options of defence and if the normal way of dealing with infection is not open, it will find another one to ward off the greatest danger, suppuration of the antrum or sinus being just one way of preventing worse developments.

You can usually recognise this complication by a copious discharge of pus from the affected side of the nose. Acute throbbing and pulsating pains in the upper jaw or forehead, depending upon which cavities are afflicted, often accompany the discharge. In chronic cases the pain may be absent and besides the one-sided discharge only hoarseness may point to sinusitis. Merely syringing the cavities will not get rid of the causes. In addition to specific natural remedies, other measures to draw the infection away must be employed. *Onion poultices*, while perhaps not very pleasant, are simple and effective. Chop an onion finely, place it between two pieces of gauze and bind it on the neck before retiring, leaving it overnight. The two homoeopathic remedies *Hepar sulph. 4x* and *Cinnabaris 4x* will help eliminate the pus and heal the affected part. This treatment usually makes syringing superfluous. For a chronic case, and when the trouble originated with a cold, *hot compresses* and *baths* always soothe and alleviate the pain.

Sore Throats

It is a fact that a sore throat, if not correctly treated or completely cured, can have serious consequences that may do permanent injury to one's health. This particularly applies to severe sore throats such as those caused by Vincent's angina, laryngitis or tonsillitis. The toxins of an improperly treated sore throat can cause an inflammation of the middle ear, rheumatic fever and arthritis. They can also be responsible for a partial paralysis of the cardiac valves, which leaves the patient with a permanent cardiac defect. This was brought to my attention not too long ago by one of my patients, a healthy woman who had given birth to several children without any complications, until the day that a neglected sore throat (tonsillitis) put an end to her good health. The doctors shared my belief that her cardiac defect was a direct result of the presence of tonsillitis toxins in her body. To make matters worse, her stomach and intestines had been affected by the allopathic drugs she had been taking. So today, this once vigorous and healthy woman is a very sick person.

Therefore, do not overlook a bad sore throat or neglect to treat it properly, for if you do, you will lay yourself open to serious consequences and relapses.

It is also dangerous to go outdoors too soon after tonsillitis when the weather is bad. You should know that tonsillitis may take a more drastic course in a low pressure system, that is, at the beginning of a warm air current. Someone suffering from calcium deficiency or a weak lymphatic system is more prone to this type of sore throat. This emphasises the need to always have a diet rich in calcium and avail oneself of the benefits of a calcium complex, such as Urticalcin.

Careful and thorough treatment of the throat and tonsils will render bacterial toxins harmless and prevent them from spreading through the body. However, it is also important to persevere and not stop the treatment as soon as the acute symptoms have passed.

Never regard tonsillitis as a harmless complaint; it is an infection that can have serious consequences. It appears that many people still do not realise how dangerous a sore throat can be; otherwise they would be more concerned about obtaining immediate treatment for, and a complete cure of, this infection. One mother wrote to me: 'My seventeen-year-old daughter had a bad sore throat eight weeks ago and she developed an inflammation of the middle ear from it.' This is the sort of letter received all too frequently. Heart problems, pericarditis and nephritis often follow in the wake of a bad sore throat or tonsillitis. This all goes to show that the toxins are far from harmless and that this complaint should receive more attention than it is usually given.

The Treatment of Sore Throats
The first measure to be taken at the sign of a sore throat is to paint the throat two or three times a day with *concentrated whey (Molkosan)*, since this may actually arrest a case of incipient tonsillitis. Whey will destroy the germs on the surface of the tonsils and to some extent even in the crypts and channels of the throat. It will prevent the formation of toxins and help the body's own defences to advance to the infected area. In fact, this condensed, natural lactic acid product made from whey has proved far superior to the strongest chemical disinfectants and is free from the harmful properties the latter may possess.

If this remedy is not handy, the *pimpernel root (Pimpinella saxifraga)* or *imperial masterwort (Imperatoria ostruthium)* fulfils the same purpose if you keep chewing it.

Thorough oral hygiene is essential. Frequent gargling with *salt water* is good, or just suck a *slice of lemon,* unsweetened, every day, for lemon juice is equally effective. Make sure that the lemon skin has not been sprayed with pesticide. In chronic cases the use of special equipment may be necessary to clean the tonsils regularly and paint them afterwards with whey concentrate. *Dr Roeder's Apparatus,* for example, is designed to suck the pus off the tonsils.

Additionally, however, it is necessary to combat the disease from within the body by taking a calcium preparation (*Urticalcin*) and *Lachesis 12x.* For external treatment apply *cabbage leaf* and *clay poultices* in alternation. The clay for the poultice should be made into a paste using *horsetail tea.* Poultices of *grated horseradish* mixed with *soft white cheese (quark)* can also be used; these are stronger and especially effective. Pure horseradish may be too strong, so mix it with soft white cheese or finely grated carrots to reduce the strength. One-third horseradish with two-thirds cheese or carrots will still give you the full healing benefit of horseradish and do the job well. With these treatments a bad sore throat can be cured fast.

If a cough or catarrh follows the throat trouble, take syrup made from raw pine shoots (*Santasapina*) or *ribwort syrup* and *Kali iod. 4x,* besides *Imperatoria.* These harmless remedies prevent the tonsillitis toxins from invading other parts of the body. But if they are already in the blood, it is essential to stimulate the kidneys to greater activity so that the toxins can be eliminated as quickly as possible. While *Solidago* and *kidney tea* are best for this purpose, *sweating cures* support the elimination process; any method of inducing perspiration is suitable, as long as the patient can tolerate the procedure.

A follow-up cure is indispensable to eliminate the toxins completely. This can be achieved by taking *kidney drops,* such as *Nephrosolid,* and *liver drops. Steam baths* also help to speed up the excretion of toxins. During the treatment the patient's diet should be low in protein and salt and high in vitamins and minerals. Never shy away from the effort and bother the thorough and careful treatment of a bad sore throat may entail. It will save you the troublesome consequences that often leave a patient with permanent damage.

Hay Fever
It is certainly miserable to suffer from hay fever while those less allergic to pollen take full delight in the beauty of flowers and blossoms. To make things worse, once an attack has started it is

difficult to stop it quickly. In fact, it is generally too late to find relief. In order to check the development of hay fever, it is necessary to begin treatment early, no later than February. If you know that you are susceptible to hay fever attacks you must start treatment in the winter before the trees and flowers begin to bloom.

A treatment consisting of ten subcutaneous homoeopathic injections of *formic acid* and a *herb complex* has brought about relief, as has been confirmed by former sufferers. To ensure a permanent cure, the treatment must be repeated at the beginning of the following year. Moreover, during the entire year do not neglect to take *Urticalcin* regularly. Urticalcin powder also has a good healing effect when drawn up the nose like snuff. Furthermore, the nose should be creamed daily with *Bioforce Cream,* which prevents the mucous membranes from drying out. At the same time take *Galeopsis, Kali iod. 4x* and *Arsen. album 4x.* Also helpful are two or three teaspoons of *honey* taken daily. Make sure that the diet consists of natural wholefoods and stay away from denatured, refined foods. Animal fats are also out of the question. *Pollinosan,* a new homoeopathic medicine made from tropical plants, has already proved to be an effective treatment for hay fever and other allergies.

If you follow this advice and repeat the treatment until the hay fever has completely cleared up, you will gradually get rid of this troublesome allergy and make your life more enjoyable even when the plant world bursts out in blossoms and flowers.

Leucorrhoea and What to Do about It
Today's fashions are responsible for an increasing number of women and girls suffering from leucorrhoea, commonly called the 'whites'. In the past, when women were accustomed to wearing warm clothes in winter, very few experienced this bothersome problem. Thick woollen stockings, warm underwear, loose woollen dresses and good shoes used to provide the necessary warmth, even if there was no central heating in the house and only the living room and kitchen were heated. Today, however, we usually live in overheated rooms and dress as lightly as possible even in winter. Add to this modern way of life our inborn vanity that appeals to our desire for a figure that is slimmer than is advisable for good health, and there you have the origin of colds and their serious consequences. What is more, the hectic pace of our times encourages us to overtax our physical strength and inner resources, and

if a person has a weak constitution to start with, colds and their consequences are an inevitable result.

Leucorrhoea is the result of catarrh (inflammation of the mucous membranes) and, as such, we should make every effort to cure it properly. This is of great importance because it is an uncomfortable condition and weakens the body. As with any other inflammation of the mucous membranes, we should persevere in the treatment until it has completely cleared up. Indeed, we should never neglect to treat the mucous membranes whenever there is something wrong with them. They are under constant threat from external influences and bacterial infections and a constant fight is called for. The mucous membranes are only able to withstand the attacks of invading harmful bacteria by calling the friendly ones to the rescue. The harmful bacteria must be killed, if at all possible. That is why we have mouth bacteria, for example, which are there to attack harmful invaders.

The mucous membranes of the genital organs in a healthy woman normally secrete lactic acid, which prevents the development of harmful bacteria. But if the production of lactic acid is insufficient, resistance against micro-organisms is considerably diminished, and it is easy for an inflammation to develop.

In this respect it is important to watch your diet, since inadequate nutrition may slow down and weaken the growth of lactic acid bacteria. As a result, invading bacteria soon gain a foothold and the body has to adopt a different defence strategy. It will secrete mucus and dispatch leucocytes and lymphocytes to combat the foreign invaders, all in an effort to expel them from the body. And that is the so-called 'whites', a white or yellowish discharge of mucous material from the vagina.

Knowing the origin of the trouble, we can successfully fight back if we use lactic acid. Women afflicted by this condition would do well to use *Molkosan* (whey concentrate), since its natural lactic acid content has indeed proved its worth as a disinfectant and antiseptic douche. Douching with an infusion of *camomile* and 3–4 soupspoons of *Molkosan* added to every litre (2 pints) of liquid, has given good results. The natural lactic acid in Molkosan is able to replace the lactic acid the mucous membranes are lacking. The treatment with Molkosan is therefore a biological method. Since the patient usually has a deficiency of calcium salts as well, it would also be wise to take the biological calcium preparation *Urticalcin*.

Another essential feature of the treatment of leucorrhoea is to take regular *sitz baths* prepared with herbs; the baths should last between half an hour to an hour, with the water being kept at a constant temperature of 37 °C (98.6 °F) adding hot water from time to time. Patients who follow this treatment will feel much better after a relatively short time. So take a sitz bath prepared with *thyme* or *juniper*, using *Juniperosan*, two or three times a week. These sitz baths will stimulate the circulation in the abdomen, which is an important factor in their effectiveness.

Also effective are the homoeopathic remedies *Sepia 4x–6x, Calc. carb., Pulsatilla, Ferr. phos., Kali sulph.* and *Calc. phos.*, in addition to the biological calcium preparation Urticalcin.

As leucorrhoea often affects the kidneys, although these will benefit from the sitz baths, they will need further stimulating. This can be achieved by taking a mild *kidney tea* together with *Nephrosolid*. It is understandable that leucorrhoea can have a weakening effect on the nerves. Hence we will want to build them up by regularly taking *Avenaforce* in alternation with *Ginsavena*. *Neuroforce* tablets are also excellent for this purpose.

On the other hand, I would advise against the use of strong antibiotic medicines. Why? Because these drugs destroy not only the harmful but also the useful and necessary bacteria, making the restoration of bacterial flora more difficult. If we want to cooperate with nature we must not first destroy its workings. Rather, we should take care and refrain from drastic medicines that destroy the beneficial organisms we want to build up, for experience shows that harmful bacteria recuperate faster than the useful ones.

The treatment of leucorrhoea, usually a very stubborn condition, requires patience, perseverance and absolute regularity in taking medication. There is no other way to achieve a permanent cure. At the same time, it is very important to avoid any detrimental habits and influences even after the cure has been achieved.

Colds

During a Change of Season
It is not unusual to hear complaints about chills and colds when seasonal changes occur. Most people accept them as unavoidable, not realising that it is really up to us to do something about them. Women seem to be more prone to catching colds, since they are usually more reluctant to exchange their elegant thin stockings for warm or, better still, thick knitted woollen ones. It would indeed be most appropriate to limit the use of elegant apparel in favour

81

of warmer clothing, or even to put it away altogether for the duration of the winter.

The change of season is the most difficult time for the body, for it is still accustomed to the warm summer and unprepared for the sudden onset of cold weather. That is why we must protect the body with whatever clothing is appropriate for the weather. Most important of all, *keep the feet warm* and, as I have pointed out already, woollen stockings and a pair of good, warm shoes are indispensable if you wish to discourage colds. It is an accepted fact that warm feet and a cool head are necessary for good health. As long as the feet are warm we will hardly ever catch a cold, because the feet are the indicators of the general warmth of the body.

People in sedentary occupations suffer to a much greater extent from cold feet than those whose work allows them plenty of activity and movement. If you have inherited sluggish circulation, you will feel the cold even more; even overheated rooms will not seem to be warm enough for you. Of course, heating does not make up for the lack of exercise and unless the feet are covered with warm stockings and adequate shoes, they will be cold. Moreover, if you leave an overheated room inadequately clothed and go out into the cool, damp air, the body will react to this drastic drop in temperature and become chilled, with an adverse effect on the mucous membranes. And there you have the best precondition for the development of the germs that cause colds, coughs, head colds, catarrh, pneumonia and other infections. So, never seek to make up for a lack of body heat by overheating the rooms; instead, wear warm clothing, take some *exercise* and try to improve the circulation. Once we become used to the cold, we will be much less susceptible to colds.

You can see that it is not at all surprising that we need to be much more careful during the change of seasons than in the depths of winter, since we become chilled much more quickly when the body is still attuned to the warmth of sunny autumn days. Therefore, do not be tempted to sit down to your work in the morning without having taken some vigorous exercise previously. Do not despise the idea of making your own bed or tidying up your room in the morning. Even this exercise will warm you up. Again, do not just hop in the car or let the bus or train take you to your place of work. It is much better for you if you can walk or bicycle to work. If you live in an area where snow falls, enjoy the new day by shovelling snow in the fresh air. You will afterwards appreciate the warmth of your room, and it is true that brain work is much easier after brisk exercise and *deep-breathing*, which invigorates and promotes good circulation. You can also warm up in a natural way by doing early morning exercises and deep-breathing in front of an open window, and by giving yourself a good brush massage. Exhaling vigorously rids the body of waste gases and deep inhalation saturates the lungs with oxygen. This is particularly important in discouraging the conditions that favour colds.

If you do have a tendency to catch colds, make sure to eat plenty of foods rich in calcium, because the body is more susceptible when it lacks calcium; especially during the change of seasons, take a biological calcium preparation (*Urticalcin*) as well. The veins should not be overlooked either, so that the circulation remains unimpaired. Heed this advice and you will acquire more resistance to the common cold and related afflictions.

Vitamin and Calcium Deficiencies
Why is it that some people catch cold when travelling on a bus or a badly heated train, when they are probably also exposed to a draught, whereas other passengers remain totally unaffected? In answer to this question we could say that some people may have better blood circulation than others. But there may be other factors involved, because susceptibility to infection varies greatly from one person to another. The germs that can cause a cold or catarrh are often already present in the mucous membranes. All it needs is for the body to become chilled and the virus is ready to attack. The result is a cold.

Of course, we usually do not take this bothersome inflammation of the mucous membranes quite so seriously, and although we may feel uncomfortable, and often rather depressed, we are not inclined to give in and interrupt our work routine. In fact, many people, for example in Europe, have acquired an inborn immunity. No one dies of a cold anymore, do they? On the contrary, the very thought makes us smile, for who could be so weak that a mere infection of the mucous membranes could kill him? In truth, this kind of reasoning is actually quite mistaken. You may be surprised to learn that when the Eskimos succumbed to the cold virus brought to them by the Americans some years ago, many of them died, even though they were well used to cold weather. In spite of their strength, their bodies had little immunity to resist the strange and unexpected infection.

Our acquired immunity cannot completely protect us from colds

83

either if the body lacks vitamins, for example. Calcium deficiency, a low calcium level, is another important factor. Furthermore, we have to look out for signs of exhaustion. Heavy demands on our energies are closely connected with a greater consumption of vitamins and calcium. Should circumstances require us to overtax our physical energies, we would need more vitamins and calcium to protect ourselves from catching colds than would be necessary if the body were rested.

The various ways in which we can build up our resistance to colds are dealt with below.

Foods that Build Up Resistance to Colds

Foods rich in *calcium* should be on your menu without fail. Eat carrots every day. Include kohlrabi (turnip cabbage) tops in your diet when they are in season; serve similar vegetables where kohlrabi is not grown. Celery leaves and roots (celeriac), white turnips, swedes, parsnips and the like are also good because of their high calcium content. So too are all kinds of fruits, nuts and seeds. Include plenty of figs, raisins, Brazil nuts, almonds, pecans and pine kernels in the diet. This diet will help you get through the difficult winter months with better health, until your own garden again produces fresh vegetables, herbs and berries rich in vitamins.

As long as there is no snow it is possible to harvest parsley and watercress to meet the body's needs for *vitamins A and C*. But if you live in a temperate or northern climate, it would be a good idea to sow cress seeds in flower pots or little boxes and raise them on a sunny windowsill. If you sow cress at regular intervals, you will have a constant supply of this healthy vegetable throughout the vitamin-deficient winter months. Every little help we can get will be to our advantage. The importance of foods containing vitamins A and C cannot be overstressed.

Other Remedies to Build Up Resistance

Much good may also be derived from taking natural remedies. Ideally suited for this purpose is *Urticalcin*, a natural calcium supplement of proven worth. Another natural medicine for colds is *Usnea* (larch moss or lichen), which builds up the resistance of the mucous membranes. To combat a susceptibility to catarrh and to alleviate colds, take *Santasapina* or *Drosinula Cough Syrup*.

As a prophylactic for the throat, use *Echinaforce* and *Molkosan*, since *Echinacea* extract counteracts infection and diluted whey used as a gargle disinfects the mouth and throat. If a throat infection is already under way, it is advisable to paint the throat with undiluted Molkosan. Also, massage the chest with *Po-Ho-Salve* every day.

Severe catarrh and even bronchitis may be tackled with *Imperatoria* (imperial masterwort), as it will help in every case. I often recommend to people who like to take walks through the woods and forests, even in winter, to chew *larch* (tamarack) and *pine buds or shoots*, as the sap has a preventative as well as a healing effect.

Guarding against the Consequences of Infectious Diseases

Toxins in the system, which stem from infectious disease, must be eliminated or they will lead to future ill health. A case of mumps that has been neglected or not fully cured can lead to pancreatitis (inflammation of the pancreas) in later life. An inflammation of the middle ear may be a result of suppressed scarlet fever. Improperly treated tonsillitis can give rise to heart trouble, for example inflammation of the heart muscle (myocarditis) or the endocardium (endocarditis), which in turn can lead to valvular defects or even pericarditis, although this is less frequent. The kidneys can suffer too, and rheumatic fever is often the consequence of toxic infiltrations from diseased tonsils. Many other diseases can arise when toxins remain in the body following an infection.

It is therefore most important that every effort be made to ensure the complete excretion of toxins in all cases of infectious disease. The following three main points must be observed:

1. *Elimination through the skin.* The patient should be encouraged to perspire by applying hot packs, taking hot showers etc. The Kneipp treatment might also be used.
2. *Elimination through the kidneys.* This can be encouraged by means of a simple kidney remedy, such as tea made from goldenrod or parsley, or any other natural remedy which acts to stimulate the kidneys. Onion poultices are also effective for this.
3. *Elimination through the bowels.* Fever usually tends to dry up the bowels. To stimulate movement, use simple natural remedies, for example linseed tea, psyllium seed, manna stick tea (*Cassia fistula*), soaked figs or prunes. A diet consisting solely of fruit juice is also excellent. While the infectious disease lasts, it is advisable to refrain from eating protein; nothing but fruit juices and vegetable juices is indicated.

If you pay close attention to these three points, you can avoid the complications often experienced as a result of ineptly treated infectious disease.

The Remarkable Laws of Immunity
Life's constant changeability sometimes presents us with rather unusual questions. For example, is it not strange that, in some parts of the world infectious diseases are declining whereas the death toll from metabolic disorders and other ailments associated with living in an industrialised society is showing a sharp increase? Could this, perhaps, be attributed to our having acquired increased resistance to certain infections? On the other hand, what is it exactly that makes us so vulnerable to metabolic and other disorders? While all this is somewhat puzzling, if we carefully review what experience and observation have taught us, we will find the explanation.

During the time I spent in the Amazon area, an outbreak of measles took the lives of thousands of Indians living there. Yet in Europe and North America, for instance, it is practically unheard of for a child or an adult to die as a result of this disease. Why should that be so? The virus is just as toxic and virulent as ever, but nature is always a step ahead of human wisdom. The layperson as well as the physician should become familiar with the body's inherent defence mechanisms and their capacity to face up to and adapt to new situations, and learn to respect them. Thanks to the wonderful generosity and benevolence of our Creator, these automatic mechanisms or 'laws of nature', given time, are able to produce an effective counterforce to any violent attack by invading organisms and substances. In the beginning a virus causes widespread disaster among people and takes numerous lives, but the very next generation is born with a degree of immunity and after a few more generations the illness has only negligible consequences. The history of tuberculosis provides a good example of this. Only sixty years ago tuberculosis was a major cause of death everywhere. Diphtheria and other infectious diseases, likewise, are no longer the scourge they once were.

Laws We Should All Take Note Of
By looking at the plant kingdom we can see similarities in the working of natural laws, there being the same powerful drive to adapt and produce forces for defence and immunity. As an illustration of this, let us consider our experience with DDT. Some

86

years ago, this chemical could kill all but two species of insects in Switzerland. Today, however, we know of at least forty species that have become immune to DDT. While I was staying in California I observed that it was necessary to keep on increasing the strength and toxicity of insecticides in order to obtain the desired results. The deplorable outcome of this process was that millions of birds and bees died, whilst the insects for which it was intended quickly became immune to the increased doses of poison. A few years ago, a friend of mine in Guatemala told me that an industrial firm near where he kept his beehives started using very potent insecticides, with the unintentional result that his bee population was decimated.

When the biological processes of nature are disturbed by chemicals, the interference is bound to bring about undesirable damage in its wake, yet the innocent victims are rarely given any compensation by those responsible for the losses.

In accordance with the laws of nature, we may presume that in fifty years from now the Amazon Indians will no longer die from measles, since by then they will have developed the immunity which we already have. As long as the Indians retain their traditional lifestyle and can avoid the detrimental effects of an ever-encroaching civilisation, they will not have to worry about many of our other so-called 'diseases of civilisation' either. The number of deaths resulting from gout, diabetes, obesity, cancer and multiple sclerosis will continue to be negligible among the Indian tribes of the Amazon.

Physicians, biologists and nutritionists who are aware of these dangers advocate a return to a natural way of life and to eating natural wholefoods as a protection against modern diseases. Like a voice crying in the wilderness, they sound the alarm again and again, appealing to us to change our life-style to a more natural one. Notable among them was the late Dr Joseph Evers, who treated thousands of people suffering from multiple sclerosis. They all hoped to find some relief from their hard lot in life. Nonetheless, it would be better to do something about preventing the illness rather than painfully trying to overcome it, because in spite of every effort made and care given, a cure is not always guaranteed. Dr Evers' book, *Gestaltwandel des Krankheitsgeschehens (Changes in the Development of Disease)*, which is published by Karl-Haug-Verlag, is so impressive that even a healthy person, after reading it, will change his life-style and diet without delay and almost subconsciously. Any reasonable person reading the book will take note of the clear and logical arguments presented by this experienced researcher. Dr Evers proves to the reader that nature has a greater share in increasing our life span than the achievements of orthodox medicine.

Why Natural Antibiotics Are Necessary

Building Up Resistance
People who have low resistance and lack antibodies, for example those who suffer from liver disorders, are rendered more susceptible to infectious diseases. Hence the need to take natural antibiotics, which will build up the body's resistance to infections. Of course, it is impossible to avoid every source of infection because we are exposed to them through the food we eat and the air we breathe. City air, especially, is highly polluted and an examination of even one cubic centimetre will reveal thousands of germs, spores and bacteria. Insects can also be responsible for transmitting diseases, flies and mosquitoes being the best-known carriers. So even with the utmost care and caution it is difficult to escape from all the adverse influences surrounding us, but we can make certain that our bodies have enough resistance and sufficient antibodies to withstand pathogenic agents, thus minimising their attacks. Certain plants, especially the medicinal herbs which contain essential oils, as well as some culinary herbs, possess antibiotic properties that ensure resistance to a wide range of germs. This will be discussed shortly, but first we will consider the effectiveness of some of the medical antibiotics, the use of which has become increasingly common in recent years.

Various Antibiotics in Practice
The discovery of such antibiotics as penicillin, streptomycin, auromycin and others which have come on the market has provided us with very potent medicines against bacterial infection. In the case of dangerous tropical diseases they have been instrumental in saving many lives. However, it is unfortunate that they are being used too frequently for the treatment of minor infections (for example a common sore throat or some other simple inflammation) which could be dealt with equally effectively by more harmless remedies.

This is where the danger lies. In the first place, the body accustoms itself to these substances and the germs develop a resistance or immunity to them until, finally, they prove useless in the fight against them when one's life is in danger. Secondly, the constant use of antibiotics, in time, harms and destroys the intestinal flora, the useful bacteria present in the intestines.

Just as certain bacteria in the intestines are necessary for the proper digestion and assimilation of food, so plants need certain bacteria to enable them to flourish as they should. For instance, it is impossible to reap a good crop of soybeans if the soil has not been inoculated with the bacteria symbiotically associated with them, or unless the beans have been grown in that particular soil before. No pine forest could grow without bacteria in the soil either. They are indispensable. A similar necessity exists in the digestive system; it, too, needs certain bacteria. That is the reason why yoghurt is highly recommended for the care of the bowels, preferably yoghurt containing bacteria of the species *Lactobacillus acidophilus*, since it encourages the normal, beneficial flora, while it hinders the harmful one, the putrefactive type, in its development. Lactic acid bacteria are good for us because they get on well with the intestinal bacteria and promote their growth. But if we take any of the various antibiotics on the market – penicillin, streptomycin, auromycin or whatever other names they may have been given – we must be prepared for their damaging effect on the intestinal flora, for it so happens that the bacteria essential to good health are also the most sensitive to drugs. No wonder, then, that the harmful bacteria proliferate and spread in the intestines after these double-edged remedies have been administered, possibly leading to chronic inflammation of the intestines. Once the beneficial bacterial flora has been damaged, the patient will have less resistance than before taking the drugs and germs can gain entrance much more easily.

If the patient then receives further doses of potent antibiotics, the body will no longer respond. In such cases even more conservative treatment may be ineffective, leaving the patient open to the gravest consequences.

Natural Antibiotics

As suggested above, persons who suffer from a liver disorder have to be cared for especially; their resistance needs to be built up with natural antibiotics. Their weakened constitution can thus be strengthened and protected. Of course, this is important not only for liver patients but also for those with weak lungs, cancer and many other crippling diseases.

Many years ago I made some interesting experiments with horseradish, watercress, gardencress and even nasturtiums. I observed that those who ate these regularly became more resistant to diseases, particularly colds and infections. At that time, I can remember how some people laughed at the idea of nasturtiums having any nutritional and remedial value, but in those days I was not able to explain why these plants have such outstanding results. This is also true of various other natural cures. Anyway, having observed the improvement in my patients' conditions, I always continued to use the treatment for their benefit, even though I could not offer any scientific explanation. To my great delight, however, I have since found in modern medical publications the confirmation that my earlier observations and conclusions were indeed correct. The research work of Professor Dr Winter, a medical scientist of Cologne, for example, has established the value of nasturtiums as a part of the diet. The thought of mixing them into a salad no longer elicits the ridicule that I had to bear years ago.

My earlier experiments had shown that the extract from the nasturtium plant was effective in killing insect pests such as aphids and others when sprayed on them. I became convinced that nasturtiums contain a very strong substance, and my assumption has since been proved by scientific research. However, there is still the question in my mind as to whether nasturtiums actually contain other substances which may have an even greater effect than their known antibiotic properties. The lethal effect on insect pests may be due to some other potent substance which science has not yet discovered. It is not only nasturtiums that yield such valuable results; the common watercress has a similar effect, as has been proved by experiments I have made over many years, especially with the cress that grows along the course of the mountain streams in the Engadine Valley in Switzerland. Eat this cress regularly and you will soon notice an improvement in your resistance to colds, catarrh and other infectious diseases.

I have made equally important observations, with even better results, in connection with another plant. Known by the names larch moss or beard moss (*Usnea barbata*), it is a lichen that grows on larch trees and its properties had not previously been analysed when I first became interested in it. During my skiing trips I would always chew some of this lichen. I noticed that deer and chamois enjoyed it too, because where there was deep snow the *Usnea* within the animals' reach had always been nibbled off. Closer investigation has now shown that *Usnea* and certain other lichens are high in carbohydrates and therefore of considerable nutritive value. The animals seem to know this and make good use of the plant as food and, incidentally, of its antibiotic properties which make them resistant to disease. There is no doubt that *Usnea* clears up catarrh. I have seen this confirmed repeatedly. On occasions, after starting out on a tour, I would feel the onset of a sore throat and runny nose. As I went along I would chew *Usnea* and by the time I arrived home again my cold would have disappeared. Such valuable experience urged me to investigate this lichen more closely, and I now use the extract in the prophylactic medicine *Usneasan*.

Observations confirm that if you have a tendency to catarrh or colds, your resistance will be considerably improved by taking this remedy regularly. So why take the risk of using manufactured antibiotics which may inflict unwanted side effects? Why not use the cultivated and wild mountain plants, whose harmless but effective medicinal properties are always present in the right composition and proportions according to the laws of nature?

Why should we subject ourselves to any dangers at all? Natural antibiotics are unlikely to have an adverse effect on the intestinal flora; neither will their regular use make germs more resistant to them. For this reason salads made from watercress, gardencress and nasturtiums are heartily recommended for healthy people as well as for the sick, and especially for cancer patients. Eat them regularly and put them in sandwiches too. Try adding some finely grated horseradish to carrot salad, or the juices can be extracted and taken in small quantities. I also recommend the seasoning salt *Trocomare* because it contains these plants. Use it as a seasoning for sandwiches and salads, and sprinkle it on hot vegetables and soups after cooking in order to avoid destroying its vitamins and minerals. When your health has been restored and you can once more think of skiing or mountaineering, do not forget to look for the lichen *Usnea*. You will find it on the bark of larch trees at an elevation of over 1,000 m (3,000 feet). Chew it while you enjoy your hiking.

Another plant which has the same potent effect is *Petasites officinalis*, the common butterbur. This plant is of special importance to cancer patients. Butterbur is a relatively rare plant, usually found near streams in mountain valleys. As it is too strong to be used in salads or as a herb, if you want to avail yourself of its medicinal value, you will have to take a *Petasites* preparation.

Improving the Value of Raw Food
Many of those people who once mocked the idea of eating 'rabbit food', raw food, are now beginning to realise that there may be something in it after all. The antibiotic properties of food are destroyed by cooking, because many substances in our food are sensitive to heat; these include not merely its vitamin and mineral content but also many other substances needed for our well-being, some of which are yet to be discovered. For the body to receive all the vital substances it needs, everyone should take a certain amount of fresh raw vegetables and fruit. As we are especially interested in the substances that help us to resist infectious diseases, if you have a garden or allotment, whatever its size, make sure to plant gardencress, watercress, nasturtiums and horseradish. Serve these plants raw in salads, chop them finely and add them to soups and stews, or mix them with cottage cheese or quark; they are also good in sandwiches. I have already mentioned that finely grated horseradish adds a refreshing flavour to carrot salad, but it can also be added to other salads. Those of you who have so far rejected carrot salad as too sweet will enjoy it with the pleasant flavour of horseradish. At the same time you will be administering natural antibiotics.

For the benefit of all who advocate health from herbs and natural foods, especially raw foods, and in defence of their convictions, let me quote the long-standing German proverb, 'You might go further and not fare so well.'

Looking After your Health – the Best Prevention against Respiratory Diseases

Various Causes
To my astonishment, when travelling abroad, I have encountered a great deal of tuberculosis even in lands which have the best climatic conditions for good health. I was amazed that even Greece, a country with an abundance of sunshine, has had to fight this disease. In Holland too, particularly in the small offshore islands, many people are affected. Doctors are probably right in blaming the damp climate of the low-lying countries, although living in such a climate does not necessarily mean that weak lungs cannot be avoided. Other factors must share the blame for such disorders, for instance a one-sided diet, especially one consisting almost exclusively of fish. Anyone who is sufficiently informed about the cause of a disease can take care to prevent it and this is clearly a

wiser course to take than waiting for a disease to strike and then trying to cure it. The following observations and hints are therefore primarily intended for those who are healthy, but they will also benefit the less fortunate to improve and possibly cure their condition.

In the first place, what you eat is of the utmost importance. This has been proved by experience gained in every part of the world. It is astonishing that people living in the healthiest mountain regions, for example the Swiss Alps, where outsiders go to be cured, may actually contract TB themselves. Some time ago I met the warden of a ski chalet who had contracted pulmonary tuberculosis in spite of the fact that he had spent whole winters at a height of over 1,800 m (6,000 feet). However, the cause was obvious: his diet consisted of too much protein, too much canned food and too many unhealthy items containing refined white flour and white sugar. The bad air in the chalet also contributed to his illness. In those days skis still had to be waxed and the fumes from melted wax naturally increased the poisons already in the stale air. Moreover, in a misguided effort to save fuel, the windows were hardly ever opened. Yet fresh air is an absolute necessity for good health.

Then again, we have to build up our immunity if we are to resist respiratory diseases, for we cannot always avoid coming in contact with infection. Research specialists are probably correct in their assertion that it is unusual to find a person in Europe who, at one time or another, has not had a mild tubercular infection that could have triggered the full-blown disease if he had not had sufficient resistance or immunity. That is why our first great task is to acquire this immunity.

These observations emphasise that the best way to prevent disease is to assure good health. How can this be achieved? By putting the following suggestions into practice. First, a natural health-food diet is essential; then we need plenty of light, fresh air, sunshine, exercise and deep-breathing. The more natural your way of life and your diet, the less time spent cooped up in small rooms, and the more you use your free time to breathe and move around in the fresh air and natural light, the less you will be susceptible to disease. Whatever else you do, these rules are basic for your health and well-being.

Adequate Nutrition

It is important that your diet be made up of foods that are rich in calcium and vitamins. You should eat plenty of salads, including, for example, white and green cabbage, carrots, beets and all greens; these are the best sources of vitamins, minerals and calcium. With regard to fruits, berries, particularly organically grown strawberries, are a rich source of calcium. This important mineral is discussed in greater detail on pages 100–1.

It is equally important to eat wholefoods and organically grown foods, for example, wholegrain or wholemeal bread and plenty of dishes made from whole wheat, whole rye and brown rice. If sugar is used at all, it should be unrefined, raw brown cane sugar, never white. Honey, grape sugar, raisins, currants and other sweet dried fruits are even better than brown sugar, which retains only part of the original goodness found in the raw sugar cane juice. Natural sugar is quickly changed into glycogen. In fact, even a weak liver is able to digest fruit sugar.

Fats, too, have to be chosen with care. Do not use kidney fat and lard, other animal fat or hardened fat, or margarine made with these fats. Instead, use unrefined oils, fresh unsalted butter, almonds and nuts. Be sure to go very easy on seasonings; use table salt as little as possible. Hot spices such as pepper and nutmeg should also be avoided, if possible. It is better to season your food with savory, thyme, marjoram, basil, coriander, in other words all the popular garden or kitchen herbs. Yeast extract (*Herbaforce* and *Plantaforce*) is a wholesome flavouring since it contains the vitamins of the B complex. Gravies and sauces seasoned with yeast extract taste like meat gravy and are welcome additions to a meal.

Another important hint is to avoid eating fruit and vegetables together at the same meal. Keep them apart and you will be able to avoid fermentations in the bowels, hence stomach or intestinal gas or wind. Have fruit and wholegrain or wholemeal bread, crispbread or flake bread in the morning and evening. Together with this, have some honey, butter and, if possible, a fruit muesli with various berries or malaceous fruits (those with pips, for example apples) according to what is in season. Stone fruits, such as plums, apricots and peaches, are likely to disagree with most people unless eaten in small quantities. For lunch, eat brown rice, potatoes and cereals, with steamed vegetables and plenty of raw salads. Cut back on fried food. If you must have meat, choose veal and beef rather than pork, sausages and processed meats. Remember, too, that instead of frying, grilling is by far the better method of preparing meat for the table.

Take *Urticalcin* as a calcium supplement. Silica can be easily supplied by the hemp nettle (*Galeopsis*). To increase immunity and resistance to respiratory diseases *Usneasan* has proved invaluable. This remedy is made from lichen (*Usnea barbata*, also known as larch or beard moss) which grows on alpine coniferous trees. Its lichen acids combined with other remedial substances have proved to be very helpful. *Petasites*, made from butterbur, and *Viscum album*, from mistletoe, are also effective remedies with tonic properties. Other herbs and plants suitable for promoting resistance are mentioned in the section on natural antibiotics (see pages 89–91).

Skin Care and Other Precautions
The body's self-healing powers can be assisted greatly by proper skin care. Every day brush the skin vigorously until it turns a rosy pink colour. Afterwards apply a good oil, for example *St John's wort oil* or another skin care oil containing this ingredient. If these are unobtainable, you can use a small amount of a good grade of unrefined olive oil. It suffices to apply the oil lightly every second or every third day.

You should also take care so as to avoid cold feet. If they do get cold, take warm foot baths, massage the feet or help to warm them up by other means. Another important body function that should be given close attention is regular bowel movement. In cases of constipation, take a tablespoon of freshly ground *linseed* mornings and evenings. For really persistent constipation use *Linoforce*, a simple and reliable natural laxative. On the other hand, diarrhoea is not a good thing either, since it drains the body of energy. Two of the simplest remedies for diarrhoea are raw, dry *oat flakes* or *Tormentavena*. The latter has tormentil as its principal ingredient, with oat juice (*Avena sativa*) added for a beneficial effect on the nerves. Intestinal disturbances and fermentations can often be relieved and prevented by thorough mastication of the food we eat. So remember to eat slowly and to chew your food properly so that it becomes well mixed with saliva. This is absolutely essential for good health.

The Importance of Joy and Correct Breathing
There is no doubt that fresh mountain air has a favourable effect on our health and those who are fortunate enough to be able to spend their holidays in the mountains should take every advantage

of it. Alternatively, if you are unable to visit the mountains, you may go to the seaside, where the air is not bad either, as long as it is unpolluted. The main thing is to get away from factories and busy roads.

Let me here draw your attention to the advice given in the sections 'Happiness Means Health' (see pages 624–32) and 'Breathing Means Life', (see pages 577–82). A positive mental attitude acts as a preventative to illness, signifying half the cure so to speak. For this reason it is good if the doctor keeps a careful eye on his patient's mental disposition, so that he can discuss this important factor with him. Moreover, proper breathing exercises contribute a great deal to the patient's improvement. Every nature-oriented doctor will appreciate the importance of these natural preventative measures and healing factors, knowing that health is not primarily a matter of taking medicines. He will thus be able to share in the patient's delight when the recovery is complete.

Asthma
Paroxysms of difficult breathing are one of the many signs of asthma. It is important to know that there are three different kinds of this disease, because if we want to select the correct method of treatment we must differentiate between nervous asthma, bronchial asthma and cardiac asthma. The symptoms must be carefully analysed and considered before carrying out the appropriate treatment.

Nervous Asthma (Asthma nervosum)
If your nervous system is very delicate, with a tendency to tension, and you suffer from asthma, it may well be that the cause is your weak nerves. In this case it will be clear that in order to cure this form of asthma it will first be necessary to treat the nerves.

Bronchial Asthma
Bronchial asthma is different from nervous asthma in that it is mainly triggered by certain climatic conditions. A change in environment generally brings about the desired cure. Living by the sea, where the air contains iodine, usually has a positive effect and asthma attacks will often disappear. High altitude often proves to be equally beneficial. An elevation of 900 m (2,800 feet) generally suffices, although sometimes an elevation of 1,000–1,400 m (3,600–4,500 feet) may be necessary to overcome the problem. The third alternative is the hot, dry air of the desert, which in many cases has helped to relieve asthmatic discomfort.

It is also possible that the spasms are caused by pollen in the air. This 'seasonal asthma' is similar to hay fever, which also results from sensitivity to pollen, an allergic reaction. If your domestic situation permits you to move to a different climatic zone you should do so, since a change of climate, together with the appropriate natural remedies, can lead to an eventual cure of bronchial asthma. Although a patient may be able to find suitable employment in an area where the climate would be more suitable, he may find it difficult to uproot himself from familiar surroundings and leave relatives and friends for a strange place, or his own family may be reluctant to move. It would, however, be a great pity if the patient could not receive the necessary support to move to a climate where he would find relief from his ailment.

Once a person has moved, if the attacks do not recur after a year or two, he can then consider moving back to his former home without misgivings. As a rule, once the asthma has been cured it is not likely to return if the person decides to live again in the area where it first occurred. Young asthmatics, especially, should be given this opportunity, since it can make a significant improvement to their well-being.

If, however, the bronchial asthma is a result of an old, improperly treated lung condition, it will be more difficult to obtain a successful cure. This is yet another reason why chronic conditions of the respiratory organs should be avoided at all costs. Negligence and indifference are dangerous. Such illnesses should be treated the moment they first arise and the treatment continued until a complete cure has been achieved, or else they may lead to bronchial asthma that is extremely difficult to cure.

TREATMENT WITH MEDICINES AND PHYSICAL THERAPY

Drugs used in the treatment of bronchial asthma are mainly antispasmodics. It is interesting to note that a patient who has been promised a cure does indeed feel better and remains free from attacks for quite some time after a course of simple novocaine injections. This goes to show that the patient's condition can be favourably influenced by the skilful use of psychotherapy. Incidentally, homoeopathic formic acid can be used instead of novocaine. As an alternative, give some other neurotherapeutic treatment.

Strong asthma tablets can bring about the desired relief in an emergency, but their long-term use is not recommended. These tablets contain ephedrine (extracted from an African plant) plus atropine, or an extract from thorn apples (jimson weed), as well as other potent ingredients. While the body may react favourably to these strong medicines, a complete cure is not obtained and, what is worse, the patient also runs the risk of becoming dependent on these drugs. That is why homoeopathic remedies are to be preferred. The following have proved excellent and should be selected according to the specific needs of the patient: *Arsen. alb. 6x–30x, Nux vomica 6x–20x, Zinc. valerianicum 4x, Antimon. sulph. auratum 4x* and a *Belladonna* preparation of high potency.

Among the herbal remedies, a preparation containing an extract from *Petasites officinalis* (butterbur) has proved effective. It can be taken in the form of drops, *Petadolor* tablets or, in especially stubborn cases, *Petaforce* capsules. These herbal antispasmodics are most reliable and, if administered over a long period of time, often give the most amazing positive results without any side effects at all. Our asthma drops *Asthmasan, Drosinula Cough Syrup* and *Kali iod. 4x* have also proved their worth in cases of bronchial asthma, congestion of the lungs and as antispasmodic remedies.

In addition to these remedies and positive psychological orientation, physical therapy has its place in the treatment of asthma. Of importance are *Schlenz baths*, hot and cold *foot baths* in alternation, *cold water treatment* according to Louis Kuhne, *brush massages, mustard packs* and *mud packs* on the chest. *Acupuncture* has also been reported as beneficial in cases of asthma, provided that the practitioner is highly skilled in performing this intricate form of treatment.

Cardiac Asthma

Even though cardiac asthma has the same main characteristics as bronchial asthma, no abnormalities of the bronchial passages can be detected. Cardiac asthma is the result of a weak heart. If the left half of the heart is affected, this means an accumulation of blood in the lung. Should the right half be affected, the result is poor blood circulation in the lungs, which in turn causes a decrease in the exchange of gases.

The face of a person suffering from cardiac asthma has a bluish tinge, and breathing is difficult when engaging in the slightest physical activity. As soon as the problem has been diagnosed, treatment with cardiac remedies and medicines that influence the vascular system should begin. Instead of medicines containing digitalis, which tend to accumulate in the body, it is recommended that *Convallaria* (lily of the valley) be taken, in conjunction with *sea squill*, also known as *sea onion (Scilla maritima)*. In order to strengthen the myocardium a hawthorn preparation, such as *Crataegisan*, is most beneficial. *Aesculaforce* and *Aesculus hipp.*, both medicines that stimulate the circulation, when taken with a calcium preparation such as *Urticalcin*, promote recovery. In any case, it is advisable to diagnose the cause of the disease and then proceed to treat each patient according to his medical requirements as well as applying the appropriate form of physical therapy.

Important Factors in the Treatment of Pulmonary Diseases

It is strange that orthodox medicine still does not pay enough attention to the basic healing factors in the treatment of lung patients. Much can be achieved by rest, light, air and sun, and their value has been proved beyond doubt. The words 'Lift up your eyes to the mountains whence your help comes' are inscribed over the entrance of a sanatorium in Arosa, Switzerland. They are an honest admission by orthodox medicine that it is primarily the air – mountain air in particular – which provides a cure for lung diseases.

Another factor must not be forgotten either, and that is nutritional therapy. The body must be supplied with the substances it lacks before it can attempt regeneration. First on the list are foods rich in calcium and vitamins – these are indispensable. Raw, freshly pressed carrot juice or raw, finely grated carrots, the freshly pressed juice of grapes, oranges and grapefruit, and other wholesome juices, should be taken slowly in little sips and well insalivated. If you observe this advice, the fruit acid will cause no unpleasant gastric disturbance.

Plenty of fresh raw vegetables should be served daily. Always dress salads with lemon juice, never with vinegar.

The intake of protein foods must be reduced. On the other hand, natural culinary herbs that stimulate the appetite are recommended. An easily assimilated calcium preparation is essential. I have always seen excellent results when patients have taken the calcium complex *Urticalcin* and herbs rich in silica, such as *Galeopsis*. In this connection *Usnea*, the moss or lichen found on larch trees, deserves special mention. The animals of the forest make good use of its tonic properties for the lungs and we, too, should take it to combat weakness of the respiratory organs. If you find it difficult to chew the fresh lichen, take it regularly as a tea or, for even greater effect, take the fresh plant extract, *Usneasan*. Plants like *Usnea* or *Galeopsis* are, in a sense, not medicinal but nutritional plants and bear out Hippocrates' principle that 'Food

99

shall be medicine and medicine shall be food'. In reality, then, remedies from the plant kingdom are curative foods. Do not forget cod-liver oil or cod-liver oil emulsions; these are of great benefit and to be recommended if the patient can take them.

Furthermore, it is of great importance to influence the patient psychologically. The glandular functions must be in good order, and this depends a great deal on his state of mind.

It is also important to stimulate the skin. Give the body a daily brush massage and afterwards apply a good skin oil containing natural herbal ingredients that stimulate the function of the skin.

That good bowel movement is necessary should go without saying. Indeed, proper functioning of the bowels and the kidneys is essential for the cure of practically any disease.

Lung patients who take this simple advice to heart will benefit greatly from their rest cures and will surprise their doctors by their speedy recovery. Always remember that it is important to try and rectify deficiencies and weaknesses anywhere in the body and not just one organ. It is then understandable why recovery is faster than usual.

Calcium

Much has been said and written about the significance of calcium for our bodies. Calcium is one of the most important minerals in the human body, and the most plentiful in it. Without calcium, neither our bones, our teeth, nor the greater number of our body cells could exist. Hence the need to eat plenty of foods containing it. What is more, calcium plays an important part in our body's resistance to infectious diseases, especially diseases affecting the respiratory organs. Children who lack calcium are prone to infectious diseases, quickly develop swollen glands and are unable to ward off primary infections. When the body is deficient in calcium there is a constant struggle to fight sickness. Nature provides us with a good comparative example. Meadows that are short of lime always have a quantity of moss growing in them. If, however, you give them a lime dressing, you neutralise the acidity of the soil and the moss disappears. Parasitic plants thrive in calcium-deficient soil. From this we can draw a parallel to what goes on in the human body. Where there is a calcium deficiency all sorts of diseases, especially the infectious kinds, will thrive. Of course, this fact has been known for a long time and various calcium preparations are on the market. But all those phosphoric, carbonic and lactic acid combinations of calcium have actually failed to serve their purpose. Calcium deficiency continues to be a problem.

Many years ago I discussed this subject with a well-known chemist in Davos, Switzerland. This man had great experience in the manufacture of calcium milk and other calcium preparations and declared that he had been swamped with orders from doctors since it became common knowledge that calcium milk played an important part in the treatment of pulmonary diseases. Yet he pointed out that this remedy was of little or no use, for in order to be assimilated, the calcium would have to come from a natural source, from plants. Now this chemist, a professional man of the 'old school', told me this years ago, yet he was evidently a man who could think 'biologically', or 'organically'. And it was his sincere conviction that strengthened me in my resolve to obtain calcium in a form that the body would be able to assimilate, so that calcium deficiency could finally be overcome.

This resolve led me to produce calcium from plants, especially from the fresh green stinging nettle. I can say that I succeeded in manufacturing a calcium preparation the body can readily absorb. A well-balanced combination with other triturated biochemical calcium salts has led to the calcium complex *Urticalcin*, which has given thousands of people exactly what could be expected from a natural organic calcium preparation. However, let me point out that nobody should come to depend on any preparation, for the purpose of the advice given in this book is to make the reader aware of what he can do to help himself without them.

How to Overcome Calcium Deficiency
I would like to tell you now how to go about overcoming calcium deficiency. First of all we have in mind the children who are born with a deficiency, but there are also many adolescents and even older people who suffer from a lack of calcium and need help.

Infants and small children should be given natural foods. Do not forget to include plenty of gruel made from unpolished *brown rice*, for it contains much goodness, especially in its bran, which infants need. Naturally, there is no better food than breast milk and no healthy mother should pass up the privilege of breast-feeding her baby, if it is at all possible. She should, by the way, begin to take particular care of her health even before contemplating motherhood.

As soon as the child starts on supplementary or bottle food, natural brown rice is the best foundation for good health. From

101

this time on, *carrot juice*, which is rich in calcium and minerals and easily digested, can also be given. Later, *almond milk* with *fruit juices* may be introduced. Be sure to obtain healthy milk, whether it is cow's or sheep's milk. Unfortunately, milk is not necessarily 100 per cent safe: in many places the cows are tubercular and judging by the way they are imprisoned continuously in stalls, it is not surprising that they become sick. Good and safe milk can only come from cows living on pasture and under natural, healthy conditions. Sheep's milk is better than cow's milk, and if you are able to obtain it from free-roaming sheep, you will have the best milk possible for your small children. It will be richer in calcium and have greater nutritional value because of the animals' healthy outdoor life. Goat's milk can also be given occasionally, but not on a regular basis. You will find more useful information in the entry on 'Infant Nutrition' (see pages 39–41).

It is important that growing children, indeed all of us, eat wholefoods and avoid white sugar and white flour products as much as possible. Food should be eaten in the same condition that nature or the Creator made it grow. In wholefoods you will find all the vitamins and minerals in the right proportions and combinations. Always bear in mind the advice to go back to natural foods and avoid those artificial refined products that human commercial greed has imposed upon us. While the manufacturer profits, the body suffers. Of course, the damage does not necessarily show up from one day to the next. The consequences of deficiencies, chemical additives and other aspects of convenience foods take time to manifest themselves, but sooner or later most people fall victim to them. Whether it is cancer, increased susceptibility to infection and disease, low resistance, a debilitation of the body, or any other known or yet unknown ailment affecting the central nervous system, they are always to be reckoned with. These frightening consequences of man's ignorance and greed are brought about by our lack of resistance, which depends on a healthy body resulting from a natural way of life and natural nutrition.

SAUERKRAUT WITH CALCIUM POWDER

If your body lacks calcium you will appreciate my special instructions on how to prepare your own home-made and excellent calcium preparation. As a matter of fact, if you live in the country this should be quite easy to do.

First of all, I realise that not everyone is familiar with sauerkraut, made from white cabbage, or knows how to prepare it. For this reason I have given the recipe later on in this book (see pages 546–7). When making your own sauerkraut, be careful to use the minimum of salt but do not hesitate to add herbs and spices such as marjoram, thyme, juniper berries and especially mustard seed, which help to preserve the sauerkraut. Sauerkraut is very high in calcium and has great medicinal value when eaten raw.

In order to increase the calcium content and actually make a calcium preparation, mix *ground eggshells* with the sauerkraut; add half a soupspoon of eggshell powder to each kilogram (2.2 lbs) of sauerkraut. You can also use washed *oyster shell powder* instead (obtainable from chemist shops or drugstores). Mix the powder with the shredded raw cabbage in the same way you would do with the herbs. The process of fermentation will then produce natural calcium lactate, which is readily assimilated. If you prepare a small wooden barrel of this 'calcium sauerkraut' every year, you will find that, by eating it regularly, in a year or two there will be no calcium deficiency in your family.

If you buy the sauerkraut in a health food store instead of making if yourself, presuming it was made with very little salt, sprinkle a teaspoonful of one of the two powders over the sauerkraut, mix it well and let it stand for another day before eating it raw. Even though this quick method of making a calcium preparation is not quite as effective as the first method, the result is still better than proprietary calcium tablets. Incidentally, you can also mix a pinch of eggshell or oyster shell powder into salad dressings if you prepare these with lemon juice. The citric acid will dissolve some of the natural calcium in the shells, making the mineral more easily assimilated.

NETTLES
Stinging nettles are another excellent source of calcium. Gather young nettles in the spring, chop them very finely or put them through a mincer, then mix into a salad. They can also be finely chopped and sprinkled over boiled and mashed potatoes or other dishes that you would normally garnish. No one will even notice that it was not one of the more common garnishes. You can also sprinkle some over soup just before serving, or spinach. It is important, however, not to cook the nettles. In these ways you can obtain your regular supply of nettles, a first-class source of calcium phosphate, vitamin D and other important minerals.

Years have passed since I gave this advice about nettles in my monthly publication *Gesundheits-Nachrichten (Health News)* and later heard from many Bernese country women who had been delighted with the way their children responded to nettles. They said that the children once again had rosy cheeks and seemed to have recovered their health and resistance – all due to this simple remedy. So why don't you adopt this inexpensive method of increasing your calcium intake? Why buy expensive medicines when there is another way that is open to everyone if only we make a little effort and give a little thought to the matter? In fact, doing so will cause less bother than giving the constant attention and treatment calcium-deficient children need, because there is always something wrong with them. Calcium deficiency makes children susceptible to catarrh, with every cold draught posing a threat. And when an infectious disease goes round they are usually the first to catch it. That is why prevention is better – and cheaper – than cure!

The Lesser Known Benefits of Calcium

Everyone knows the importance of calcium as a structural component of our bones and teeth. A low calcium level indicates a calcium deficiency that will, in time, be detrimental to the teeth and bones. The effect of this deficiency is especially dangerous in pregnant women, and generations ago they used to say in parts of Switzerland that every child cost his mother a tooth; in other words, calcium deficiency was the price a mother had to pay for bearing a child. We also know that a calcium deficiency in the blood may bring about tetany-like conditions characterised by cramps and spasmodic contractions.

However, calcium is not only a building material, but also one that combines with harmful metabolic wastes, particularly acids, which are then eliminated through the urine. One example of these is oxalic acid, which plays a part in the formation of kidney stones. When combined with calcium it becomes calcium oxalate, a substance that can be disposed of easily by the kidneys.

An adequate balance of calcium in the body protects one against scrofula and the tendency to tuberculosis. Doctors are able to tell us a great deal about this. If the calcium level in our blood is normal, it can protect us from the harmful effects of radioactive strontium 90. This discovery, while still new to many of us, is reassuring, since it is not very difficult to build up our calcium level. Thus, the reasons for maintaining a normal level of this vital mineral should be sufficiently clear to make us remember its importance to our health.

Wholegrain foods, raw vegetables and dairy products are all excellent sources of calcium, and we should make daily use of them. Unfortunately, our body is unable to assimilate calcium contained in water, or in any other inorganic form. That is why we must make sure to obtain organic calcium, that is, calcium of plant origin. Since this important mineral is readily assimilated only in this form, organic calcium alone is to be preferred. But if, in spite of a proper diet, a person still suffers from a deficiency, then regularly taking a biological calcium complex such as *Urticalcin* is indicated and, of course, the need to eat foods rich in calcium is obvious. Urticalcin contains calcium obtained from nettles and is ideal for maintaining a normal calcium level in children as well as adults. Once you have tried this simple and pleasant preparation you will no longer wish to do without its benefits as a natural source of calcium. Those who are in a state of exhaustion, over-worked or whose health is low, so that no remedy seems to do them any good, will be able to improve their general condition by taking Urticalcin. The body will then soon be able to utilise other remedies too. Given that the mineral balance in the body is so important, we should heed the advice given in this section and take great care to ensure that it is achieved and adequately maintained.

Our Blood – a Mysterious Fluid
The Bible tells us that 'the soul is in the blood'. A poet of long ago also sensed the mysterious composition and working of the blood when he called it a very special fluid. He was aware of this long before his assertion was supported through the findings of various research experiments conducted in modern times. Still, it was the declarations made recently by well-known scientists that made me stop and think. They claimed that a single drop of blood reveals everything about the condition of a person's health. However, a proper diagnostic method has yet to be found which can support this assertion. Scientists must first discover this before they can properly evaluate it. The method of blood crystallisation has already taken us one step further and certainly merits our attention. No doubt other methods will be worked out and the time seems near when diseases such as cancer, tuberculosis, rheumatism, gout and many others will be detected in their early stages long before the more obvious symptoms manifest themselves.

Even though the blood has been subdivided into groups, the Rh factor has been discovered, and we know already that the texture of our blood may be either coarse or fine (similar to the skin with its coarse or fine pores), there are many singularities of the blood that remain unknown. Just think of the mysteries surrounding the content and structure of an individual's blood. It is left to the scientists to lift the veil as time goes by.

If the blood, this truly mysterious red fluid of life, had already been sufficiently researched, there would hardly be some 20,000 deaths a year due to blood transfusions in the United States alone. In the future, it is probable that surgeons, having been made aware of the great risks involved in transfusing human blood, will only make use of the much improved and effective non-blood plasma and blood replacements that are now available. Let me also mention that hepatitis, a much feared inflammation of the liver with infectious jaundice, has frequently resulted from blood transfusions. The prevention of serum hepatitis as a consequence of blood transfusions is a problem that has not yet been solved. In more recent times, AIDS too has been passed on through blood transfusions. Considering that even the medical director of an American blood bank has expressed serious concern over the risks involved in transfusions and that many surgeons, as a result of unsatisfactory experiences, prefer to work with substitutes, is there any wonder that the patient should wish to express his personal preference, talk it over with the surgeon and then make his own decision?

How could we possibly know all the secrets of blood, not having had a part in its formation? But to Him who made it, blood is no mystery. He, the caring God and Father who knows what is best, strictly prohibited the consumption of blood to the survivors of the great Flood. Eventually, this command was incorporated into the code of law of God's chosen people. Later still, the governing body of the early Christian Church in the apostle Paul's time chose not to cancel this law, but restated it as being valid and binding upon their members. The law regarding the abstinence from blood has remained valid and applicable for the entire Christian era right down to our own time. Sexual morality is another divine commandment laid down in the Bible and those who respect it are assured of greater protection from AIDS.

If we look closely at these laws, we should find that they are beneficial to our health, whether we realise this or not. The obedient observation of the divine commandments can act only for the protection and good of the individual. The person who refuses to take blood in any form into his body, whether for the sake of his obedience to God's command or for reasons of health, will receive an increasing amount of support and recognition as time goes on and research progresses, confirming the validity of his conviction.

The Lymphatic System – the White Bloodstream

Even though the lymphatic vessels are much longer than all the red blood vessels together, our knowledge of the white bloodstream is still very limited. The lymphatic vessels, which are much finer than those of the red bloodstream, are distributed throughout the entire body. In contrast with the blood, the lymph flows only in one direction and the fluid is returned to the bloodstream after its task is completed. The body can be divided schematically into four parts in the form of a cross, starting at the navel. Each of these four fields more or less corresponds to a lymphatic network, with a centre located at the right and left side of the groin area and in each of the armpit regions. Smaller centres are also located below the lower jaw, at the right and left side. Leading to these centres, the lymph glands form little nodes, which reach their maximum size in the centre itself.

Functions of the Lymphatic System

The lymphatic system is responsible for keeping the body fluids, the blood fluid and cerebrospinal fluid, in order. The total amount of fluid accounts for approximately 60 per cent of our total body weight. But the lymph has yet another important and vital function. Not unlike a police force, the lymph cells (lymphocytes) must combat and destroy all invading organisms that enter and endanger the body tissue. We are referring here to bacteria, which are more or less injurious or dangerous, depending on the type. For example, if you cut yourself, or a rusty nail penetrates the skin, millions of bacteria enter the body through the wound as if through a broken trap door. The fine, outer lymph vessels are perhaps not strong enough to resist the intruders and the bacteria continue their advance into the nodes of a centre. The centre then calls up the defences; the vessels expand and we feel a swelling in the area of the armpit or the groin, for example. The swelling can become as large as a hen's egg. If the lymphocytes, phagocytes, wandering cells, and whatever other names the defence forces may have, cannot handle their task, the lymphatics become inflamed and swollen. They become very sensitive to pressure and can be seen as red lines. This condition is called blood poisoning (septicaemia, toxaemia), even though the toxins are actually still contained in the white bloodstream of the lymphatic system. In fact, if all toxins and bacteria were passed on to the red bloodstream, no one could survive his childhood because of the many poisons that would enter the blood.

The tonsils and the appendix (see below) are also allied to the lymphatic system and have the job of cleansing the body and destroying germs. Both can be regarded as filtering systems, which explains why we should never have them removed unless it is strictly necessary. Their removal constitutes a weakening of the forces in the fight against harmful bacteria.

In the event that cancer cells escape during a biopsy or because of incomplete removal of malignant tissue in an operation, the lymph generally catches them and the centre harbours them with the intent of destroying them. If the attempt to destroy them fails, these giant cells begin to grow and multiply, and the result is the much feared lymphoadenoma, or Hodgkin's disease (see page 111), a form of cancer of the lymph nodes. That is why surgeons remove all lymph vessels and nodes during a cancer operation, especially in cases of breast cancer.

Another function of the lymph is to absorb emulsified fat and pass it on in small, tolerable quantities to the bloodstream. All so-called antibodies, which ensure immunity against infectious diseases, are formed in the lymphatic system. You can therefore understand how important it is for this system to function properly. Certain disorders of the heart, the kidneys and the blood vessels can be attributed to a partial failure of the lymphatic system.

THE TONSILS AND APPENDIX

Not everyone may know that the tonsils and the appendix possess a well-defined lymphatic network. As they also serve to filter out and destroy bacteria, they may be called sister organs. Since their importance to the body is so great, these organs should not be surgically removed as long as they do their work. Even if something is wrong with them, it would be better to see what could be done with a view to healing them and so keeping them in the body.

THE LYMPH NODES

The lymph nodes are small masses of tissue situated along the course of the lymphatic vessels. Their purpose is to filter out and kill bacteria as well as to neutralise toxins. Should one filtering station prove insufficient, another one will be called upon to help. As the bacteria advance, we notice hard red lines, rope-like and tender, leading to a swelling, for example on the inside of the elbow. As noted earlier, the swelling may grow to the size of a hen's egg and will become sensitive to pressure. This condition is caused by an accumulation of lymph cells which have become embedded in connective tissues and muscle fibres, presenting the symptoms of blood poisoning. It is possible that in such a case the centre will not be able to cope and will call on the lymphatics in the armpit as well. If the septic injury is in the foot, the patient will feel the tight lymphatic course right along the leg and the swelling will be found in the groin.

THE SPLEEN

Although we do not yet know everything the spleen does in the body, it is nevertheless referred to as the largest lymph gland. It is located to the left of the stomach just opposite the liver, but has nothing to do with the digestive system; nor is it allied in any way or related in function to any other organ. The spleen is connected directly to the bloodstream and not to the lymph. It could therefore be located anywhere else in the body, the only explanation for its actual location on the left side being that there seems to be room for it. To this day, the spleen continues to puzzle scientists. One could go on living after its removal but the production of anti-bodies without the spleen would be so small that one could not survive a massive attack of micro-organisms, as might occur in a case of malaria, for example.

WANDERING CELLS

Lymphocytes and leucocytes are wandering cells; they leave the lymphatics as well as the bloodstream and, being so minute in size, pass through the capillary walls. Their movement is similar to that of starfish circulating through a coral reef. Whenever and wherever they are needed they are ready to attack, just like a special branch of the police. It is truly astonishing to note that they number in the billions, so that there are more itinerant cells in our body than there are people on earth.

How to Keep the Lymph Healthy

Despite the excellent organisation of the lymphatic system, as we have just seen, the lymph often needs help. For example, a deficiency of calcium or vitamin D creates a problem for the lymphatics. Swellings in children, notably in the region of the groin and at times on the neck or behind the lower ear, can be attributed to this deficiency. Lack of calcium and vitamin D is marked by susceptibility to colds and catarrh, sore throats and other infectious diseases, as well as loss of appetite, irritability and constant fatigue.

Plenty of exercise and fresh air are a boon for our lymphatic system. Mountain sun and sea air, if enjoyed in sensible measures, have an excellent effect on the lymph.

A proven botanical remedy especially recommended for building up the lymphatic system is the subtropical plant *Echinacea. Echinaforce*, the tincture from this plant, can be taken internally as well as applied externally, and brings speedy relief in cases of swollen lymph nodes and blood poisoning. For external use the freshly squeezed green leaves can be made into a pack or poultice, or a cotton swab can be soaked with the tincture and placed on the affected area. If the condition is an acute one, take ten drops of the tincture with a little water every hour. Because of its effectiveness, Echinaforce should be kept in the medicine chest of every home.

In most instances a *proper diet* can bring relief. White sugar, sweets, biscuits, pastries and other sweet snacks must be cut out. The same goes for refined food items made with white flour, refined sugar and highly processed or refined oils and fats. In their place, serve and eat more vegetables and salads. Then one is on the road to recovery. A vitamin supplement, for example *Vitaforce*, together with *Urticalcin*, has been proved to give good results. For best effect, give children this form of calcium as a prophylactic measure, long before any of the above symptoms ever appear.

Horseradish has a favourable effect on the lymph and is one of the best remedies available. Often the most stubborn disorders and ailments of the lymphatic system disappear when a teaspoon of horseradish is taken daily. It is very tasty and less pungent when mixed with cottage cheese or finely grated carrots.

Tuberculosis and Cancer
When the lymphatic system is working efficiently, it is impossible for tuberculosis or cancer to develop. As regards cancer, the proper functioning of the liver is essential too. That is why special attention should be given to both the lymph and the liver. Long before tuberculosis can be diagnosed, careful observation will disclose the presence of painful lymph nodes when pressure is applied to them. These early symptoms are often observable years beforehand and call for our special attention if trouble is to be avoided later. In order to keep the lymph in good condition, we must receive sufficient oxygen and sunlight. Dark apartments, facing away from

the sun, are veritable breeding grounds for TB bacteria and should be shunned when choosing a place to live.

Lymphoadenoma
This malignant disease of the lymph nodes, also known as Hodgkin's disease, afflicts more men than women. As early as 1832, the English doctor Thomas Hodgkin described it in detail, but to this day its origin is unknown. Since the disease begins with a high temperature, some doctors believe that it is an infectious disease. However, as yet, no virus responsible for it has been identified. Other physicians consider it a type of cancer and treat it with radiotherapy (with X-rays and cobalt rays). As a rule, the success of this kind of therapy is of short duration. In cases where only a few nodes are affected by the disease their removal is recommended, until a better method can be found to deal with it effectively. On the other hand, a complete changeover to a *natural wholefood diet* consisting of plenty of raw vegetables, soft white cheese (quark) and horseradish, as well as brown rice, has proved beneficial. Hodgkin's disease is often accompanied by anaemia. This condition can be counteracted by drinking daily one tenth of a litre (100 ml; about 3½ fl. oz) of both *carrot* and *beetroot juices* and, in addition, an infusion of nettles, flowering oat plants and alfalfa. *Petasites* preparations taken with *Galeopsis* often give good results too.

Looking After our Capillary System
Few people may know that the capillary network of the human body consists of 100 million metres (over 62,000 miles) of blood vessels. This would be two and a half times the circumference of the earth if all the tiny hair-like vessels were put together in one long line. This calculation made by scientists clearly illustrates one of the many wondrous things the Creator put in our bodies. But it is not enough to be familiar with the structure of these tiny vessels; it is equally important to know and understand their functions in the body. The exchange of metabolic waste material, the passing on of carbon dioxide to the venous blood system, and many other functions known and unknown to us, take place in the capillaries.

The body as a whole, including the capillary system, can be adversely affected and harmed by an incorrect diet and life-style. Foods that produce too much uric acid, such as meat and eggs – instead of vegetables and fruit – cause a degeneration and dilation

111

of the capillaries to a degree that capillary photography can detect it. When magnified, dilated capillaries have the appearance of small varicose veins. Excessive alcohol consumption has the same harmful effect. Chemicals absorbed from medicines and nicotine alter and damage the capillaries and impair their function of nourishing of the cells, thus disturbing the entire metabolic process. Of what good is our marvellously equipped body if we disregard its working order and eat the wrong food, as well as follow an unnatural way of life, with insufficient exercise and deep-breathing?

Defects of the capillary system cause degeneration, slackening and aging of the muscle and nerve cells due largely to their not receiving sufficient nourishment in time. It is important to know about this when we are young, so that we can guard our health carefully. If we fail to realise it until we are old, it will be of little worth by then, and we will be like the person who wasted all his fortune in his youth. In his old age he lived in poverty while contemplating, with pain and nostalgic sorrow, the bygone luxury of his youth. We can compare youth to the seven fat years in Egypt referred to in the Bible. We should act wisely, just as Joseph did, storing up good health to be able to, figuratively speaking, live off the 'savings' during the 'lean' years of advanced age. By adopting a healthy, natural way of life, from our youth onwards, we also show the greatest care for our blood vessels.

Our All-Important Circulation

In order to illustrate the function and purpose of the blood circulation, let us for a moment consider the mail train travelling from Basel to Lugano and back, making scheduled stops to unload on the way to Lugano and picking up mail on the way back to Basel. Imagine the confusion if the train did not keep to its timetable. At each station we can see the postmaster impatiently pacing up and down the platform looking for the train to arrive and trying to calm down the people who are waiting for their mail. Such a relatively small mix-up in the commercial world could trigger undesirable delays and upset everyone.

We can draw an analogy between the mail train and the circulatory system. Let us compare the outward-bound train on its way to Lugano with the arterial network, which has the job of supplying the millions of body cells with nourishment so that they are able to perform their functions. All the necessary minerals, vitamins, enzymes, amino acids for the manufacture of protein, all the sugars and fats, and even oxygen are being transported via the arterial network on a strict schedule, every day, every hour.

Every cell is a miniature factory and needs raw materials and fuel for its processes. Only if it is supplied with all it needs, on schedule, can it be expected to perform as reliably and marvellously as it does. Shortages of the required quantities and flaws in the quality of raw materials force the cells to find a make-shift solution. It is only under the most trying conditions that the cells look for shortcuts and thereby suffer in their performance. A case in point is seen when the body begins to build giant cells, known as cancer cells. Of course, the cell itself cannot be blamed for the defect, for it fights and resists desperately to the point where failure can no longer be avoided.

We must, therefore, ensure that the 'mail trains' of our arterial system can keep their schedules by stimulating circulation through exercise and proper breathing. Furthermore, we must see to it that all the necessary raw materials are provided in the right quantities and quality. Only then can the laboratories of our cells perform their wonderful work in harmony with the divine purpose and programme assigned to them. We can then reap the full benefits of the cells' willing performance on our behalf.

Thus far we have spoken of only one function of the circulatory system, the supply. But, as in every manufacturing plant, we must also concern ourselves with the waste products the body produces. They must be promptly eliminated if congestions, in other words breakdowns, are to be avoided. The train on its way back to Basel may be compared to our venous system, which is responsible for returning all the waste products resulting from burning-up processes, for example carbon dioxide and uric acid. Some of these waste products are recycled by the liver or eliminated with the help of the kidneys. If this process of transportation becomes obstructed, problems will be inevitable, since the accumulation of waste causes tension and pressure. The train may be derailed and the mail scattered, lying undelivered on the rails. In terms of our body this means the formation of varicose veins. Advice on treating varicose veins can be found on pages 132–6.

The Marvellous Design of the Circulatory System
The Dutch scientist Dr Hoorne once said that the body is made up of blood vessels. It was he who discovered a method of making the vessels visible by injecting them with a red dye. Tsar Peter the Great, who happened to be visiting Holland at that time, was so

intrigued by the experiment that he arranged to take some of the dye home with him. Unfortunately, however, on his arrival in Russia he found that it was no longer useable. The sailors had consumed the alcohol in which it had been placed to preserve it!

Truly a wonder of creative design, every single one of the billions of cells in our body has access to the uninterrupted flow of the circulatory system. It takes the blood only about one second to move from the arterial capillaries to the venous capillaries. And it is during this second that the metabolic process takes place whereby oxygen is withdrawn from the blood and carbon dioxide from the tissue is permitted to enter. At the same time, the nutrients from the blood enter the tissue and the metabolic products from the tissue enter the bloodstream. Having fulfilled its task, the blood then flows back to the heart via the venous system.

The circulation of the blood between the heart and the lungs and back to the heart again takes about six or seven seconds. The circulation through the heart, which supplies the myocardium by way of the coronary vessels, takes place in about three or four seconds. The supply of blood to the brain takes eight seconds and to the tip of the toes, about eighteen seconds. One blood cell can make about 3,000 round trips in the course of a day. The cells are moving about incessantly, day and night. It seems that nothing in the world is more fond of travelling than our blood cells. Beginning at the heart, a cell reaches the loop of the capillaries with a swift motion. The further away it gets, the slower the motion becomes because of the thinner vessels. At last it delivers its load, as an express messenger would do, and begins immediately its return trip through the venous system. Physical stress, cold weather, excitement and fever make the blood cell speed up its pace. On the other hand, depression and psychological upsets cause it to slow down. In these situations, billions of cells receive inadequate nourishment and illness may result if the situation is not remedied by means of a positive psychological influence on the individual. This goes to show that depression and similar psychological problems may lead to physical illness if they continue for any length of time.

The Important Function of the Arteries
When I think about the enormous amount of traffic that passes incessantly over the highways leading to and from major cities such as New York or London, I must say that the expression 'arterial roads' indeed seems appropriate and justified. If for some

reason those traffic arteries were paralysed, life in those large cities would soon come to a standstill. The importance of the 'arterial roads' in our bodies, the arteries, will only begin to dawn on us when we study them closely. Even the most attractive human body, with shapely limbs and perfect muscular build, will begin to deteriorate and degenerate, just as the gifted and trained brain will begin to fail, when the walls of the arteries thicken and harden and thus lose their elasticity.

Even the anatomical structure of the arteries tells us a great deal about their importance. Imagine a pipe made up of various layers, the inside being a smooth, elastic tube. This tube is covered with other layers that consist of elastic, or loose but tensile, connective tissue. The tube can withstand a pressure of about 20 atmospheres (1 atmosphere equals 14.72 pounds to the square inch).

These few details give us at least some idea of how our arteries work. Like the heart, the arteries have their own blood supply. For this purpose a network of vessels, the so-called *Vasa vasorum*, is ingeniously built into their walls. Furthermore, the walls of the arteries have their own network of lymphatic vessels and nerves. The further removed the arteries are from the heart, the more branched out they become, and consequently their total cross section becomes proportionally larger; pressure decreases and the walls become thinner. A cross section of the capillaries, at the very tip of the arteries, is about 50 times smaller in diameter than that of the finest human hair.

Narrowing and Hardening of the Arteries
A narrowing or hardening of the arteries has serious, in time even incurable, consequences. The victim literally degenerates, both physically and mentally. To this day more people in the civilised, industrialised world, especially in Europe, the United States and Australia die of diseases of the arterial walls, and the number of deaths is on the increase. The length of our life is often determined solely by the condition of our arterial walls.

Hardening of the arteries (arteriosclerosis) begins with a small alteration, which looks like a flat sore or ulcer. This sore then develops into a growth of the connective tissue, followed by a deposit of calcium salts, with the result that the inside of the artery becomes gradually narrower and the blood has less space in which to circulate. The artery loses more and more of its elasticity, eventually becoming hard and brittle. The blood pressure then rises and the victim may eventually suffer a thrombosis or embolism of the brain or a cerebral haemorrhage. Dilation of the heart or haemorrhage of a blood vessel near the heart, as well as nephrosclerosis (nephritis due to a hardening of the kidney blood vessels) may also occur.

WHAT ARE THE CAUSES?
1. A diet high in fats, especially animal fats, which causes an increase of cholesterol in the blood, can contribute to the disease.

2. Nicotine is another contributory factor to a narrowing of the arteries, especially the coronary vessels.

3. A rich diet, with too much animal protein, especially too much meat, eggs and cheese, may lead to arteriosclerosis.

4. Overindulgence in alcohol is harmful to the capillaries and thus may indirectly contribute to this disease.

PREVENTION AND CURE
1. A diet consisting of *brown rice, soft white cheese* (quark) and *salads* can have almost miraculous results if adhered to consistently. By lowering the blood pressure in a natural way, it becomes unnecessary to take any radical medicines. This simple natural treatment makes it possible to rehabilitate the blood vessels right from the beginning. As I have seen from experience in Asian countries, rice bran positively influences the regeneration of the arteries.

2. Plants rich in natural *iodine*, such as seaweed, contribute largely to the prevention and cure of arteriosclerosis. The curative properties of these plants of the sea can easily be made available by including them in seasoning salts or foods; for example, they are contained in Kelpamare, Trocomare, Kelpaforce and Kelpasan.

Other medicinal herbs and spices are also beneficial, such as watercress and other kinds of cress, horseradish, garlic and leeks. A natural remedy that is to be recommended is *Rauwolfavena*, a combination of rauwolfia and oats. Further excellent remedies for the blood vessels and arteriosclerosis are *Arterioforce* capsules (containing mistletoe, garlic, hawthorn and passionflower) and *Ginkgo biloba*.

3. Plenty of *oxygen* is necessary and this means taking long walks through woods and forests, hills and mountains, or by the seaside, always deeply inhaling the fresh air. But a word of caution is necessary for those who already suffer from arteriosclerosis, such people should avoid higher altitudes because the thin air could lead to a stroke.

If you spend most of your time sitting in an office, the above advice and simple remedy is especially recommended. If you do not wish to be a doddery old man who shuffles along and has to be led to his office, you should give careful consideration to how you spend your time away from it. Make sure you don't spend your free time with friends in a bar instead of outdoors.

HOW TO AVOID POSSIBLE HARM
One does not have to be a fanatic in order to admit that modern, civilised man is living somewhat dangerously. Just think of all the conveniences we have gained from technology in our age of motor cars and mechanisation. They bring with them less activity out-doors and cause pollution of the air. Our indulgence in refined food products does not exactly contribute to good health either. The arteries degenerate as a result of the drawbacks of our life-style; symptoms of old age appear much too early, decreasing our efficiency and productivity and sometimes bringing an early end to our lives. The average increase of our life span, due to a reduction in infant mortality, does not change this picture either. It is not a question of reaching an advanced age by artificial means, by the use of drugs and special therapies, while our body is ailing and vegetating. Rather, it is much better to live to a ripe old age and still be in good health. Our life-style and what we eat should be governed by the laws of nature and not by the dictates of society, which have gone awry and, at best, contribute very little to our physical well-being.

Arteriosclerosis, Coronary Thrombosis and Heart Attacks
While I was spending some time in the Far East, I paid special attention to the occurrence of the above illnesses. It was quite evident that among the people living in the countryside of Japan, Korea and the Philippines, heart-related diseases are seldom heard of. If they do occur it is usually among the better off who have a higher standard of living. In all these Far Eastern countries the country people eat very little fat, generally not more than 50 g (a little less than 2 oz) of fat and oil a day. And let me add that these 50 g consist of mainly home-made fats with a high content of unsaturated fatty acids. Equally significant in terms of their healthy diet is their habit of eating rice to meet the need for carbohydrates. This is a custom worth copying, since rice has the quality of keeping the arteries young for a long time. Among those people whose staple diet consists of rice, I have noted that the blood

117

vessels, particularly the arteries, are in much better condition than in those who have a different diet.

And another thing. The benefits derived from a regular intake of seaweed are still a secret which may offer many answers to our questions in the future. It is the custom in Korea, Japan and many Chinese provinces to eat rice served with thin wafers of pressed seaweed. During my stay there, I adopted this habit and I must say that it made me feel very well indeed. So, if you are concerned about preventing these three illnesses, or if you are already a victim of one or more of them, you should consider the following rules, which are basic to preventative as well as curative treatment.

1. It is, above all, essential to reduce the consumption of protein and fats. If possible, avoid animal fats altogether and use natural unrefined oils such as sunflower, safflower, poppy seed or corn oil instead.
2. Make brown rice the basis of your diet.
3. Raw vegetables and soft white cheese (quark) should supplement the rice diet. Be sure to eat fresh salads every day, preferably dressed with Molkosan (whey concentrate) and unrefined oils.
4. For their curative properties, include in your diet wheat germ oil or wheat germ oil capsules, Sojaforce and Kelpasan, as well as any foods that contain seaweed. However, keep off Kelpasan if your blood pressure is high.
5. Instead of any other favourite cheese, eat only mild white soft cheese (quark) or cottage cheese. If it is difficult to give up the old habit of eating meat, eat very little of it and infrequently. The same advice holds true for eggs, which should never be eaten hard-boiled.
6. For seasoning, use salt very sparingly, It is best to change over to sea salt and Herbamare herbal seasoning salt.
7. It is of the utmost importance to provide the body with plenty of oxygen. So take long country walks at a good pace to stimulate deep breathing. If it is not possible to do this on a daily basis, at least use the weekend for that purpose. Instead of spending time in one's favourite café, bar or restaurant, sitting in front of the television or behind the wheel of a car, get out and exercise your legs in the countryside, in the woods and through the meadows.

If you try to be conscientious in living according to these seven rules, you will definitely increase your life span and help yourself to avoid many health problems in your advanced years. For example, hardening of the arteries will not incapacitate you, neither will coronary thrombosis, and you will have no need to fear a sudden end through a heart attack. It is simple to obey nature, and doing so will reward us in turn with good health and long life.

Embolism and Thrombosis
Women especially suffer from swollen veins, which often occur after surgery or just after childbirth. Generally, the blocking of venous blood vessels happens sometime between the third and the eighth day following surgery or delivery. In such cases a physician will usually give anticoagulant and vasodilator injections. However, more appropriate and helpful than this medical intervention is the following prophylactic treatment, which is to be recommended to all those who show a congenital or acquired tendency to embolism and thrombosis, and in particular to people with varicose veins.

Preventative Treatment
First of all, take proper *care of the bowels*, because intestinal disorders such as insufficient bowel movement or the retention of a faecal matter causes the blood, and hence the whole body, to become affected by metabolic toxins. Going on a juice diet for one day a week usually helps to improve regularity. The question of diet or nutrition for the rest of the week is no less important; only natural, unadulterated, unrefined foods will contribute to the eventual correction of irregular bowel movements.

Secondly, it must be remembered that regular *sweating* cures have an important place in the prevention and treatment of embolism and thrombosis. Sweating, of course, is easy for people who engage in strenuous physical activity. It can also be induced by mountain climbing, or by hiking, digging, gardening and the like, if you do not live near hills or mountains. Whatever the means, make sure to change wet or damp clothes quickly. If you happen to be one of those people who are unable to sweat even when engaging in physical activity, you have yet another way open to you. Take a sauna (up to 60 °C/140 °F) once a week. This will be of great help in reducing the tendency to embolism and thrombosis.

Thirdly, take the appropriate *medicinal herbs*. But I must point out that pregnant women should not wait until shortly before childbirth to take the herbs. They should begin to take them

119

months ahead of time in order to improve the condition of the blood and exert a positive influence on the entire vascular system. An excellent remedy is *Hamamelis*, an extract from witch hazel, a shrub known to the North American Indians as a 'miracle plant'. As early as the Middle Ages women realised that embolism and thrombosis could be prevented by taking arnica, yarrow, St John's wort and *Pulsatilla*. More than thirty years ago I began to use these herbs as a basis for a well-known fresh plant preparation, *Hyperisan*, that has since proved helpful to thousands of women in many countries around the globe. Many women have told me that serious complications at the time of delivery were prevented because they had been taking this herbal complex during their pregnancy. Much to their surprise, delivery was easy and without subsequent complications, which had not been the case for them before, when they had not been taking the preparation. A qualified midwife once wrote me an enthusiastic letter about a perfect delivery, which, according to her, could only be attributed to the fact that the mother had been taking the preparation. As a midwife of many years' experience, her observation and assessment can hardly be questioned. In addition to Hyperisan, it is recommended to take *Urticalcin*, because biological calcium is good for the vascular system. Another good supportive remedy, called *Aesculus hipp.*, a fresh plant extract from horse chestnuts, should not be overlooked either.

These are simple remedies for the vascular system, but they act in a preventative way, and this is no doubt better, simpler and less painful than leaving the problem untreated and suffering the subsequent discomfort. Once the trouble has taken root it is not always easy or possible to effect a cure, so it is more sensible to follow the advice given in good time.

Calcification and Calcium Preparations
Many people have a totally mistaken idea about calcium preparations, calcification and, in particular, calcification or hardening of the arteries. Quite often a patient tells me, 'I can't take calcium, I suffer from arteriosclerosis, and I'm sure it would be bad for me to take any more calcium; it would only be deposited in the arteries.'

But this view is entirely wrong. Biological calcium preparations such as Urticalcin have nothing to do with calcification. On the contrary, someone who is suffering from hardening of the arteries can take such a preparation without any problems, for it is easily

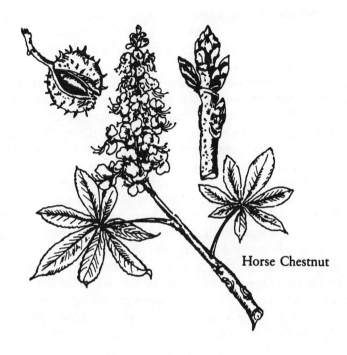

Horse Chestnut

assimilated. This calcium is used to repair worn out parts of the body and is never deposited in the vessels. In fact, the 'deposits' we are talking about are not really pure calcium; the term is used in the sense of arterial degeneration whereby the arterial walls gradually lose their elasticity.

First of all, fat-like substances called lipoids are deposited on the lining of the blood vessels and only later is calcium added. According to some research workers, the thickening takes place as a natural necessity so as to strengthen the walls of the arteries. It is thought that the body, as a defence measure, deposits calcium when the blood vessels have lost a degree of elasticity and stability and can no longer cope with the changed conditions of pressure. Other researchers, however, are of the opinion that it is just because of these deposits in the vessels, the so-called arteriosclerosis, that they become hardened.

Whatever the case, calcification is a sign of ageing which appears as a result of a disturbance in the general metabolism and an unhealthy diet, primarily one containing too much protein. But by no means can we hold the calcium in food or a biological preparation responsible for the pathological process of calcification. The bones of the skeleton contain reserves of calcium that would be quite sufficient to calcify all our blood vessels, yet in practice, such a contingency never arises.

As far as possible, naturopathy treats arteriosclerosis with remedies that restore some elasticity to the vessels. The blood pressure will thereby drop, for it previously had to rise because of constriction, with the lack of elasticity of the vessels compelling the heart to generate greater pressure to keep the circulation going. Of course, for arteriosclerosis we do not prescribe any medicines containing calcium. What we do indicate are *arnica* and *Crataegus*, as well as *Viscum album, garlic perles, Arterioforce* capsules and *bear's garlic tonic*. These remedies have an excellent effect. At the same time care should be taken to minimise the salt and protein intake. One of the best foods for preventing hardening of the arteries, or helping to reduce an existing condition, is *brown rice*. For this reason, anyone with arteriosclerosis should eat brown rice several times a week; it can be served morning, noon or evening and prepared in various appetising ways. The blood pressure will then fall, because a diet of fresh fruits and vegetables, together with plenty of brown rice, will gradually halt the disease and improve the condition.

If you should have to take a calcium complex such as Urticalcin for some other physical problem, remember that this preparation will not have an adverse effect on the blood vessels: on the contrary it will be beneficial. These details should reassure the patient who shies away from taking a good calcium preparation. He must by now realise that such a preparation is in no way associated with the hardening (calcification) of the arteries and positively supports rather than hinders a cure.

Older People and Calcium

Older people often raise the question of whether it is advisable to take biological calcium preparations, for example Urticalcin, or even to eat foods high in calcium, since it is known that in later years the potential danger of the hardening of the arteries and other body tissues is greater. It is an indisputable fact that during old age calcium is being withdrawn from the bones and deposited in vessels and tissues. This process causes the bones to become porous and fragile and the tissues, blood vessels and scar tissue to accumulate calcium deposits. At a quick glance, this argument would appear to favour a reduced intake of calcium. However, experience has proved that a diet low in calcium, surprisingly enough, can even promote osteoporosis, the loss of calcium from the bones.

How can this problem be solved? Calcium is a basic mineral that compounds easily with acids. If during the latter part of life the body accumulates certain acids, for example, oxalic and other acids, which should have been eliminated with the urine, the body compounds these with calcium to form calcium salts. When reduced to an unsaturated state in this way they are rendered less harmful. If we do not permit a deficiency to develop in the mineral metabolism, and we see to it that the calcium level remains normal, we can be sure that there will be no abnormal decalcification of the bones, even during old age. For this reason, too, there will be no calcium deposits in the blood vessels and tissues. This leads us to the question: what can be done to prevent premature aging?

RECOMMENDED PREVENTATIVE MEASURES

An older person, first of all, needs plenty of *oxygen*, in other words, plenty of exercise and deep-breathing in the open air. It would be beneficial to engage in some light sport; light gardening is another good form of exercise. Long walks through a forest or wood, or walking and climbing in the soothing tranquillity of hills and dales will also provide enough refreshing exercise for the body and the lungs.

Secondly, an older person should eat foods that have a high *iron* content, which assures the proper oxygenation of the blood and normalises the metabolic processes. This can be achieved by simply enhancing our meals with plenty of raw vegetables and salads every day. Of course, this is easier to do during spring, when many kinds of cresses and the tender leaves of spinach are available. Add these to your salads without fail. Also, do not forget the young shoots of stinging nettles which provide exceptional benefits. Indeed, there are many alternatives to ensure that we can meet our daily requirements of iron and other vital substances.

Thirdly, it is essential to look after and stimulate the endocrine glands. Daily *brush massages and showers*, alternating between hot and cold water, are helpful; after using hot water, douse the body briefly with cool or cold water. But be careful not to become chilled. You should feel comfortably warm after the alternating hot—cold shower; if this is not the case, it would be wiser to refrain from using the cold water.

Another basic rule is to get plenty of *sleep* in the hours preceding midnight. Sleep does much for our health, especially during these hours. What is more, if you go to bed early sleep will come more easily, as you are less likely to be overtired. Take *kelp* to supplement the mineral content of your diet. And, as previously stated, it does not affect one adversely to eat foods rich in calcium and to take a biological calcium preparation as well. On the contrary, this will be beneficial. Finally, it is helpful, from time to time, to stimulate the kidneys in order to ensure the adequate elimination of uric materials by taking a natural herb preparation, for example *Nephrosolid.*

If you follow these rules, and eat and drink sensibly, you will reach your old age without having to become stiff and doddery. Interestingly, the preventative measures that need to be understood and followed are few and simple, but they will protect you from much greater problems.

Diets for Hypertension, Arteriosclerosis and Other Signs of Old Age

It is important to determine whether hypertension, or high blood pressure, is caused by a kidney disease or by the diminishing elasticity of the blood vessels. If the latter, it may be easily corrected through a rice diet, as this is effective in practically all diseases attributable to the aging process. Rice is a medicinal food, which provides surprisingly good results, but you must be sure to use brown unpolished rice, for this is more beneficial and valuable than the more common refined white rice. If you cannot obtain brown rice, although this is unlikely, two commercially prepared rice packages, 'Uncle Ben's' and 'Avorio' may serve as a compromise, because both of these brands still retain many of the important minerals found in brown rice.

It is not easy for everyone in countries where rice is not produced to stick to a rice diet. In many areas people are used to eating mainly potatoes and local cereals, but in the Far East rice is a staple food. In this respect people in Far Eastern countries are better off, for if they adhere faithfully to the simple brown rice diet of their forefathers, they will never have to worry about high blood pressure.

Since high blood pressure is usually associated with eating too much protein, patients would be wise to cut out from their diet all animal proteins such as meat, eggs and cheese; if they think they cannot live without these, they should at least reduce the quantities to a bare minimum. In other words, the basis of the diet should be rice, cottage cheese and salads, if high blood pressure is to drop.

The reason rice is of such importance in this diet is that it helps to restore the elasticity of the blood vessels. Soft white cheese (quark) is a good source of protein, goes well with vegetables, especially salads, and is tasty. By adding various seasonings, for example horseradish, curry and all kinds of herbs, as well as vegetable juices, you can enrich its content and taste and provide some variety. Salads, by the way, supply the body with the necessary vitamins and essential mineral salts.

A doctor in the United States has helped many people suffering from hypertension by means of a diet similar to the one suggested below. These patients would probably not have been so successful had they tried the treatment alone at home, as the temptation to lapse back into old habits may have been too strong. Through the treatment the high blood pressure was reduced, but with it went a considerable sum of money too.

As a rule, the results of this treatment begin to be seen after 3–4 months. So, if a patient can only spare four weeks to attend a clinic, he does not really have to give up when the time comes to leave, because the experience gained may be used at home and he can continue the regime. True enough, it does take a little willpower to be consistent and not revert to one's old eating habits. Of course, family members can help tremendously by showing understanding and giving encouragement. Success will not fail to come in time. In the paragraphs below we are glad to give valuable hints and directions for a recommended diet.

A Recommended Diet

BREAKFAST

Even without meat, eggs and cheese, breakfast can still be varied from day to day. We can make Bambu Coffee, have rye bread, crispbread, wholegrain or wholemeal bread, butter or a good vegetable margarine and honey or jam without additives. A dish of muesli with seasonal berries or fruits completes the breakfast menu. (Muesli, the famous Swiss breakfast food, is a mixture of rolled oats and other cereals, nuts and dried fruit.) This breakfast is tasty, nutritious and invigorating.

Instead of having fruit every morning, you may wish to introduce some variety and take your Bambu Coffee together with wholegrain or wholemeal open sandwiches. Spread the bread with butter

125

or cottage cheese, cover it with slices of radishes in springtime, and top it with fresh seasonal herbs or tender leaves of lettuce. Finely chopped ramsons (bear's garlic) are also wholesome and, incidentally, very popular as a salad or steamed vegetable; they are especially good for people suffering from high blood pressure. When tomatoes are in season, use these in sandwiches too. At certain times of the year when horseradish and cress are available, they too will enrich our breakfast.

MIDDAY MEAL

The meal we eat at noon is an essential part of the treatment. It can indeed be curative if prepared according to the following suggestions.

Prepare rice, cottage cheese enriched with horseradish, and a salad of four or five different fresh vegetables, not forgetting to season with a little garlic in order to benefit from its healing properties. In springtime you can replace the garlic with fresh ramsons (bear's garlic). If you do not like the strong aftertaste or smell of garlic, be assured that this can usually be eliminated by eating parsley afterwards.

If you think up different ways of serving rice, it will not become tiresome. For example, it is possible to prepare tasty vegetable rice dishes, as they do in the Far East. This idea has endless possibilities, such as rice with courgettes, with tomatoes, with mushrooms, with aubergines, with chillies and with soybean sprouts. To all these dishes add creamed curds or cottage cheese with herbs, and don't forget the salad.

For the sake of variety we may want to prepare a sweet rice dish with grapes and almonds, and eat this with a fresh fruit compote. Finish off the meal with Bambu Coffee and cream.

The rice should be cooked so that the grains do not stick together. If you overcook rice it will lose its tastiness and become starchy. It is true, the Japanese usually prepare it that way deliberately, but the Chinese take care to keep the grains separate. To enhance the flavour of a rice dish sprinkle it with finely chopped parsley and a little grated cheese and brown in the oven. This will make a welcome change.

EVENING MEAL

It is advisable to take only a light meal at night and refrain from eating any hard-to-digest foods in order to ensure a good night's rest. We recommend some fruit and wholegrain or wholemeal bread, spread with butter or vegetable margarine, and a cup of Bambu Coffee. The fruit may be in a dish of muesli, or served as a fruit salad made with fresh fruit only. Fruit as a diet food has to be fresh, so that you will have to limit your choice to the varieties that are in season.

If vegetables rather than fruit are preferred, make a dish of cold buckwheat gruel (see below) and serve with any salad as an evening meal. Or in lieu of that, make some fresh vegetable soup accompanied by wholemeal sandwiches and a mixed salad.

In order to avoid flatulence, it is best to avoid eating vegetables and fruit at the same meal. If you did not know about this, it may be difficult to change your habits. But observing this rule is worthwhile, because your digestion will improve, gastric disturbances will disappear and your body's energy reserves will last longer.

WHAT TO DRINK

If we want to to have a suitable drink with our vegetable dishes, we should choose something that contains lactic acid, for example diluted Molkosan, or juices, such as beetroot and carrot juices. However, it should be remembered never to make a practice of drinking while there is food in the mouth as this prevents proper mastication and hinders the pre-digestive process.

THE ART OF SEASONING

When suffering from high blood pressure it is important to consider the type of condiments used. Since too much salt can increase the blood pressure, the diet should be very low in salt, just as is necessary in the case of kidney trouble. Instead of using salt without thinking, you must learn the art of proper seasoning. This is something that every cook should know, especially if diet meals have to be prepared. Food should never taste dull or else it will be unappetising. Instead of salt, the following spices and herbs, if used moderately, are better for your health: horseradish, parsley, marjoram, thyme, and if you like, also chillies, paprika, and curry. Garlic adds a pleasant flavour to rice dishes too.

The popular herbal salt Herbamare makes seasoning easier and is economical to use.

BUCKWHEAT

In the past buckwheat was more popular than it is today. Since this cereal, just like rice, serves as a remedy for high blood pressure, it should appear on our table for a change. It may be prepared in the same way as rice and can take its place along with cottage cheese and salads. One method of serving buckwheat is by cooking it in a vegetable broth to which has been added home-made tomato purée and finely chopped seasoning herbs. Leave to cool, then serve cold for supper, together with tomatoes and lettuce. Another variation is to mix cooked buckwheat gruel with onion, garlic and a little marjoram, let it cool and then fry like rissoles. *Bon appetit!*

Normalising the Blood Pressure through a Wholegrain Rice Diet

WHITE OR BROWN RICE?
In the United States it has been the custom for quite some time to treat high blood pressure with a rice diet. A Swiss sanatorium has employed the same diet to combat hypertension with the satisfactory result that the pressure decreased significantly, but at the same time the diet produced a bad side effect – the patients became anaemic. What could have caused this unfortunate result? Well, it was quite simply due to a lack of knowledge. No one took into consideration that white rice is not at all suitable for diet purposes; having had its goodness to a large extent removed, it gives rise to typical deficiency symptoms. Did not the outbreak of beriberi make the world aware of this fact?

A mono-diet of rice is indicated only if it is based on the whole grain; it must be *unpolished brown rice*. Only then will the patient benefit and the blood pressure drop without any accompanying deficiency symptoms. It is a good thing to observe this in everyday cooking as well, because brown rice is far more nutritional than the refined white kind, as brown rice contains 9.5 times more minerals (nutritive salts) than white rice. During the refining process, not only is the external cellulose husk removed, but so too is the tasty silvery membrane and the germ. While this process makes for a nice white rice grain, it devalues it at the same time. It is an open secret that the removed 'wastes' of the rice grains are not thrown away but are bought by the pharmaceutical companies to be included as ingredients in their tonic medicines. It is always good to look behind the scenes if you can, because you often discover some useful hints for better health.

What Can You Expect to Achieve?
It is a proven fact that a diet of wholegrain rice promotes normal blood pressure. As it regulates low as well as high pressure, it would be wrong not to give it a chance for either of these problems. Not long ago I received a letter from a friend in Germany to whom I had recommended a wholegrain rice diet for his very high blood pressure. He had followed my advice and was able to report excellent results.

He remained on the recommended diet for ten weeks and found that he had lost weight and that his blood pressure had gone down from 230 to 190. This result alone was most encouraging. He then took a two-week vacation, at the end of which his pressure had fallen even further, this time to 170. Let me add that this patient is already sixty-three years old and it is especially interesting to note that he obtained such splendid results without the aid of any medication – simply by following a diet of wholegrain rice, cottage cheese and salads. If he keeps to this diet he will experience a further reduction in blood pressure and, with it, the elasticity of the blood vessels will improve.

Even though my friend did not make use of any medicines – and still achieved a noteworthy result – it would not be wrong to supplement a diet of this kind with certain preparations which would make it even more effective. For example, *Viscum album tincture*, a mistletoe preparation, is able to lower the blood pressure. Additionally, *hawthorn (Crataegus)* and *arnica* should be taken, both remedies having a positive influence on the blood vessels. Another helpful remedy is *bear's garlic tonic*, since it is a specific for regenerating the vessels. In spring, gather bear's garlic (ramsons) and prepare it as a fresh salad, or steam it as a vegetable. For the rest of the year, take bear's garlic tonic and *garlic perles* or *Arterioforce* capsules.

If, as a result of this treatment, the arterial pressure falls, this signifies not simply a lower reading but the welcome fact that the elasticity of the blood vessels has improved – that is, a genuine rejuvenation of the vessels has taken place. If we realise the consequences of high blood pressure, we will feel it is well worth the effort to persevere with the recommended diet until satisfactory results have been obtained.

Low Blood Pressure (Hypotension)
High blood pressure as a disease has been extensively discussed and written about. All attention is focused on it in the fight to cure

it, and this is often possible by means of medication, therapies and a proper diet.

But much less is known about low blood pressure, or hypotension, and many questions are asked: 'What causes it? How does it develop? What can be done about it?' These questions are not adequately answered even in literature written by naturopaths, despite the fact that many people complain of low blood pressure.

A person with low blood pressure may be subject to dizziness or even occasional fainting spells at high altitudes of 1,500–1,800 m (4,500–6,000 feet). Every little exertion may upset the blood circulation or the normal heart activity. A change in locale is often necessary to permit the patient to live in a lower, and therefore more suitable, altitude. It must be added, though, that some patients actually feel better at a higher altitude than they do in the lowlands. In 90 per cent of all cases, the symptoms appear as a result of insufficiency of the gonads. In a woman the ovaries do not function correctly and in a man it is the male sex glands that are out of order.

What Relief Is Available?

As soon as medication that stimulates the glandular activity is given, the blood pressure returns to normal. Let me point out, however, that it is not advisable to take powerful hormone preparations, since their remedial effect is usually not permanent and can result in unpleasant side effects, or the blood pressure may be forced up too quickly. So would it not be better to stimulate the sex glands indirectly? It is possible to do this with potassium iodide preparations containing organically bound iodine from seaweed. Although all kinds of seaweed can be used, kelp is especially appropriate. No wonder *Kelpasan* tablets have for this reason gained such wide popularity. *Rauwolfia root*, which is grown in India and Sri Lanka, has also acquired a good reputation for its effectiveness and patients are also given the tincture to reduce high blood pressure. *Ginkgo biloba* drops are another splendid remedy, since the active ingredients obtained from the leaves have a beneficial effect on the circulatory system. For women, a very good homoeopathic remedy for the ovaries is *Ovarium 3x*. This excellent remedy regulates the function of the ovaries without any side effects.

Another good remedy for low blood pressure is *hyssop*, a plant that has been known and used since biblical times. Bible readers will recall God's instruction to Moses in connection with the sacrifice of the lamb at Passover. At that time the Jews were commanded to paint the door posts and lintels of their houses with the blood of a lamb, using bundles of hyssop to do so. Even today, the Samaritans use hyssop to prevent the curdling of blood of the sacrificial animal. There is a simple reason for this effect: the juice in the hyssop plant has the property of preventing blood from coagulating or clotting. In the 51st Psalm hyssop is mentioned in connection with spiritual cleansing. This singular plant does indeed possess a peculiar and mysterious power. It is most likely that its benefits in affecting blood pressure favourably and raising it are due to its influence on the gonads or sex glands.

Other Remedies and Treatments
In order to raise low blood pressure it does no harm to drink a glass of natural, unadulterated *red wine* now and again. '*Buendner meat*' (slightly salted and air-dried beef) is also indicated for this purpose. Vegetarians, however, will no doubt prefer to take *bee pollen*, which helps to increase low blood pressure due to its stimulating effect on the sex glands. The combination of *Auroforce, Kali phos. 6x* and bee pollen has been found to be effective. But here is a word of warning: bee pollen is so effective in raising the blood pressure that people who suffer from hypertension should not take any at all since doing so could provoke a stroke. I remember the case of one patient who had taken some pollen and could have had a tragic end if immediate counteracting measures had not been taken in time. You can see from this experience that even natural remedies are not always harmless if improperly employed.

Another natural remedy that increases the blood pressure is *raw carrot juice*. People with high blood pressure must therefore abstain from drinking carrot juice, but those with low pressure will benefit from it when taken in addition to the other indicated remedies. However, if carrots are eaten whole or as a salad, they will have no effect on the blood pressure; only the pure juice is curative. This applies also to *beetroot juice*.

If high altitudes make you feel dizzy and you wish to overcome the spell quickly, you might like to try *caffeine*; have a strong cup of coffee and the symptoms will quickly pass. If you live in a coastal area and have low blood pressure, *oysters* are excellent for regulating pressure and improving, at the same time, an insufficiency of the sex glands. Of course, you will have to eat them regularly.

A downward fluctuation of the blood pressure indicates a lack of vitality. It is therefore not enough simply to treat the symptoms of dizziness; a means must be sought to improve the overall condition of the person, restoring lost strength and the energy needed to keep up with the daily routine of work and life. This is much more desirable than having to force ourselves to do justice to our daily duties and chores. If the sex glands do not function properly the result is not only a loss of sexual potency, but also of vitality and energy in general. This translates itself into a lack of desire to work and a lack of creativity in physical, mental and artistic fields. A condition like this should not be left to linger on, unless one has already retired from active involvement in life and is quite happy to lead a leisurely life with no greater exertion than short daily walks.

Varicose Veins

If you reflect on the significance of the blood vessels and the blood, you can benefit from the Bible's statement that 'the soul of every sort of flesh is in the blood.' Goethe's words in *Faust*, 'blood is a unique fluid', express a similar thought. Everything in the body, its development and functions, depends on our blood and its quality, even our perceptions and feelings. If the blood is sound, our feelings and attitudes will also be healthy. We often hear about hormones, the glandular secretions present in the blood in minute concentrations, and how they influence the functions of the body and its physical activities. But this is not their only influence. They also affect our mental and emotional state and even have a bearing on our character and personality. Hormonal disturbances have been known to cause changes in character. Such thoughts make us feel very uncomfortable about taking another person's blood through a blood transfusion. Not without reason did God strictly forbid the ancient Jews to take in blood in any form.

If the blood is to fulfil its task properly, it must contain all the minerals and vitamins the body requires to maintain itself. The circulation has the important function of carrying these elements to the tissues. Thus, on the one hand, the blood itself must contain the necessary nutrients, and on the other hand, the circulation must be in good working order so that these nutrients will be taken to every cell in the body. More than that, even if the cells received everything they need they would still die if the metabolic wastes were not removed. The cells would inevitably be poisoned by their own waste matter.

If you are reasonably well acquainted with the body's functions, you will know that the arteries carry oxygenated, nutrient-laden

132

blood to the cells, while the veins carry the depleted blood back to the heart after the tissues have received what they need. Thus, the arteries and veins are complementary to each other. Everything our Creator has made was designed so that normal function and activity can take place.

Disturbances in the venous system are much more frequent than in the arterial system, and women especially suffer from stagnation of blood in the veins. When young people complain of cold feet it is usually a sign that the circulation is malfunctioning. Lack of exercise or inadequate clothing are generally responsible for young women and girls feeling cold. And cold feet often leads to ailments of the abdominal organs and the kidneys. In this way, young girls frequently ruin their prospects of good health later in life. Their parents ignore the fundamentals of appropriate clothing and the girls themselves know little or nothing about them anyway. They are usually more interested in fashion and fads than in matters of health and what is necessary to maintain it. Their periods are frequently accompanied by cramps and all sorts of upsets, and much of this is due to stagnation of blood in the veins. Even chilblains are not warning enough for such people, because they have no idea of their cause. So chilblains are simply treated locally, where it hurts, and no thought is given to treating the veins, the origin of the trouble. In such cases alternating *hot and cold foot baths* and *long baths* would be indicated and should be complemented by taking herbal remedies.

The fashion for wearing trousers would be better for many women and girls because they would hide their knotted and swollen veins. However, if some women follow fashion blindly to the point of wearing high-heeled shoes, with the heels often pencil thin, then I am afraid to say that we lose our pity for their condition. High heels, tight clothes and underwear with tight elastic help to promote varicose veins. For this reason it would be much more prudent to dress in accordance with sensible rules for good health. Surely it would be more reasonable to find out and meet the requirements for good health, would it not?

Sclerosing
When the veins cease to function efficiently the circulation becomes impaired and varicose veins develop ('varicose' is derived from the Latin word *varix* – a dilated vein). This frequently happens during pregnancy and immediately after childbirth and should be tackled at once, for neglect at this stage will, slowly but surely, lead to

further trouble. Lack of care of the venous system can bring on thrombosis and embolism. If a good pregnancy is desired, an easy labour and a trouble-free time after birth, look after the veins!

It is understandable that one would like to get rid of varicose veins as quickly as possible. This is sometimes done by injecting a strong hypertonic saline or sugar solution into the affected vein, sclerosing it, so that it ceases to function. Each calf possesses two deep and two superficial veins, and each thigh has one of each, with smaller communicating veins. If one of these veins is put out of action, the other will have more work to do. It is obvious that this one may, in time, also become defective, for how can one vein manage to do the work of two, especially when the work was evidently too much when shared by two veins? Eventually, the second vein will also have to be sclerosed and the circulation will depend on the subsidiary veins. True, these can indeed expand a little and become stronger, but not enough to save the circulation from being impeded. Insufficient circulation will lead to further problems. Circulatory disorders, especially among the elderly, are common and often cause grave ailments, such as can be seen in senile gangrene. In many instances such afflictions can be traced back to an earlier interference with the venous system when the patient was young. Indeed, even young people can be affected. The danger of embolism and thrombosis is accentuated by meddling with the blood vessels, as many patients can confirm.

Surgery

It is, of course, also wrong to put up with varicose veins without doing anything about them. For one thing, with advancing age the condition will deteriorate and the prospects of curing it become slimmer. In very serious cases it may be impossible to avoid surgery. Such serious cases are rare among Africans, except their older women. Where a medicine man is still practising, he will cut the affected vein with a sharp piece of broken glass and then squeeze out the stagnated blood. This method, which perforce is less hygienic than an operation in a hospital, is all that is needed as far as surgical intervention is concerned. Although we in the West may not submit ourselves to this kind of treatment, nevertheless, in grave cases an operation is better and less likely to be followed by serious complications than treatment by sclerosing. It is a fact that the injected saline solution reaches not only the demarcated vessel but also adjoining cnes. As a rule, no one talks about the adverse consequences of sclerosing.

Perhaps 10 per cent of all cases of varicose veins justify surgery. The other 90 per cent of venous disorders in the legs can be treated successfully, or at least with partial success, by other means, such as those outlined below.

Natural Regeneration

It is imperative that people should be warned against any harmful, unnatural treatment of varicose veins. Why go in for dangerous methods when the veins can be regenerated by natural means? When varicose veins appear, the body is in need of a good calcium preparation, for example *Urticalcin*, as well as a preparation called *Aesculaforce*, made from horse chestnut, witch hazel, arnica and yellow melilot (sweet clover). *Hypericum perforatum* and *Millefolium*, too, are very good for this condition. The veins are regenerated in a wonderful way by means of these remedies. To alleviate a painful inflammation, take *Lachesis 10x* and *12x*. Moreover, pay attention to an appropriate *natural diet rich in calcium*. In this way, even where heredity plays a part, varicose veins can be made to recede and can sometimes be completely removed, or at least regenerated to such an extent that they will not give you any further trouble. This advice is especially important for expectant mothers because it is not only helpful to the circulation but also prevents complications during confinement. These remedies stimulate the venous system and remove obstructions so that there will be no danger of embolism or thrombosis.

Thus the veins, like other organs of the body, should be regenerated rather than removed. As has already been pointed out, the solution to varicose veins first of all requires that sensible clothing is worn, shoes with normal heels no higher than 2–3 cm or 1½ inches, and reasonably loose dresses and lingerie so that the circulation is not constricted or otherwise impaired.

A second factor worth mentioning is the detrimental effect on the veins of standing for long periods. In particular, you should strictly avoid standing for any length of time on stone or concrete floors.

Thirdly, watch what you eat. Your diet must be rich in vitamins and minerals. That is why plenty of raw vegetables and fresh fruit are important.

Rule four is to stimulate the circulation by supplying the blood with sufficient oxygen. Plenty of outdoor exercise in the fresh air will do this for you.

Then consider the general care of the legs. Put them up for a period every day and carefully empty the veins by gently stroking upwards, not massaging, as doing so may be a little too drastic. The best time to do this is in the evening before going to bed, but if you have enough time during your lunch break, you can repeat it then. Oil the legs once a week with St John's wort oil or massage oil containing this ingredient. For a change you can use a lanolin cream, such as Bioforce Cream.

At the same time, I am happy to repeat that there are some excellent natural remedies for stimulating the circulatory system. Would we have a certain number of veins, tonsils or an appendix if these organs were not vital to our well-being? Surely then, every interference and anatomical change presents a risk that is more often than not accompanied by unpleasant consequences. How strange it is that we are inclined to show more confidence in surgery than the meaningful purpose of our Creator's design! Unfortunately, the damage only becomes evident later, after the person has been considerably harmed.

Some time ago it was considered fashionable to remove the appendix, even if it was healthy, whenever the surgeon had cause to open a patient's right abdomen. Their justification for this was that it might become diseased one day and would have to be removed then anyway. Fortunately, the profession is more enlightened today and such short-sighted decisions have been abandoned so that an appendix is removed only when absolutely necessary. The same goes for the tonsils; they too can be treated and regenerated long before they are beyond repair. Really, then, there can be no excuse for neglect. We usually know our physical weaknesses. If we give immediate attention to even slight physical signals, and with persevering care and patience treat them in a natural way, the body will respond. We have the remedies; you only have to use your intelligence, understanding and willpower to apply them, and the results will be rewarding.

Anyone who suffers from varicose veins should treat them by natural means, and with perseverance. There is no immediate cure; it is impossible to blow them away from one day to the next, for it took a considerable time for the veins to become diseased in the first place. Healthy veins play such an important part in our bodies that the patient attention and care we give them to ensure their proper function will be well worth our while.

Phlebitis (Inflammation of the Veins)

Alcohol compresses are very good for phlebitis. Better still are *compresses* with tinctures from plants such as *St John's wort*, *yarrow* or *marigold*. These are always indicated for phlebitis. If you take *Aesculaforce* at the same time, or an infusion of St John's wort, yarrow, and *arnica*, the problem will be treated from the inside as well. The use of yet another plant, *Echinacea*, is also important for effecting a cure. The fresh herb preparation *Echinaforce* supports the body's efforts in combatting bacteria, which are always present in phlebitis. *Usneasan* and the homoeopathic medicine *Lachesis 12x* have a similar effect. By taking these remedies it will be possible to prevent blood poisoning, which sometimes accompanies phlebitis.

Changing one's eating habits will be of further benefit, bringing faster relief. A *natural diet* should be followed, preferably a vegetarian one, and plenty of fruit and vegetable juices should be included.

Leg Ulcers

Those who suffer from ulcerated legs usually are unaware that it is wrong to attempt to heal the ulcers externally without also improving the general condition of the blood. Even though a good ointment or other natural remedies may be used, it is advisable not to try to heal the ulcer too quickly. If the secretions with their metabolic toxins cannot drain away freely before the blood has been purified, the condition will give rise to increasing discomfort. This has been confirmed by many whose leg ulcers have been healed too quickly.

You must understand that, according to the principles of natural therapy, the body uses just such an ulcer, or similar afflictions, as a kind of safety valve through which it can expel material which otherwise cannot be disposed of. If this valve is closed, the toxins will remain in the body. The patient's general condition will worsen and he will feel unwell. When he begins to feel dizzy and weak it is the body's urgent plea for help to open another valve. This help is given when the patient is treated internally, with a view to restoring the efficient working of the veins.

As a rule, it will be necessary to stimulate the kidneys, since in such cases they are usually weak. If the patient takes, in addition, the special remedies for the veins as they are included in *Aesculaforce*, a complex made from horse chestnut, witch hazel, arnica and yellow melilot, as well as a course of biological calcium complex *Urticalcin*, do not be surprised if the ulcer breaks open again. Neither should you be surprised if the patient begins to feel much better. This treatment is designed to attack the problem from inside, to purify and vitalise the system by acting on the kidneys and veins. As a result, the internal condition will be improved and the ulcers will soon heal up outside without any fear of further disturbance to the patient's general well-being.

If the patient is constipated, prompt action should be taken to relieve this condition. In less stubborn cases *psyllium seed* will help, as will *soaked prunes or figs*.

If high blood pressure is noted, indicated by a feeling of dizziness, do not neglect to treat it. *Viscum album, Crataegus* and *arnica* are well-known remedies that have a regenerating effect on the blood vessels. Further advice is given in the section on hypertension (see pages 124–9). It may be that the heart requires strengthening too. All these factors have to be assessed according to each case.

It goes without saying that an appropriate diet is essential for any healing process, if it is to be successful. If by now you have come to terms with the meaning of natural therapy, it should not be necessary to re-emphasise this fact. Cleansing the body from inside requires a diet that is low in salt and protein. Meat consumption should be reduced to a bare minimum, or better still, eliminated altogether until a complete recovery has been achieved. Pork, sausages and all other processed meats, eggs, cheese, white sugar and flour, as well as canned foods, should all be avoided. In their place eat plenty of natural wholefoods, including steamed vegetables, raw salads and wholegrain products.

The above recommendations are intended to help all those who suffer from leg ulcers. If you recognise and follow these important principles of natural therapy, your recovery and future well-being will be within your reach.

Circulatory Disorders

Chilblains
Red–blue skin patches that hurt with every movement are known as chilblains. They mainly affect the hands and feet and are caused by prolonged exposure to severe cold. However, this complaint can be easily prevented if we maintain a constant effort to keep our circulation in good order.

If you have a tendency to develop chilblains or already suffer from them, you will find the simple home remedies and preventative measures outlined in the first part of this book (see pages 3–4) of great benefit. If you also take *Hypericum perforatum, Aesculaforce* and *Urticalcin* at the same time, your circulation will gradually improve and the tendency towards chilblains may disappear.

Gangrene

Gangrene is a term associated with the death of tissues due to failure of the blood supply. The condition requires immediate attention. If neglected, the skin of the legs or feet turns a bluish-red colour, becomes shiny and hard and makes the patient feel extremely uncomfortable, especially at night, when the patches begin to burn to the extent that relief can only be obtained by moving the feet from under the blankets and exposing them to the cool air.

The symptoms usually appear in older people, but have their beginnings earlier in life, possibly when the person has been repeatedly exposed to cold and rain. Gangrene can also result from untreated frostbite. This is dangerous because the tissues and vessels of the feet suffer permanent damage. Another possible cause of gangrene is the sclerosing or drying-up treatment applied to varicose veins. Prolonged standing or sitting is harmful to an older person who suffers from gangrene because the venous blood circulation slows down. Sufferers usually benefit from having an occupation which allows them to move around; with increased mobility the pain will sometimes subside altogether. Even though the disease cannot be cured completely, it is possible to alleviate it with the help of natural remedies, to the extent that the patient may go without serious complications for many years.

For an effective external treatment, add five drops of *Arnica 1x* to a little warm water and use this to make a wet pack. Take the two remedies *Echinaforce* and *Lachesis 10x* in a little water; they should be taken separately on alternate days, in the morning and at night, over an extended period. *Aesculaforce* and *Ginkgo biloba*, if taken regularly, also give satisfactory results.

The patient should not expose himself to the cold and should wrap up warmly against the weather. He should also adopt a light vegetarian diet. These measures are not difficult to follow, when he takes into account that by doing so he can find a measure of relief from his unpleasant condition and be spared much discomfort.

Haemorrhoids

Haemorrhoids, commonly known as piles, are often associated with chronic constipation. A dense network of blood vessels runs through the intestinal lining. When the stool in the rectum becomes hard and accumulates there these blood vessels become stretched. The resulting obstruction causes the walls of the vessels in the anal canal to become dilated, turning them into varicose veins in and around the rectal opening – haemorrhoids. The pressure needed to force out hard stools makes the veins in the thin membrane rupture; blood leaks out, and we have what are called bleeding haemorrhoids. At the time of evacuation, light-coloured blood will usually be noticed in the stool. If this condition is not remedied, the tissues will become inflamed and hard, resulting in the well-known piles. Hard stools can push the piles outwards so that they hang out of the anus; these can sometimes grow as large as a plum. This description alone will give an indication of the great discomfort this problem can cause. Anyone suffering from piles will therefore be most grateful for relief and a cure.

Women frequently get haemorrhoids after childbirth. Even during pregnancy the entire venous system is subjected to greater pressure than usual, often giving rise to varicose veins or enlarging those already there. In the weeks just before delivery the baby's head presses on the vessels in the pelvis and this, in turn, affects the vessels in the rectum. During delivery this pressure increases even more so that piles often appear after giving birth. Specific advice for expectant mothers is given on pages 26–9, but what can be done about this problem in general?

The Treatment of Haemorrhoids

First of all, you must take up the fight against constipation, for as long as you remain constipated any treatment will have only partial success. It must be said, however, that the cause of constipation is often more than the lack of a proper diet – one made up of wholegrain or wholemeal bread and plenty of fresh fruit and raw vegetables – and good herbal remedies such as Rasayana and Linoforce; an additional factor can be the mental and emotional stresses and tensions many of us experience as a consequence of unsolved problems in our life. An 'uptight' attitude can be an outward sign of a similar tension in the bowels, which, incidentally, are governed by the sympathetic nervous system. Once constipation has been remedied, it is relatively easy to treat the haemorrhoids successfully.

For this purpose there are some fine natural medicines available. *Aesculaforce* and *Hypericum perforatum* are good for the circulation and have aided many people in their effort to get rid of varicose veins. For this reason they are equally effective for the treatment of dilated veins in and around the anus. These remedies help to reduce the pressure in the veins and thus have a healing effect on the entire venous system.

Of great benefit also are *Millefolium*, a fresh plant extract from yarrow, *Hamamelis virginiana* and *Calcarea fluorica* (calcium fluoride). In cases of heavy bleeding, treat with *Bursa pastoris* (shepherd's purse) or *Tormentavena*. For local treatment and to ease pain, use haemorrhoid suppositories containing *cocoa butter* and *Hamamelis*. Teas made from *bloodwort* and *stinging nettles* are also beneficial. Spurge applied externally also helps to ease the pain. Although this plant is poisonous when taken internally, when crushed and applied to the anus as a poultice, it will soon help to make the pain subside.

A good way to prevent haemorrhoids is to bathe the anus with cold water every morning. The same water treatment should be given when piles have already formed.

The Heart – an Indefatigable Organ
Even before we become conscious of our existence, before birth, the heart begins to beat and continues to do so day and night throughout our life. It performs its work unflaggingly until the body is worn out and we close our eyes in death. Are we really grateful to the heart for serving us so faithfully during our lifespan of maybe 60–90 years, without even stopping for one hour, or do we take the heart for granted and neglect to look after it?

The Heart's Matchless Activity
Where could we ever find a machine that would work as efficiently as the heart? When we begin to study the structure of the myocardium we cannot help but be overwhelmed by this astounding example of divine Creation. Just look at the design of the muscle fibres. They are made up of fibrils, laid down in criss-cross layers, giving them marvellous elasticity. The cardiac wall consists of thousands of such fibres. Interwoven with this fibrous tissue we find a network of blood vessels providing nourishment and a network of nerves to register the stimuli. On reflection, we must admit that this living miracle in our body deserves more consideration than we are wont to give it. Is it not true that young people and

athletes tend to treat the marvellous heart in their trust in an irresponsible and careless manner? Yet it is not only physical over-exertion that can tax and damage it. Worries and anxieties also weaken and harm the heart. The sympathetic nervous system serves to stimulate the heart and the parasympathetic slows it down. Both of these impulse conductors work in a rhythmic fashion, which means that the heart beats either slower or faster according to demand. Between every beat the heart stands still for about one-sixth of a second, the only rest it ever indulges in. But this rest in no way compensates for the amount of work we expect it to do throughout our lifetime. The heart, with all its capabilities and untiring service, is truly a miracle.

Nevertheless, it is not at all surprising to learn that about 50 per cent of all people today show some sort of abnormality in their heart function. Modern man always seems to be under stress and hurries even when there is no need, while at the same time he may be careless about attending to other responsibilities. This imbalance certainly does not make for peace of mind, as we still find it among those who enjoy their work as opposed to viewing it as a necessary evil. 'Haste makes waste', so the saying goes. Haste may indeed be harmful, but a steady pace is good for the heart.

The endocrine glands, especially the thyroid, influence the heart, a fact that can be noticed in patients with hyperthyroidism (Graves' disease). If the heart rhythm, the pulsation, is traced on paper by means of an electrocardiograph, a heart disorder can be detected. If the recording, called an electrocardiogram, shows two entwined curves, this indicates that two hearts are beating simultaneously. How can that be possible? The answer is simple if you are a pregnant woman! And if there are three curves, the happy mother-to-be can be told that she may expect twins.

Complications Deserving Attention

It is interesting to note that the heart may continue to beat even when the person is already dead. On the other hand, it is also possible for the heart to stop beating although death has not yet occurred, as in the case of suspended animation (apparent death, or asphyxia). A strong electric shock, for example, causes a spasm in the heart which may temporarily suspend its function, but death itself does not occur until later, when the oxygen supply is cut off completely and carbon dioxide accumulates because it is no longer eliminated.

Vesalius, the father of modern anatomical research, wanting to determine the cause of death of a nobleman he had treated, performed an autopsy during which he noticed, to his horror, that the heart was still beating. Witnesses who were present at the autopsy took him to court. He was found guilty of having performed a post-mortem examination on a living person and he was sentenced to death. This illustrates that life does not always coincide with the activity of the heart. So, even if death has occurred, the eyes are glassy and breathing has stopped, the heart may nevertheless continue to beat for a little while.

On the other hand, the opposite phenomenon, where the heart stops beating before the person is actually dead, has been observed in criminals who have been electrocuted. Being aware of this fact, a doctor was permitted to give a 'dead' man an injection in order to ease the spasm, because the doctor had attributed the sudden cardiac arrest to a spasm induced by the electricity. His diagnosis proved to be correct; the executed man who had appeared to be dead came back to life and had to undergo a second time the distressing procedure of the electric chair.

Many other astonishing incidents and facts connected with the functions of the heart could no doubt be cited. New surprises still come to light, some being discovered accidentally and others as a result of medical research.

Interesting Help for the Heart
The discovery of the so-called 'heart hormones' was made accidentally. A Hungarian professor was conducting experiments that involved injecting an old sheep over a long period of time with an extract derived from the heart of a young lamb. As a result of this treatment, the vitality of the old sheep increased; its heart rhythm gained in strength and it was once again able to climb around the hills as if it had been rejuvenated. When the old sheep was killed, the assumption that a rejuvenation had taken place was proved correct by the presence of new heart cells and cells which showed the nucleus to be in the process of dividing. Yet this dividing process is normally only found in young sheep during their growth period. The heart of a young animal is therefore somehow able to cause the nucleus of the heart cells to divide and form new cells. However, this process ceases to occur once the animal has reached maturity.

The cause of the observed rejuvenation, which is still unknown today, was attributed to a heart hormone, a term that seemed to be the most appropriate to designate the unknown factor. Since the substance concerned was perfectly harmless, researchers thought it might benefit humans too, and their subsequent experiments gave satisfactory results. It has since been used as an effective treatment for dilation of the heart, athlete's heart, and in cases of a tired or exhausted heart.

Nevertheless, this should not lead us to believe that if we abuse the heart and cause damage to its muscles we can always have recourse to heart hormones, which can easily correct any defects. This is not the case. Indeed, the most sensible way to ensure the proper functioning of the heart is to give it normal care and consideration. This faithful pump works wonderfully and is fully automatic if it is not constantly overtaxed. The heart hormone treatment, like any other good plant or homoeopathic medicine, is helpful in a case of real need. In such cases, there are various plant remedies available to us, for example *tincture of arnica root, Crataegus, Cactus grandiflora, Strophanthus, Spigelia*, the heart nutrient *Avenaforce*, the homoeopathic remedy *Calcarea carbonica* and homoeopathically diluted *gold*. A heart tonic made up of these ingredients will alleviate a whole range of problems. In certain cases, individuals will benefit from taking *Convallaria* and *Scilla maritima*, or a tea made from the woody partitions found inside a *walnut*, separating the two halves (see pages 153–4).

If you make sure not to overstrain your heart when you are young by engaging in very strenuous sports, you need not fear that you will have to suffer any ill consequences in later life.

Lycopus europaeus – a Remedy for Palpitations

Lycopus europaeus, commonly known as gipsywort or bugleweed, is a little known but efficacious medicinal plant. In Switzerland it is found in some parts of the Churfirst mountains at an elevation of up to 1,000 m (3,280 feet). In the valleys of the Ticino and in Pusciavo it is more abundant. European *Lycopus* is very similar in content and effect to that found in Virginia, in the United States.

Lycopus produces excellent results in the treatment of mild over-active thyroid conditions (hyperthyroidism) and the accompanying heart palpitations. Even in cases of very strong pounding and nervousness, doses of 5–10 drops have a tranquillising effect. If a hyperthyroid condition has existed for some time, *Urticalcin* is also recommended, since patients who suffer from palpitations usually lack calcium. I have often been able to achieve excellent results with people who thought they were suffering from a severe heart ailment simply by giving them *Lycopus* and calcium. It is also interesting to note that a somewhat increased basal metabolism can be normalised with these remedies if they are taken together with a homoeopathic seaweed preparation such as *Kelp 4x*. However, it is important that patients avoid the use of iodised salt. *Lycopus* and Urticalcin are also a helpful combination in cases of rapid heart beat due to over-excitability, a frequent complaint in our hectic times. Even though a calming effect can be felt almost immediately, the two natural remedies should be taken over a longer period of time for a more permanent result.

It is also important that the patient find out what is an appropriate dose of *Lycopus*, since this depends on the individual's sensitivity and response. For extremely sensitive people, five drops of *Lycopus* taken three times a day will suffice. Since the preparation is harmless the dose may be increased, if necessary to twenty or thirty drops at a time.

If a heart specialist can find nothing organically wrong, even though the patient may believe that he has a bad heart, I am confident that following the above advice will be of great benefit.

Modern Heart Poisons

Stress – Pace and Haste

The ever-increasing pace that characterises our modern way of life is one of the worst poisons for our heart. Even though, for the most part, individual productivity has not exceeded that of former times, it has become the custom to cram too many activities, especially those connected with our job, into a short space of time. Related to this, of course, is the shortened working week which has become so popular. The resulting free time is hardly ever used in a wholesome recreational or relaxing way such as pursuing a hobby, say working on an arts and crafts project, listening to good music, acquiring more knowledge through a study course or some other favourite subject or activity. Instead, we continue at the same hectic pace we use for work and seem to find enjoyment at weekends in the midst of the mad world of crowded motorways.

No wonder the result is a state of complete exhaustion instead of recuperation from the week's work. Driving at high speed creates anxiety and inner tension and affects the heart like a poison. Not only is the speed of the drive harmful, but the exhaust fumes are equally dangerous to the heart and blood vessels, particularly the fumes caused by leaded petrol. How much more sensible it would be to take a short leisurely ride to a nearby forest or the hills, get

145

out of the car and go for a relaxing walk or hike. This kind of exercise would be invigorating for the blood vessels and, of course, the heart. The time spent in a clean environment would then permit us to return to work and our duties on Monday morning refreshed and relaxed, instead of tense and irritable as is so often the case today, when we misuse our leisure.

A similar tendency that should also be mentioned here is that of senselessly abusing our energies by allowing too little time to get to our place of work. We should always leave the house early enough so that it is not necessary to make a dash for the bus or train. Even a short run with a briefcase, bag or basket can be more taxing on the heart than most people realise. Obese people should be especially careful and remember the warning contained in the old proverb, 'Haste makes waste'. It has become a habit with many to rush around as if they have no time to lose, even though the gained time may be wasted later on in an idle telephone conversation or an insignificant chat with a neighbour. This is really most unwise, for the heart is not like a modern engine that can be accelerated from a standing start to 60 m.p.h. in seconds; the heart cannot be driven at top speed without suffering some damage.

Even young people who participate in overstrenuous sporting activities can develop dilation of the heart or other heart trouble. Sadly, modern athletic competition no longer attaches importance to purity and style of performance but requires the athlete to give his all, and it is exactly this excessive speed measured in split seconds that is dangerous. The excesses will act like poison to the heart, particularly for those athletes who are not in constant training. More often than not the damage is permanent.

The shorter working week mentioned earlier is also detrimental to the heart, since the work must be done faster if the number of working days is reduced without a proportionate reduction in the workload. The heart would only benefit from such an arrangement if the former, more sensible pace of work could be maintained. If a shorter working week depends on increased speed to produce the same results, the health of employee and employer alike will suffer.

Smoking

Smoking is harmful to the heart. We should none of us be in any doubt about this fact, especially women. The question of why women smoke if it is so dangerous to the heart, has many possible answers. One may be found in the assumption that it helps to assert their liberated status and strengthen their self-image; or it may be the need to imitate whatever is currently popular, for no one wants to be out of step with the prevailing trends. Another reason may be the mistaken idea that smoking calms the nerves and helps to take one's mind off things. It is a fact that even fifty years ago very few women were smokers. In those days, if a woman lit a cigarette she was eyed with suspicion and dismissed as frivolous, or worse. The relatively new trend of women smoking, and thus exposing themselves to the dire consequences of this habit, may be attributed to the general change in life-style that we have undergone since then. Abundant proof exists that nicotine is harmful, as it constricts the coronary blood vessels and really has the same effect as a slow-acting poison. It is unfortunate that the tragic consequences to a smoker's sensitive vascular system do not become evident until twenty or thirty years later, so that it is all the more difficult to convince young people to stop smoking or not to start in the first place.

There is no question that nicotine is harmful to men also, but it is more so to women whose bodies are more sensitive to its effects. Also, statistics suggest that more men today smoke pipes, which are not quite as harmful as cigarettes since the toxicity is somewhat reduced due to a filtering system and a different way of preparing pipe tobacco. Nevertheless, whatever one might argue, it is more sensible and much easier to refrain from punishing the heart while there is still time.

Only One Heart!
Never forget that we have only one heart, from which we expect faithful service during our entire lifetime. It is a miracle in itself that the heart is capable of rendering this service unremittingly, and we should show our appreciation by caring for this marvellous gift. But we are failing this responsibility if we hasten its deterioration by careless overexertion and wilfully feeding it with poisons we know to be harmful. Such abuse will serve only to cut short the peaceful twilight years of our life. It is sad when proper understanding, regrets and a change of life-style come too late to save a person from an early grave.

If you are willing to make the effort to break bad habits early enough, you can bring about a restoration and strengthening of the heart with the help of natural remedies. For example, *Crataegus*, an extract from hawthorn, acts as a tonic for the heart muscles and *Auroforce* strengthens the nerves of the heart. A calming effect on

147

the heart is obtained from *Lycopus*, a harmless plant which is native to Virginia and also grown in Switzerland. If *wheat germ oil* is taken at the same time, a weak and neglected heart will soon be stronger and healthier. Nevertheless, no matter how good the natural remedy, the cure will not be lasting unless we stop subjecting the heart to harmful influences. Taking great care of this vital organ should be our first priority.

Beware of Heart Attacks

An elderly physician once told me, to my amazement, that he never came across a case of heart attack among his patients during the early years of his practice. And this was despite the fact that country people had to work much harder physically at that time because modern labour-saving machinery was not available. Why then, we might ask, do heart attacks rank as one of the most frequent causes of death today? Obviously, it cannot be linked to physical exertion from everyday labour, because modern technology has reduced the need for us to work as hard as our fore-fathers had to.

This question reminds me of a talk I heard during my stay in Vermont, the United States. Professor Raab, the famous research scientist who specialises in blood circulation, spoke about the 'loafer's heart' of our generation. He did not mean, however, that the 'loafer's heart' is a result of 'loafing around'; this certainly would not be true in today's increasingly busy world. Rather, it is the result of one-sided activity and a lack of exercise outdoors in the fresh air. The proper balance between exertion and relaxation has become distorted, disturbing the harmony of the rhythm of rest and activity.

We have all developed the bad habit of using the motor car for every little errand instead of walking. It is most unusual for a person who owns a car to take regular walks, not even when it is just a stone's throw to the corner shop. We have become a generation spoiled by the many inventions that make life easier: we no longer want to walk, we no longer want to use our limbs, and our muscles suffer from disuse. Many people are not aware of the danger that results from this way of life. Our circulation suffers and there may even be a deterioration of the entire vascular system as well as of the heart. Monotonous mental activity may lead to tensions, stagnation in the circulatory system, spasms, high blood pressure and many other problems. All these things are potential causes of heart attacks, especially for people in their late fifties.

Finding a Happy Medium

Many times of late I have received obituary notices concerning dear friends and acquaintances whose busy and productive lives had been suddenly cut short by heart attacks. An analysis revealed that, in every case, these people had long ago ceased to engage in any regular programme of physical activity or exercise. They would not make time for long walks or hikes in the forest or woods, or along country lanes. They had stopped participating in outings with a hiking club, which had always benefited their health in the past, and could not find time to do a little gardening. Neither did they have the time, or interest, to continue with some sport that they had enjoyed in their youth. They never stopped to think that they were actually shortening their life expectancy by twenty or thirty years, even though they may have had plenty of vitality.

This may sound contradictory, but it is a fact that the unbalanced use of one's energy, under constant stress and strain, is very taxing. Limiting our responsibilities and duties and reducing the pace of life would guarantee our heart more years of faithful service. Thus, we can conclude that a heart attack, in a sense, is often a self-inflicted blow. Every organ that is not regularly utilised or exercised degenerates and the body itself cannot exist if all activity ceases.

There is a happy medium between the over-taxed heart of a professional athlete and the under-taxed 'loafer's heart'. Anyone who does not want to end his life prematurely should certainly try to achieve this medium. It is extremely dangerous to give up physical exercise around the age of forty, because by doing so you may run the risk of having a heart attack fifteen or twenty years later and perhaps dying as a result. So, if you practise therapeutic exercises early enough and always make sure to take plenty of exercise in your daily life, you will avoid the need to go on strophanthin medication in later life.

There are times, however, when certain symptoms appear as an advance warning, making us aware of a potential problem. This happened to me several years ago when I began to have severe heart spasms. A subsequent examination showed there was nothing wrong with my heart, but I was prompted nonetheless to take a closer look at my life. In doing so I found that for some months I had been doing only brain work, with little physical activity. What made things worse, during this time my life was filled with problems and worries. It did not take much persuading to make me resume my interest in hiking and climbing in the mountains. And sure enough, within a short time I felt fully recovered.

Recommended Changes

A change of life-style would be of benefit to thousands of over-worked businesspeople, office workers, politicians and others holding sedentary positions – all executives and managers under stress – before it is too late. They should realise that it is much wiser to take some form of preventative action rather than to be concerned solely with the financial benefits, which is all their young families would be left with in the event of an untimely death that could have been prevented.

Let us not be deceived: nature has its own hard and fast rules which we cannot disobey with impunity. If an assessment or analysis of your life shows that you are in danger of having a heart attack, would it not be sensible to change your life-style and modify your daily routine? It would be wise to buy less petrol, for example, and use your legs more to make sure that your body cells receive enough oxygen. As far as diet is concerned, eat smaller quantities and stick to natural wholefoods of high nutritional value. The body will welcome such a change and show its gratitude by increasing its efficiency. Moreover, no unexpected heart failure will suddenly cut your life short. People under stress should make it a point to take the tincture made from the taiga root, *Eleutherococcus*, as well as *Ginsavita* tablets. These natural remedies, when taken regularly, with the recommended changes in life-style, will help to combat the harmful effects of stress.

Athlete's Heart

When winter arrives it brings with it the chance to partake in a whole range of snowsports, increasingly referred to as 'pleasure sports'. Some of these, however, may present a danger to the heart, because not everyone is sensible enough to choose a sport that has a beneficial effect on the health; instead, they become enslaved, body and soul, to movement and speed. Yet everything in nature is based on a wholesome rhythm of movement followed by rest. We were not created with wings, so we were not intended to dart through the air like birds. Our heart was designed to be close to the earth and we should observe its human, earthly potential.

There is a great difference between the pleasure of movement and the slavish pursuit of a competitive sport. Some light exercise after an occupation that demands a lot of sitting down is beneficial, indeed essential. But if you force yourself beyond your endurance and strength, you must not be surprised if your heart muscles become dilated because they have lost their elasticity. Yet it is still possible to do something about such a condition and, to a certain extent, regeneration can be achieved, although it is much better to take note of the old proverb, 'Prevention is better than cure.'

Athletic people usually have strength and resistance, but they must not make the mistake of thinking that their resilience and ability to spring back from overexertion has no limits. Thoughtless waste of any of our potentialities will be followed by loss of fitness. Why sacrifice to sport the energies that could serve you for many years to come? Why dash with abounding strength into overstrenuous sports and come out with chronic ill health?

Many may think that I am painting a rather pessimistic picture, but this is not so. Now and then I receive sad letters from sports men and women who were once famous champions; one, for example, was from an athlete who many years ago won the Swiss pentathlon and decathlon. For years now, this once energetic athlete has been suffering from loss of breath when climbing stairs, a weak heart beat, low blood pressure and ear and head noises (tinnitus). At his age he should be full of vitality.

So this is a warning not to carry any sport to extremes, yet is is a warning difficult to heed on the part of those who have already sold themselves 'body and soul' to this unrelenting taskmaster. The passion for winning in competitive sports consumes a tremendous amount of strength and energy. And who benefits from this useless drain of energy? Nobody really, and certainly not the athlete's heart, or why would it become defective so early in life?

Angina Pectoris

There are different forms of angina pectoris, the peculiar disease that produces something like heart spasms. It is caused by an insufficient supply of blood to the walls of the heart, which in turn induces oxygen starvation. The serious symptoms do not appear all at once, but increasing instances of acute heart cramps accompanied by a feeling of tightness across the chest – called cardiac insufficiency – should be a warning that immediate action must be taken.

The newest treatment with hormones has yielded comparatively good results. There are, however, various homoeopathic and herbal remedies that should not be overlooked in the treatment of this disease. Correctly employed, they are invaluable. For serious acute cases *Tabacum 6x* is helpful, and *Tabacum 12x* for chronic conditions. The cramping heart pains which induce fear, dizziness and nausea, an irregular pulse and cold sweat will be relieved by

151

Tabacum. It is noteworthy that this remedy also works well in cases of nicotine poisoning, thus proving the homoeopathic principle, like cures like. *Tabacum 6x* will greatly improve the patient's condition if he suffers from nicotine poisoning, which constricts the coronary vessels and causes the symptom-complex of angina pectoris.

Imminent collapse, with cold sweat on the forehead and a cramp that travels far down the legs, invariably requires the use of *Veratrum album 6x*. Heart hormones are very effective in cases of genuine angina pectoris as a consequence of a heart condition, in which dilation of the heart and gradual loss of tone occurs. In fact, heart hormones actually regenerate the heart. In arteriosclerotic conditions *Arnica 30x* is often extremely effective, and can be given as an injection or taken orally. Add ten drops of tincture to a glass of hot water and sip this during the day. Five to ten drops of *Crataegus* mother tincture or *Crataegisan* taken daily will strengthen the heart generally. Should asthmatic symptoms manifest themselves, *Galeopsis* mother tincture and *Cactus grandiflora 2x* will provide effective help. If the patient has a high colour, slightly bluish, and his veins are somewhat dilated, the homoeopathic remedy *Naja 12x* would be indicated. High blood pressure calls for *Viscum album*, an extract from mistletoe. *Rauwolfavena*, a preparation made from rauwolfia, has also proved its worth.

Correct breathing, with slow, sustained exhalation, can often stop an attack in its early stages, especially when the blood is then drawn away from the heart by bathing the arms. These arm baths, as recommended by Sebastian Kneipp in his water cures, have a particularly good effect when used for incipient attacks.

If congestions are also present, do not forget to take *Aesculaforce* and *Ginkgo biloba*. Moreover, a warm bath to which an infusion of *lemon balm* has been added will have a calming influence on the nervous system.

Massaging the body regularly with a good oil that stimulates the skin functions is good for relaxation of the nerves and induces a feeling of well-being.

The proper functioning of the bowels, ensuring the elimination of all waste materials, is as important with angina as it is with other diseases. If necessary, use *psyllium seed*, or a *linseed* preparation or any other natural herbal laxative to promote good bowel movement.

As regards foods, a diet rich in natural grape or fruit sugar, but low in protein and salt, is recommended for angina pectoris.

An Old Country Remedy

In general, bad heart cramps in cases of angina pectoris are relieved by radical medicines, usually amyl nitrite or Trinitrin (nitroglycerin). There is, however, an old and exceedingly simple remedy which is quite easy to come by. It relieves the spasms without any side effects or complications. The same remedy is also good for asthma attacks. This old country remedy has been in use for centuries but has now, alas, been practically forgotten even in rural areas.

Here is what you do. Take some *fermented cider*, the older the better, heat it until it reaches boiling point and quickly remove it from the heat. Then soak some towels in the hot liquid and place them, as hot as the patient can bear, on both arms, covering each arm completely. The heat plus the fruit acids of the hot cider will decongest the heart circulation, soothe the blood vessels and the nervous system and relieve the cramps. The effect of this simple natural treatment can be reinforced by placing a hot linseed, hay flower or lemon balm *compress* over the heart at the same time. Linseed is the best choice for this purpose.

Cramp-like conditions brought about by angina pectoris or other similar causes follow the course of the sympathetic nerve. They often start in the pit of the stomach near the sternum and move up to the throat, leaving a feeling almost amounting to strangulation. Such distressing conditions, if treated as described, will be relieved to the patient's greatest satisfaction.

The Woody Partitions inside the Walnut

An infusion made from the woody partitions inside the walnut is excellent in cases where the coronary vessels have become hardened, and for cardiac pains and fever. A narrowing of the coronary vessels can often be attributed to chronic nicotine poisoning. The doctor and knowledgeable friends may have encouraged the patient on more than one occasion to quit smoking because of his heart trouble, the so-called angina pectoris. Unfortunately, the nicotine addiction often triumphs over health considerations, and severe chest pains will continue to plague the smoker. Would he continue to smoke if he knew that every severe attack of angina pectoris leaves a small scar in the muscle tissue of the heart? I wonder. Still, his unreasonableness may compel him to carry on smoking and the final result will be a myocardial infarction, death of the tissues in the myocardium. Many weeks resting in bed may bring about an improvement in his condition, but it is not to be mistaken for a cure. For once again, instead of healthy pink muscle tissue,

153

the patient will be left with yet another white scar on the heart. Even so he must consider himself fortunate, as a 'heart attack' can sometimes lead to a rupture of the heart, which would be fatal.

Needless to say, the scars themselves are far from negligible. One day, the last attack will come. A post-mortem will then reveal countless tiny scars which bear witness to the pain that accompanied each seizure and to the folly of refusing to give up smoking, preferring instead a smoker's death. If you would rather not let it come to that sad ending, stop the dangerous habit that puts your life in jeopardy – give up smoking. Moderation in alcohol and meat consumption is also indicated, and if you are able to abstain from these altogether, so much the better for your heart and general health.

The woody partitions inside the walnut contain an excellent medicinal property from which you can benefit when taken as an infusion. Remove the dividing walls of four or five nuts, soak them in water for one day, leave overnight and then boil them for a few minutes the next morning. Drink the resulting tea in the morning on an empty stomach. When taken regularly it will alleviate the feeling of constriction and pain in the chest.

This infusion is also effective in cases of high temperature accompanied by pains in the heart. Some relief is frequently noticed after the first cup, but if the pains continue, the tea should be sipped frequently until they and the fever have disappeared.

Sick without a Sickness

If you own a car you may at times hear a noise when you are driving, a noise that comes and goes. To find out what it is, you decide to take the car to a garage for a check-up, but just at that time, the noise is not there, and naturally the mechanic cannot find anything wrong with it. A few weeks later, however, your car stops in the middle of the road because the defect that had not been found and therefore not taken care of, has developed into a serious fault.

It is even harder to detect a disorder in the human body, especially if it is not a question of an actual organic disease. At times, all possible methods of examination used by the physician or naturopath do not disclose any clue of a malfunction. Intuition can be a great asset in the medical profession, but it is not enough to help those patients who feel very unwell yet the doctor is unable to put his finger on what ails them. Indeed, it often takes many years of experience to understand such patients. Many of these patients are women, whose complaints are often simply attributed to a hysterical nature or their imagination, as in psychosomatic illnesses. However, this diagnosis will only force them into deeper despair.

Hyperthyroidism

Not long ago, I was consulted by a girl who had just returned to the Engadine Valley from a trip to Italy. Her big, shiny, bulging and staring eyes showed unmistakable signs of an overactive thyroid. She explained that her doctor had practically taken her apart without finding anything wrong, although she complained of frequently feeling very ill and weak.

When staying at the seaside this 'sick person without a sickness' could sleep for twenty-four hours at a time if no one woke her up. Long sleeping periods are a typical effect of the iodine contained in sea air on those suffering from a thyroid condition. Some patients become very active, vivacious and highly strung, others feel an unnatural desire and need for sleep. It is essential for such people to be aware of what the problem is, for it will enable them to adjust to their environment and to take the appropriate remedial measures.

Some years ago I sent a patient suffering from the same symptoms to her doctor to have him check her basal metabolism. Since he felt there was nothing wrong with her thyroid, he was reluctant to check her out. But she insisted, and to his astonishment the results of the test revealed a substantial increase in her metabolism.

This condition, in almost all cases, is associated with a calcium deficiency in the blood. For this reason these patients need to eat plenty of food high in calcium. Taking a calcium-complex preparation, such as *Urticalcin*, is also highly recommended, in addition to a homoeopathic *iodine* preparation, preferably made from sea kelp, as well as *Lycopus*.

It is a source of great satisfaction to see the unpleasant symptoms disappear when the body is given the things it lacks and resumes its nature functions once more.

Neurodystonia (Autonomic Nervous Disorders)

Many disorders of the nervous system are purely psychological in nature, or they may be caused by a malfunction of the endocrine glands. Doctors call this type of problem 'neurodystonia', a descriptive term that does not really tell us much. It encompasses all disorders of the autonomic nervous system, except those of organic origin, and is therefore a rather broad and complex concept. All of the following symptoms, not attributable to organic disease, can be classified under this term: vascular spasm, sudden sweating, cramps in the vascular system and gallbladder, spastic stomach aches, intestinal and heart disorders (including organic neurosis).

Since this all-embracing term was first coined, there have been fewer people with unidentifiable illnesses. So, if the doctor cannot find an explanation for a certain complaint, he simply attributes it to 'neurodystonia'. This is convenient and benefits the doctor as well as the patient, at least from a psychological viewpoint. For to be suffering from an illness without a name is a rather uncomfortable affair. By giving it a name the doctor satisfies his patient, if only for the sake of his not being called a malingerer, one who is simply pretending to be sick.

In such cases, a skilfully handled psychotherapeutic treatment has always produced good results, especially if combined with certain tonics for the nerves such as *Neuroforce* and *Ginsavena*, as well as antispasmodics, like *Petadolor*.

Visible and Invisible Goitre

Many people, and more particularly women, often complain about a pounding of the heart without being able to explain its cause. Naturally, when climbing stairs rapidly everyone becomes aware of a faster heart beat. However, if you frequently experience a rapid heart beat without prior physical exertion or emotional upset, it would be wise to undergo a thyroid test.

A hyperactive thyroid has certain characteristics. Besides a faster pulse rate there is generally a loss of weight and an inner vibration in the chest area. Other symptoms are loss of hair, diarrhoea, and often a feeling of tension and anxiety. The basal metabolic rate is increased and the eyes take on a distinct shine. The doctor's examination will usually reveal a swelling of the thyroid gland, a goitre.

Goitre, as a result of either an overactive or underactive thyroid, is much more frequent than many people are aware, particularly in land-locked countries such as my native Switzerland, or the central plains of the United States. Many sufferers simply resign themselves to a constant state of nervousness and hypersensitivity, two of the unpleasant symptoms of this complaint.

Causes and Cures

Although iodine deficiency always plays a part in causing goitre, other minerals and trace elements are essential for successful treatment. Experience has shown that calcium is as important as iodine, so for treating and preventing goitre I recommend a diet high in calcium. White cabbage salad and sauerkraut are rich in this mineral, as are kohlrabi (turnip cabbage) – especially the leaves – turnips, carrots and beets. The latter two can be taken as juice or included raw in salads. A good calcium preparation, for example *Urticalcin*, is an excellent supplement.

On the other hand, be very careful with commercial products containing iodine. In cases of unduly sensitive people, those who suffer from hyperthyroidism, the use of iodised salt alone will sometimes cause palpitations and upsets. A person who is sensitive to mere traces of iodine should avoid such products altogether.

A calcium therapy does not cause any complications, neither does the minute amount of iodine found in some plants. For example, watercress and all the other varieties of cress contain homoeopathic amounts of iodine which even the most sensitive person can tolerate. Seaweed prescribed in homoeopathic doses, such as *Kelp 6x, 5x and 3x*, is an excellent source of iodine. When a seaweed preparation is prescribed it is best to begin with Kelp 6x, then after a few months change to Kelp 5x and continue reducing the potency until, after about two years, the patient responds well to the tablets in uncontrolled strength. The herbal seasoning salt *Herbamare* contains freshly processed cresses in addition to all the trace elements found in kelp, and is therefore a useful prophylactic.

If goitre is present and is not caused by a hyperthyroid condition, *kelp tablets* will help the patient, since they contain all the minerals found in seaweed. These tablets also help to reduce obesity without any side effects. I have also found that goitre due to hypothyroidism reacts favourably to treatment with *potassium iodide*.

Goitre not only detracts from one's appearance and is physically annoying, but it also places a burden on the mental processes because of its detrimental effect on the memory and nervous system. It is therefore advisable not to put off the treatment of goitre but to do something about it quickly. Surgery can be avoided in many cases if the proper treatment with natural remedies and therapies is administered early enough. Natural treatment will restore the normal body functions and physical strength, which is not always the case after surgical removal of a large part of the thyroid.

Post-Operative Treatment of Goitre

Where surgery is necessary, it should not be considered as a complete cure, making further treatment unnecessary. On the contrary, post-operative treatment is essential in order to eradicate the cause of the disease. Iodine remedies, especially in the case of exophthalmic goitre, are not at all indicated and should be carefully avoided. Instead, choose foods that contain traces of organic iodine, for these definitely serve to cure goitre. Once again, the two herbal seasoning salts *Herbamare* and *Trocomare*, both made with sea salt, are recommended first of all. Furthermore, effective post-operative treatment of goitre includes plant products rich in fibre and iodine. *Watercress* is high in iodine and should be eaten in salads when it is in season. It is also good for exophthalmic goitre and will not harm the patient. In addition, homoeopathic and herbal remedies can be used to good effect.

Cabbage poultices, alternating with *clay poultices*, preferably prepared with a decoction of oak bark, have been found excellent for the treatment of goitre. If the cabbage poultices prove too strong in their effect, leave them on only as long as the patient is able to stand them. In time, the period of application may be extended as the patient becomes accustomed to them. Let me add that *kelp* in combination with *Urticalcin* have given good results in post-operative treatment too.

Goitre and Iodised Salt

Many years have passed since Dr Eggenberger of Herisau first advocated the idea of iodising cooking salt and it was partly due to his initiative that iodised salt began to be used in Switzerland. The knowledge that iodine deficiency is responsible for the development of certain forms of goitre also made other countries decide to add iodine to salt. But let us examine whether this blanket arrangement makes sense.

Admittedly, iodised salt benefits those who suffer from thyroid deficiency (hypothyroidism), that is to say, tending to myxoedema, and those people can take it without it doing any harm. However, iodised salt has exactly the opposite effect on people whose thyroid is overactive, with tendency to Graves' disease (hyperthyroidism, exophthalmic goitre). Experience shows that if such people take the slightest amount of iodine they experience palpitations. So these unfortunate people think that something is wrong with their heart and run to the heart specialist to find out what is the trouble. In any case, because of the lack of a warning on the salt package, or their failure to understand the implications of iodised salt, they will have been harmed by what appeared to be a harmless salt.

This example goes to show that not everything that is meant to be good for us is necessarily good or safe for everyone. Indeed, it is incomprehensible how this salt can be offered as something that is wholesome for everyone without distinction. It should be recommended only for those whose complaint has been diagnosed as hypothyroidism, never for people with an excessive secretion of thyroid hormones, who cannot tolerate iodine.

Of course, it is an undisputed fact that a deficiency of iodine plays a part in the development of goitre, for the thyroid needs iodine for its normal function and development. But it can be found in sufficient quantity and an easily assimilated form in the food we eat, provided our diet consists of wholefoods. Such foods cause no disturbances or damage. However, if you throw away the edible skins from fruits, and vegetables, apple cores, the outer layer of cereals, such as bran, in short, anything that is part of the naturally grown whole, then you will sooner or later have a mineral deficiency. This includes, of course, a lack of iodine, which ultimately will encourage the development of goitre. Instead of recommending the use of iodised salt, it would be far better to educate people to give up eating white flour, refined sugar, canned foods and all other products of our 'civilised' way of feeding, and eat only nutritive natural wholefoods.

The introduction of iodised salt was prompted by the observation that people who live by the sea hardly ever suffer from thyroid problems. The iodine of the sea, especially in sea salt, was rightly taken to be the reason for this. Even though the cause of the problem was correctly analysed, the wrong solution was adopted. A manufactured product simply does not have the same effect as a substance found in nature. Sea salt is an excellent source of iodine and everyone in 'goitre areas' should use only natural sea salt for seasoning. (The vast stretches of the mid west in the United States, for example, are commonly known as the 'goitre belt'.) Although sea salt contains iodine, nature has included it in such combinations and proportions that you need never fear any of the disturbances iodised salt brings about. Moreover, when fresh herbs are added to sea salt you get the perfect herbal seasoning salts known as *Herbamare* and *Trocomare*. A great number of people have come to appreciate these salts because of their taste and goodness.

Do you have a garden? If so, there is another way to help prevent

159

or overcome thyroid problems. The answer lies in fertilising your garden. Feed the soil with iodine-rich bone meal and other iodine-containing fertilisers. The plants grown in such soil will be richer in iodine and thereby satisfy the body's requirements, for they are able to process the mineral iodine in such a way that our body can absorb it without any trouble and damaging effects. For the same reason iodine in sea salt can do no harm. It is a biological solution that is therefore much to be preferred to the orthodox medical way of taking iodised salt.

If you have been using iodised salt and are experiencing a faster heart beat, other disturbances of the heart, palpitations and excessive anxiety, you should definitely stop adding it to your food. This salt may be effective, though not always in the desired manner, but one thing is sure, it is by no means harmless, judging by the debates its usage has caused. Iodine is one of those medicines for which one cannot establish general rules. In the same way as one cannot say that alcohol is harmless because most people drink it, nor can one argue that nicotine is not harmful because so many people smoke. It may be true that a number of people do not succumb instantly to the bad effects of alcohol and nicotine, showing visible signs of damage right away; others, however, who happen to be more sensitive by nature do not get off so lightly and soon suffer the usual consequences of these poisons. Does this not convince you of the necessity to observe nature and abide by its rules? In accordance with your sensitivity and inherited disposition, the final effects, one way or the other, cannot be avoided. In fact, one cannot even conclude that if certain things are harmless to one person they are harmless to everyone. So, if you are a sensible person you will consider your own individual nature and reactions and let these be your guide, never making your condition worse by taking potentially hazardous substances. However difficult this may be, if you prefer to remain healthy and active rather than having to suffer unnecessarily, abstinence – the effort to cut out certain things – is no doubt the course of wisdom. After all, your health is at stake!

Iodine
Iodine is a peculiar substance that still puzzles research scientists. Taken in great quantity it is a dangerous poison; on the other hand, the body cannot exist without it. Iodine is one of the elements that the body needs only in minute quantities, a trace element; at the same time, it is of such importance that it may be compared

to the push button that is needed to start and stop a sophisticated piece of machinery. The human body contains approximately 0.05 g of iodine, half of which is found in the muscular system, one-tenth in the skin and a large portion in the endocrine glands, especially the thyroid. Here we find iodine attached to an amino acid, forming the hormone called thyroxine.

It is interesting to note that the so-called iodine level, that is the amount of iodine contained in the blood, is the same for all healthy people, no matter where they live, whether in the mountains, by the sea, in the polar regions or at the equator.

Where Iodine Can Be Found

Iodine is present in rocks, from which it is released when the rocks decompose during the process of weathering. It is dissolved in rain water and is carried to the oceans by the rivers. This, no doubt, is one of the reasons why the ocean is so rich in iodine, as well as other minerals which are carried to it in a similar way. While various other salts remain in the sea, iodine evaporates and is returned to the soil by means of rainfall, dew, fog and snow. Every year hundreds of tons of iodine are thus returned to replenish the soil.

In mountain valleys, however, a deficiency of iodine is often found in the population. The explanation for this may lie in the fact that the water rushes along so rapidly that it carries away large amounts of dissolved iodine instead of restoring it to the soil, as it is able to do in the flatlands.

The Effects of Iodine Deficiency

It is possible to become mentally retarded due to a deficiency of iodine. The thyroid fails to produce enough hormones, and in severe cases myxoedema can result. The deficiency may cause physical and mental lethargy. It can deaden all initiative and result in extreme lack of interest in anything, especially in work or job-related activities, while it may increase the desire to eat. The entire metabolism is affected, normal heart function is slowed down considerably, with low blood pressure following. When sexual potency is also low or lacking entirely, liveliness and emotional feelings will be missing. It is not infrequent to observe a miraculous change in a patient if he is given iodine in the form of seaweed tablets, for example, *Kelpasan*, and if he is put on a natural whole-food diet.

The formation of goitre is in almost every case connected with an iodine imbalance. This subject has been discussed in great detail in the preceding sections (see pages 156–60) and the reader is advised to refer to these for further information.

Iodine is also indirectly responsible for obesity. The thyroid and sex glands work together and if an obese person is given iodine as contained in plants, for example, *kelp tablets*, the thyroid steps up its hormone production. This, in turn, activates the entire metabolism. The gonads become more active and, as a result, the deposits of body fat decrease.

You can see that iodine is more important than one might think, because this mysterious element, even though present in minute traces, is responsible for operating the 'gears' of our body, not unlike the illustration in the proverb, 'Big oaks from little acorns grow.'

Although the effect of *watercress* is less marked than that of seaweed, nevertheless it contains a modest amount of iodine and can thus be of good service to the thyroid. Other excellent remedies are the *Topinambur* tincture *Helianthus tub.* and homoeopathic *Graphitis 6x*.

Menstrual Problems
Excessive and insufficient bleeding can both be a source of great discomfort. A heavy menstrual flow means an unnecessary loss of blood, which may even lead to a slight case of anaemia. It is important that women who suffer from this condition make sure that they do not engage in any strenuous physical activity beginning a few days prior to the period. This may be especially difficult for women who have to do physical work, because it is not easy to find someone to help and the work still has to be done.

In these circumstances, *Tormentavena* has proven to be a simple, reliable, natural remedy. It is a combination of fresh tormentil root and the juice of the green flowering oat plant. This remedy also has a tonic effect on the nerves. *Sherpherd's purse tincture (Bursa pastoris)* is also very helpful.

A very light flow of blood can cause an emotional upset. *Sea kelp* from the Pacific Ocean is very beneficial in cases of this sort because of its potassium iodide content. Generally, taking one kelp tablet in the morning and at noon suffices to normalise the flow. Do not take in the evening and continue only until the period is regular again. However, women suffering from hyperthyroidism must take kelp only in homoeopathic doses. Women who have been suffering for some time, or frequently, from the discomforts of insufficient menstrual flow should also take a preparation that stimulates blood circulation, for example *Aesculaforce*. In addition, to cure the disorder, another preparation, *Ovarium 3x*, is necessary in order to influence the ovaries and establish a regular period.

Take regular *sitz baths* (hip baths) to which an infusion of thyme or camomile has been added, to complement the treatment with the above-mentioned botanic medicines. The baths help to normalise the functions so important to women. Since the cure of menstrual malfunction goes hand in hand with the relief of emotional depression, every woman in need will be glad to follow the advice given.

Menopausal Problems

During the menopause practically every women experiences hot flushes and other distressing symptoms to a greater or lesser degree. At times a woman may be affected so severely that her nerves and emotions become totally upset, and any relief is always welcome. It is important to take even better care of the body than usual during the changes of life. Excellent benefits are obtained by *exercising* regularly out-of-doors; the importance of activities such as walking and hiking and the practice of taking deep breaths of fresh air cannot be emphasised enough and will bring about a striking improvement.

Physical therapy may also contribute to improving the condition. For example, daily *brush massages* and twice weekly *sitz baths* (hip baths) with a decoction of hay flowers or lady's mantle added to the water are recommended. Extreme emotional depression may be relieved through *Kuhne's cold water treatment* (see pages 436–8). As with menstrual problems, physical exertion as well as occupational stress should be avoided at all costs. In addition, learn to do without coffee, tea and alcoholic beverages, as it is indeed best to leave them alone altogether during the menopause.

These precautionary measures will make it easier to sleep at night and improve the patient's general health. The following remedies help to give relief and eliminate the symptoms causing discomfort: *Salvia, Ovarium 3x, Ignatia plus Sepia 6x, and Aconitum 10x*. Sounder and more restful sleep influences the mind and nerves, restoring emotional balance to people of a normally happy disposition and thus relieving constant depression and moods.

It is certainly good to know that the discomfort and upsets experienced during the menopause can be alleviated in such simple ways. For this reason, now you are acquainted with the various remedies and treatments available, use them to the full and enjoy better general health.

The Kidneys

If we were to compare our body to a modern chemical plant, the air-conditioning unit responsible for getting rid of poisonous exhaust fumes would correspond to our lungs. In the case of a prolonged breakdown of such an air-purification unit, the workers would die from poisons released into the air. The result would be just as tragic if our lungs stopped functioning. Furthermore, in order to assure the workers' well-being, it is of utmost importance to get rid of the poisonous solid waste materials too. In the body this is accomplished by the kidneys, with some help from the liver. If the kidneys were to stop operating for only two days, thus causing a retention of metabolic toxins, uraemia would set in. The accumulation of waste products, normally excreted in the urine, would cause metabolic poisoning.

This can be observed in cases of an enlarged prostate, hypertrophy of the prostate. If the enlarged prostate blocks the urethra completely – a not uncommon occurrence in older men – every effort should be made to correct the obstruction within forty-eight hours. This can be done with the help of *hot herbal steam baths* or by means of a *catheter*, a rather uncomfortable treatment. If immediate attention is not given, uraemia may develop, as already mentioned, and endanger the patient's life.

Kidney stones may bring about the same condition, that is, when they block the ureter. In such cases, prolonged *hot baths* are very beneficial. They should be accompanied by a light underwater *massage* of the kidney and bladder areas. To prevent the formation of kidney stones *madder root (Rubia tinctorum)* is still the best remedy. (For further advice on treating kidney stones, see pages 167–70).

Noteworthy Characteristics of the Kidney Structure

The structure of the kidneys is truly marvellous. All design problems have been solved with such perfection that the ancient anatomists called the kidney a '*viscus elegantissimum*', meaning 'most elegant organ'. The kidney is really a complicated filtration plant consisting of about a million cup-shaped individual filters. Each of these filters is surrounded by a two-walled capsule and is separated by small conducting tubes which supply blood and filter out the urine simultaneously. Every day about 1.7 litres (about 3 pints) of this diluted filtrate are transported to the bladder by way of the ureter and then expelled. The remainder is reabsorbed by the bloodstream so that the entire activity takes care of about 175 litres (about 38.5 gallons) of filtrate in one day.

The human kidney is bean-shaped. The filtering units are located in the outermost layer, the cortex. The inner structures form the medulla, consisting of the collecting tubules. The size of the tubules increases towards the inside; the large vessels and the beginning of the ureter are inside the pelvis of the kidney which, by the way, has nothing to do with the basin-shaped cavity formed by the bones in the hip region.

Harmful Influences

Aside from the heart and the liver, no other organ suffers more from the consequences of our modern life-style and refined foods than the kidneys. In my practice I have been able to observe time and again the extent of the damage white sugar has done to them. Often a kidney patient has been relieved of his pains simply by abstaining from all foods containing sugar. Just to prove the point, the patient would again be given sugar on a test basis and, sure enough, the pains would return. However, this holds true only for products made with refined sugar, whereas natural sugars as contained in dried grapes (for example raisins), figs, bananas and other fruits never cause any such complications.

It is also generally known that the kidneys can be rendered a great service and protected if the intake of salt is reduced to a minimum. Bacterial poisons, likewise, have a detrimental effect on them. That is why infectious diseases such as measles, scarlet fever, diphtheria, tonsillitis and others, always have an adverse effect. Permanent damage can be prevented if proper care is taken to cure these diseases fully, and by making sure that the kidneys function properly during and after an illness. This is best done by taking the excellent plant extract of *Solidago*, as contained in *Nephrosolid*, a remedy that should be kept in every home.

Very dangerous for the kidneys are metallic poisons such as lead. This is why painters and decorators, as well as operators of hot-metal printing machines, and compositors, traditionally risked kidney problems unless precautions were taken (although these risks have since diminished as technology has advanced).

Moreover, the kidneys will function better if we protect them from getting cold. For example, when hot weather makes us feel like a cold drink, we should make it a habit to sip slowly instead of gulping it down. If you bathe in cold water or feel cold after having been caught in the rain, for example, you should immediately restore the body's proper temperature balance by taking a bath or a shower, or by applying warm water packs or any other warm water therapy. Otherwise, the cold shock to the kidneys may have adverse effects.

How to Detect Kidney Disorders
Close attention should be paid to the kidneys because kidney problems do not always manifest themselves immediately by acute pain. If the amount of water passed is less than normal over a period of time, we should have a urine analysis made. This is also indicated if the colour of the urine changes and for some time is either too dark or too light, almost colourless. If we notice the presence of blood, cloudiness, or any other residue in the urine, this is also a cause for concern. A sediment of tiny crystals indicates that the person has a tendency to develop kidney stones or gravel. Do not wait for pain or a colic before doing something about it. Seek treatment at once.

If we examine the urine sediments under a microscope, we will be amazed at the diversity of the crystalline formations nature is able to produce even in the urine. All sorts of prismatic forms and bundles of needle-like crystals can be seen. They are in fact the crystallised forms of uric acid, sulphuric acid and benzoic acid. The amino acid leucine crystal is especially interesting, forming a bundle of 'needles' more compact than a snowflake.

Such observations turn an inspection of the uric sediments into a fascinating and meaningful study. Indeed, the trained expert can draw valuable conclusions from the pictures revealed by the microscope during a urine analysis. It is even possible to find out whether the patient has adhered to a prescribed diet. For example, if numerous sulphuric crystals are present, it is evident that the patient has eaten foods containing sulphur, such as eggs, beans, peas, lentils and radishes, even though he may have been instructed not to do so. If the test shows any oxalic acid crystals, the patient has been eating spinach, rhubarb, lettuce or sauerkraut. If a large number of creatinine crystals are in evidence, the patient obviously did not abstain from eating meat.

Thus, an analysis of the urine can be most informative, often more than even some doctors may think possible. We may learn something about metabolic disorders, certain organic diseases or other functional disorders.

Having been made aware of the value of a urine test, we should not consider it extravagant to have a comprehensive examination at least once a year. On several occasions I have been able to detect diabetes through a urine test. In these cases the patients have complained for years about tiredness and thirst but no one had ever linked these symptoms with diabetes. The urine analysis, however, proved it beyond a doubt.

In view of the demands of today's ever-increasing pace of life, it is of paramount importance to care for our body at least as much as we look after our car. We all understand that it is more economical to rectify a problem with the car when it first shows up, before a major repair job becomes necessary through sheer neglect. Does our body not deserve the same consideration? Take, for example, our kidneys and think of the great demands they are subjected to; much pain and discomfort can be avoided later if prompt attention and constant care are given them.

Kidney Colic
Many people have kidney stones without being aware of the fact. The same goes for gallstones. Their presence is only noticed when the stones enter the ureter (or in the case of gallstones, the bile duct) and can move neither forward nor backward.

When a kidney stone becomes stuck in the ureter the resulting pain is so excruciating that the patient may end up in a state of delirium. It is not unusual for him to lose all control, knocking into things around him, screaming in agony and, of course, causing great concern to those around him. The pain can last for hours and there is great danger if the proper treatment is not given.

The patient must be placed in a *hot bath* and with light, careful *massage*, the stone must be made to move from the ureter into the bladder. The hot water itself will make the patient feel more comfortable. Should the heart start to give trouble or if he suffers from hyperthyroidism (exophthalmic goitre), he must also be assisted with cold compresses. The best way to do this is to apply a 'heart tube'. Place a tube in a circle around the heart area and let cold water flow through it. This will cool the heart down and bring relief. If necessary, put cold compresses on the wrists and forehead, renewing them frequently to keep them cold. With this treatment the patient should be able to remain in the hot bath for half an hour without fainting.

Internal treatment should also start at the onset of a colic. *Magnesium phos. 6x* and *Atropinum sulph. 4x* should be given. If the patient brings everything up, then the remedies must be given by means of an enema.

If, in spite of all precautions, the patient loses consciousness anyway, there is no need to panic as the spell will pass off without doing any harm, and perforation can be prevented.

Keep the bath hot by adding hot water; it should last half an hour, the patient being massaged all the while and the cold compresses being renewed. After the bath apply hot packs and give frequent herbal enemas. If blood comes instead of urine, this means that the stone has become stuck in the ureter and has damaged it. At this stage, it would be beneficial to give *Solidago* by enema in order to stimulate the kidneys, for if he has a severe attack, the patient will usually be unable to retain anything given by mouth. Continue the packs and enemas for half an hour and then follow up with another hot bath, with massage and compresses.

This treatment is to be repeated, in alternation, for half an hour each time. As soon as the stone begins to move toward the bladder the pain will move from the back to the front and then slowly diminish. The moment the stone enters the bladder the patient will be more or less free from pain. It may take several hours to accomplish this, but once achieved, the patient can then lie quietly and rest without any further danger. If he is thirsty, give him diluted *Molkosan* (concentrated whey) to sip as this reduces the internal heat and replaces the liquids lost by perspiration in the bath. It will also provide the liquid essential to eliminate any further toxins that are still in the system. Additionally, give the patient plenty of *knotgrass (Polygonum aviculare) tea* because this too helps to dissolve the stones.

However, this is not yet the end of treatment. A thorough followup cure, including *sitz baths* and *massage* is necessary, as the stone must not be allowed to remain in the bladder where it could give rise to irritation and bleeding.

Taking everything into account, this is still a simple method of treatment and will avert a ureter blockage with its serious consequences or even the need for an operation. It is clearly worthwhile, because the patient will recover astonishingly fast after the cure, whereas an operation can often have complications, requiring a great deal of after-care. However, should the size of the stone prevent its elimination through the natural, physical therapy outlined above, it is not too late to resort to an operation. I would add, however, that there is very rarely a need for this. In most cases it will be possible to effect a successful cure if the treatment is given with great care and thoroughness. Of course, stones can also be gradually dissolved by taking natural remedies. *Rubiaforce*, made from the madder root, is such a remedy, and one that has been tested and proven in practice. If taken over a longer period of time, Rubiaforce will dissolve even larger stones, especially if the patient also drinks a lot of goldenrod tea.

TREATMENT WITH RUBIAFORCE
Many patients whose kidney stones were dissolved by *Rubia tinctorum* (madder root) have attested to its excellent therapeutic effect. In addition to taking this remedy, however, it is most important that the patient avoids catching cold and becoming exhausted. To ensure its success, a *special diet* should be followed during and after the treatment. The patient must avoid all denatured or refined foods containing white sugar and white, bleached flour. Nor should he use salt or any sharp condiments in the food. Furthermore, the kidney patient should not eat Brussels sprouts, spinach, asparagus, rhubarb or, especially, pork, luncheon meat and other cold meats. Since vitamin A deficiency promotes the formation of gravel and stones in the kidneys, it must be counteracted by eating plenty of carrot salad and drinking carrot juice. If bleeding is noticed in the urine, no meat should be eaten, the only animal protein allowable being soft white cheese (cottage cheese or quark). For the best results the patient should stick to a diet of brown rice, vegetables and raw salads.

Physical therapy is also beneficial. For about half an hour each night a hot and moist *compress* made with hay flowers and camomile should be applied to the kidney area. Hot *sitz baths* will also help. If the stones should cause bleeding, the patient should take *Millefolium, Hamamelis virg., Echinaforce, Tormentavena and Cantharis 6x.*

While carrying out these recommendations take the *Rubiaforce* treatment. Drink less liquid when taking Rubiaforce tablets. After completing one box of tablets wait a week before starting on another, but during this interval drink as much liquid as possible in order to thoroughly flush out the kidneys and prevent the formation of new gravel or stones. At the end of the week begin to take another box of Rubiaforce tablets; drink limited amounts of a weak *kidney tea* with *Nephrosolid.* Follow up with a further week without medication but drinking plenty, as before. The treatment is completed after the third week on tablets and a further week when, again, plenty of liquids are consumed.

Even though the stones will have disappeared after this treatment, it would be wise to repeat it in a shortened form every three months, just to be on the safe side. However, the diet must be watched all the time. If available, a tea made from *Chanca piedra*, a plant found in the tropical jungles of Peru, will enhance the effectiveness of the Rubiaforce treatment and can be taken in conjunction with it.

The Urinary Bladder

The urinary bladder is a hollow organ made up of muscle fibres and lined with mucous membrane. Ordinarily, the bladder has the capacity to hold about 750 ml (almost a quart) of fluid. Since the fibre cells are elastic, like rubber, the bladder is able to expand greatly without suffering any damage. According to the amount of fluid collected, pressure is exerted on the walls of the bladder and, as it mounts, this triggers the feeling of needing to pass water. However, the amount of fluid present in the bladder is not the only force causing the urge for elimination. External influences such as exposure to cold produce it too. Having cold feet or stepping barefoot onto cold tiles or a cement floor cause a contraction of the bladder wall and a strong need to pass water, even if the bladder is only partially filled. A bladder infection creates the same urge, but often the patient is able to produce only a few drops of water while suffering pain and discomfort. The bladder is one of the body's most sensitive organs, and one that reacts to physical as well as emotional stimuli in an unusually strong way.

Inflammation of the Bladder (Cystitis)

Generally, inflammation of the bladder, or cystitis, is a result of a cold. 'Whatever results from a cold can only be taken away through heat' is an ancient law of natural therapy. Since it also applies to the bladder, *hot herbal packs, compresses* and prolonged *sitz baths* are very successful aids in treating cystitis. The water used to prepare a compress should be as hot as the hands can bear when wringing out the cloth. The sitz bath should have a temperature of 37–38 °C (98–99 °F) in order not to cause any congestion. This should be carefully observed, particularly if the patient has high blood pressure or a weak heart. The sitz bath should be continued for half an hour, with hot water being added from time to time to maintain a constant temperature.

Certain bacteria such as staphylococcus, streptococcus and sometimes colibacillus can often be responsible for bladder infections. In rare cases the bladder may be affected by tuberculosis, a condition more likely to occur if the patient already has a kidney tuberculosis, which permits the bacillus to enter the bladder through the kidney and manifest itself at the slightest irritation. Chronic cases of cystitis may be connected with any of the above-mentioned causes and would need special treatment.

The symptoms of cystitis are pain or burning sensations on passing urine. Due to the infection and irritation a strong urge to pass water persists. The urine generally contains some red and white blood cells, is cloudy and forms a white, often slimy sediment when left standing.

ADDITIONAL TREATMENT

The treatment with warm wet packs can be greatly supported by the use of several biological remedies. One of the best medicines with which to counteract any kind of inflammation is *Echinaforce*. Doses of 5–10 drops should be taken every hour. Also, *Nephrosolid* has healing properties and stimulates the kidneys; *Cantharis 4x* takes away the unpleasant irritation and burning sensation experienced when passing urine and *Usneasan* contains natural antibiotic substances and fights off harmful bacteria. Meanwhile, it is advisable to stay in bed until the inflammation has completely subsided.

If at the same time the urethra (the duct through which the urine passes) is narrowed, or an enlargement of the prostate gland or bladder stones exist, the treatment must be adapted accordingly and some other remedies added. In cases where the patient is unable to control urination due to a weakness of the sphincter muscle, *Cystoforce Bladder Drops* should be taken additionally. The same drops are usually excellent for the treatment of enuresis in children too. *Galeopsis, Sabal 1x* and a tea blend made up of *marigold, yarrow and St John's wort* are also recommended.

Bed-Wetting (Enuresis)

Bed-wetting is a real problem that affects mother and child alike. Even though it may be the result of some emotional upset or nervous tension, certain remedies, physical therapy and a bland diet may greatly assist the organism and even help to overcome the emotional problems as well.

Bed-wetting in normal older children, if they do not have a cold or some other physical complaint or weakness, can generally be attributed to a psychological conflict. It can be a very unpleasant

171

home atmosphere, or the child may have simply been spoiled by indulgent parents.

What steps should be taken to help? First, create a happy environment in the home, a pleasant relationship between parents and children. The home should be free from anxiety and the accelerated pace of modern life. It should then not be too difficult to isolate the cause of the emotional problem. Empathy and patience on the part of both mother and father will help reveal it. There may be a variety of reasons, such as fear, jealousy, ambition, over-exertion, or exciting television programmes that the parents allow the children to watch until late at night, or some other emotional upset.

Being a bed-wetter is always upsetting for the healthy, intelligent child, as well as for the handicapped one. Hence, no effort should be spared to cure the child's problem. A child whose health leaves much to be desired and who may not be so quick mentally has enough to put up with and will feel even more helpless when nothing seems to go right. Bed-wetting also means an added burden to a child suffering from cerebral palsy. So there are sufficient reasons to make use of all available natural remedies to strengthen the bladder and kidneys. In addition to these, the child must be given biological calcium and silica, but only from plants.

In order to treat the various factors involved in bed-wetting, the following remedies are recommended: *kidney tea, Cystoforce Bladder Drops, Galeopsis, Usneasan and Urticalcin.* The treatment must be supported by an appropriate *diet*, low in salt and fat. The diet should consist of brown rice and millet, together with vegetables and salads. At the same time a glass of fresh carrot juice should be taken daily. As with all types of liquid, it should be sipped slowly and well insalivated. Train the child to chew well so that the food becomes properly mixed with saliva so as to promote good digestion. No fluids should be given to the child after 4 p.m.

Considerable improvement can be brought about in time through physical therapy. A warm and moist *compress of hay flowers* placed daily on the lower abdomen stimulates the blood circulation of the urinary organs. From time to time the child should be given a *sitz bath* with a decoction of hay flowers or horsetail added to the water. But make sure that the child does not start shivering or even get cold. His whole body should be kept warm by covering the tub with large towels, protecting the parts of the body that are not under the water, or by heating the bathroom.

Also take care that the child does not get cold feet or feel chilled

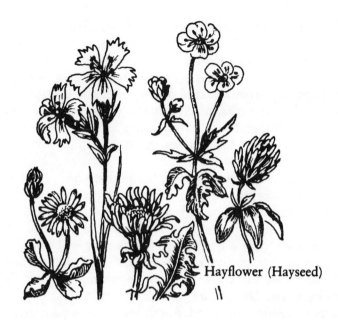

Hayflower (Hayseed)

or cold. For this reason see to it that he has adequate footwear, warm socks and warm clothing to protect his body in cold weather. Moreover, make sure that he gets plenty of exercise out-of-doors, as this will stimulate the circulation and make him feel comfortable and warm. Take him on hikes or walks, possibly through a forest or wood, and encourage him to breathe deeply in the aromatic air. This will do much to build him up.

At all times the child should grow up in an atmosphere of soothing tranquillity since it will help him to relax. A happy home is the main factor that contributes to his speedy recovery; it induces a sense of balance by helping to overcome the emotions that have been a basic cause of the problem. Where there is happiness there is no room for tantrums, a defiant spirit, sullenness or depression. Engrossed as we often are in our daily routine, we tend to forget how much health, in particular the health of a child who is weak for some reason, depends on the feeling of being wanted and loved in an environment of calmness and harmony.

Prostate Trouble
It is not always possible to cure prostate problems, in fact, there are cases, especially with cancer of the prostate, where treatment

173

is difficult and sometimes in vain. Operating is not always the answer either, and if it can be prevented, so much the better. In cases of benign enlargement of the prostate good results have been achieved with *Prostasan*, a preparation containing *Sabal, Staphisagria, Populus, Echinacea* and *Solidago*, in conjunction with *herbal steam baths*. However, when urination has become easy again, do not take it for granted that you are now rid of your problem. Prostate conditions are seldom cured so completely that they do not recur sooner or later.

The trouble may be alleviated, but perhaps not completely cured. And do not forget, you do not get any younger either. If the enlarged prostate can be softened and brought back to its normal size, the passing of urine will once more be painless; however, it is quite likely that a degree of enlargement will remain. A slight cold, a cold beer, or anything in the nature of a temporary disturbance can cause the gland to swell somewhat, so that the trouble flares up again. Once more you may resort to steam baths and the remedies already mentioned. But to avoid disappointment you must be aware that although the treatment will probably bring you relief, it may not actually eliminate the possibility of relapses. As a matter of fact, you would fare better if you were to continue to take the remedies after the attack has subsided, reducing the quantity to half or a third of the usual dose. In this way the gland continues to be favourably influenced and the problem is kept in check, so to speak.

Prostate trouble is not unlike hardening of the arteries in that it is a condition brought on by the aging of the body and since this process is unavoidable you must remember that removing the problem once does not mean that it cannot crop up again. By using the appropriate remedies and precautions you can support nature in its own healing efforts and prevent the trouble from recurring as far as is possible.

Inflammation of the Testicles (Orchitis)

Inflammation of the testicles (orchitis) is a fairly prevalent condition yet its treatment tends to be neglected because embarrassment makes the patient reluctant to see a doctor. For this reason I would like to explain the causes and treatment of this inflammation. To begin with, never ignore this condition hoping it may correct itself. By simply trying to forget the inflammation and not caring for it properly you may invite infertility later, which can result in serious psychological problems, especially for younger men.

Orchitis is generally caused by germs that are carried in the bloodstream. They need not be of the venereal type, however; in fact, tuberculosis of another organ could be responsible for orchitis. A complication of mumps or some other infectious disease may also be the cause and the resulting inflammation can be painfully awkward for young men. Obviously, then, the correct treatment of the basic problem is called for.

For internal use, massive doses of *Echinaforce* have proved successful in cases like this. Take 10–20 drops every hour. During the night, apply a *mudpack* to the inflamed area. In order to increase its healing power and to keep the paste from drying out and breaking up, mix it with *horsetail tea* and a tablespoon of *St John's wort oil*. A helpful alternative is a poultice made from crushed *cabbage leaves*. However, if the cabbage increases the soreness, stop using it and revert to the mudpacks, which are always soothing. Finally it is important to keep the bowels open. These suggestions will work if you follow them conscientiously.

Skin Disorders

Eczema – and Other Skin Eruptions
In treating eczema it is of primary importance to discover the cause of the disease. It is usually to be found in faulty metabolism or an allergy to certain foods or other irritants. Naturally, these factors will have to be taken into consideration. In many cases a complete change of diet may be necessary. Without question, the bowels and kidneys should be stimulated so as to enable them to function adequately. Then we must find out if it is a chronic or acute skin eruption. External irritation, such as that occasioned by certain occupations, can play a part in the development of such skin diseases, but frequently it may be a hereditary condition.

For external treatment *Molkosan* (concentrated whey) has always given the best results. Molkosan is a biological lactic acid preparation which destroys harmful bacteria, stimulates the circulation and regenerates the skin by virtue of the minerals and enzymes it contains. As a rule, however, Molkosan alone is not sufficient, especially when treating psoriasis. It is then usually necessary to also powder the skin with a biological calcium preparation. For the best results use a calcium complex with *Urtica* (*Urticalcin*) in powder form. The third essential remedy is a lanolin cream, *Bioforce Cream*, which contains St John's wort oil, being ideally suited for this purpose. The complete external treatment for eczematous skin is therefore as follows:

In the morning swab the affected parts with undiluted Molkosan. If it is too strong and makes the sore places smart or burn excessively, dilute with a little boiled or distilled water. After this, powder the affected areas with Urticalcin powder. Make sure that it gets well into the cracks and scales. In the evening, dab the area once more with Molkosan, but instead of then using the powder, rub the affected parts with a little Bioforce Cream. For a change occasionally use *St John's wort oil* on its own. Repeat these applications daily.

Any skin eruption requires internal as well as external treatment; therefore the following advice is also useful for skin disorders other than eczema, particularly psoriasis. It is important to improve the condition of the blood and the lymph. First of all take a kidney remedy, either *Solidago virgaurea* (goldenrod drops) or *Nephrosolid* in daily alternation with *Violaforce* (heartsease drops). Secondly, take *Biocarottin* as a liver remedy and vitamin supplement. And thirdly, as a specific treatment, there is the *'formic acid therapy'*. This acid has to be given in form of injections, because if taken orally, it is partially transformed into carbonic acid on contact with the gastric secretions. The best results are obtained by giving hypodermic injections in the sixth and twelfth decimal potency, in alternation. During the first two weeks an injection should be given every third day, and then once every fourteen days, till the cure is complete.

Even the most difficult case will yield to this treatment, providing the proper diet is maintained and very little salt and protein is ingested. When it comes to skin disorders, salt is a poison and the metabolic toxins resulting from an excess intake of animal protein aggravate these diseases in general and psoriasis in particular. Further advice on diet is given on pages 180-1. If there is a discharge of pus from the eruption, *Hepar sulph. 4x* should be taken. If the trouble is connected with an acid condition of the body or if there is an oozing, burning, blistering rash with painful itching, then *Rhus tox. 4x* to *6x* will be the best remedy. *Arsenicum alb. 4x* to *6x* is good for both dry and oozing eruptions which burn and irritate especially by night. In cases of chronic eruptions the homoeopathic sulphur remedies *Sulphur 6x* and *Sulphur iod. 4x* to *6x* have proven their worth, particularly if the eruption is of a scrofulous nature. Finally, if the disease is the result of a tendency to rheumatism or gout, then *Calcarea carb. 4x* alternated with *Lycopodium 6x* would be indicated.

Whatever the cause, it is useful to add a calcium preparation which incorporates nettles, for example Urticalcin, to the other medication. And do not forget that Violaforce (heartsease drops) is an especially effective remedy for skin disorders.

When a Tendency to Eczema Runs in the Family

Cradle cap (*Crusta lactea*), commonly found in young infants, is often associated with a genetic predisposition to eczema and other skin disorders, passed on from one or other of the parents. Experience has shown that if cradle cap is not properly treated the child may become very susceptible to infections due to low resistance. For example, let us consider such a child suffering from whooping cough, which in turn is suppressed or wrongly treated. For this reason the bacterial toxins are not completely eliminated and it is likely that the child's heart will be affected or he will develop asthma, two conditions that are very difficult to put right.

Any kind of skin disorder, including cradle cap, must therefore receive proper treatment from the outset in order to effect a complete cure. This is the reason why I aim to direct attention in my books to combatting skin diseases by means of an appropriate treatment of the liver. The first step in this direction is a low-salt, or better still, salt-free liver diet as described in my book *The Liver, the Regulator of Your Health*.

IMPORTANT RULES FOR NUTRITION AND RELIABLE NATURAL REMEDIES

If we are careful in our choice of protein we can count on rapid success. Lactoprotein, as found in soft white cheese (quark), buttermilk and sour milk, is a good form of protein to take when skin disorders have to be treated. It is preferable to mix in finely grated horseradish, because fresh horseradish has antibiotic properties. People suffering from a skin disorder often cannot tolerate full-cream milk and should therefore abstain from it. On the other hand, they can take protein as contained in almond milk or soya milk. However, stay away from eggs, especially boiled eggs, and egg dishes, which cause strong reactions in persons suffering from eczema and similar skin disorders. The same holds true for all kinds of cheese with the exception of curds, cottage cheese, quark and most soft white cheeses made from skimmed milk, if they cause no upset.

The recommended diet consists basically of *brown rice* and foods rich in *calcium*. White cabbage salad and raw sauerkraut are among the vegetables that should be eaten regularly. Kohlrabi leaves (turnip cabbage) also have a high calcium content and should always be eaten, not thrown away.

Urticalcin, a proven biological calcium complex, makes the assimilation of calcium from food much easier and helps to prevent deficiency. Medical advisers sometimes prescribe calcium injections, which in theory may seem the correct way to supply the patient with sufficient calcium. I do not, however, recommend these, since I believe that the only healthy way of supplying the body with sufficient amounts of calcium is by eating vegetables that are rich in calcium, for example white cabbage and carrots.

When suffering from eczema it is important to keep off sweets of any kind. White sugar is harmful and may even create allergic reactions in some people. White flour, although not quite so drastic in its effect, should also be avoided. It is recommended for therapeutic reasons to confine one's diet to wholegrain or wholemeal products and wholefoods.

A kidney remedy, such as *Nephrosolid*, and *kidney tea* should be taken to stimulate the kidneys. Additionally it is recommended to drink more liquids than you are accustomed to, preferably natural fruit juices, for example bilberry or blueberry juice, blackberry juice and grapefruit juice. If you wish you may dilute these juices with mineral water, either the still kind or one with only slight natural fizziness.

Detailed recommendations on the appropriate remedies for eczematous conditions were given on pages 12–13. However, it is useful here to summarise the most important ones with a general application.

We have learned from experience that the most effective natural remedy for eczema, including cradle cap, is *Violaforce*, an extract from the wild pansy. *Urticalcin* should always be given too. This biological calcium preparation helps to heal the lesions when used as a powder. *Molkosan* and *Echinaforce* have the same effect and should definitely be incorporated in the treatment, not only externally but also internally. Eczema is generally associated with defective sebaceous glands and it is necessary to supply the skin with sufficient oil. *St John's wort oil* or *Bioforce Cream*, a lanolin cream, will accomplish this purpose very well.

When treating skin problems, as with most other diseases, it is important that emotional upsets and difficulties be dealt with promptly and in the right way, otherwise they tend to aggravate the condition. That is why I have devoted a whole section in this book to 'Happiness Means Health'. Special attention has been given to the same question in my book about the liver, since this organ is notably sensitive to emotional influences.

Knowing how to deal with your illness is a step in the right direction, as it is clearly important to maintain mental balance in approaching any problem. One must be determined to elect for natural treatment rather than chemical therapy. By adhering strictly to a natural diet you can be sure you are on the right track. To complete the cure, it is absolutely necessary to carry out the treatment for six months to a year. The treatment need not be expensive since it is mainly a question of correcting one's dietary habits. Adverse reactions and side effects are usually minor or do not crop up at all if the treatment is undertaken correctly.

In summary, I would like to stress that in cases of eczematous skin disorders the liver needs special attention and care. The same applies to the kidneys, which must be protected from exposure to damp and cold. Furthermore, take care that the skin does not come into contact with strong detergents, floor wax and other products containing turpentine. When the kidneys and liver are functioning properly the strain is taken away from the skin and the unpleasant, often unbearable, itching will subside. At the same time the lesions will also disappear.

For those who follow my suggestions conscientiously an eventual cure is certain, but those who think that drugs and chemicals alone will suffice may go for years without finding any relief. The more stubborn the case, the more patience is needed to obtain satisfactory results.

Psoriasis
This is one of the skin diseases which is extremely difficult to heal. One successful treatment, however, is with *Formic Acid 30x* and an external application of *graphite* powder. Although orthodox doctors consider psoriasis incurable, natural therapy, especially with the help of homoeopathy, can claim a considerable number of cures. I remember the case of one girl who was almost completely covered in scaly patches, with the exception of a few small areas on her body. Anyone afflicted with this disease knows what

179

a terrible strain it is on the nerves. Once the awful irritation starts up very few patients can bear it without scratching themselves until they bleed. It was just like that with this unfortunate girl, who was suffering from one of the worst cases I had ever seen. Often, by the morning she had scratched herself to such an extent that she was bleeding under the breast, on the legs and on the stomach. After three months of intensive treatment the girl was cured, although two follow-up treatments were later necessary to cope with a few minor relapses. Despite having been treated before, her skin was not so badly damaged that it could not be healed. For some patients who have undergone an extensive tar and sulphur treatment and have perhaps even used grey mercury ointment, achieving a cure can be much more difficult.

The chances of healing the disease are also very poor if the patient has been given radiation treatment, and I would warn patients never to resort to this particular therapy.

Skin eruptions, including psoriasis, are generally curable if the patient perseveres with the treatment until the disease is completely healed. However, if you handle skin irritants, such as terpenes, turpentine, turpentine floor wax or other strong turpentine products, the stimulus can provoke a relapse.

Psoriasis is not infectious and cannot be spread from one person to another. It is, however, possible to pass it on to one's children through the genes. For this reason such children should be given prophylactic treatment. Make sure that they have plenty of calcium and vitamins in their diet and take proper care of their skin. For further advice on treatment follow the recommendations outlined in the section on eczema.

RAW FOOD DIET FOR THE TREATMENT OF PSORIASIS
Proof of the regenerative power a raw food diet has on psoriasis is given in the following interesting letter from a patient. She writes:

'Just now I am in B., where I am on a strict raw food diet. For 23 years I have suffered from psoriasis and have had all kinds of treatments; but so far, all have been without success. After arriving here I had to fast for seven days, then I was put on fruit juices; next I was given fruits, nuts and corn bread. For several weeks now I have been eating raw salads and potatoes for lunch, and fruit morning and evening. I feel quite well and I am glad to say that the eruptions have gone. True, now and again the sun brings an occasional blemish to the surface, but it never gets big and disappears within a day or two. This does tell me, however, that

I am not yet completely cured and that I must continue the treatment. It does not really worry me, though, for I enjoy the fruit and salads. I can't quite put into words what it means to me to know that I am on the way to recovery and that I shall have the strength to work and be useful again. I only know that I shall be eternally grateful.'

The reply to her letter read as follows:

'I am truly glad and rejoice with you, knowing that with a simple raw food diet you have been able to overcome psoriasis. Now we must achieve a complete cure and you need to be patient for a little while longer. The raw food diet has stimulated the various body functions, including that of the kidneys, and has given the body sufficient vitamins and nutritive salts. This proves that psoriasis is associated with one's diet and that the function or malfunction of the organs has much to do with its development. Psoriasis is usually given external treatment only, and in various clinics this receives primary attention, which is fundamentally incorrect. In this regard orthodox doctors are, unfortunately, quite wrong in their opinion and approach. Psoriasis, one of the worst skin diseases, is not merely a visible problem, for which reason external treatment should be of secondary consideration. Of course, it is important to keep the skin clean, supply it with sufficient oil and disinfect it properly so that further complications are avoided. Nevertheless, internal treatment is far more significant, and your letter is proof of this. If you wish to improve your health still further, then let me recommend kidney tea as well as goldenrod (*Solidago*) and sufficient calcium. These remedies will be of great benefit to you.'

Nettle Rash (Urticaria)
Nettle rash, also known as urticaria, is a peculiar and very unpleasant condition. Although easily diagnosed, the actual cause is another matter. The itching variety of urticaria is accompanied by small pink eruptions on the skin. Identifying the cause of the complaint is often difficult. As a rule, it is recognised that a sensitivity to certain substances or foods is responsible for nettle rash, the kind of hypersensitivity generally referred to as an allergy. Where such a tendency exists, certain foods, such as strawberries, fish, cheese, eggs, seafood, pork and salami may be the allergens that cause such a reaction. There could also be a reaction to certain medications, even if these are biological preparations such as arnica, to cite just one.

181

What can you do if you are susceptible to attacks of urticaria? The first and obvious thing to do is to avoid every agent that could be a possible cause. Your careful observation over a fairly long period may be necessary to determine exactly what is causing the allergy. Sometimes the sensitivity may be hereditary, which unfortunately makes it all the more difficult to overcome. Still, it is possible to train the body to slowly get used to the agents that have been causing problems and eventually to eliminate the annoying symptoms. This can be accomplished by regularly taking very minute quantities of the allergens in question. Another way to successfully treat the sensitivity is by raising the calcium level, which can be achieved by taking plenty of calcium in the form of *Urticalcin*. A further remedy for nettle rash is *Violaforce*, a fresh plant extract from wild pansy. This little plant blooms in mountain pastures before haymaking time and if you suffer from urticaria, you can also make a decoction from these to wash yourself with or add to the bath water.

Simple Remedies for Neuritis
The pain of neuritis can be eased by repeatedly applying *hot water compresses*. Still better results are obtained by using *herbal poultices*, well heated before application. For an even more intense effect, put the herbs in a linen or cotton bag, immerse this in hot water, wring it out and apply it to the affected area.

Another alternative is to pour slightly warmed *St John's wort oil* onto a piece of woollen cloth and apply this. If you mix *potter's clay* with St John's wort oil, again, slightly warmed, and apply the resulting paste, not forgetting to place a hot water bottle on top to retain the heat, the effect will be intensified.

A very simple, old-fashioned method, though perhaps rather unpleasant, has also proved beneficial. Soak a piece of cloth or cotton wool in hot paraffin, place this on the inflamed area and cover with more cotton wool or a woollen cloth. This treatment is useful for pain in the back, arms and legs. There is nothing cheaper or simpler, even though it may be rather smelly. Take care to remove the compress as soon as the skin begins to turn red and feel warm, because paraffin can burn and blister the skin. Anyone living in a rural area where paraffin lamps are still used can easily take advantage of this method of treating neuritis.

An old doctor who served in the Austrian army once told me that they used petrol compresses for the same purpose and sometimes even treated lumbago in this way with good results.

The use of *formic acid* has also proved very successful in cases of neuritis and sciatica. If a sufferer knows where there is an anthill in the woods, he should go there, expose his leg to the ants and let them 'work' on it. After a while, he can wipe off the insects with a cloth and will soon begin to feel the benefit of this inexpensive 'injection' of formic acid. Of course, the patient will achieve the same effects by applying spirit of ants, an alcoholic solution which also contains formic acid. Alternatively, if you know a homoeopathic doctor you could ask to be given injections of homoeopathic formic acid. This will be sufficient to relieve neuritic pains in most cases.

If, however, yours proves to be a very stubborn case, you can combine the various treatments described above, but you may have to persevere a little longer before experiencing relief.

It is also to your advantage to rid the body of toxins. Especially in the spring, if you live in a temperate zone, the blood can be cleansed by taking *bitter herbs*, followed by a *juice diet* that will facilitate the disposal of metabolic waste products. In order to help the body eliminate the toxins, it is important to stimulate the kidneys, bowels and skin at the same time. After the juice diet, adopt a sensible natural diet so as to avoid accumulating more poisons which may start up the neuritic pain again.

What is an Allergy?
This question is easily answered if we think of an allergy as a hypersensitivity to a certain kind, or variety, of different substances – allergens. This hypersensitivity may cause such drastic reactions that it seems as though the patient has been poisoned. For example, I am acquainted with the son of a pharmacist who becomes ill if only the smallest amount of egg is present in his food. A late friend of mine in New York would react in a similar way to wheat. Whenever he ate a piece of bread or pastry made with wheat flour he became critically ill. Professor Abderhalden once told me of one of his assistants who suffered with head swellings every time he ate white beans. Other people may have allergic reactions to daffodils, primulas, strawberries, rhubarb and even blueberries.

Merely touching certain flowers can cause skin eruptions, urticaria and other skin disorders in people who are allergic to them. Fruits can have the same effect, or they can cause a person to vomit. It is also known that some people are allergic to certain animal proteins and fats. Others I have observed become violently ill when eating seafood, such as crabs, lobster or any other shellfish.

183

However, that anyone should be allergic to wheat or rye I still find astonishing.

What Can Be Done about Allergies?

Many people have asked this question, but so far I have not been able to give them an answer that completely satisfies me. True, it is possible to undergo a series of tests carried out by specialists, which I understand is increasingly becoming a standard practice in the United States, for example. As a rule, however, this approach is rather expensive and requires an additional sum of money in cases where immunisation with antibodies is subsequently performed. Moreover, the effectiveness of this kind of treatment is by no means guaranteed.

The best thing is to test yourself in the following way. Every time an allergic reaction is noted write down everything that was eaten, touched or smelled. In time, a study of these notes should reveal the recurrence of a certain substance, perhaps a food item, a fruit or a flower. This may be a clue as to the cause of the allergy. Then, of course, the most obvious thing to do is to avoid the responsible agent or agents at all costs.

People who have allergies often suffer from calcium deficiency, which makes it necessary to take a good calcium preparation and eat calcium-rich foods. This will help to control if not eliminate the allergy. The homoeopathic drops *Pollinosan* have also given good results in cases of allergic colds and other allergies.

A Fast Cure for Shingles (*Herpes zoster*)

It is not easy to treat shingles and a cure often takes a long time. So it is good to know of the excellent results that can be achieved with the natural methods of treatment combined with homoeopathic medicines. For speedy relief injections of *Formisoton 6x* and *Rhus tox. 12x* are given and *Mezereum 4x* (daphne, spurge laurel) is taken orally. To stimulate the kidneys, drink goldenrod (*Solidago*) tea and an infusion of *rose hip kernels*. Locally, dab the affected area with a fresh plant extract of *Melissa off.* (lemon balm) and *Calendula* (marigold).

Attention to the diet is important. Cut down on salt and concentrated proteins such as eggs, cheese, fish and meat; they are best avoided. Fruit should only be eaten if well mixed in with flakes of wheat, millet or barley. Eat plenty of vegetables and drink carrot juice. Wholegrain cereals are also indicated, for example wheat

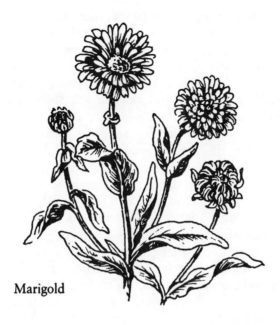

Marigold

grains, brown rice, barley and buckwheat. Since shingles affects the nerves, good remedies for building up the nerves are a valuable support to the treatment of this disease. Highly recommended are *Ginsavena* or *Ginsavita* tablets and *Neuroforce*, also *Kali phos.* *6x*; these should be taken three times a day.

Spasms and Cramps

There is a variety of fairly severe cramps that may be caused by a nerve or brain disease such as encephalitis, or may be brought on by an infection such as tetanus. Severe cramps may also be the result of urine poisoning, as in the case of uraemia and eclampsia. Each of these conditions requires specialised treatment. However, what we want to deal with here are the simple, frequently occurring muscle spasms. Sometimes these are experienced as twitching, or clonic, cramps, brief in duration but returning in quick succession; they can also be continuous cramps, known as tonic contractions.

These simple cramps can be successfully controlled by applying *hay flower or camomile water packs* on the affected area. Alternatively, a long hot *shower* can be taken, directing the spray onto the affected area. On hot summer days, if there is no hot water available, cold water will bring relief too.

185

Depending upon the person's constitution, physical exertion may cause severe tonic contractions in the rectal region. These cramps can be so violent as to make the afflicted person cry out in pain. He may well believe that he is suffering from some malignant disease. In reality, however, it is nothing but a temporary cramp that can easily be relieved by taking a hot shower, as described above, for one or two minutes.

Menstrual cramps, which cause great discomfort to many women, fall into the area of cramps caused by spasms. Many different kinds of headaches may also be brought on by spasms, particularly migraine and the much-feared headache caused by the föhn, a warm dry wind blowing down into the Alpine valleys. Such a headache is worse when accompanied by a stiff neck, but the stiffness can usually be alleviated by massage.

It is a relief to know that there is no need to take hazardous medication that may even lead to addiction in order to alleviate severe pain and cramps. Instead, *Petadolor*, a preparation derived from butterbur (*Petasites officinalis*), is usually all that is necessary. This wonderful herbal remedy has proved very reliable in controlling cramps without causing harmful side effects. In addition, *arnica flower tincture*, when rubbed on the affected area, has an antispasmodic effect, and *Kali phos. 6x* builds up the autonomic nervous system.

Our 'Nasty' Sympathetic Nervous System

Our sympathetic nervous system is a greater marvel of technology than, for example, a telephone system. But if something goes wrong with it the consequences can be dreadful, which is why I call it our 'nasty' sympathetic nervous system.

Never in my life had my sympathetic nervous system troubled me as much as it did recently, during a period of much stress and worry. It was in such a state that I left St Gallen and headed for the Engadine. Shortly after I had started my journey, I felt severe spasmodic pains in the stomach area, so that I could hardly bear to continue sitting any longer. Unfortunately, I had not brought any *Petadolor* with me, which would have relieved the cramps. Usually I have a good stomach, but on this occasion it was so upset that I brought up my whole lunch. In spite of the beautiful weather, the otherwise enjoyable ride up to the Engadine was agonising. All night long I had severe pains in the stomach, which felt as if it were tied in a knot. After my arrival in the Engadine I was able to control the nausea with *Nux vomica 4x*, and *Crataegus* helped to calm my agitated heart.

Even though I did not eat a thing the next day, the cramps reached up to the breastbone and did not subside until the evening, after I had taken a prolonged hot shower.

It was this experience which helped me understand why one of my friends, who had been very worried about the sale of his business, had to undergo surgery several weeks later because of extremely painful stomach ulcers. Doctors and physiotherapists seem to be correct in assuming that practically all stomach ulcers are the result of spasms caused by worries, upsets and anxiety. This does not mean to say that the acute symptoms need be as drastic as they were in my case. Constant spasmodic cramping of the stomach muscles can, and usually will, lead to ulcers.

Prevention is Better than Cure
Since prevention is better than cure, the laudable quality of self-control should help us to overcome unexpected anxieties and problems as quickly as possible, to conquer difficulties rather than letting them conquer us. Of course, this is often a question of experience and practice, for even if we know how to react in difficult situations, old habits may prevail and prevent us from making correct decisions in a calm and collected state of mind. People with a placid nature find it much easier to remain composed when facing unpleasant and distressing events than those who are prone to making split-second decisions without giving sufficient thought to the outcome. The sympathetic nervous system, unfortunately, is not subject to control or reason, but rather to our feelings and emotions. That is why it is always important to remain composed, so that unforeseen situations may be taken in our stride. When the wise King Solomon advised us to take better care of our hearts than of anything else he made a valid and valuable point. We should heed his advice, since 'out of the heart are the sources of life', as he said. By keeping our emotions under proper control we are able to reap many benefits, not least with regard to our health. Of the utmost importance is the fact that we thus will be rendering a service to our sympathetic nervous system.

Insomnia
It is certainly annoying when you cannot get to sleep in spite of being tired. But it is even worse to lie awake for hours because the tensions of the day simply do not leave you, and are transformed

187

into problems of insurmountable magnitude. Unpleasant daytime experiences prevent sleep and create a state of depression and the 'wheels' which are supposed to stand still during the night turn faster and faster. The restless individual tosses from side to side and finally, because he knows no other way out of his predicament, he reaches for a sleeping pill.

This, of course, is the worst thing he could do, because in no time at all, if he continues using such help, he will find he cannot do without it. He tends to forget that drugs destroy the body's ability to react and respond in a natural way and that their continued use has a destructive effect that can be far-reaching. It is far more sensible to isolate the cause of the problem that keeps you awake. Then, by resolving it, you will eventually restore your natural ability to fall asleep and rest.

If you suffer from insomnia, therefore, it will be necessary to discover and eliminate the cause of it. You may have been drinking strong coffee for years and should replace it by a cereal or fruit coffee. Should you find it difficult to give up your favourite drink, wean yourself away by mixing both kinds of coffee, gradually reducing the proportion of real coffee as your palate becomes accustomed to the new taste. In the end you will be taking a harmless drink that will permit you to rest throughout the night undisturbed.

A good drink to have before you go to bed is *lemon balm tea*, the relaxing effect of which may be increased by adding *hops*.

The homoeopathic remedy indicated for sleeplessness is *Avenaforce* (oat extract). Lemon balm, hops and *Avena sativa* taken together are sleep-inducing and a ready-made preparation containing these ingredients is *Dormeasan*. *Passiflora* or *Valerian* may be added to these sleeping drops for an even stronger effect. Valerian is often prescribed on its own, but as its effects are narcotic it does not provide lasting help.

Mountain guides in Switzerland know of and use another good remedy, namely *marmot oil*, and a teaspoonful of this taken daily is said to induce sleep. Since it is not too palatable it is best taken in the form of gelatin capsules, or followed by a strong herbal drink.

Of course, do not forget the habit of going to bed early, perhaps going even earlier than usual so as to be in bed well before midnight, because sleep during these hours will conserve your health and energy.

Remember, too, that retiring on a full stomach is not conducive

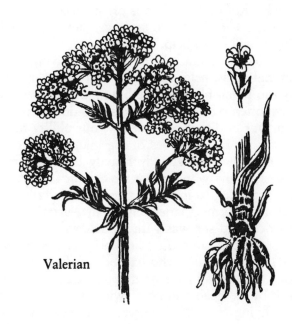

Valerian

to a good night's rest and is usually responsible for bad dreams. It is important when we eat, and how much and what we eat. Supper, as the last regular meal of the day, should not be taken at 8 or 9 p.m. or even later in the evening; that would be asking for trouble. If at all possible, we should have a light, easily digested meal shortly after 6 p.m. After supper, take a short walk and breathe deeply. This will aid the digestion and ensure a good night's healthy sleep.

Some Reliable and Inexpensive Remedies for Insomnia
In addition to the measures outlined above, a number of other simple approaches to inducing sleep have been found helpful by many people.

You may find it possible to put the cares of the day out of your mind when in bed by *reading* an upbuilding book or a magazine article. If one reads for long enough, it will usually lead to drowsiness and sleep.

In cases where you have overtaxed your brain, making the back of the head feel tense and painful, it is helpful to *massage* the aching area with the fingertips. This gentle massage generally relaxes the tension and induces sleep. Cold water can also help to dispel tension, and a *Kuhne treatment* is often successful in relaxing the body (see pages 436–8). *Brush massages* can also be effective, and even *fresh air* will often help.

Anything that stimulates the circulation, driving the blood back to the external areas, helps to induce sleep, since insomnia is often caused by too much blood in the brain. Our busy life today lacks balance; we often overtax our minds and do not provide enough exercise for our bodies. Consequently, our ability to relax diminishes. We cannot rid ourselves of the many problems that haunt us and thus subject our already heavily burdened mind to even more stress. Is it any wonder that we cannot fall asleep?

Another approach to inducing sleep was described in a letter I received from a former patient living in Australia. She wrote to tell me how thrilled she was with a book written by Kneipp. Her enthusiasm led her to introduce her entire family to *Kneipp's cold water cure*. Her husband, who had been suffering from insomnia for months, was cured by the brief application of cold water packs to the back of the head and neck (without drying off afterwards) just before going to bed. The treatment resulted in a deep and undisturbed sleep. One of their daughters, who could not sleep either, also tried her father's method and had been able to fall asleep without any trouble ever since. Sufficient sleep had also bucked up her spirits and benefited her general frame of mind in every way.

How gratifying it is to know that books on health have a wide circulation in every country and continent. There can be no doubt that their influence is very beneficial. The thought that my own health books, which are available in many languages all over the world, will continue to provide good advice for those who read them even long after I am gone, is enough to put my mind at rest and let me sleep peacefully.

OTHER WATER TREATMENTS

Sauna baths, once popular only in northern European countries, are now accepted in many other areas of the world. In northern Europe it is common for people to take a sauna and then roll in freshly fallen snow in winter. This exercise is said to build up the body's resistance. *Walking barefoot in the snow* as well as *snow-and water-stamping* are all favourite activities. All of these activities cause the blood to be drawn from the brain, so if practised before going to bed, they make restful sleep possible. Information on variations of these methods as practised in different countries can also be useful and enlarges the list of water treatments already known to us.

Years ago I was greatly surprised to find a sauna when I visited a colony of Finnish people in Brazil, of all places. Ask yourself, what purpose is there in having a sauna in a place where the temperature reaches 40 °C (104 °F) in the shade on hot days? The answer to this is that old habits die hard and become a necessity, which was certainly true for those Finnish people who built their sauna in a hot and humid foreign land. Perhaps it even helped them to overcome their homesickness for the old country. Moreover, in the tropics the evenings are cool and I remember that the sauna gave us a pleasant feeling of well-being. After the sauna we found a nearby jungle creek for a cool dip, which stimulated the circulation and helped to make for a restful night. Perspiring in a sauna differs from perspiring in the heat of the day in that it relaxes the mind and body and enables one to sleep soundly.

In summary, it is always useful to work out which one of the different natural treatments will be the most appropriate for overcoming your insomnia. Often all it needs is a little determination to do something about the problem and you will find what is required to give you a a full night's wholesome and restful sleep.

Epilepsy – New Views concerning its Treatment

Epilepsy, formerly known as 'falling sickness', is frequently mentioned in old writings and even in the Bible, yet although it has been around for thousands of years the therapy employed today still entails little more than a simple treatment of the symptoms. Bromine, used in various combinations, as well as Luminal, Cominal and other dangerous drugs prescribed to reduce the severity of the seizures, can hardly be called satisfactory by either the patient or the doctor.

If the patient is sensible enough to avoid alcohol, nicotine and other harmful stimulants, it may be possible to obtain more satisfactory results. Following a diet consisting of raw foods, rich in vitamins and minerals, is of definite advantage. Experience has shown that attacks are less frequent and less severe when the patient adheres to the right kind of diet.

It also appears that a new road to successful treatment has been found in positively influencing the patient's mineral metabolism. As a rule, epileptics have a low calcium level and often eliminate a lot of calcium, especially that bound to phosphorus, through the urine. For this reason a *calcium therapy*, together with an

191

appropriate diet, is advisable and beneficial. In addition to eating foods high in calcium, the patient should take *Urticalcin*, a biological calcium complex, as well as other supplements as described below. Besides being very effective, this treatment has no harmful side effects. The same cannot be said for treatment with bromine because over a period of time the patient's emotional and mental health invariably begins to suffer.

Reasoning on the Evidence
Not long ago I received good news from a patient in South Africa whose epileptic seizures had formerly occurred almost daily, but had diminished to only one a month – and the monthly attacks were milder than before. The improvement had been attributed to the patient's taking *Urticalcin, Vitaforce* (a vitamin supplement) and *kelp tablets*. It is likely that the organic potassium iodide contained in these seaweed tablets was responsible for the strong influence on the endocrine glands. No doubt other minerals found in kelp had also helped to produce the desired result.

In any case, as various studies have shown, epilepsy can now be treated with less harmful medications than bromine. As suggested above, the diet should consist of mild, alkaline-based foods, supplemented by a biological calcium preparation such as Urticalcin. Vitaforce should be taken at the same time, since its vitamin D content will make it easier for the body to assimilate the calcium. The main remedy, however, is kelp in tablet form, one tablet to be taken in the morning and one in the evening. None of these are specific remedies, but nutritional supplements giving the body what it needs most. Another plant which has helped in the treatment of epilepsy is the *oak mistletoe (yellow-berried mistletoe), Loranthus europaeus*, which is native to the Balkan region.

It is unfortunate that to this day specific medicines are prescribed which treat the symptoms, the external signs, without giving due consideration to what the body may lack internally. As a result, the condition cannot be improved or cured. Hence the need to find out the cause of the deficiency and then endeavour to rectify it.

Not everyone needs the same amount of every substance. Depending on the individual's nature, his temperament and hereditary disposition, his specific deficiencies and affections, the need for a particular element may be greater than normal, requiring more vitamins, mineral salts or other substances to restore the proper balance in the system.

A report from an acquaintance in the United States, an epileptic since her youth, confirms this assumption. She wrote to me saying that she was well aware of the excellent effects of kelp for epilepsy and had been using it for more than ten years. But she also mentioned in her letter that she believed that taking a biological calcium preparation in addition to the kelp had helped her even more. Since her attacks had been severe and frequent, it was a source of great satisfaction to learn that she was able to overcome them by taking these supplements and by adhering to a diet rich in calcium.

Biologically-oriented doctors have come to the same conclusion, as a letter from one of my friends in New York indicated. He related the example of an eighty-year-old doctor who is totally nature-oriented. This well-known doctor also emphasises the excellent effect of calcium on the general state of health, especially when combined with vitamin D if the patient does not normally receive sufficient exposure to sunlight.

Although already pointed out, I would like to reiterate the importance of following a non-irritating or bland diet that is low in salt. No doubt some patients will be happy to learn that their condition can be treated by natural means, but others may find this too difficult and prefer to take a less demanding approach. Such people do not want to make changes to their life-style and prefer to lose a chance of improving or even curing their disease. What a short-sighted and unreasonable attitude! And how can help be given if it is rejected?

Tragic Hereditary Factors

When young couples decide to get married they rarely stop to think about their health and what they may pass on to their children. It is understandable that their happiness in having found each other is based on emotion rather than reason. True, they may talk about certain things before marriage, but these are usually more of a material rather than a spiritual nature. However, even though the emotions may be ruling, it is still of paramount importance to take stock of the make-up of the two individuals involved, because this factor will have strong implications for the health of their future children.

None of us is perfect and few feel so strong and healthy as not to be aware of some weakness of a physical or mental nature. If any unfavourable hereditary factor should exist, it would be better if one partner did not possess the identical genetic weakness, but instead had a positive predisposition to offset the severity of the defect in the other. For example, if the parents of both partners

193

have poor nerves and experience great difficulty in maintaining a healthy balanced life, it often needs only minor emotional stress for their children to suffer an emotional defect for the rest of their lives. Let us take another example. If there is a history of diabetes in both families, some basic mistake in the diet of the young couple will be enough to double the inherited predisposition in one or the other of their children and insulin treatment may become necessary. For it is the case that susceptibility to tuberculosis, ulcers, cancer, arthritis, rheumatism and many other diseases may be transmitted genetically.

With this in mind, it is not unreasonable for young people, before they think of getting married, to make a point of examining their particular genetic predispositions in order to determine whether starting a family appears to be advisable, bearing in mind the possible problems concerning their children's health. If, however, they should choose to take the risk anyhow, it is even more important to consider the question of health very carefully, since much harm can be avoided through adopting a reasonable approach and by taking the appropriate action. Naturally, if the persons involved are inexperienced and have no idea whatsoever of the possible consequences, they will not be able to take any precautionary measures.

Basic Qualifications for Starting a Family
Many young people, even though properly brought up and otherwise responsible, hardly ever think about health as being a prerequisite for marriage. Their topics of conversation are often limited to the obvious: questions of where to live, how to furnish the home, holidays and excursions, leisure activities and hobbies, and perhaps the question of whether to have children and how they might bring them up.

As we all know, most employers require job applicants to complete long and detailed questionnaires. The answers help the employer to determine whether the applicant has all the necessary qualifications for the job. It would be just as informative and certainly appropriate with regard to starting a new family if the prospective marriage partners were to complete such a questionnaire. Any good physician or psychologist could easily recognise from the answers what medical risks, if any, the couple might expect to possibly affect their children.

For example, if two people who were both suffering from hypothyriodism were to marry, it is possible that some of their children might be myxoedemic and mentally retarded. The risks involved in cases of epilepsy are generally known, and epileptics are advised to forgo having children. Laws prohibiting marriage between close relatives have been made because the transmission of negative hereditary factors becomes stronger the closer the blood ties are between the two people.

Mature people, who are conscious of their responsibility towards their children, will not overlook the problems and precautions discussed above, but will give them due consideration. Only in this way may they be spared much possible suffering later on. And thanks to their reasonable and sound attitude they will have the opportunity to bring healthy children into the world.

The Treatment of Psychosomatic Illnesses and Mental Disorders

The Meaning of the Word 'Soul'

If we are to understand the meaning of the word 'soul', we shall have to turn to the Book of Books, the Bible, and ponder over a marvellous passage in the account of the Creation: 'God proceeded to form the man out of dust from the ground [one might say of the elements of the earth] and to blow into his nostrils the breath of life, and the man came to be a living soul . . .' or as another translator paraphrased it, 'a sentient creature'. Elsewhere we read: 'He poured out his soul to the very death', and yet again, 'the soul of the flesh is in the blood'.

If we pause to analyse these scriptures, we must conclude that the 'soul' (in Hebrew, *nephesh* and in Greek, *psyche*) refers to the whole person, with all his complex emotions and senses, not an immaterial entity within him or only his mind, or psyche, as defined by psychiatrists. In fact, with every pint of blood he loses, it could be said that he loses part of his soul and his sentience. If too much blood is lost, as in an accident, sentience and feeling progressively diminish, until life ceases altogether.

First God created the lifeless body, made up of billions and billions of cells; he caused the cells to live, to have in them the force of life (in Hebrew, *ruahh*). But for the life force to continue in the cells they needed oxygen, so God provided the body with the breath of life; man began to breathe because his lungs started to function. He was now alive, breathing, and began to feel and think – his existence as a living soul had begun. Thus the integrated whole of the body and mind, according to the Bible, is the living, sentient soul. Medically speaking, we must therefore treat man as a whole if any therapy is to be successful. Mental and emotional health go hand in hand with the physical, and vice versa.

The Interaction of Mind and Body

Psychological problems and disturbances lead to reactions in the physical body as well. Knowing of this interaction, it is necessary to treat the body, the physical problem, in order to relieve the psychological disorder. The reverse is also true, in that physical afflictions leave their mark on the mind of the patient to such an extent that his mental balance may be upset. Every psychotherapist will confirm that mental conditions can be responsible for physical ailments, and that organic problems can affect the mind so severely that the patient becomes mentally unbalanced. For example, a malfunction of the ovaries or the male sex glands frequently gives rise to mental disturbance, which will disappear when the physical disorder has been corrected.

Generally speaking, the field of psychosomatic medicine is still mysterious and little explored, so that it is impossible to establish doctrines and principles that are valid in every case. Nevertheless, experience and observation have clearly shown that one-sided treatment is insufficient and often fails to achieve good results, whereas the treatment of the patient as a whole, a unit, is more likely to succeed.

Natural Treatment

Electric and insulin shock treatments could be a step in the right direction. Although these treatments cannot strictly be termed natural methods, the principle behind them may be based on observations from life; for example, the shock brought on by a fright, an accident or other emotionally 'shocking' experience can jolt a person back to reason.

A change of climate, environment and latitude, long walks and hikes, breathing exercises (especially diaphragm-breathing), physical training, singing, vocal breathing exercises, etc., are all beneficial and may help to change the patient's mental outlook. Hydrotherapeutic treatments such as baths, cold or hot showers, Schlenz baths (see pages 433–6), underwater massage, walking or stamping in cold water, walking barefoot, also walking barefoot in the early morning when the dew is still on the grass, are further sources of help which can be employed according to the doctor's advice and bearing in mind the individual's needs.

In accordance with the patient's condition, doctors and nurses should try various approaches and watch and note the patient's reactions to each treatment, however small the influence of the shock effect may be. Moreover, anything contributing to a happy atmosphere should be encouraged by the nursing staff, as physical therapy and cheerfulness alone can quite often work small miracles.

From my Own Experience

Some years ago, when I still had my clinic, I had to deal with a very interesting case. A friend of mine, whose 24-year-old daughter suffered from hysterical fits that caused her to bury her head in a pillow and cry for hours at a time, asked me to treat her. I might add that her doctor's diagnosis was schizophrenia and that her sister, who was herself a doctor, could only stand helplessly by her bedside.

I took on this patient and my initial approach was to ensure the proper functioning of the ovaries by means of a *Baunscheidt treatment* to stimulate the weak menstrual flow. When this began to take effect, the patient at first became unruly, but as soon as the elimination of the leucocytes had started, a most extraordinary change occurred. The girl, now completely in her right mind, said herself that it was just as if a veil had been lifted from before her eyes. One single treatment had sufficed to bring about a complete cure and even later, after she got married, there was no relapse.

I remember another instance of such an illness, where the patient was not having any periods at all. I prescribed *mustard hip baths*, and *Ovarium 3x* for internal use. The periods were soon re-established and the emotional crisis completely disappeared.

New Approaches to these Problems

Psychological problems are not always easy to solve, but there are instances where the solution could be quite simple if only the right method of approach was first sought and then used. Every improvement in the body functions, even if it is perhaps only relief from constipation, can help or even lead to a cure. The use of physical therapy in its many forms can open up new avenues in the treatment of such patients.

As usual, diet plays an important part, for we know that pure, natural wholefoods keep a healthy person fit for daily work and help maintain general balance. Is it therefore not reasonable to expect that a proper nutritional therapy would be necessary and useful for the sick person too? Indeed, you should see to it that all denatured or refined foods are avoided. Make sure you eat only

197

food items that still contain their full nutritional value, that is, wholefoods, and that fruit and vegetables have not been contaminated by chemical sprays and fertilisers. This careful attention to diet, in conjunction with physical therapy and a healthy psychological influence, will provide real help for both body and mind, giving the patient the chance to recover.

It is also important that circulatory disorders are taken care of, by means of natural remedies such as *Aesculaforce* or *Ginkgo biloba*, and that the patient's calcium level is raised by taking an easily assimilated calcium preparation such as *Urticalcin*.

Nursing Patients with Mental Problems
It often happens that the immediate family treat the patient with a mental problem either too gently and indulgently or else too strictly. Even qualified nurses do not always find it easy to adopt the right approach in dealing with emotional and mental illnesses.

It is true to say that strong nerves are needed to deal with such cases and the attendant's own weakness, occasional helplessness and feeling of being 'fed up' must be carefully hidden. Patients must have confidence in the one caring for them, as they are exceedingly sensitive on account of their weak nervous system and they can react very quickly. If you become annoyed because the patient has done something wrong, or if you are unhappy because his progress is slow, be careful not to irritate him for this does not encourage him to get better; rather, it will throw him back once more into mental confusion and lead to unpleasant reactions and tensions that will have both physical and mental repercussions. On the other hand, the patient is likely to abuse your kindness, so it is better not to be too gentle, soft or even indulgent; be firm but kind at all times.

Nursing staff need tremendous self-control and self-confidence, also a measure of composure and vast reserves of strength, in order to help a patient with neurasthenic or mental problems to progress. If the patient is conscious of a strong hand supporting and guiding him he will come through the wilderness of his distraught emotions and thoughts with confidence in both himself and his future. He will then cooperate with his helper and begin to think, feel and behave quite normally again.

A TYPICAL DAILY PROGRAMME
The patient should start the day early in the morning by walking barefoot on dewy grass, as recommended by Kneipp. This exercise

draws the blood down to the feet and takes into the body the energy obtained from the earth. The result is a wonderful feeling of relief. If the weather does not allow this, paddling or stamping in cold water followed by physical exercises, preferably in the open air, can be done instead. In the course of the exercises, rhythmic movements, singing and vocal breathing exercises will help to disperse any mental blocks and free the inner self.

Breakfast should consist of pure, natural foods: various fruits, wholegrain muesli, wholewheat bread, butter and honey. Avoid the customary breakfast of milky coffee, white bread or rolls, and choose only natural wholefoods which contain the nutrients the body needs.

After breakfast a period of occupational therapy should follow. The purpose is to capture the patient's interest, concentration and attention by doing something practical. This distraction is an essential part of the treatment, for the patient must not be left alone and to his own thoughts, which have a tendency to become more depressing as he broods. If his attention can be diverted to everyday realities, depressing thoughts and feelings will have less chance to assert their influence on his mind. In the field of emotions an analogy can be drawn with the working of two transmission wheels: while the belt drives only one wheel, no power is transmitted to the other one. Applied to the patient, this means that we must see to it that he continually occupies himself, mentally, spiritually or physically, with the realities of life. If we succeed in this, he will gradually be lifted out of his condition marked by morbid sensitivity and imaginations, unhealthy fantasies and dreams. For those who have an artistic nature, arts and crafts projects are especially indicated as they divert and satisfy the patient without the need for constant encouragement. They also constitute a pleasant bridge between the worlds of fantasy and reality.

The midday meal should mainly consist of raw vegetables, with the addition of steamed vegetables and potatoes, brown rice or some other wholegrain dish. All highly spiced foods must be scrupulously avoided. A further period of occupational therapy should follow the meal, even if it is only washing and drying the dishes.

During the afternoon some form of physical therapy should be given, perhaps a Schlenz bath with sweat-inducing packs (see pages 433–6). Such a bath may be repeated two or three times in a week, depending on the degree of benefit derived from it. Instead of the hot bath, alternating hot and cold showers may be taken, starting with the hot, then cold, then hot again.

In cases of insufficient menstrual flow, a hip bath lasting about half an hour at 37 °C (98.6 °F), if possible with herbal extracts added, can be of great benefit.

After any one of these treatments some form of physical relaxation is called for, such as a walk in the fresh air, which will give an optimistic turn to the patient's thoughts. If some time is left before the evening meal, it should be employed with further occupational therapy.

Supper should be eaten at about 6 p.m. and be a light, easily digestible meal that will not disturb the patient's sleep. Highly recommended are muesli with fruit or a fruit salad, together with wholegrain bread, butter and honey.

As the patient's day began with the first rays of sunshine, so it should end with the fading light and he should get ready for bed as it begins to get dark. If he has trouble getting to sleep, give him *Dormeasan drops* taken in water sweetened with honey. This will help soothe the nerves.

Also, during the day the patient should be given the nerve tonic *Ginsavena*, made from oats and ginseng. In more serious cases a combination of *Rauwolfia* and *Avena sativa* is indicated (*Rauwolfavena*). The use of these natural remedies and therapies will help the patient overcome his condition. They will make it possible for him to control his morbid thoughts and depression, helping him towards mental and physical improvement. If the suggested daily programme is adapted to suit individual needs, many a patient can be helped to recover.

In all cases it follows that the diet should be planned on a natural basis and should be rich in vitamins and mineral content. If the patient's condition allows it, a juice diet or a short fast could be tried too. It is important to have his understanding and cooperation, for such diets demand the kind of effort on his part which often proves too much even for a healthy person. Never lose sight of the necessity to help him mentally by acknowledging, in a matter-of-fact way, that he is sick. He has to be cared for but at the same time the illness should not be given undue importance. The idea is to show and convince him, without pressure and almost imperceptibly, that there is a better, more favourable and simpler way out. Having gained confidence, the patient will be able and willing to follow our direction little by little. His mind will gradually begin to think correctly, coherently and, above all, logically again.

Weight Control (Underweight and Overweight)

In the past it was thought that being underweight was caused by an insufficient intake of food and that eating too much resulted in obesity. However, there are some people who eat a lot and remain extraordinarily thin, and others who eat very little and still put on weight. Everything, they say, turns to fat!

Meanwhile, research has shown that dysfunction of the endocrine glands, the glands with internal secretions, is largely responsible for both excessive corpulence and thinness. These glands are, primarily, the pituitary, the ovaries, the testicles and the thyroid. Their overactivity or imbalance usually leads to thinness, while their insufficiency (or underactivity) leads to corpulence. It has been observed that removal of the ovaries, or a disease causing ovarian insufficiency, causes a person to put on weight. Obesity following the menopause confirms the truth of this statement. Typical examples are the inhabitants of southern climates. How slim and supple the Italian or the Latin and South American girls are in the early prime of life. But as soon as the glandular secretions diminish, which is usually at a much earlier age in hot countries, they become plump. If the older generation is stout, stolid and comfortable, the reason for this can be traced to the insufficient functioning of the endocrine glands and, more than anything else, the sluggishness of the ovaries. In such cases *sitz baths* and other therapies which stimulate the ovaries (see below) would be of immense help towards reducing corpulence.

Pituitary obesity, however, is not so easy to deal with, because the pituitary is less amenable to corrective treatment than the ovaries. There are, of course, glandular preparations on the market which do act on the pituitary, but their administration is still a delicate matter. Nor do these preparations always produce positive results with the pituitary, though they often do with the ovaries.

A more effective way to reduce obesity is to take the seaweed ocean kelp. Two *Kelpasan* tablets taken twice a day are usually enough to reduce excess weight slowly but surely. Additionally, take *Helianthus tub.*, a fresh plant extract made from *Topinambur*, over a long period of time. Where the ovaries need stimulating, *Ovarium 3x*, in combination with a good diet, has given good results.

Another simple method, particularly for stimulating the ovaries, is to take various foods that contain vitamin E. The most important of these is *wheat germ*. There are some people who will not eat wheat germ for fear of getting fat, because it has also been recommended to thin people who wish to gain weight. Women need not worry about this, since wheat germ and its vitamin E content only regulate the function of the ovaries. In fact, wheat germ stimulates their function in the case of fat people and reduces their overactivity in the case of thin people; in this way it actually helps the obese to lose weight and the thin to put it on. In addition, wheat germ contains other valuable nutrients, such as vegetable protein, phosphates and natural sugar, all of which have a good effect on the body without the danger of causing an abnormal weight increase. So if you suffer from obesity, do not hesitate to eat wheat germ, for it will not increase your weight but regulate or control it.

Then there are those people who do not eat any food rich in vitamins because they are afraid they might overdose themselves. This fear is only justified where synthetic vitamins are concerned, for, indeed, they can produce an overdose. However, such a thing cannot happen with natural vitamins contained in biological remedies and organically grown food. Being an integral part of organic compounds they are never present in harmful concentrations. The body absorbs from the food only what it needs, while any surplus of certain natural vitamins is stored up or disposed of. For these reasons synthetic vitamins can never equal the natural ones. According to the Book of Books, human inability and lack of understanding bring the wisdom of the 'wise' to nothing. We may be able to analyse things, but when it comes to synthesising a biological equivalent we often fail. We simply do not know all the secrets hidden in these plants. How much more desirable it is, therefore, to turn to natural, biological sources, because the things the Creator has made for us can never be surpassed or equalled with synthetic products.

In recent times, artificial vitamin preparations have been strongly promoted by their manufacturers; before that, mineral salts ruled the scene. Fortunately, far-sighted researchers like Dr Schuessler and Dr Hahnemann found that the body requires various minerals only in minute amounts and that they can only be assimilated in triturated form, that is, ground into a fine powder.

At one time it was believed that gold could be made artificially; indeed, alchemists even tried to make an artificial man, a so-called 'homunculus', in their laboratories. Our age has become less ambitious in that it has merely attempted to produce a tablet or pill which contains all the nutrients the body requires and thus would make artificial nutrition possible, replacing our usual way of feeding. But even these efforts have been abandoned and now only elicit a smile. Before too long, synthetic vitamins will also go the same way, since they can never replace or equal those forces the Creator has put into plants, our natural food source. A return to these natural principles will prove much more profitable than all the theories the human mind has ever conceived. In this way, the natural way, the problems of obesity, thinness and metabolic disorders will be solved much more effectively.

Guidelines for Slimming without Danger
Obese people must never let themselves be persuaded to take a commercial slimming preparation. Except for seaweed, never take an ordinary preparation that contains iodine, since iodine is a dangerous element and should be used only in homoeopathic potencies and with the greatest caution. So if you do not know the contents of a slimming product, be sure to find out and reject it if it contains iodine. One should be very sceptical of any highly publicised weight-reducing remedies. Remember, the safest way to lose weight is by means of a suitable diet and a well-planned programme of physical therapy.

All chemical slimming preparations should be completely avoided. They are dangerous not only to the health but to life itself. Some people who have taken these preparations have met a tragic end. If you feel you must lose weight, take nothing but natural remedies.

When deciding how to approach a problem of obesity it is first necessary to identify its cause. It is no doubt true that excess weight is often caused by an improper diet or by eating too much. The unfortunate consequences in that case have their origin in too good an appetite. However, as discussed in the preceding section, there are some people who gain weight despite the fact that they eat very little. These people cannot reduce their weight simply by cutting down on the amount of food they consume. Advice on safe approaches to both types of problem is given below.

DISORDERS OF THE ENDOCRINE GLANDS
Those who put on weight although they eat very little suffer from impaired functioning of the endocrine glands. In my medical practice I have observed cases where the gonads as well as the pituitary gland and even the thyroid were responsible for obesity. If such functional disorders have been existing since youth, the gonads are generally underdeveloped or retarded as far as proper activity and

hormone production is concerned. In such cases, fat is often deposited on the hips and waist only and never on the arms and legs, so that these limbs are not excessively big. In women the breasts show considerable fat deposits instead of being the shapely glands they normally are. Sagging breasts, due to a malfunction of the ovaries, are often an additional worry of overweight women.

This type of obesity cannot be dealt with successfully either by dieting or any other kind of slimming course. Weight loss may be possible only if the causes are treated. This means that the gonads must be stimulated and the thyroid as well as the pituitary must be given attention. When choosing medication we will certainly want to turn to seaweed, especially as contained in *Kelpasan*, for reliable results. For detailed recommendations on regulating the functioning of the endocrine glands, which includes stimulating the ovaries and pituitary gland, please refer to the section on 'Weight Control' on pages 201–3. Bee pollen will be of additional help, since it is known to have a stimulating effect; but do not take it if your blood pressure is high.

The diet should be low in protein and all white flour products should be avoided, as well as white sugar. Instead, stick to a natural wholefood diet and take plenty of juices, including beetroot, carrot and celery. Horseradish and young nettles should be eaten daily and, as a supplement to the diet, oysters, shrimps and squid have great therapeutic value.

A carrot juice diet is beneficial. Juices of grapefruit, grapes and oranges are also excellent. Experience will tell which juice suits you best, because certain acids, although harmless to people in good health, do not always agree with someone who is not quite so well. If you want to achieve good results without complications, follow the reactions of your body and take care. Also, drink only reasonable quantities of the juices, because you could do more harm than good by overdoing it. Caution is recommended even when the juices and remedies which are to help reduce weight are natural.

Extracts from animal glands may be helpful, but only if given in the appropriate doses, because they may otherwise do more harm than good. Exercise and deep-breathing, preferably in mountain or ocean air, are among some of the best remedies for stimulating the glands.

UNCONTROLLED APPETITE

Where the appetite is a contributory cause of obesity it requires attention too. People whose digestion works well or whose body metabolises food efficiently have a tendency toward a ferocious appetite. For them the most effective remedy is to follow the old and tested principle that you should stop eating when the food tastes best! A diet prescribed for this situation must follow certain rules: it must be low in carbohydrates and fats and high in raw and fresh produce, that is, raw vegetables either as salads or as juices.

It is most important to avoid all kinds of sweets and white flour products. If you like soups, forget cream soups and leave them to those who want to put on weight! Since beer is one of the worst things an obese person can drink, the need to avoid it may be a real stumbling block for some men. As regards meat, limit your intake to lean muscle-fibre cuts. What is more, it is best to remove all animal fats from your kitchen lest you be tempted to use them. One exception is fresh butter, which may be eaten in limited quantities. Season your food with the various kinds of cress, horseradish, paprika, curry and yeast extracts, as well as *Herbaforce*. These herbs and spices have a stimulating effect on the endocrine glands and the metabolic processes.

Medications claiming to melt down fat are highly dangerous and should be avoided at all cost, for one's health is more precious than a trim figure. Preparations containing seaweed and cellulose, which expand in volume, are tolerated for a short period of time, but after a while the patient gets tired of them. The best weight-reducing plan is one that utilises kelp, since it contains minerals in concentrated form and potassium iodide. Kelp not only stimulates the function of the endocrine glands, as mentioned earlier, and consequently helps to reduce weight, but it also induces a positive feeling of well-being. A word of caution, however: people suffering from exophthalmic goitre must take kelp only in homoeopathic doses.

Kelp is known to be one of the richest of all seaweeds. It will suffice, therefore, if the person takes one or two *Kelpasan* tablets in the morning and at noon, and *Helianthus tub.* A steady reduction of weight will be noticed from month to month, and the general condition of health and vitality will improve at the same time. Many patients have been helped to lose weight by taking Kelpasan and can testify to the truth of this statement.

The Stomach

As is true of any other organ in our body, the stomach is a miracle of divine Creation. The mucous lining of the stomach, like all other mucous membranes, consists of elastic rubber-like connective tissues permeated by a network of arteries, veins, lymphatic vessels and nerves. All of these minute vessels and nerve bundles taper off towards the inside into extremely fine, microscopic end loops surrounding the stomach glands. The inner lining of the stomach is not smooth, but drawn up into folds, the larger rugae, or folds, being subdivided into many smaller ones. When magnified under a microscope they look like the fins of an old-fashioned central-heating radiator. The rugate inner wall of the stomach is covered with about five million tiny secretory cells. The microscopic nozzles secrete in precise amounts the enzymes pepsin and rennin making up the gastric juice, according to the particular requirements of the kind and quantity of the food that has been eaten. A sufficient amount of hydrochloric acid has also to be secreted because pepsin is activated only when there is acid present.

Hunger and Appetite

Whenever we are hungry or fancy a particular food, this natural reaction stimulates the secretion of gastric juice. If, however, we eat without appetite, forcing ourselves to consume whatever is set before us, we will have poor digestion, which in turn can lead to other disorders. It is therefore important to ensure that we always have a healthy natural appetite. This is possible, not by working non-stop, but by taking sufficient exercise and by deep-breathing in the fresh air. So, if you work fairly near to your home, walk there instead of using transport. You can also whet your appetite by taking bitter herbs such as centaury, or artichoke tincture.

Our emotional and mental state may either stimulate or suppress the appetite through its influence on the secretion of gastric juice. So, if you easily give in to anger or annoyance, do not be surprised if this makes you go off your food. It should now be clear that happy people, who are always in a good mood, digest their food much better than those who are very serious, or worried and upset. Nor is the process of digestion helped by sitting down at the table when plagued by problems, or when the situation is aggravated by an animated discussion about them. If you are not hungry because of being too tired, it is wise to rest a little and unwind before eating. The manner in which the food is prepared and the dishes arranged on the table tends to make the meal more or less desirable.

206

When prepared with love, food tends to taste better. By the same token, a nicely set table which does not reflect the haste of the daily routine, but which does show care and attentiveness, most certainly promotes the desire to eat by stimulating the flow of gastric juices, encouraging good digestion and the assimilation of the food. It goes without saying that the atmosphere at the table likewise contributes to better digestion. Every meal should be a family party where not only is the good food enjoyed and appreciated but also where stimulating conversation takes place.

Skilful seasoning of food is of great importance too. This is not accomplished by simply sprinkling salt on everything, but by using different herbs, the effects of which we should endeavour to find out. Most seasoning herbs serve to stimulate the stomach lining to increase its secretions and thus aid the digestive process.

It is too bad that in modern times we have lost much of what used to be known as table manners and the pleasures of sharing a meal with family and friends. Modern man is glutted with the hurried pace of life, always on the go, confronted with an endless choice of newspapers, radio and television programmes, so that even such things as TV dinners, eaten in front of the screen, are now becoming a way of life. Is it any wonder that so many people are suffering from gastric ailments, indigestion and ulcers?

Stomach Disorders
Stomach problems, while not the number one category of illness, have been on the increase. This is especially true in the United States, where people are in such a hurry all the time that they literally gulp down their meals, often not even taking time to sit down at a table because they do not want to lose time away from their place of work. If one has acquired the habit of eating food that is too hot or swallowing it too rapidly, it should not come as a surprise when gastric problems surface. It is just as harmful to hurriedly eat ice-cream on top of a hot meal. The extremes of hot and cold can lead to gastritis. And once the lining of the stomach has become chronically inflamed, one need not be surprised if this condition develops into ulcers. How ulcers are formed and some suggestions for their treatment is discussed in a later section (see pages 210–12). Although ulcers can be cured, it is clearly preferable to treat gastritis in good time, before it reaches the ulcerous stage.

For this purpose *St John's wort oil* is excellent when taken in the morning and at night, a teaspoonful each time. And do not

207

forget the help that can be obtained from natural remedies such as *Gastronol, Centaurium, Hamamelis* and *Solanosan.*

Whenever the stomach is upset we immediately blame it for the problem, but very often the liver is actually at fault. If fruit acids and fatty acids cannot be digested, causing discomfort, the liver is not functioning as it should. Since in such cases the stomach is not the basic cause of the problem, but only indirectly connected with it, the disorder will be corrected as soon as the liver is treated. A diet without fruit acids and fatty acids, but with plenty of brown rice, will soon achieve this. Brown rice is easily digested and does not burden the liver in any way, which is why it is so ideally suited for the necessary diet. You can also serve millet, buckwheat, whole rye or whole wheat for a change. Eat one of these wholegrain cereals together with salad; as a condiment use *Molkosan* (condensed whey) rather than vinegar, which is not really good for the stomach lining. Vinegar can upset the liver or the stomach juice, causing a burning sensation that results from excessive gastric secretion. Of course, this burning may also stem from some other adverse influence on the secretion of the mucous membranes of the stomach.

If you want to get rid of this burning sensation quickly, take a little *wood ash* in warm water. Should you not wish to take the ash like this, place it in a soft cloth, tie it up, pour boiling water over this and drink the lye you have just made. *Charcoal* is also good as a neutraliser and is available where wood is burned. But if you also find this treatment unpalatable, drink *raw potato juice* which has been diluted with a little warm water. *Dry rolled oats,* when chewed and insalivated well, are another good remedy to neutralise acid. *Centaury tea or drops (Centaurium)* are marvellous for heartburn and have a healing effect at the same time, whereas raw milk, although beneficial too, only treats the symptoms. If you follow the suggestions given here, it will be easy to stop the burning sensation that results from eating the wrong things.

Gastric Acid

Gastric acid is a peculiar wonder fluid, consisting of 0.5 per cent hydrochloric acid, which in some inexplicable way does not damage the mucous membranes or cells. The hydrochloric acid is produced from the chlorine or the saline solution circulating in the bloodstream. The healthy stomach lining is saved from digesting itself by anti-enzymes which to this day have not been fully identified. If, however, the mucous lining has suffered some damage or

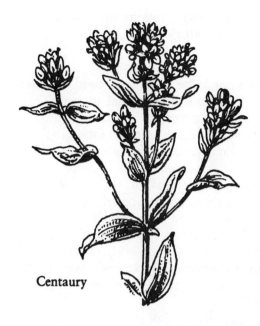

Centaury

a chronic inflammation gains a hold, the protection given by the anti-enzymes is no longer fully effective and the gastric juice begins to eat away the mucous lining, with the result that gastric ulcers develop. When the strong acid reaches the ulcerous parts the so-called 'hunger pains' set in.

As soon as the patient drinks a little *milk* or chews some *dry rolled oats* the acid is neutralised and the pains temporarily subside. Even more effective is *wood ash*, taken as described in the preceding section, as this is able to neutralise the acid immediately because of its alkaline content. Ashes from birch wood or grapevines have proved to be excellent. The remedy *Gastronol* contains this ash, as well as condurango.

Hydrochloric acid acts like a disinfectant and kills the germs that cause fermentation and putrefaction. Where there is little hydrochloric acid present, fermentation accompanied by gas formation and bad breath is more likely. It is peculiar, too, that cancer of the stomach generally develops when there is a great lack of hydrochloric acid; the reason for this has not yet been satisfactorily explained. When we come to think of it, how difficult it is for man

209

to find answers and explanations for that which we receive from the hands of our Creator!

Gastric Ulcers

It is common knowledge that more men than women suffer from peptic ulcers (gastric and duodenal ulcers). The explanation for this fact may be that women are seldom affected by anger and tension to the same degree as men. Emotional stress, anxiety and annoyance are known to be the main causes of the development of gastric ulcers. But irritation of the stomach lining, especially when the condition persists or recurs frequently, may also be responsible. It is therefore important to isolate the causes of the irritation, since only then can they be effectively avoided. On no account should you eat very hot food and, at the same time, beware of ice-cream or iced water, unless you warm it sufficiently in the mouth before swallowing. And remember that hot spices, strong alcoholic drinks and potent medications can cause unwelcome irritation.

Ulcers at the cardiac end of the stomach are rare; they are much more frequent in the region of the outlet of the stomach, the lesser curvature. As mentioned earlier, the first thing to occur is an irritation of the stomach lining. This irritation alone may cause some pain, but generally the patient ignores it and hence it goes untreated. When 'hunger pains' set in, which are so called because they characteristically appear when the stomach is empty and disappear when some food is ingested, the lining is already affected and there is a strong possibility that an ulcer is beginning to develop. The stomach wall, now no longer protected, is being eroded by the action of the gastric juice and it is this which causes the pain. Normally, the walls of the stomach are saved from self-digestion by a protective enzyme. If the mucous membrane of the stomach is already damaged, causing pain, the patient need only eat a little food and the discomfort will be relieved at once, because the gastric acid must now act on the food and is simultaneously absorbed by it.

If the pain sets in about half an hour after meals, this is an indication that the ulcer is located in the duodenum, generally 4–5 cm (about 2 inches) away from the outlet of the stomach.

A neglected ulcer, one that has not been treated, continues to grow and in time becomes a crater-like formation. Even though the wall of the stomach becomes thicker, the ulcer may eventually perforate it and allow the chyme to leak into the abdominal cavity.

This sets off an acute inflammation of the peritoneum (peritonitis), a very painful condition accompanied by vomiting and a racing pulse rate. The abdomen then becomes swollen and tight like a board. The patient's life will be in danger and he must be hospitalised without delay. Provided his general health is good and he is treated by a skilful surgeon, he has a good chance of pulling through.

It is possible for peptic ulcers to grow to the point where they eventually affect other organs, endangering particularly the pancreas, possibly even the liver and the transverse colon. Simple gastric ulcers are generally associated with a high acid content in the stomach, and the patient may experience belching or a sour-tasting regurgitation. If ulcers are not properly treated they may turn to cancer.

A malignant ulcer is more difficult to diagnose, since it is not normally accompanied by pain and thus not often detected until a later stage. Experience shows that malignancy is almost always connected with a lack of gastric acid, whereas a simple ulcer develops in a hyperacid condition.

THE TREATMENT OF ULCERS

Fasting has proved to be an effective treatment for stomach ulcers, provided the patient is physically strong enough.

Raw *potato juice* is recommended as a specific remedy and, taken regularly, it has a marvellous healing effect. Likewise, raw *carrot juice* and raw *cabbage juice* are excellent. Drink the juice of a small raw potato three times daily before meals and 50 ml (approximately three tablespoons) of cabbage juice, either in soup (see below) or after eating. For the best results the potato juice should be taken raw, but if the patient finds it difficult to drink these raw vegetable juices by themselves, they may be added to a minestrone or oatmeal soup. The soup should be cooked and allowed to cool a little before adding the juice. The soup makes the juice lose its strong flavour and the patient will be more likely to eat it and benefit from its goodness. These juices are indeed wonderful remedies at your disposal right in the home; all you have to do is to use them. Of course there are other useful medications, such as *Hamamelis*, *Solanosan* and *Gastronol*, but it is not necessary to buy something expensive from the pharmacist if the remedies are already in your garden or kitchen.

Condensed *bilberry (blueberry) juice* has given excellent results, also condensed *liquorice juice*. These juices should be taken daily

211

in doses of 20–40 g (0.7–1.4 oz). Before swallowing, they should be kept in the mouth for a minute or two to ensure proper insalivation, as this will hasten the cure.

All spicy foods and every kind of roughage should be excluded from the patient's diet, in order to prevent further irritation of the stomach lining. Provided the overall physical condition is excellent, one or two days of fasting per week will achieve good results. The diet should consist largely of milk, soft white cheese (cottage cheese or quark), cooked cereal porridge and cereal gruels. Even when the patient is completely cured and the pains have totally subsided, he will have to refrain from alcohol, nicotine, pork, cold meats, animal fats and hot spices for a long time. In fact, it would not be a bad idea to eliminate these items from the diet altogether. It would certainly be the best preventative measure possible and, considering that there are many other palatable foods which are not harmful to the body, the sacrifice involved seems small indeed.

Gastric ulcers are often the result of nervous tension, or stress. It is therefore advisable to free oneself from worries and anxieties. It is not really difficult to get rid of stomach ulcers if the simple methods outlined above are carefully followed. You are at liberty to combine the various simple remedies indicated or to conscientiously follow only one treatment until you are cured.

Poisoning of the Stomach and Intestines

Causes
It is alarming to think how easily we can be poisoned, especially today when the use of chemicals on farms and in food processing is so commonplace.

Cold meats and processed luncheon meats pose a particular risk, as do commercially prepared, precooked meals. So if you are in any doubt as to the freshness of such foods, do not eat them; they may have gone bad.

Anyone who has visited or lived in a tropical or subtropical climate knows how dangerous it is to eat fruit that has not been thoroughly cleaned. In the tropics, a cucumber salad made with unpeeled cucumbers can actually endanger your life. To be on the safe side, it is better to eat fruits that can be peeled, for example bananas and oranges.

The possibility of poisoning greatly occupied my mind when I myself fell victim to it and had to stay in bed as a result. One day I had been in search of certain herbs and while in the woods I crossed a clearing in which there were some wonderful specimens of deadly nightshade (*Atropa belladonna*). As the ground just there was very steep and slippery I involuntarily held on to the strong plants. Later, I came upon some poisonous prickly lettuce (*Lactuca scariola*), which I broke off and examined more closely. Shortly afterwards I found some wild strawberries under a luxurious growth of herbs and, forgetting I had not had the opportunity to wash my hands, I began to eat the delicious fruit. And then, to crown it all, on my way home I picked some poison ivy (*Rhus toxicodendron*) and held it in my hands. I remembered all these details later that night when I woke up with violent abdominal pains and tried to puzzle out their cause. On the whole I am not particularly sensitive to poisons, and I am sure that the poison ivy had little to do with my discomfort since it usually causes a rash in sensitive people, but I had no such symptoms. I had also eaten vegetables which we had bought from a store, since those in our own garden were late due to inclement weather and a late spring. This, too, could have contributed to the disturbance. Whatever the actual cause, the results were most disagreeable!

Successful Treatment
Intensive diaphragm-breathing eased the pain considerably, but it kept returning and woke me up again and again. At the break of day I tried to obtain some relief by going out into the open air. While there I collected some giant dock leaves which I placed on my abdomen to alleviate the pain. For a short time I did experience some relief, but later that morning the pain returned. My bowel movement was good, but I passed very little water. This surprised me until I began to realise that the body was retaining the liquids so that it might eventually help to expel the toxins. And so it was. A violent bout of diarrhoea set in, recurring several times during the morning, yet in between trips to the bathroom I did try to get on with my work. At the end of five hours, however, I had to give up.

I took sips of my medicine made up of *Lachesis 12x, Echinacea* and *clay*. Later, I decided to take *Belladonna 4x* as well, in the hope that it might do some good since I had handled deadly nightshade the day before and this could have been to blame for my condition. The remedies were indeed helpful, stimulating my system well, and at midday I was able to vomit. Strangely enough I brought up my lunch from the day before. I had not noticed such sluggish digestion before, since my system is usually quite efficient.

213

Unfortunately, by now I was much too tired to look around for a remedy to relieve the nausea, although *Nux vomica 4x* and *Ipecacuanha 4x* would have served me well. I had worked too hard during the previous week and this probably contributed to my feeling of utter weariness. But when I began to experience cramping pains in my heart I added a few drops of *heart tonic* to my medicine mixture and within five minutes my heart had calmed down. When the bowels were quite empty, discharging nothing but water, and the medicine which I kept sipping continued to work in the body, I soon began to feel better. By this time, deep-breathing caused only a slight feeling of soreness in the bowels and my otherwise healthy body had triumphed over the poison.

Special Guidelines
Many people become seriously ill from poisoning because they suffer from constipation, the bowel movement being weak or arrested, at the same time. It is therefore of the utmost importance to empty the bowels immediately to eliminate the toxins. If the bowels do not function and it is not possible to vomit either, then the body is forced to deal with the decomposing material in some other way. If it cannot render it harmless, a very serious condition might result and under certain circumstances could prove fatal, the simple reason for this being the retention of poisonous material. Hence it would be negligent not to take steps to empty the bowels when the first sign of poisoning becomes evident.

Should the patient bring up the remedies as well, then an enema to which a laxative has been added will be helpful. Do not worry about vomiting up a laxative, for the stomach will be cleansed in this way and this in itself will be of value. If the bowels are helped to function, hardened stools will dissolve, even if there has previously been constipation. Dragging, cramping pains will be a sign that things are beginning to move. The body itself may react to the situation by vomiting in order to get rid of the poison. Indeed, the body will do its part if only we give it the help it needs. Frequent diarrhoea is a symptom of poisoning, and if this natural reaction of the body should be absent, an enema is called for.

After the bowels have been cleaned out, the patient should fast for a time. If the heart is not in good condition, take a natural *heart tonic*. When you feel ready to eat again, start with light cereal gruels. In case the liver is still a bit sensitive, sip *raw carrot juice*. After two or three days *clay* mixed with water should be taken; then fast a second time for a little while, providing your heart can stand it. As soon as the feeling of hunger returns, proper meals can be enjoyed once more.

Such a case of poisoning is similar to the common children's diseases; when properly treated they promote better health. A fever and strong reactions in the stomach and bowels both help to eliminate wastes from the body, resulting in greater vitality. Even a case of poisoning can thus provide an opportunity for a thorough cleansing. The intestinal mucous membranes and the stomach lining will be cleansed, benefiting the whole body.

Never take chemical medicines which suppress the symptoms and impede the natural functions, for such a course would prove detrimental in the end. Rather, do everything you can to support the functions of the body. If you cooperate with nature you will not make any mistakes in treating illness, because nature is our best teacher. It is only we humans who tend to make mistakes.

Appendicitis

The appendix is a worm-shaped offshoot from the caecum, the blind intestine at the beginning of the ascending colon. It is this small tube which can become inflamed, the condition referred to as appendicitis, and is often removed surgically. The vermiform appendix is located exactly half way between the navel and the right iliac crest, the highest portion of the ilium and the pelvis. Imagine, for a moment, the face of a clock; if the navel were the centre, the small hand when it is on eight o'clock would then indicate the direction in which the appendix is located, exactly in the middle between the navel and the protruding hipbone.

Occasionally, an inflammation of the ovary (ovaritis) on the right side is mistaken for an attack of appendicitis. When the area of the appendix is depressed by the hand and suddenly released, the sensation of pain is radiated to the right, whereas in the case of ovaritis the pain would be local and of a dull nature. Appendicitis may also be diagnosed through the rectum. It generally makes itself known through severe, sudden pain in the right lower portion of the abdomen, appearing without warning and usually accompanied by malaise and vomiting. As a rule the tongue is coated and the patient runs a slight temperature of 37.5–38 °C (99.5–100.4 °F). If the diagnosis is difficult, the physician may also take a blood test to determine whether the number of white blood cells has increased. In cases of inflammation the usual number of 6,000–9,000 may have jumped to 15,000, and the pulse rate also climbs above 100.

215

Years ago the surgical removal of the vermiform appendix was considered hazardous and often ended in death. But today, with highly developed surgical techniques, it is a safe and simple matter, generally free from complications. If difficulties do arise they are usually caused by other existing circumstances rather than the operation itself. For example, the risk of thrombosis or embolism is naturally higher in people who have varicose veins or who show a tendency toward venal stagnation. However, this condition may be greatly improved or even eliminated with the help of simple natural remedies. For effective precaution, it is useful to take *Aesculaforce* before and after the operation. *Echinaforce* decreases the susceptibility to infection and also promotes and speeds up the healing process after surgery.

The danger of infection is much greater in tropical areas and if at all possible a visitor should avoid having to undergo an operation because of a sudden attack of appendicitis. An operation performed under primitive conditions could be a real problem for the traveller and his friends may later hear that 'the operation was successful but the patient died'. So, if you intend to visit the tropics and are suffering from a chronically inflamed or grumbling appendix, it may be better to have it removed before your departure, a precaution that will make the trip safer and more enjoyable.

Non-Surgical Treatment
Conservative treatment of appendicitis, that is, without operating, is primarily based on a *juice diet* and *bed rest*. Carrot, beetroot, bilberry and grape juices are particularly recommended for the cure. One part of juice should be diluted with two parts of good spring water. Sip the liquid slowly, allowing it to become well insalivated before swallowing. Add to 100 ml (4 fluid oz) of juice about 20–30 drops of *Echinaforce*. The burning sensation can be relieved by applying *cold milk packs* and nausea can be controlled with *Nux vomica 4x*, five drops to a glass of water, taken in small sips.

From the beginning it is very important to empty the bowels. For this purpose, take a harmless laxative tea or herbal laxative such as *Rasayana No. 1* or *Linoforce*. If the bowels fail to react quickly, an *enema* is called for. Either *camomile, mallow (cheese plant)* or *sanicle tea* can be used, preferably with twenty drops of Echinaforce or *Symphosan tincture* added.

Although we now know that the appendix is there for a purpose and is not just a vestigial structure of no real importance to the body, it is generally advisable to have it removed when it becomes inflamed, rather than run the risk of a perforation and resultant peritonitis. On the other hand, surgeons who routinely remove a healthy appendix merely because the abdomen has been opened for another operation are, from nature's standpoint, guilty of an incomprehensible action. Every scar carries with it the possibility of subsequent irritations and disturbances. Anyone who lives sensibly, keeps his bowels working well and makes sure that infectious diseases are completely cured, will generally be able to keep his appendix throughout life without any danger of inflammation.

It has been discovered that once the appendix has been removed the bowels become more sensitive. This alone indicates that an operation should be resorted to only when really necessary. Even then, a person should proceed with caution and seek a competent and conscientious surgeon, to be sure that the operation will be performed with the utmost care, because second operations have at times been necessary when an instrument or a piece of bandage was left inside the patient. However, such carelessness and negligence can only happen if those responsible for the blunder are not equal to the high standards of their profession.

Diarrhoea

Is Constant Diarrhoea Harmful?
Probably some 50 per cent of the population, particularly women, suffer to some degree from constipation. We hear again and again that it is bad to allow constipation to go on for any length of time, and there is no lack of good advice for its treatment. In contrast with constipation, not many people suffer from constant diarrhoea, a condition that prevents normal evacuation over long periods of time, even years, as opposed to the occasional bout of diarrhoea that passes quickly. Very little has been written about this kind of diarrhoea, even though it is more harmful than constipation.

THE FUNCTION OF THE SALIVARY GLANDS
If we are to understand this condition, we must first familiarise ourselves with the functions and processes of the salivary glands. These glands secrete a fluid called saliva which is mainly alkaline in composition and contains a variety of minerals; the body secretes these substances in accordance with the need determined by the type of food consumed. Since enzymes are important to the digestive process, these are also present in saliva. Few people may be

217

aware of the fact that the different glands – the salivary glands in the mouth, the mucous membrane of the stomach, the liver and the pancreas – together secrete several litres of saliva every day. Saliva begins the chemical processes of digestion, making the food ready for assimilation. When the saliva has finished its task, the colon reabsorbs its valuable substances. Once again they become part of the body fluids, and through them they eventually return to the salivary glands, ready to start all over again in the digestive process.

When diarrhoea strikes, however, the valuable salivary fluids are lost. The body is depleted of important minerals, which cannot be replaced quickly enough through food intake. As a consequence the body is weakened and the mineral metabolism becomes greatly disturbed. This does not mean to say that a temporary attack of diarrhoea lasting two or three days will occasion the loss of a great amount of valuable fluid, but if the condition continues for several months it could have serious consequences and must be treated.

Effective Treatment

To correct this condition, the patient must change his diet. Avoid all fruit, raw vegetables, sweets, cooked cabbage, and every other food that may cause fermentation and flatulence. Raw, unprocessed milk is recommended. The diet may include soft white cheese (cottage cheese, quark), any of the mild cheeses, rolled oats, crispbread, rusks, potatoes boiled in their jackets and brown rice. Not all fruits are forbidden; apples, blueberries (bilberries) and bananas have a constipating and healing effect. It is important, however, not to eat fruit and vegetables at the same meal, a precautionary measure which prevents fermentation. Make sure that everything you eat is well chewed and insalivated before swallowing. A short fast is beneficial, too, because it gives the digestive organs a rest during which time the bacterial flora can be restored and regenerated.

One of the best remedies is *tormentil tincture*, prepared from the fresh plant. It is most effective when taken in conjunction with sedative oat juice, *Avena sativa*, the combination being known as *Tormentavena*. By taking five drops in a little water every hour and preferably also refraining from eating, this excellent preparation stops even chronic cases of diarrhoea, usually within a day or two. This is a simple, completely harmless, yet most reliable botanical remedy and can be given even to infants without any danger. Temporary relief may also be obtained from *raw rolled oats* if masticated well and nothing else is added to them. *Wood ash* or *charcoal* made from lime wood have a beneficial therapeutic effect. *Clay*, white healing earth, is also recommended and is very effective.

When diarrhoea has been brought under control and can be considered arrested, it is necessary to consolidate the normal condition and complete the healing process by creating a new bacterial flora in the intestines. Two remedies are available that will help to achieve this: *Acidophilus* in powder form and the lactic acid preparation *Molkosan*. It generally takes a long time for the intestinal flora to become sufficiently established so that the intestine can once again function normally without assistance. Much care and patience are the key to beating this problem.

Chronic Constipation

The Dangers of Leaving Constipation Untreated
'Death resides in the bowels' is a warning the meaning of which we should carefully take to heart. It is an undisputed fact that constipation is the cause of many ailments. People who have been complaining about headaches for years never think that their discomfort could be caused by a transfer of accumulated metabolic toxins from the intestines to the bloodstream. Stomach, liver and kidney disorders may also stem from constipation or irregular bowel movement. Skin eruptions, spots and various eczematous conditions may be due to it. It is even possible for certain diseases or disorders to fail to respond to any kind of natural remedy until constipation, which poisons the system time and again, has been completely eradicated. Women are generally more affected by constipation than men.

If the condition is allowed to go untreated, it may have grave consequences. So never shrug it off lightly; constipation is a dangerous thing. A malignant growth leading to obstruction of the bowels (ileus) may be the result of constipation that has existed for thirty years. An artificial rectal exit (anus) is certainly not a desirable answer to the problem. We often fail to appreciate the automatic devices of our body until it is too late, that is, at the moment when these natural functions fail. They should never be taken for granted and every consideration must be given to nature's requirements. Even the most skilful surgeon can produce nothing but a makeshift solution, in comparison to the original. Only someone who has had to put up with the burden of an artificial rectal opening is able to appreciate and comprehend the marvellous working of our anal sphincter. So, never let things get to the point of neglecting proper movement of the bowels.

Some people complain about having spent a small fortune on laxatives, but all in vain. This should not be surprising when we consider the many chemical medicines sold over the counter, which, at best, offer only temporary help. It takes more to remedy the condition than just making it disappear for a few days. Just as a tree needs the right kind of fertiliser and pruning in order to grow strong, the natural functions of the human body need to be supported instead of suppressed. Instead of heeding the direction of nature, man has become too dependent on modern scientific research and reasoning.

The tribespeople in various parts of the earth would not know what to do with the best herbal laxatives, even when offered to them free. Neither the Berber tribes in the Atlas mountains, the Incas in the Cordilleras, the Vedda in the north east of Sri Lanka, nor many other aboriginal people would have any use for them. And why not? The answer is quite simple: their diet is not as opulent as ours in the developed world. Those people usually eat just enough to satisfy their hunger, whereas most of us tend to overeat.

Then there is another reason. The more primitive peoples usually have more fibre in their diet, and this provides the necessary roughage to stimulate the intestinal muscles. We gorge ourselves on white bread, rolls, pastries, puddings and all kinds of sweets and dishes made from bleached flour and refined sugar, which all contribute to a slowing down of the bowel movement, causing constipation.

Natural Remedies
If we want to understand why these aboriginal peoples have a better digestive system than we do, we must not overlook the fact that they still live close to, and in harmony with, nature and enjoy a relaxed pace of life. We, however, who live in an 'advanced' society have come to accept a way of life where speed and bustle are the norm. We have come to feel that this is appropriate for our modern times. How wrong we are! Restlessness, anxiety, vexation and constant hurrying affect the sympathetic nervous system, resulting in spasmodic constipation. If we then take strong laxatives we only make the problem worse. It is much wiser to change our pace, try to find peace of mind and calmness, refuse to accept more

tasks than we can deal with and rather than pursuing every so-called pleasure keep a proper balance in our lives. We will then have enough time to get the necessary rest and relaxation. Furthermore, we will use our legs much more, walking instead of sitting around. Remember, walking helps to stimulate the bowels. Early morning exercise, massaging the stomach and brush massages, if done daily, will be of particular help to those in sedentary occupations.

We can profit from the experience of a farmer, who knows what to do when his livestock shows signs of constipation. He will take *linseed*, prepare a gruel and feed it to the animals. The linseed promotes the formation of mucous in the intestines, which in turn relieves constipation. Linseed has the same effect on humans. Another oil-bearing seed, *psyllium seed* is very effective and easy to take, even whole, because of its small size. These seeds do not have to be boiled as is the case with linseed and are more palatable than linseed gruel. If you do take linseed, it should be freshly ground each time as it goes rancid in a short time. Of course, there are ready-made linseed products on the market, for example *Linoforce*. Linseed serves as an excellent stimulation to the bowels when it is taken together with muesli and walnuts. It is interesting to note that walnuts stimulate the bowels, whereas other kinds of nuts often have the opposite effect. One reason for this is that constipation is frequently caused by malfunction of the liver. Walnuts stimulate the function of the liver and in so doing influence the bowels. Even in severe cases of constipation good results have been obtained by taking various liver remedies, for example *Rasayana No. 2, Chelidonium 4x and Biocarottin*, as well as *Podophyllum 4x–6x*, which aids the flow of bile.

There are a number of different basic causes of constipation. Nervous tension may be responsible for it, malfunction of the liver has already been mentioned, and pancreatic insufficiency can also contribute to poor bowel movement. However, diet is probably the main factor. The various causes of constipation require specific treatment.

The farmer knows that he cannot keep his animals in the stable all the time; they need exercise and a change of diet from time to time. We can take a lesson from this and make sure we get enough exercise and pay attention to our choice of food and its variation. Avoid all constipating food items and particularly chocolate and sweets. Likewise, we would do well to keep off cheese, eggs and egg dishes. Instead, eat plenty of carrots, raw sauerkraut, and bitter salads such as dandelion and chicory. Over a long period of time, it is beneficial to eat soaked prunes and walnuts for breakfast, together with a slice of wholegrain bread. Alternate this breakfast with muesli and ground linseed. During the berry season eat plenty of muesli with fresh berries added, instead of bread. As far as possible, avoid dough products made with bleached white flour and any other starchy foods. On the other hand, natural brown rice causes no complications when boiled so that the grains do not stick together. Potatoes, however, may turn out to be constipating.

By observing these guidelines, you will be able to overcome constipation, especially when you are determined to adopt proper eating habits, not gulping down your food, but masticating it well before swallowing – and always in a calm and relaxed frame of mind.

Another beneficial approach to the problem is to take a warm *hay flower sitz bath* every evening just before retiring. Relief may also be obtained from a special blood-cleansing programme, the *Rasayana Programme*. According to Indian doctors, this treatment has a stimulating effect on the entire metabolism and increases the efficiency of the kidneys, liver, bowels and pancreas. Hundreds of people have been able to get rid of chronic constipation with the help of this programme, which serves to cleanse the body fluids especially in the spring. Nevertheless, in spite of the many excellent natural remedies available today, lasting benefits can only be achieved if our many mistakes in diet and life-style are corrected. If you get to the root of the problem, make the necessary changes, and use the natural remedies and treatments suggested, you will be able to find relief from constipation.

Whether you suffer from constipation or any other functional disorder, foods that tempt the taste buds but contribute to constipation should be firmly rejected. There are plenty of delicious natural foods that are good for the digestion and the bowels, so why not choose these instead? You simply cannot eat and live just any old way and then hope to overcome the resulting discomforts by means of pills and drops. This approach will only hurt you, and eventually lead to chronic ailments. We must subject ourselves to the demands of nature and only then, with the use of good natural remedies as well as appropriate adaptations to our life-style, will we achieve the desired results. There is no other way.

Do Starchy Foods Cause Constipation?

Many people suffering from constipation claim that a diet high in carbohydrates makes their condition worse or perhaps even causes it. Looking at this argument closely, we are inclined to agree, for in such cases the pancreas does not produce enough enzymes to break down starch. Hence it is indeed true that starchy foods can lead to constipation. Potato starch is particularly binding, so that it would be advisable to restrict one's intake of potatoes or forgo them entirely until the pancreas is back to normal. Too many patients make the mistake of not finding out which foods are known to cause problems, in order to avoid them until a complete cure is achieved. They have the mistaken belief that there must be some kind of miracle cure that will do the job without any sacrifice on their part. But would it not be wiser to avoid all foods that could trigger the disorder instead of waiting until we have the problem and then depending on a remedy to overcome it? Abstinence from such foods is often the only action required to rectify the condition.

Besides potato starch, grain starch may also cause or promote constipation. However, this is only true of denatured or refined cereals. The whole grain, on the other hand, neutralises the constipating effect because of its bran content. Rice starch is the least constipating of all; it is also easily digested and therefore recommended for infants and children. Since white rice has a depleted mineral content, only unprocessed brown rice should be included in a healthy diet. Moreover, brown rice can be most palatable when well prepared.

The cooking time for rice depends on the variety used. Italian rice cooks faster than the Asian variety. If you like the grains nice and firm, which is most beneficial for the digestion, do not overcook or soak for long periods of time. A variety that does not go soft during the usual cooking time can be briefly brought to the boil the following morning and left during the morning to soak in the rest of the water. All you need to add is the seasoning of your choice. Steam a clove of garlic, finely chopped parsley and a peeled, chopped tomato in a little oil and add to the rice to enhance its flavour. Or sprinkle with grated cheese and prepare *au gratin*. Placing sliced tomatoes on top is another tasty variation. When well prepared, brown rice is so palatable that even those who have always rejected it will enjoy it. This is apart from the fact that it is very nourishing. Before long you will find the taste of white rice insipid and will become accustomed to the darker colour of natural brown rice. If, however, you should still prefer a light-coloured variety, at least choose one that still contains most of its minerals, for example, the brands Avorio and Uncle Ben's.

THE RIGHT WAY TO GO ABOUT IT
Another advantage of brown rice is that it is nutritious and can sustain one over a long period of time. It is filling too, so that even a small quantity is satisfying. This is good for the pancreas, an organ that is often weakened through eating excessive quantities of food. If we stick to a natural diet, chew well, eat slowly and insalivate the food before swallowing, the pancreas is being helped to recover and efficient intestinal activity is more likely. Even small mistakes in eating habits can rob us of the vital elements so necessary for good digestion. At any rate, it is advisable to limit the intake of starchy foods and supplement the diet with vegetables and salads. Sesame seeds, eaten daily, are also helpful. And let me remind you once again, when choosing your menu, be sensible and avoid items or combinations that cause fermentation and flatulence.

So, if the pancreas should be too weak to digest starchy foods, we must take good care of it and do everything we can to restore it to its normal and full capacity. Only then will it be able to help us digest a reasonable amount of starchy food in the future.

Two Soups to Open the Bowels
There is a special soup which stimulates sluggish bowels if eaten every morning with a little crispbread or wholegrain (wholewheat) bread. The recipe is as follows. Cook freshly ground whole wheat, a small chopped onion and a crushed clove of garlic in some water. After taking the soup off the stove, add a little finely chopped parsley and a spoonful of pure olive oil.

This simple breakfast has cured many of their constipation. For more stubborn cases, psyllium seed or ground linseed should be added.

Alternatively, if you are bothered with intestinal sluggishness, have been overdosed with laxatives, if even natural plant laxatives no longer give relief, or if you simply want to normalise your bowel movement, the following recipe will be helpful.

First, make a herbal infusion. For sensitive people use cassia stick (*Cassia fistula*, also known as purging cassia) tea; for those less sensitive, use senna leaf, senna pod or some other herbal tea to stimulate the bowel movement. Brew and strain the tea, then for each person add one small raw potato, diced, with the skin. Mix in a teaspoon of bran and one of linseed. Simmer for fifteen minutes. Eat this herbal soup in the morning and also at night, if necessary. If it does not appeal to you, put it through a sieve and drink the liquid. You may eventually become used to eating it without it being strained. The effect of this soup on the bowels is astounding and it works when no other laxative does.

It is noteworthy that people who normally do not tolerate senna leaf tea respond well to this rather strong mixture if it is prepared in the way I have just described. The alkaline substances in the raw potato bind certain acids and resins which sometimes cause griping pains when senna tea is taken. I should add that horsetail (shave grass) tea is also easier to take if it is made in this way. Horsetail tea has a strong effect and it is not recommended to drink it on its own. Anyone who intends to take it regularly should remember to avoid excessive doses because of its possible side effects, which are equivalent to the symptoms of poisoning.

Dysbacteria

Much is being written and talked about the modern principles of proper nutrition. Wholegrain products, brown rice, wheat germ, natural honey, buttermilk, soft white cheese (cottage cheese, quark) and vegetable oils high in polyunsaturated fatty acids are being recommended as nutritionally sound food, and rightly so.

But it is also interesting to note that in a family of five, all eating the same healthy natural food, not every member benefits to the same degree. One member of the family may be strong, healthy and in good physical shape, whereas another may be skinny and weak, and a third member could even be anaemic and pale. Only when one of them suffers from such a marked calcium deficiency that he experiences constant cramps and spasms and can only keep free from pain by taking antispasmodics does it begin to dawn on us that nutrition involves more than simply giving the body a certain quantity of good food with a high nutritive content. Nutrition also means making sure that the body can absorb this good food, thus enabling the cells to receive all the nutrients they need.

Dysbacteria is one of the new diseases that lead to a debilitating loss of strength in thousands of people. Some degenerate totally without knowing what is the matter with them. The main causes of dysbacteria are two modern groups of medicines, first sulphonamides and second, antibiotics. To counteract their detrimental effects, it is suggested that the patient be given the liver remedy *Boldocynara*, which also stimulates production of bile. But to combat dysbacteria successfully he must take *acidophilus powder, Biocarbosan* and *Molkosan* as well.

A few days after taking these remedies, the normal appetite will return and the bowels will begin to function properly again. The patient will feel much better and notice a definite improvement in his physical condition as a result of his energy and strength returning. Once the intestinal bacteria have started to recover, the assimilation of food will improve and, in turn, the leaden tiredness caused by the illness will disappear. The body will once again be adequately nourished.

Patients with dysbacteria who are not too weak will find that going on a *juice diet* for two or three days brings excellent results. Besides other juices, beetroot juice is especially recommended. The juices should be diluted with half the quantity of spring water or slightly effervescent mineral water. If, while dieting, your stomach feels empty, eat a little crispbread.

I have often recommended a weekly 'juice day' because of its excellent effect on the general condition of health. The digestive system is able to rest, resulting in an improved absorption of food. Remember, nutrition does not depend on how much food we eat, but rather on how well the body assimilates and utilises it. These requirements can best be met when we eat unrefined, natural wholefoods.

Intestinal Parasites
In the old days, when grandmother would take a good look at her grandchildren and conclude from the symptoms she saw that they had intestinal worms, she was usually right. The children would have shadows under the eyes, be constantly picking their nose because it was itching, manifest a nervous demeanour and a lack of interest in playing and would restlessly toss and turn in bed at night instead of sleeping soundly. So what would grandmother do? She would give the children tansy or wormwood tea to drink. When tiny white threadworms appeared in the stool, she would make the children drink milk to which crushed garlic had been added. Even though the children may have hated to take this concoction, it was usually effective, but if the results were not entirely satisfactory, the garlic milk was also used as an enema. Thanks to their elders' close attention and care, the children were rid of the bothersome worms in no time, and it was a good thing

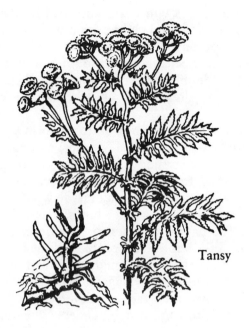

Tansy

too, because these parasites can do a lot of harm to a child's organism.

The same precautions grandmother exercised should be followed today. A child who is pale, always tired and moody could have worms and should be carefully examined. Otherwise, years may pass until someone is alerted to the problem and an examination of the stool and blood reveals their presence. What a pity, though, that these poor children meanwhile have had to suffer for years because of sheer negligence. Such lack of care can have serious consequences for the children's normal growth and development, since the worms are responsible for their discomfort and their unhappy, moody state of mind, making it difficult for them to show willingness and be obedient.

Threadworms and Roundworms

Intestinal worms should never be considered harmless or their presence accepted as a necessary evil. Although in most cases we are dealing only with threadworms and roundworms, these intestinal parasites can still be quite harmful. The tiny threadworm (*Oxyuris vermicularis*) is often the cause of much discomfort. These worms, as well as the roundworm (*Ascaris lumbricoides*), secrete

227

toxic metabolic substances which are absorbed by the body. The result is a change in the blood composition and an adverse effect on the general condition of the person afflicted. Children with calcium deficiency are especially prone to infestation with worms, which constitutes a double dose of trouble for them since their power of resistance is already low and the damage will thus be magnified.

The roundworm, which resembles an earthworm in appearance, reaches a length of 25–40 cm (10–17 inches) and has other detrimental effects besides its poisonous metabolic secretions. The eggs, which are transmitted from vegetables that have been fertilised with liquid manure, develop into small larvae which penetrate the intestinal wall and are carried into the lungs, where they settle and develop further. The patient appears to be suffering from a stubborn case of bronchitis, but the real problem is the infestation with worms. From the lungs the worms migrate through the bronchials and back into the digestive tract again, but eggs emerge in the stool only 70–75 days after the initial infection. Even so, the migration of these worms has not yet ended. When fully mature, they are found not only in the intestines, but sometimes they come down the nose and into the mouth, much to the horror of the victim. At other times they may bore their way into the bile ducts, causing jaundice. Or they may creep through the intestinal wall, which can precipitate peritonitis. Both cases are serious and dangerous. Their number may increase to many hundreds, a bunch of worms actually being able to cause an obstruction of the bowel and endanger the victim's life. I could go on enumerating the many ways in which worms can pose a danger, but what I have explained already may suffice to convince you that intestinal worms are not harmless. Their elimination must receive our attention.

Today it has become much easier to eradicate these intestinal parasites, in as far as non-poisonous plant remedies are readily available. So do not let them settle in the intestines. Papaya preparations greatly facilitate the eradication of threadworms in the colon and of roundworms which inhabit the small intestine. *Papayasan* is made from the tropical plant *Carica papaya* and is actually able to digest all kinds of worms that settle in the small intestine and the colon. Papaya is a palm-like tree with leaves similar in shape to fig leaves, but much larger. Its fruit, also called papaya, resembles a melon. When ripe it contains only a tiny amount of the vermicide enzyme papain, so it is from other parts of the plant that Papayasan is made.

Although ordinary worm medicines can sometimes have a bad effect or none at all, the Papayasan treatment is quite different. While it is an excellent anthelmintic, it is quite safe to take. Whereas other modern worm medicines kill the worms by poisoning them, leaving the body to expel what is left of them, the effect of Papayasan is based on a different principle. It does not poison the worms, but the protein-splitting enzyme papaya contains, called papain, attacks them and digests them in the intestine. It is true that the stomach, pancreas and intestinal walls produce enzymes to break down protein in the digestive tract, but the worms are immune to them. On the other hand, papain is able to literally digest the worms without harming the intestinal lining in any way. In fact, the intestinal lining is neither affected by the plant enzymes nor the body's own enzymes. It is important to maintain a low-protein diet while taking Papayasan, otherwise the proteins from meat and eggs use up the worm-dissolving enzyme for their own digestion, so that it will not be available for its intended purpose.

Sometimes it appears that worm remedies have been ineffective, because after a short time the parasites may be noticed again. However, it does not follow that the remedy was necessarily at fault; it is more than likely that reinfection has taken place. This happens during the night in a warm bed, when the tiny worms leave the body and deposit their eggs in the minute skin folds near the anus. Itching sets in and naturally the child begins to scratch, only to get the eggs under the fingernails. Since children have the habit of putting their fingers back into the mouth, the eggs are transferred back into the digestive tract. It is also possible that the microscopic eggs had been shaken from the sheets when the bed was made, dispersing them into the air, from which they were inhaled together with the dust from the room.

For this reason, the need for scrupulous cleanliness cannot be emphasised enough. During a worm treatment, the room should be dusted daily with a damp cloth. It is also imperative to change the bed linen frequently. Tight-fitting pants should be worn under the night gown or pyjamas to avoid involuntary scratching whilst asleep.

Fortunately, not everyone becomes infected when worm eggs are swallowed, because the body's natural resistance and good digestion do not permit them to develop in the first place.

Tapeworms

Tapeworms are more dangerous than the smaller nematodes. A tapeworm is extremely difficult to get rid of because of the barbed hooks on its head by which it remains firmly attached to the mucous-membrane lining of the intestines. When small segments, 7–10mm (¼–⅓ inch) wide and 10–20 cm (4–8 inches) long, are seen in the stools, this is no reason to think that the victim is now rid of the tapeworm. Rather, these are merely sexually mature parts containing eggs, which the full-grown worm casts off. Moreover, even though the tapeworm drops off segments from the end of its body, it does not become any shorter, because it continues to grow at the other end, the head, where the individual body segments begin. A tapeworm can produce hundreds of thousands of eggs which, through the excrement, eventually find their way into the cesspool. Of course, this is also true of the eggs of threadworms and roundworms. You can see why it is a hazardous thing to fertilise the vegetable garden with cesspool manure. In a heavy downpour the worm eggs may be spattered up from the ground onto the vegetables, thus providing a source of reinfection. The same danger arises when using liquid manure on a pasture where sheep and cows graze, as these animals stand every chance of becoming infected with tapeworm eggs.

There are various kinds of tapeworm. When eating meat that has not been properly cooked it is possible to become infected with the so-called bladderworms (*cysticerci*) of the cattle, pig or fish variety. The bladderworms or larvae then develop into tapeworms in the human host.

Even more dangerous than the cattle tapeworm, which can reach a length of several metres, is the dog tapeworm, of the genus *Echinococcus*. It is only about 5–6 mm (¼ inch) long but its size bears no relationship to its danger, for this little worm is capable of causing greater damage than the much longer cattle tapeworm. Although called the dog tapeworm, it has been known to infest sheep, goats, pigs and even cattle. When this happens, blisters the size of a walnut form in the lungs of cattle, and in the case of swine, these formations are found in the liver. The Swiss Information Service to Physicians reported that in 1963, for example, 508 cattle and 62 swine brought into the Zurich abattoir were infested with the *Echinococcus*. As far as domestic animals and pets are concerned, extreme precautions need to be taken, especially with dogs and cats. Adults who are otherwise meticulously clean, are often offended when reminded to be careful when handling pets. They think nothing of patting their pets while eating. But it is unwise to do this. Neither should we allow a dog or cat to lick the hand or the face, because of the danger attached to it. What is more, young animals, puppies and kittens, should be trained not to do so. To minimise the risk of infection, dog owners would be wise to abstain from feeding raw lungs or liver to their dogs. After a long journey, perhaps abroad, check your dog's faeces, since 7–8 weeks after infection small flecks with thousands of eggs may be seen. You certainly cannot be called over-fussy for taking such proper care and precautions in the interest of your health.

Since field mice can be infected from the faeces of dogs, the eggs can be transmitted to people from the cats that catch the mice. The larvae of the dog tapeworm can cause small blisters in the human liver. This is quite dangerous since worm remedies are only effective in the intestine and not in the liver.

There is another danger. The eggs can develop into minute larvae in the intestines, bore through the intestinal wall and then migrate via the bloodstream to various organs of the body, where they form blisters or cysts varying in size from that of a pinhead to a little child's head. This condition can be fatal. Do not, therefore, ignore the warning to exercise due care when handling your pets. There are no doubt many ways of playing with them and enjoying their companionship, without endangering your health.

Because international travel has now become a way of life, yet another danger presents itself. In our travels we come into contact with strangers and their animals. This is an area in which there is always a possibility of risking infection through the transmission of eggs and parasites. Being aware of this danger should make us more conscious of the need for meticulous cleanliness and hygiene.

Getting rid of a tapeworm is not as simple as one might think. I once helped a young man lose one by means of a diet and special tapeworm medication, although previous treatment with chemical medicines had done him no good whatsoever. My instructions for the diet and the remedy were as follows.

Diet: No meat, but plenty of vegetables and fruit, especially raw carrots, no bread, no potatoes, and nothing made of flour. For lunch: a stew made up of lentils, carrots, onion and garlic. Cook all the ingredients together in one pot. It may be seasoned with a little fresh horseradish. Twice a day a small dish of sauerkraut (4–5 forkfuls). In the morning, on an empty stomach, a handful of peeled pumpkin seeds and a handful of unsweetened cranberries, chewed well. Follow this up an hour later with one or two cups of tapeworm tea, without sugar. It is also helpful to sip a glass of garlic milk as well.

Recipe for tapeworm tea: Take 5 g (⅙ oz) powdered aloes, 20 g (⅔ oz) alder buckthorn (bark), 20 g (⅔ oz) senna leaves, 25 g (1 oz) valerian root, 30 g (just over 1 oz) peppermint leaves. Mix them together and use to make an infusion, one tablespoon for every cup of boiling water. Leave to brew for ten minutes, but do not boil.

Another, more radical, remedy to get rid of a tapeworm that does not seem to yield to any treatment is a teaspoonful of *Kamala powder*, taken just once. This remedy is good for adults and pets alike. Less radical but equally effective is *Papayasan* if taken over a period of time.

It is very important to avoid becoming constipated. If you tend to do so, *Rasayana No. 1* will solve the problem. And do not forget to help the body expel the tapeworm by drinking *Biocarottin*.

When examining the stools make sure that the head as well as the body of the worm has been expelled. If the head remains, the treatment will have to be repeated within two or three weeks. Should the first day of treatment produce no results, continue for another day. An *enema* with *garlic milk* given once a day can be very effective and is recommended too.

A word of caution is required at this point. The expelled tapeworm must under no circumstances be thrown on the compost heap but should be burned or buried deep in the ground.

Finally, if no treatment whatsoever is able to shift the worm, there is yet another remedy that has been successfully used in Africa, namely the *root of the pomegranate tree*. One teaspoonful of this root in powder form should be taken in a little warm water every morning and evening. Alternatively, a tea can be made by boiling the root, in which case two cups should be taken daily.

Dangers of the Tropics

Overseas travel has become commonplace since large airliners have conquered the problem of distance. It is not surprising, then, that in the more temperate regions of the earth travel agents keep issuing glossy brochures and leaflets, tempting us to travel to far-distant exotic countries. If you live in an area where glittering snow and majestic mountains predominate, it is hard to resist the call to experience the peculiar charm of the tropics; to enjoy a walk in the balmy air under palm trees or amid banana trees, laze around in the shade of huge avocado trees, watch the crocodiles from a canoe, follow an elephant herd in a jeep driven by a watchful guide, or perhaps admire some lions roaming in absolute freedom. An added bonus would be the prospect of getting to know the customs, habits and life-style of the natives. In reality, travelling in tropical countries is often arduous and not always as pleasant as some might make us believe, even though it may be interesting. The people who encourage us to visit faraway places are usually so enthusiastic about them that it does not occur to them to alert us to the dangers the tropics can have in store for us. Not even the travel agencies see fit to do so, but as you will see from what follows below their suggested precautions and insurance are really not enough in every case.

Unseen Dangers – Parasites and Micro-organisms
For most people who visit the tropics, big game seems to be the main thing to be feared. Elephants, lions, tigers and crocodiles figure especially in our imagination and we may be fearful enough to believe that there is a wild animal lurking behind every bush. And of course we dread the snakes. However, the well-informed traveller will reassure us, knowing that wild animals are not really the great danger they are generally thought to be.

This knowledge is certainly a relief but it should not make us drop our guard. There are other threats, generally unnoticed but far more perilous than adventures with wild animals, and these stem from a variety of micro-organisms. What really makes the tropics dangerous are the things the scientist can see under a microscope and the doctor in a blood test, when examining an unfortunate traveller. A European, for example, may never have had an experience with certain micro-organisms, but what an unpleasant shock they can cause if through ignorance and carelessness he allows them to invade his body. How easy it is for a traveller to become infected and suffer the consequences of amoebic dysentery, a persistent and sometimes fatal disease. Yet one does not have to travel all that far to be in danger of contracting amoebic dysentery, as it can be caught in southern Italy, Greece and the Middle East. So if you live in a temperate zone and travel to such subtropical lands or islands, be very careful to avoid getting infected with amoebas.

In many other areas, for example in North Africa and Egypt or

233

Sri Lanka and India, travellers are exposed to the ever-present danger of hookworms. This dangerous worm is so widespread that Professor Dr Nauck, one of the foremost specialists in tropical diseases, believes that over 500 million people are infested with it. According to his estimate, every fifth person in the tropics is a carrier of this dangerous parasite.

Not only are roundworms and the tiny threadworms or pinworms extremely widespread in tropical lands and islands, but the even more dangerous whipworms are abundant in some areas, so that practically all the inhabitants are infested with one kind or another of these parasites.

REASONS FOR THE WIDESPREAD INFESTATION

If you are at all familiar with the conditions in the countries to which I refer, you will not be surprised at the widespread problem of parasites and the great number of people infested with them. The main reason is the glaring lack of sanitation and sewage systems. There are often no sewers at all; nor, in many cases, are there proper lavatories or toilets. The consequence? Human excrement lies around on the ground, even in the beautiful palm groves among all the tropical plants, and this waste matter is riddled with thousands of worm eggs. As a rule there is no safe drinking water supply either, and this of course is very dangerous. Another extremely hazardous factor is the lack of meat inspection, so that the people consume meat full of bladderworms and various other parasites. This circumstance makes it possible for the dangerous dog tapeworm to be transmitted, while filariae, another variety of parasitic worm, are spread through mosquito bites. One type of these filarial worms is known to be the cause of the dreadful disease called elephantiasis (see the following section).

Tropical Diseases
Paddling in a canoe through the dense jungle is no doubt an unforgettable experience many a nature-lover dreams about. The untouched character of nature has a special attraction, and indeed, where man has not yet created order, or disorder, the tropical environment is a unique experience. You think you are in a different world when the sun's last red-golden rays shoot through the fan-like palm branches in the evening or when the vines hanging from jungle trees appear to take on eery forms. At night, lying on a bamboo mat in a native hut under a mosquito net, never hope to find undisturbed sleep. In the solitude of the jungle unusual

234

noises and animal sounds, often terribly frightening, reach your ears. We get the uncanny feeling of adventure, realising that what we have let ourselves in for is actually more interesting than it is pleasant. Nevertheless, we soon become accustomed to things, and what seemed strange and exotic to begin with becomes gradually more familiar. We begin to recognise plants and animals, and every day new experiences occur in the jungle. Comparatively soon we get used to snakes and wild animals and even the lack of sanitary arrangements, as well as all the discomforts connected with it.

The true dangers only begin to dawn on us when we have to lie in a hut because a cold or hot fever, vomiting and diarrhoea have laid us low, weakening us to such an extent that days later we have hardly any energy and desire to live left in us. The dangers of tropical diseases have risen drastically in recent years, especially in countries where the sanitary and health inspection is now in the hands of people who still lack sufficient training and understanding. The Congo and other African countries are typical examples. In some towns in Central Africa, where malaria had previously been eradicated, the visitor has no longer any guarantee of escaping infection. The efficiency and effectiveness of inspection and control of breeding grounds in those countries that only recently acquired independence have not been possible to maintain in areas that previously had been made safe.

It is very sad that the results of many years' efforts are being relinquished due to a change in circumstances. Malaria, typhoid fever, paratyphoid fever, elephantiasis, amoebic dysentery and dysentery are, unfortunately, once again on the increase and the danger of infection in many tropical areas can be expected to continue to grow before it falls. The white colonial powers were responsible for many wrongs, but as regards hygiene and the control of epidemics they also did a lot of good. Human weakness is often responsible for 'throwing out the baby with the bath water', particularly where childish naivety or the blindness of nationalism predominates.

It is indeed regrettable that all the good progress achieved in the course of many years of effort and work should come to nothing. It is a step backwards when tourists are exposed to greater dangers and risks of infection. So if your health is not exceptionally good and your powers of resistance are limited, or if you are very sensitive, think twice for the present before you decide to go on a safari or other holiday in tropical countries. Despite all kinds of vaccinations, you will not be immune to all tropical diseases.

For one thing, vaccines are not available for every disease; what is more, vaccination in itself can often pose a problem for the traveller, because it can weaken his general condition. And do not forget that for many serious tropical diseases prophylactics do not exist. What comfort will the most beautiful and tempting colour brochure depicting glorious beaches and colourful surroundings be if the unsuspecting tourist comes down with something serious? Moreover, the treatment of tropical diseases is not always a simple, easy or safe matter. Strong medication is required and this affects especially the liver, often inflicting great harm. I have been shocked many times when browsing through travel brochures, to see that they give no hint whether the travel agencies, tour operators and their guides have any idea at all of the dangers in the destinations advertised. One such brochure planned to take the travellers to an area in Sri Lanka, to the south of Colombo and Mount Lavinia, an area where the dreaded tropical disease elephantiasis has not yet been fully eradicated. In spite of this knowledge, the agents chose exactly that place for an overnight stay.

THE REALITY

Elephantiasis is transmitted by a mosquito. The female bites an infected person, sucks in the blood and transmits the parasite to a healthy person's bloodstream by another bite. Once the parasites, which we could call minute worms, are in the human blood, they multiply into the millions, causing fever and extreme enlargement of the lymphatics. Given time, the limbs may enlarge to the extent that they are two or three times their normal size. In fact, the disease got its peculiar name from this condition, for the legs come to resemble elephants' legs in their bulk. But it is no laughing matter: elephantiasis is a sad affliction and one that is difficult to cure successfully.

I have also heard from doctors specialising in tropical diseases that malaria has not yet been fully eradicated in all parts of Sri Lanka. It is therefore advisable to sleep under a mosquito net and to take preventative medicines. There is, however, no danger in the mountainous areas of Sri Lanka where the strikingly beautiful tea plantations are to be found. Yes, tropical countries and islands might present an especially exciting and tempting attraction and no doubt offer plenty of beauty, yet caution is definitely called for because of the unknown dangers. As I have said before, I would not recommend a tropical vacation to just anyone; weak, sickly and especially older people should not even think about visiting the tropics.

The beauties of Switzerland, in a wider sense also Europe in general and other temperate zones, have much to attract the enthusiastic traveller and holiday-maker. That is why I would like to remind the prospective traveller of the old proverb, 'You might go further and not fare so well.' Why do I recommend that you take these words to heart? Because on my many travels I have met some Europeans who had been laid low by tropical diseases and became physical wrecks as a result. So, may the foregoing words of caution serve as a warning to all those who want to travel in the tropics but have no idea of the existing dangers to their health.

Precautionary Measures
Below are listed several precautionary rules that everyone should heed when travelling in the tropics.

1. Never eat raw meat. Even meat roasted on the outside but still rare inside should be rejected. The same warning applies to raw fish of any kind. In the Far East raw fish prepared by a process of fermentation is extremely tasty and prized by many as a delicacy. Nevertheless, however tempting it may be, it can be very dangerous and should not be consumed.

2. Do not eat raw vegetables. Salads of any kind must be totally eliminated from the diet when travelling in the tropics. If the vegetables are grown in the fenced garden of a friend where you can be sure they were raised under sanitary, safe conditions, you may perhaps take a chance. Vegetables may be washed in a solution of potassium permanganate, but this does not afford 100 per cent protection either.

3. Do not eat fruit that cannot be peeled. True, it may be difficult to resist the temptation to eat strawberries or cherries in January in certain tropical regions south of the equator, but it is not worth taking the risk of exposing yourself to the great danger of possible infection with some tropical disease. Wait until you return home and pick them in your own garden.

4. Drinking water constitutes a high risk. Make sure it has been boiled before drinking it. This point applies to drinking water anywhere in the tropics, including in restaurants; it is unsafe, and so is ice, which is probably made from the same water. You must either take the trouble to boil it or try to quench your thirst by eating juicy fruit which you can peel, being careful not to transfer

any bacteria from the skin of the fruit to its fleshy part. In the jungle you can drink palm water, which is contained in the marrow of the palm tree. Even for those who normally do not drink alcohol, it would be better to quench the thirst with beer, if available, rather than run the risk of drinking contaminated water, for a little alcohol is less harmful than a dangerous tropical disease. Remember, unboiled water can be dangerous – do not take any chances.

5. Walking barefoot, although a pleasant and healthy habit in temperate zones, is hazardous in the tropics. Various parasitic larvae may stick to the skin, penetrate the sole of the foot or the skin between the toes and travel via the lymphatics and the bloodstream to various parts of the body where they can wreak havoc. If you are a nature-lover, who cannot resist the impulse to walk barefoot in these warm areas, make sure you do so only on beaches where the sand has been cleansed by the ocean tides. Even the sand dunes farther back from the beach and which are not in direct contact with sea water are a danger and must be avoided. In tropical and subtropical regions the sand farther back is often contaminated with human excrement, releasing hundreds of thousands of worms and other parasites that can be easily transferred to the foot – and their new host – while walking on the dunes.

6. In hot, humid, tropical or subtropical regions, it is advisable to take with you, and sleep under, a mosquito net at all times. A net is an excellent protection and prevention from insect bites that could result in malaria, elephantiasis, sleeping sickness, and many other tropical diseases.

Many an enthusiastic traveller may find the joys and expectations he is looking forward to dampened by so many precautionary measures and warnings. However, it is better to be sensible and take precautions, because being forewarned one can guard against any perilous circumstances to which one might otherwise fall victim. Among my closest friends I can count many who have had to pay dearly for their inexperience and ignorance of the hidden dangers awaiting the innocent traveller in the tropics, especially in recent years. Others, who have been obliged to live in the tropics for extended periods, have returned home with serious diseases or have died prematurely.

The precautionary measures mentioned in this section are not meant to spoil your expectations and joys of travelling; rather, they should serve as warnings and guidelines to help you to be adequately prepared before undertaking a trip. Preparation does not mean cumbersome equipment added to the weight of your already heavy baggage. In fact, it is only a question of some valuable advice upon which you can draw when the need arises. The old adage 'An ounce of prevention is worth a pound of cure' is of special importance to the traveller in the tropics. For further hints and suggestions on this topic see my book *Health Guide Through Southern Countries, Subtropics, Tropics, and Desert Zones.*

The Liver and Gallbladder

Causes and Symptoms of Liver Disorders
More and more people are beginning to realise that the liver is one of our most important organs and needs to be kept functioning properly. Since the liver does not send out an alarm until a disorder has made considerable progress, it is to our advantage to be especially aware of certain symptoms which can serve as early warnings. If we know and understand the various causes of liver trouble, we will be in a good position to take precautionary measures and protect this vital organ.

Almost 50 per cent of the people in Switzerland, my native country, are ill because they are overfed. The variety of things available to satisfy their palate is too great. So overindulgence is largely responsible for their disorders, whereas the opposite is true in the Far East where malnutrition is the cause of liver problems. It is astonishing to find that even in countries where rice is grown and is the staple food, only white rice is sold at the market. The only exceptions are in rural areas where the peasants prepare their own natural, or brown, rice. Generally, however, the people like only white rice and prefer to buy and cook it. The majority of the population is totally ignorant of the nutritional value of brown rice and of the many benefits it offers in its natural state as compared to denatured white rice. True, in Switzerland and elsewhere ignorance prevails as well, but at least rice is not our principal food.

If certain eating habits in Japan, Korea and China were not adhered to, the resulting deficiency of minerals would be disastrous. One habit in those countries that contributes to their good health is that they eat kelp (seaweed) as part of their daily diet. The minerals contained in ocean kelp are able to counterbalance to a great extent the deficiency caused by eating white rice. Calcium and fluoride, however, are not contained in kelp. A deficiency of these two minerals affects the teeth and this accounts for the widespread tooth decay among those people. It is only in rural or primitive areas where the people retain their teeth because of a natural wholefood diet. For instance, I have seen really beautiful teeth among the Fiji islanders.

WORMS AND LIVER DAMAGE

Unadulterated, unrefined, natural food helps to keep the liver healthy and efficient. If natural wholefood has been replaced by denatured, refined food, the cause of liver disorders may be attributed partly to this unhappy change. However, if refined food is not the reason, then a damaged liver can be the result of an infection, possibly caused by the widespread problem of parasitic worms.

In Japan, Korea, and other lands where the bad practice exists of fertilising vegetables with human excrement from a cesspit, the majority of the population are infested with worms. One of these parasites, the dangerous hookworm, can even kill its victim. Another species settles in the liver and also ruins one's life, albeit slowly.

In other areas amoebas are a constant danger, and this goes not only for the Far East but also the Near East. Amoebas can be transmitted when eating salads or other raw vegetables and fruit. They can also be passed on by people who are themselves infested with these insidious parasites. Uncleanness is only one way in which their transmission to healthy persons is possible. It is important to establish if these dangerous parasites have invaded our organism as quickly as possible, and do something about them before they are able to get to the liver via the intestines and the bile duct. Because once they have reached the liver they can destroy their host, slowly but surely. So, when travelling in the Far and Near East, never eat uncooked food or drink the water. Even fruit that can be peeled should first be thoroughly cleaned so that the parasites which stick to the fruit skins do not attach themselves to your hands while peeling it. If you fail to do this the amoebas can be transferred from the hands to the peeled parts and enter your system. You can therefore appreciate the great risk you are exposed to and it would be wise to always carry some disinfectant for cleaning the skin of fruit. I am sure you will agree that this precautionary measure is better than contracting some disease through carelessness, or even dying from the consequences. Friends I have visited in these areas often complained about a typical pain on the right side in the liver region. You cannot be too careful, for even a common attack of dysentery can permanently damage your health.

UNMISTAKABLE SYMPTOMS

It is an unmistakable symptom that the liver is somehow out of order when the patient can no longer stand the sight or smell of fatty or fried food. For instance, if you cannot tolerate fried potatoes any longer although they used to be a favourite dish, you can be sure that you are suffering from a liver disorder, which will need careful attention. Another symptom of a liver problem is an extreme sensitivity to fruit, for example, oranges or orange juice suddenly upset you, or stone fruits no longer agree with you. In this case your liver has lost its ability to digest the fruit acid. A further liver symptom may be seen in an irksome itching that can turn out to be so unbearable that you would like to scratch until you bleed. An insatiable sensation of thirst can also be considered as a symptom of liver disorder, unless, of course, it is a sign of pancreatic insufficiency or even diabetes.

On the other hand, emotional breakdown is a typical symptom of liver trouble. We feel depressed, everything seems dismal, without our really knowing why we feel that way. Nothing cheers us up anymore and we are usually morose and in a bad mood. Instead of seeking the cause of the problem within ourselves we are more of the opinion that the whole world is against us. So, when others in the family confirm that we are often quite unbearable, we can be sure that our liver is out of order.

CHANGED ENVIRONMENT

What has contributed to our having become much more sensitive than our forefathers were? Well, was not their life very different before the advent of fast-developing technology? And is it not true that two world wars have made our life more restless and less secure? Air pollution caused by various exhaust fumes is no basis for good health; neither is the threat of increasing radioactivity in the air, a relatively recent peril.

In spite of greater affluence in some parts of the world, we are burdened with greater anxieties than in the past. Although modern technology has made some heavy jobs easier and even takes care of them altogether, we seem to have less time than ever before. The paraffin lamp disappeared long ago; in those days its dim light did not allow anyone to work late into the night. Years ago people enjoyed the few hours after coming home from work, whereas today artificial light makes the day longer. Years ago people went to bed early and got up in the early morning to start a good day's work with renewed strength. Today, however, work or pleasure

241

continues late into the night, resulting in overtiredness. Our quota of sleep is cut short and is far from invigorating, and the next morning we wake up feeling in a bad mood, remaining so all day long. Is there any wonder that our liver will be affected by such a life-style? Constant hassle and worry, anxieties and fear, the mad rush of our daily lives are all bad for it. The old, traditional customs and habits needed to remain healthy have all gone.

Indeed, we do not even make the time to sit down and eat our meals in peace anymore. But if you are not willing to take your time when eating, you will one day have to take it being ill. For it is inevitable that we will harm our health if we do not learn to relax in spite of the daily hustle and bustle around us. Instead of listening to an exciting news item on the radio or, worse, reading the newspaper while eating, we should relax and make every meal a special occasion with the family. Instead of gulping down our food in a hurry, we should enjoy it calmly, eat it slowly, insalivating well and chewing everything thoroughly. In fact, every fast eater should be condemned to eating with chopsticks, as it is the custom in the Far East. You see, this technique takes more than just practice and skill, it takes patience, because if you are fidgety and restless you will hardly be able to keep any morsel between the sticks and pass it to your mouth. I am convinced that eating with chopsticks is a wonderful method for learning how to eat in a relaxed and quiet way!

Worries, anxieties and fear engender nothing but agitation – and upset the proper secretion of digestive juices. A simple illustration will prove this point. An angry, aggressive dog will not digest its food properly. It will lie around listlessly, discontented and sullen, unwilling to eat its food when it is time to do so, actually refusing to touch anything. The dog's organism is influenced by the mood forced upon it. Newfoundlands are known to lose their appetite when they feel sad or upset. But the animal takes a much more natural approach to the problem than we do. Instead of looking for some favourite food, the dog simply fasts; it does not eat at all until the disturbance has passed and it is well again. Years ago, fasting was customary for many people, but today most of us think we would die if we did not get our meals at the usual times. Only in times of privation do such people prove that their health is actually better than they had believed it to be. If it were not so, the enormous streams of refugees from war and famine would have few survivors. No, believe me, sensible fasting will not kill but benefit us, and will benefit the liver in particular.

Even if we are knowledgeable in matters of nutrition and diet, and a day's fast presents no problem, the liver may still give problems when we are constantly under pressure because of worries, anxieties and frustration. Do not be surprised if you begin to suffer from a liver disorder when constant stress and anxieties assail you. A sensible attitude toward questions of nutrition is only helpful if our mental and emotional attitude is also right. Of course, it is not always easy in today's world to keep one's balance. There is really no better help in our daily struggle with worries of one kind and another than a calm and collected spirit. If we remain calm we will be able to shut out of our minds all distractions, retain our mental tranquillity and thus provide the best protective remedy for the liver.

Liver Disorders and Nutrition
What conclusion about the liver can we draw from what has been said above? No doubt we are more aware of the need to protect it and if some disorder should arise, we can treat it properly if we are well informed about the right kind of food to eat. For if we ignore the question of diet, we should not be surprised if deficiencies and weaknesses will not respond to treatment. Furthermore, we must be willing to continue observing the basic requirements of a sensible liver diet even after having achieved a significant improvement in our condition. It must be remembered that the liver, despite having recovered from the disorder, is usually still quite sensitive and not immediately as strong as it was previously. That is why it is advisable to be sensible. After all, it should not be all that difficult to keep up a good habit rather than give it up and have a relapse.

THE PROBLEM OF FAT
It is generally known that the liver is highly sensitive to fats when it is suffering from some disorder or disturbance. However, one cannot cut out fat altogether since the liver needs some unsaturated fatty acids in order to function properly. It is therefore important not to use any fat in which the unsaturated fatty acids have been destroyed. Heated fat should also be avoided. In fact, the basic rule for liver patients is eliminate all fried foods from your diet.

If you understand and observe this rule, you will have come to grips with a liver diet. You will then abstain from potatoes and onions fried in butter, oil or any other fat; this includes sauté potatoes and French fries or chips. If you want to help your liver recover, you will not indulge in such food however delicious it may be. Meat fried in fat will also be off your menu. As a matter of fact, any kind of dish requiring frying or baking in fat is out. Butter must no longer be used in cooking. Natural oils such as sunflower, sesame, linseed or any other cold-pressed oils may be used in limited quantities in the preparation of salads, because, strangely enough, a moderate amount of these natural, unrefined and unadulterated oils is actually good for the liver. The problem of fat is therefore one that needs careful consideration and the right solution.

This does not mean that a healthy person must be just as careful as a liver patient, but it certainly would do him no harm to heed the advice given regarding oils and fats. A little less fat would mean less strain on the system, although this fact may be disputed by those cooks who adhere to the old-fashioned opinion that we need plenty of fat to keep healthy and fit. This is untrue because the body benefits more from a modest intake of fat, since it is able to produce its own anyway. People who become obese even though they consume very little fat will confirm the truth of this statement. Just think of those who drink a lot of beer. The malt supplies the carbohydrates, which in turn produce unwanted fat deposits. We do not need much fat, although we think we might. In fact, we could reduce our fat consumption by half and still be well nourished. It would not cause a deficiency, nor would it lead to ill health. On the contrary, it would increase our chances of maintaining good health. It is an excessive intake of fat that is responsible for ill health.

THE PROTEIN PROBLEM

Once we have learned what kind and how much fat we need, we should take a closer look at the question of protein, because the liver needs a supply of good protein for maximum efficiency. Pulses, that is, peas, beans and lentils, as well as milk, are excellent sources of protein. Milk protein is the best type for the liver. Not only the sick person benefits from protein taken in the form of sour milk, yogurt, or cottage cheese and curds, but anyone who is healthy too.

If a patient suffering from a liver disorder wishes to eat some meat protein, the meat should be grilled, never fried. Avoid fatty cuts or meat that was cooked in its own fat. Very lean, muscular meat, preferably veal or beef, is the best for the patient who thinks he cannot do without it. Since pork is the most harmful of all meats, it should be eliminated from the diet. Among the divine laws given to the Israelites was one forbidding them to eat pork and, as it so happened, this abstinence proved to be in the interest of their health.

Fish protein is a food that should not be overlooked. It is important, however, that only fresh fish is used and that it is prepared with the utmost care. If fish is slightly tainted the danger of poisoning is very high, and if fish is not carefully cleaned there is the additional danger of poisoning because it may have swallowed some toxic dead matter that still remains in its entrails. Fish poisoning is especially damaging to the liver. Be particularly careful in southern regions where food goes off relatively quickly. Since fish tend to consume anything they see in front of them, they represent an immediate danger if eaten by the unsuspecting. I once watched a sick man spit into a lake somewhere in Switzerland. At once a trout surfaced and swallowed the unusual bait. Yet it could well have been the sputum of a consumptive. And it is not impossible to imagine that the fish might have been caught and served up on one's table the next day! Well, that's enough of that. The final point to remember is that should a liver patient want to enjoy some fish for a change, heed the advice given and either grill or poach it.

Eggs are also a source of protein and many people like to include them in their diet. But hard-boiled eggs, omelettes and egg salads are hard on the liver and should be avoided by anyone with a liver problem; indeed, it would be better for them to have meat rather than eggs. It is important to make sure that the eggs we consume are fresh and come from healthy chickens raised on natural feed. An egg is better for you when eaten raw, since in its liquid state an egg can be considered a valuable source of nutrients. This can also be said of soft-boiled eggs (for 2–3 minutes). Eggs are harmful, however, for anyone suffering from rheumatism or arthritis. Acting on this knowledge can only be of benefit to you.

I would like to stress the importance of making sure the eggs are safe, if you like to eat them raw, because the diseases chickens suffer from can be transmitted through their eggs. This is a problem that has received considerable publicity in recent years, particularly in the United Kingdom, and people should not forget the fact that it poses a very real danger to their health.

It is a good thing that there are other, even better sources of protein than eggs. Soybeans, for example, are an excellent supplier of vegetable protein. In certain areas of China soybean protein is the single most important protein available to the population. The lack of animal protein from milk and meat is critical in many tropical regions. Years ago the need for protein presented a particular problem for the growing population of China. Since meat was not produced in sufficient quantity to supply over 500 million people, China's population at that time, it became necessary to find a vegetable substitute. The soybean was selected because it is an excellent source of protein, able to take the place of animals as the prime supplier. In many parts of the world today the Chinese custom of germinating the soybean has been adopted and the resulting product, 'bean sprouts', has become a popular and palatable vegetable dish rich in protein.

Remember, then, that liver patients need protein too; vegetables and cereals alone are not enough. As mentioned before, milk protein, especially in the form of cottage cheese or curds, is the best protein source available in this case.

HEALTHY SEASONING

The proper seasoning of food prepared for those who suffer from a liver disorder is very important, since the liver is influenced by it for good or for bad. I must warn against certain Indian dishes because the spices are so hot that they affect the mucous membranes of the stomach. They begin to play up and may actually stop working for a few days. The palate does not necessarily like the spices either and may still feel on fire half an hour after eating the strange food. Does it not go to show that even herbal spices need to be used in the right amount? It is not good to use excessive quantities, which will only affect the liver adversely. Many Indian people have yellow mixed in with the white of the eyes, no doubt a symptom of an affected liver. Indeed, their blood sometimes contains a yellowish-red bile substance. The two main causes of this can be found in their spicy food and widespread infestation with worms. This shows that one should use spices sparingly.

Of course, if we did not season our food at all we would soon lose our appetite. It is true that bland food does not appeal to our tastebuds; instead, it can make us go off food altogether. The herbs we can sow or plant in the garden are sometimes also sold at the market. They are the basis for mild yet tasty seasoning. However, be careful with pepper, nutmeg and similar spices; better still, avoid them completely, since they are able to cause a lot of upsets. Peppers are an exception, if they are eaten only occasionally in small quantities and do not upset your digestion.

A suggested diet for the liver patient is given below. Further details about diets and care of the liver are given in the well-known book *The Liver, the Regulator of Your Health*. This book contains some excellent menus for meals, recipes and, of course, dietary instructions.

DIET FOR LIVER PATIENTS

As a good diet for the liver we suggest the following:

Morning: one glass of carrot juice; a slice of toast or crispbread with a little butter or yeast extract; a soupspoon of wheat germ, either dry or in the carrot juice.

Midday: vegetable soup; brown rice or potatoes boiled in their skins; chicory and raw carrot salad, or any other raw salad vegetable, preferably the bitter kind. Steamed vegetables may also be added. All fried and sweet dishes and desserts must be avoided.

You can vary the lunch menu as follows:
First day: brown rice; fennel root; mixed salad.
Second day: potatoes boiled in their skins, with a little cottage cheese and fresh butter; mixed salad.
Third day: vegetable soup; sandwiches made with rye or wholewheat bread or crispbread, spread with a little butter and yeast extract, topped with onion, garlic, sliced tomatoes; mixed salad.

A little while after the meal you can have a cup of cereal coffee (*Bambu Coffee Substitute*) with milk but no sugar.

Evening: soup made with oats, barley or brown rice with a few vegetables added; mixed salad, seasoned with lemon juice or sour milk, but never with vinegar. For the sake of variety, sandwiches and different salads may be served, followed by cereal coffee with a little milk.

Always remember that fruit is taboo while the liver is out of order.

SESAME SEEDS — EXCELLENT FOR THE LIVER

Modern life with its restlessness and worries, as well as all other detrimental influences, puts a great strain on the liver, this important organ in our body. To allay our concern, it is always good to be reminded of some simple remedies, one of which is *sesame seed*. There is nothing easier than eating sesame seeds every day for the sake of your health. You will never tire of this delicacy if you sprinkle it on your bread. I recommend this practice to all who suffer from liver problems and depend on high-quality oil and vegetable protein, but also to anyone else who wishes to protect and care for his liver and keep it sound.

In addition to eating the seeds you can also use *sesame oil*, a good source of highly unsaturated fatty acids, as well as vitamin E, which is good for the glands. It definitely benefits our health if we eat sesame seeds regularly. They contain a protein with eight essential amino acids and vitamins of the B complex which are important for cell oxygenation and thus have a favourable influence on the liver cells.

The neutral flavour of sesame seeds makes them useful for fruit salads, if sprinkled over the salad or mixed in with it, or they can be used in a similar way for vegetable salads and vegetables in general. These varied uses increase our opportunities to benefit from their goodness.

Cracked sesame seeds can also be added to wholefood muesli. And if you suffer from some kind of internal inflammation, you can still benefit from the seeds by taking them finely ground and made into an emulsion. This preparation will cause you no trouble whatsoever, however sensitive your system may be.

The sesame plant grows in subtropical soil and contains the region's abundant energy from the sun. In temperate zones you can usually buy the seeds from healthfood stores. Once you have come to appreciate their excellent effect on the bowel movement, you will never want to do without them. Unfortunately, the benefits of sesame seeds are still not as widely known as they should be. So do not only use them yourself, but recommend them to your friends, especially to those who suffer from some type of liver disorder.

Everyone in the Near East, particularly in Palestine, knows the sesame plant, uses and cherishes it. There, the seeds are sold under the quaint name 'sumsum'. Seeds have always played an important part in the nutrition of primitive or aboriginal peoples. The gathering of all kinds of seeds has always been vital in areas of the world where there is limited variety regarding food. Sometimes it is the little things that provide supplementary benefits, and this can certainly be said about sesame seeds. Let us therefore not ignore the seeds because they are so small, but enjoy them to the full.

Treating Infectious Diseases of the Liver and Gallbladder
There are a number of liver and gallbladder disorders that can come about through infection. The patient feels sick and brings up bile; he has diarrhoea and sickness and in some cases develops a slight attack of jaundice. Such symptoms call for great care.

The first thing the patient should be given to drink is *clay water*; either white or yellow clay will do, a teaspoon of clay to a small wine glass of warm water (100 ml glass, about 3½ fl. oz). Add several drops of *Lachesis 10x* or *12x* to the clay water. The effect is greater still if 10–20 drops of *Echinaforce* are also added. The patient needs to go without any food for two or three days, drinking nothing but clay water. After this time he will perhaps feel a little hungry and can then try a peeled and finely grated apple, or he can eat it whole but chew it well. To quench his thirst he can take sour whey – one teaspoon of *Molkosan* to 100ml (about 3½ fl. oz) of water – or he can drink fruit juice, such as grapefruit, raspberry, blackberry or non-alcoholic grape juice. Sip and insalivate well before swallowing. If the patient is still very sensitive he may not be able to drink anything but freshly pressed carrot juice. But let me repeat, the juice must be sipped slowly.

Solid food should be avoided at this stage, because the disturbance will be cleared up much faster if the patient fasts. Rehabilitation will only be delayed by burdening the digestive system with food. In cases where the patient vomits bile, be sure to give him liquids afterwards. *Horsetail (shave grass)* or better still, *dandelion tea* will be excellent. You can use dandelion leaves and roots to make the infusion. An extract of dandelion called *Taraxacum* will be found most effective in such cases. Avoid cereal gruels, because they always contain some fat and in the digestive process the liver will be irritated. Taking solid food can serve no useful purpose and, again, the value of fasting during the first few days cannot be overemphasised.

Once the grated apple and any of the various fruit juices can be digested and the patient feels hungry again, try giving him wholefood muesli for breakfast and supper. At midday, a little salad may be eaten, taking care that the dressing contains only a little cold-pressed, unrefined vegetable oil, or no oil to start with, just lemon juice or Molkosan. For several days after recovery fried foods of any kind should be avoided, because a certain degree of sensitivity will remain. Even slightly heated oil or animal fat will soon cause the feeling of congestion in the back of the head or in the forehead to return. A peculiar feeling of nausea may manifest itself also,

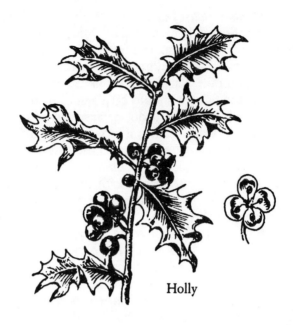

Holly

even though it may be slight. Until all germs, which may or may not be known, have been eliminated from the system, the normal diet should not be reintroduced.

No liver complaint should be treated lightly, but if the patient follows the advice given, he will soon be on the mend. *Solidago*, as usual, should be taken to stimulate the kidneys. *Horsetail* and *witch grass root tea* are alternatives. If the patient runs a temperature, and it is not unusual for it to reach 39 °C (102 °F), then *Ferrum phos. 12x, diluted holly infusion, Aconitum 4x* or any other good fever remedy is called for. A daily dose of one or two tablets of *Podophyllum 3x*, and according to the circumstances, three or four drops of *Chelidonium 4x* or the combination remedy *Boldocynara* should be taken. Condensed carrot juice, *Biocarottin*, is also beneficial.

My book *The Liver, the Regulator of Your Health* answers all questions relating to the liver and gallbladder in full detail.

Oil Cure for Gallstones
Serious thought should be given to trying the oil cure for the elimination of gallstones if the patient is willing and thinks he can take 300–500 ml (½–¾ pint) of oil in one go. Some might assume

that this treatment works by the oil entering the gallbladder and cleansing it, but this is not so. The oil merely stimulates the profuse secretion of bile. It could be said that it causes a flood of bile which carries the small and medium-sized stones with it.

The oil used for this treatment should be unrefined. Whether it is the highly unsaturated fatty acids that make it more effective than refined oil has not yet been determined, although it seems quite possible. Unrefined olive, walnut, sunflower and poppy seed oils are all suitable.

Before carrying out the cure, it would be useful to take a natural plant remedy that helps to liquify the bile, for example *Boldocynara* made from artichokes and other medicinal herbs.

For the best results, it will also be necessary to give the bowels a good clean-out beforehand. Soaked *prunes or figs*, freshly ground *linseed* or *Linoforce*, and *psyllium seed* will serve this purpose very well. But if they do not move the bowels sufficiently, give an *enema* with a warm *camomile infusion* in addition. To help even further, *hot packs* should be applied to the liver area for a few hours before and after drinking the oil. As soon as the bowels have been emptied you can take the oil. That accomplished, lie down, turn over on your right side, relax, and remain in this position for two hours. If you find it difficult to drink the oil by itself, try to take it in alternation with a cereal coffee (*Bambu Coffee Substitute*). Should even this prove to be obnoxious, you will then have to ingest the required quantity of oil spaced out, a little at a time taken over several days. This method will not be quite so effective, but at least the smaller stones may be eliminated and the remaining bigger ones may not cause any trouble for a while. However, anyone who is capable of drinking the whole quantity of oil at one time should not be surprised if all the stones are eliminated from the gallbladder. Of course, this is more likely to occur in cases which have not become chronic and where no large stones are present.

If a chronic condition suddenly flares up again, accompanied by a high temperature and an increase in the number of white blood corpuscles, there is most likely an inflammation. In that case, the patient unfortunately has no alternative but to undergo surgery to remove the gallbladder. This is not the ultimate solution, however, because after the operation condensed bile will no longer be available; it cannot accumulate as it previously had done in the gallbladder that now no longer exists. The bile entering the duodenum will always be thin and fresh and if digestive disturbances are to be avoided, a protein- and fat-restricted diet will have to be

251

adopted thereafter. Thus, if the oil treatment can bring the desired cure, the patient will escape the need for surgery and the undesirable consequences it brings with it.

Jaundice

Jaundice is much more dangerous than is generally assumed. People who have suffered from it confirm that once they have had it, they never feel the same again. They also notice that fried foods and sweet things no longer agree with them.

A case of jaundice must not be taken lightly. There are two types of jaundice: one is caused by an obstruction or blockage of the bile duct and the other is a result of infection. Both are serious. As part of the treatment the patient must abstain from fats and fried foods for quite some time. The bowels must be thoroughly cleansed and the bile must be liquified by taking the following remedies: *Chelidonium 4x* and *Podophyllum 4x*, or *Boldocynara*, as well as *Biocarottin*, condensed carrot juice. Moreover, take plenty of fresh *carrot juice* daily, at least 100 ml (3½ fl. oz), but preferably more. *Warm water treatments* will help considerably and should always be given, either by placing a hot herbal compress over the liver or directing a shower of warm water onto the liver area. Afterwards, apply *cabbage leaf poultices*, alternating daily with *clay poultices*. At the same time the kidneys should be stimulated by drinking *kidney tea* and taking *Solidago* or *Nephrosolid*. Besides goldenrod, other suitable herbs to stimulate the kidneys are *horsetail, couch grass root, birch leaves* and the mildly acting *rose hips*. Even when the doctor pronounces the patient well, the treatment should on no account be stopped. The special diet must be continued for some time, likewise the use of poultices and warm water treatments.

When treating a case of jaundice it is always important to take care of the bowels. If regular movement is lacking, *herbal enemas* should be given to open the bowels. The bile must be removed from the blood as quickly as possible, for the longer it remains in the system and the more concentrated it is, the greater the harm that will result.

Beware of modern proprietary medicines for the treatment of jaundice. They invariably only serve to mask and suppress the symptoms and serious complications can follow their use. It is much wiser to let the illness take its normal course and assist the body with natural remedies. Even so, the healing process takes time and cannot be unduly hurried. Most cases under the supervision of an allopathic doctor will take 6–8 weeks of treatment. But if you employ the recommended natural therapy with its various measures, a cure can be achieved in two weeks in some cases. However, it must not be considered complete until the follow-up treatment has been carried out conscientiously as well. If these measures are neglected, the patient may be left with some permanent damage.

Anyone who has had jaundice should, especially in the spring, eat plenty of *dandelion salad. Artichokes, chicory*, and all bitter herbs and salad vegetables are also excellent for the liver. The various kinds of *radish* are considered medicinal and should for this reason be taken in moderate amounts, but too many can do more harm than good. And never forget to drink carrot juice, as I have already mentioned on different occasions.

If this advice is followed and the follow-up cure is faithfully adhered to, the jaundice patient will fully recuperate and suffer no unpleasant consequences.

The Pancreas
Next to the liver, the most important organ in our digestive system is the pancreas, yet it weighs only about one-twentieth of that of the liver. This small, elongated gland is located above the navel between the posterior stomach wall and the spine; below it lies the horseshoe-shaped loop of the first part of the small intestine. The left end touches the spleen and the left kidney. Small it may be, but it performs two important functions, producing an external secretion to be poured into the duodenum and an internal one to be poured into the blood.

The pancreas secretes only about one-fifth of the amount of juice produced by the much smaller salivary glands, yet its secretion is much more concentrated and important. As many as four enzymes are secreted into the small intestine immediately adjacent to the bile duct. One of these enzymes, rennin, is also produced in the stomach. It turns milk into curds, a job that is mainly done by the stomach. When the stomach fails to function effectively the pancreas has a marvellous capacity to take on part of the stomach's work load, since it can produce rennin just as efficiently as the stomach. Diastase, or amylase, changes starches into sugars, such as glycogen, dextrin and maltose. Trypsin, like pepsin, breaks down proteins into peptones and finally into the basic building blocks of protein, amino acids. The fourth enzyme, lipase, together with the bile, hydrolises fats into fatty acids and glycerol. In fact, the body cannot break down, digest and assimilate proteins, starches and fats without the enzymes secreted by the pancreas.

Neither the bile nor the pancreatic enzymes are fully efficient if the juice in the small intestine and the bacterial flora are not normal. So you can see that the digestive process involves a complicated series of relationships between many individual factors. If everyone understood this fact and fully appreciated the implications, they would no doubt make a greater effort to live more carefully and watch what they eat and drink. Excesses endanger the wonderful interplay of the digestive organs and the glandular functions.

What makes us marvel most in our quest to understand these fascinating relationships is the fact that these organs are fully automatic in their functions. We eat something and immediately the message is sent via the nerves to the cerebellum; at once another message is sent back to the intestine, the liver and the pancreas. The necessary enzymes are immediately made ready for the arrival of the food. Of course, the entire process goes on without our having to think or do anything about it. What a marvellous thing! No wonder the Bible psalmist once gratefully acknowledged that 'in an awe-inspiring way we are wonderfully made'. Anyone who fully understands this will, and can, never accept the theory of evolution. The wisdom and intelligence of a Creator's design, even in the smallest detail, is much too obvious. No sound reasoning could ever deny Creation. So let us continue our research into the wonderful secrets of the human body, for the more we understand them the stronger the proof of the Creator's power.

Embedded in the pancreas we find some peculiar cell formations, shaped rather like blackberries. They are actually small glands, but not in the least connected with the other glands. Like islands in the bigger gland, they are called the islets of Langerhans, after their discoverer, Paul Langerhans. The vital substance insulin is produced in these small glands and sent straight into the blood, not the small intestine. If these islets do not manufacture sufficient insulin, the glycogen, the sugar stored in the liver and passed on to the blood in accordance with the body's need, will not be burned up, so that the blood sugar level rises. The excess is excreted through the kidneys, which is why sugar is found in the urine. This is a symptom of the disease known as diabetes.

Proper Care of the Pancreas

Diabetics and anyone who has bad digestion need to know what to do to help the pancreas function efficiently. Since the blood carries nutrients and remedial substances to the parts of the body it can reach, the primary requirement is to stimulate the circulation. Take *hot showers* or apply *moist hot packs* for this purpose; herbal packs are especially good. As regards medicines, only few are known to act specifically on the pancreas. One such, sour whey as contained in *Molkosan*, is rich in rennin and lactic acid and gives good results. Years ago, *fermented bedstraw (Galium aparine* or cleavers) used to be prescribed with modest success. Of course, *papaya* preparations can be used to good effect, since their papain content helps to digest protein. *Lycopodium 6x* (club moss) is useful too.

You can also set aside days for *fasting* and *raw vegetable diets*, their effect being very encouraging. My book *The Liver, the Regulator of Your Health* contains instructions for diets that are good for the pancreas as well as the liver. A number of food items must be avoided completely, for example all boiled protein foods and the combination of fat, protein and sugar, either cooked or fried. Hot spices should also be avoided; use culinary herbs from the garden instead. The protein foods best tolerated are sour milk products. Prepare salads with a little cold-pressed oil and Molkosan. Of curative effect are bilberry (blueberry) juice, blackcurrant juice, weak herb teas, and occasionally a little buttermilk.

As already stated, fasting is an excellent means of resting the pancreas. Moreover, whatever the patient eats, it is important to ingest small quantities, chew everything thoroughly and insalivate well before swallowing. These are inexpensive ways and means of supporting the pancreas in the healing process. If you feel a slight pain after eating, you have probably had something that did not agree with you, did not chew your food well enough, drank too fast or ate too much. The answer to the problem is in the patient himself; he should watch himself carefully to avoid unpleasant reactions.

Regular deep-breathing exercises, with diaphragm-breathing, practised in the open air are also effective and promote the healing process at the same time. In conclusion, then, breathing exercises, together with a proper diet, warm water therapy and moist hot herbal packs, will help to rectify any condition where the pancreas is weak or upset. Many a serious, chronic ailment can be prevented if its proper function is restored. All it needs is a little understanding and perseverance with the treatment.

A Diet for Diabetics

Diabetics need to pay special attention to their diet. In contrast with most other diseases, diabetes makes the patient want to eat more. To solve the question of diet, we must therefore see to it that he eats an adequate amount of food but with the proviso that it does not consist of too many carbohydrates. This can be achieved by giving the diabetic primarily vegetables, which are rich in vitamins but low in carbohydrates.

Lacto-vegetarians obtain their protein requirements from milk products, especially sour milk, buttermilk and soft white cheese (cottage cheese or quark). If the patient is used to eating meat, he must restrict himself to only small quantities of lean, muscular cuts of meat. The following menu for one day can be taken as a model.

BREAKFAST

Take your pick from buttermilk, sour milk or cereal coffee (*Bambu Coffee Substitute*). For a change, you can sometimes have yogurt.

Make sandwiches using rye bread, flake bread, wholemeal bread or crispbread. There is also a special diet crispbread available for diabetics. Spread the bread with soft white cheese, maybe 'Gervais' fermented skimmed milk cheese or cottage cheese.

Garnish the sandwich with tomato slices or culinary herbs, such as parsley, chives or freshly grated horseradish.

If you prefer fruit for breakfast, follow my second menu:

Bambu coffee with cream, fruit muesli with rye flakes, whole rice flakes or All Bran, a well-known commercial cereal product. Use only fresh fruit in season. Bilberries (blueberries), blackcurrants and apples are particularly beneficial. Add some sesame seeds or grated almonds, but no sugar. When the berry season is over, use natural fruit juices with no additives.

MIDDAY MEAL (LUNCH)

Soya mix rissoles, creamy cottage cheese or curds with horseradish and a seasonal vegetable, either steamed or au gratin.

In addition, a large plate of salad made up of various raw vegetables is most important. Make your choice according to what is seasonally available. White cabbage, raw sauerkraut with no additives, lettuce and, above all, plenty of cress, as well as nasturtiums are all excellent. Prepare the dressing from *Molkosan* and cream; whey is very good for activating the pancreas.

For this reason diluted Molkosan is also recommended as a drink. For a change, have a cup of *Bambu Coffee Substitute* with a little cream after your meal. What you should avoid, however, are beverages containing chemical additives.

If you like meat, another typical menu is as follows:

Grilled veal or beef; steamed vegetables; and a mixed salad, as explained in my first example. Choose either diluted Molkosan or sour buttermilk to drink.

EVENING MEAL (SUPPER)

You would do well to eat only a light meal at night. For this reason, follow the suggestions given for breakfast. For a change, you might try the following:

Vegetable or sesame soup; a vegetable baked in the oven or steamed tomatoes; and a small plate of mixed salad or raw natural sauerkraut.

INTRODUCING VARIETY

You must provide for a little variety, however, so that the diet does not become monotonous and one tires of it. This can be achieved by varying the combination of the items mentioned or varying their preparation. If loving hands prepare the food, it is always possible to find new ways of presenting it. For instance, diet pasta for diabetics can be used instead of soya mixes, bran mixes or sesame dishes.

Horseradish and cress have a healing effect on the pancreas and should be used as often as possible. From time to time, mix in a little finely chopped mugwort, another herb which has a beneficial effect on the pancreas. Diabetics can also use onions to season their food. Another good seasoning is yeast extract. Spread *Herbaforce* extremely thinly on bread and cover with onion slices. This is excellent for the pancreas because it includes both yeast and onion. A word of advice for diabetics is to make a conscious effort to eat slowly, to chew everything well and insalivate properly. This will help to utilise the food more effectively and to satisfy one's hunger more quickly. Even though the diabetic has a greater craving for food, it is not advisable to eat too much, since the excess will only place a greater demand on the digestive system. For this reason it is extremely important that the patient eats only natural whole-foods that are rich in nutrients.

Multiple Sclerosis

Just hearing the name of this disease can inspire fear. It is a strange disease, progressive and insidious, and it can have tragic consequences for the rest of one's life. Multiple sclerosis, often abbreviated to MS, is not known among people in less developed parts of the world, where the diet is still 100 per cent natural and unadulterated. Hence it must be a disease of our modern civilised world, a typical disease caused by civilisation.

The Real Cause

It is understandable that we want to know the cause of an illness, and it is no different with multiple sclerosis. Unfortunately, however, the cause of this dreaded affliction has not yet been conclusively pinpointed despite continuous research. Although there is no certainty, the symptoms seem to suggest a pathogenic agent, but it has not yet been identified. It is also thought that the reason that some people are susceptible to this agent is probably a deficiency of some vital substances.

The Symptoms

The symptoms of multiple sclerosis are not always the same, so that the identity of the disease sometimes escapes diagnosis, especially in its early stages. One of the earliest symptoms is often the absence of the abdominal reflex. A fairly reliable diagnostic sign concerns the optic nerves. In this case, by using an ophthalmoscope the eye specialist will observe demyelination where the optic nerve enters at the back of the eye.

There is no doubt that multiple sclerosis is a progressive disease of the central nervous system. It rarely strikes before the age of twenty or after the age of forty. Women sometimes fall victim to it after giving birth and men after an accident or a neglected infectious disease. The first signs of illness may also be a disturbance in the sensory nerves, especially in the feet. The patient gets the feeling of walking on cotton wool and runs the risk of stumbling on uneven ground. After the attack on the sensory nerves there follows a disturbance of the nerves controlling movement, a paralysis of the limbs. A little while later, the patient begins to drag his legs, walking stiffly. In accordance with the focus of the disease, the feet and lower organs or the arms and hands, perhaps even the jaw muscles and facial muscles are involved. When the intestinal muscles or the bladder sphincter are affected or put out of action, the condition is indeed serious. As the disease progresses, the muscles of the mouth and the vocal cords can become involved, causing impairment of speech. Pain is not always present and when it is it is rarely unbearable. There may be inexplicable periods of remission, with the symptoms subsiding; or there may be a sudden worsening of the condition, a relapse. The disease may go on for decades and it is not surprising that a lot of patience and mental energy is needed, both on the part of an MS patient as well as his family and those who take care of him.

It is important to begin treatment as soon as the disease has been diagnosed, since the chances of success are then better than if it is neglected, although many orthodox medical doctors do not agree with this view, or do so only reluctantly. Years ago, a lady from eastern Switzerland came to me for treatment. Three or four doctors and a professor had diagnosed multiple sclerosis. The symptoms of paralysis were only slight to begin with. About three months later, when the lady went to see a specialist, he did not believe that she had suffered from multiple sclerosis, since she was found to be in good health. If she had had multiple sclerosis, the doctor contended, she could not be well again, because there was no cure for it and no one had so far been cured. The treatment she was given is the first of those outlined below.

Various Approaches to Treatment

TREATMENT NO. 1
This treatment is a nutritional therapy, similar to the one employed by Dr Evers. Even before Dr Evers became well known, I had based my approach on the view that the patient's diet should be kept the same as that enjoyed by the primitive people who were not affected by multiple sclerosis. That means eating plenty of raw foods and only boiling those vegetables which cannot be eaten raw. The basic diet plan includes brown rice with soft white cheese (cottage cheese or quark) and horseradish, and mixed salad. Eggs are allowed very occasionally and only when raw. Meat is left out of the diet entirely and in its place milk and soya protein are consumed. White flour products are also cut out completely. Bread is only permitted in limited quantity, and nothing but wholegrain, wholemeal and crispbread. Since canned foods cannot really be called natural or a wholefood they, too, must be avoided alto-

gether. Fruit must be natural, organically grown fruit that is in season; it can either be eaten whole or added to muesli. Honey and fruit sugar as obtained from grapes, also chopped currants, raisins and grapes are the only sweeteners permitted.

TREATMENT NO. 2

This is a stimulation therapy according to the *Baunscheidt method* or *Chinese treatment*. First the upper half of the back is treated and about ten days later the lower part. After about twenty days the treatment is repeated; once again treat the upper half of the back first and then the lower part. The same treatment is given three times, so that a total of six applications are performed. The dietary treatment will not achieve the same results in a year that this stimulation therapy can bring about in a matter of a few months. However, it is advisable to let an experienced therapist give this treatment.

A CASE HISTORY SPEAKS FOR ITSELF

Some years ago, when I was still operating a clinic, one of my patients was serving in the armed forces. He had consulted a neurologist and was given little hope of improvement. This diagnosis shattered the man's interest in life. One of his colleagues noticed his state of mind and asked him to consult me. We accepted the patient and gave him both treatments outlined above. About three months later we discharged him and I can still see the young man's happy face when he, for the first time, was able to walk with feeling in his feet.

During the course of his illness the patient described how the feeling in the nerves was returning. He noticed that it returned in the same sequence in which he had lost it in the limbs. Shortly after going home he had to surrender his military equipment and the army doctors were most surprised to see him do this personally. They asked him about the treatment he had received and one of the younger doctors was rather disparaging when he heard of it, but another doctor present, an older man, spoke up in defence of the treatment on the basis of the obvious results. The young man was very happy when he told us about the incident later on.

TREATMENT NO. 3

There is now another method of treatment available which was unknown in those earlier days. I am glad to say that it also helps considerably towards achieving a successful result. It is a fresh hormone treatment. As with the treatment of poliomyelitis, it is necessary to obtain the fresh testicles of a healthy young bull. Take off the skin and chop up the tender inside with a sharp knife or put it in the food processor. Then apply the mixture to the whole extension of the spine, from the nape of the neck to the coccyx, massaging it in vigorously. This massage treatment should be given once a week in two stages, in the evening and early the following morning. The portion to be used in the morning will need to be kept in a cool place during the night.

A TESTIMONIAL OF SUCCESS

On 31 March 1964 I received the first letter from a patient in Brussels who had been suffering from multiple sclerosis for sixteen years. A year later, on 30 April 1965, he wrote again, about the effect of the recommended treatment. His letter read as follows:

'I have been taking your reliable medicines for one year now and have very much improved. It is exactly a year since I started taking Petasites, Usneasan, Echinaforce, Aesculaforce, Urticalcin and Biocarottin regularly. Every week I receive a massage with fresh bullock testicles. My nurse always waits at the slaughterhouse when a bull is killed, so that she can get the testicles quite fresh. The massages are indeed excellent for me. But let me give you a few details of my progress. All symptoms caused by the illness – cold feet, problems with the bowel movement, insufficient urination, bad eyesight, half the head going numb – have completely disappeared. However, I am not yet able to walk. True, I can stand up now and my right foot is already 60 per cent active; only the left foot does not respond yet. But considering that I have been ill for seventeen years, I have made very good progress in just one year. May I add that I had not been able to hold a long conversation without getting tired out; but this is no longer a problem.

'Now I can watch television for hours without any difficulty, participate quite normally in conversations, and I read a lot.'

Letters like this one from our Belgian patient are indeed encouraging. They show that if we support nature it has the power to bring about a regeneration even in serious cases of illness. The patient in question had been ill for many years and I am sure that his progress and success would have been better still if the treatment could have been given right from the start. The remedies mentioned by the patient are good for raising the calcium level and curing circulatory disturbances, inflammation and spasms.

However, the remedies alone could not produce the fine results he experienced.

Considering the mental anguish multiple sclerosis patients are subjected to, it should not be too much work or trouble to apply the treatment described. It should be followed conscientiously even when the healthy person, who still has full use of his limbs, finds it hard to understand what it means to the sick to wait for years, perhaps decades, seemingly without any hope, until he is relieved of his affliction.

Arthritis and Gout

It is estimated that 4–7 per cent of the world's population are afflicted by the dreadful, painful scourge called arthritis. Two to three hundred thousand people in Switzerland have fallen victim to it and millions of people elsewhere in Europe and the United States can speak of their personal experience of arthritis, many of whom may have suffered from it for decades. Arthritis and gout mar the sufferer's happiness and can be sheer agony. It is the purpose of the following discussion to help as many of these people as possible.

Arthritis often has its origin in a chronic infection somewhere in the system. It may be the tonsils, a dental abscess or some other purulent inflammation which keep discharging minute quantities of toxins and poisonous waste products of the protein metabolism into the bloodstream. The effect is damaging to the joints and the internal organs such as the heart and kidneys. Apart from that, arthritis is definitely a disease of civilisation, the outcome of eating the wrong kinds of food and a wrong life-style. In many cases we may also have inherited a predisposition to it; we suffer the consequences of what our forefathers passed on to us, in the words of the Bible, 'Fathers are the ones that eat unripe grapes, but it is the teeth of the sons that get set on edge.'

A disturbance of the mineral metabolism makes it mandatory that we change from a diet that produces too much acid to one yielding an alkaline surplus. In the first place meat, especially sausages, cold meats, all kinds of processed meat and beef soups, as well as foods cooked with eggs and cheese, should be avoided wherever possible. If you feel you cannot give up meat entirely, at least confine yourself to freshly prepared unprocessed meat and keep off all preserved meats, sausages and processed meats.

Secondly, stay off all processed foods, white sugar, white flour products, canned foods, in other words everything that is no longer in its natural state or original form. The diet should consist of potatoes, cereals, unpolished brown rice, fresh vegetables and fresh fruit or naturally dried (unsulphured) fruit and vegetables containing no chemical additives or preservatives.

The simpler and more natural the diet, the greater will be its contribution to our all-round health, well-being and long life.

The most important remedy for arthritis is *potato juice.* It is not only its alkaline constituents which contribute to curing arthritis but possibly other, as yet unknown factors. Patients should take the juice of a potato daily and in severe cases the amount should be slowly increased. Grate the potato, squeeze out the juice and take it first thing in the morning before breakfast. It can also be taken in warm water or added to soup if you feel you cannot drink it neat. This is the most important remedy and should be taken every day. There should be no difficulty at all in obtaining potatoes anywhere on earth. Additional curative juices which should be taken daily are those of *white cabbage* and *kale,* as well as *carrot.* These principal medicinal juices should be taken every day without fail, even if only in small amounts, in addition to following a simple, natural diet. If you do not like the taste, mix the juice in with vegetables after they have been boiled or otherwise prepared. The best way to take the juices is, of course, undiluted. Sip them slowly so that they are insalivated before swallowing.

Externally, apply crushed *comfrey root* to the affected parts and you will find that the pain will gradually subside. Tincture of comfrey (*Symphosan*) is excellent also, and *butterbur (Petasites officinalis)* is a good supporting remedy. For further supportive medicine you can prepare an infusion made of *birch leaves, imperial masterwort (Imperatoria), restharrow (Ononis spinosa), anise (Pimpinella anisum), goldenrod (Solidago virgaurea), dandelion (Taraxacum)* and *meadowsweet (Spiraea.)* Naturally, the fresh plant extracts of these herbs are of excellent help too. Further recommendations are *Juniperus, Berberis vulgaris, Urtica* and, in addition, attenuated doses of *Colchicum.* These ingredients are all contained in our excellent remedy *Imperarthritica,* which should be taken as follows: five drops in a little warm water, or for better results, in potato juice, three times daily before meals. Add an extra drop every day until you reach twenty, or perhaps thirty drops if there is no sign of a severe reaction. Then reverse the procedure and decrease gradually to five drops, before increasing again to thirty drops. The dose must be adjusted to suit individual requirements even if it means reducing it to only two drops, if the effect on the respective parts or joints is strong. Imperarthritica can be used externally too: put a few drops on the hand and rub gently into the affected area. Finally, if an infection is the cause of the trouble it must be either healed or removed by other means.

Can Tomatoes Cause Cancer and Arthritis?
One often hears or reads in the newspaper that eating tomatoes encourages cancer, meaning that tomatoes could cause malignant growths. Even doctors often voice this opinion, which is based on various erroneous conclusions of certain researchers. Many patients, especially those whose parents or grandparents had cancer, ask me: 'What about tomatoes? Can I eat them?'

Cancer mortality has absolutely nothing to do with eating tomatoes. Research carried out by careful investigators has shown that cancer mortality is highest in those countries where the intake of protein, particularly animal protein, is excessive. A diet in which protein predominates can ultimately lead to the development of cancer and arthritis, especially when a predisposition towards these conditions, either inherited or acquired by inadequate nutrition, already exists.

Another factor is the constant irritation of cells through medicinal or mechanical, that is, physical, action. Chronic ailments and conditions, even constipation, can irritate the tissue to the extent that degenerative changes in the cellular system appear, which may sooner or later become malignant or cause arthritis, if the other two factors are present. Experience shows that cancer and arthritis may have the same basic causes, especially as far as incorrect eating habits and our modern life-style are concerned; it is only in their detail that they differ.

Many women say that after having received a blow or similar injury to the breast or other delicate part of the body, it has led to an induration of the tissues involved, which was later diagnosed as cancer. Needless to say, not every blow results in a tumour. If the person has no predisposition to malignancy, the immediate results of such an injury to the tissues will naturally disappear without leaving any ill effects.

Of course this has nothing to do with tomatoes! In fact, there are hundreds of cancer patients who have never eaten tomatoes in their life. If tomatoes were responsible for the disease, we should find the greatest incidence of cancer in the area around Naples, in Southern Italy, for instance, where people consume immense quantities of them. Yet I have come across few cases of cancer in this district and, indeed, mortality from this disease is extremely low there because great emphasis is put on fruit, vegetables and pasta, with very little protein other than fish being eaten. No doubt, the diet is a contributory factor to the low incidence of cancer in this area, despite their appetite for tomatoes.

Sufferers from arthritis or gout are often frightened by the same argument, that tomatoes encourage their development. This view has been propagated by researchers whose experiments have been confined to laboratories, without the necessary field work. It is true, however, that green or unripe tomatoes are not good for the health, since they contain toxic substances that are only rendered harmless by the process of ripening. But is it not also true that unripe apples, or any other unripe fruit for that matter, are detrimental to the health for exactly the same reason? Of course it is. However, it is wrong to argue that such toxins are contained in ripe fruit merely because they are found in the unripe ones. In reality, tomatoes that have fully ripened on the plant are wholesome and contain at least five different vitamins which are essential for the human body.

Rheumatoid Arthritis

Rheumatoid arthritis belongs to the category of rheumatic-arthritic diseases called 'Polyarthritis' in German, literally 'multiple arthritis', for it occurs in several joints at the same time. Did you know that it imposes by far the greatest financial burden on the social welfare and health institutions of most developed nations? Few people realise that each year huge sums of money are spent in an effort to help the millions who suffer from this terrible disease. Since I have had cause to treat many patients with rheumatoid arthritis, I would like to write a few words on this subject.

THE NATURE OF THE DISEASE

Academic debate about the real origin of this illness still persists. It can be caused by micro-organisms, perhaps in the wake of an infection, or by any of a number of toxins. More often than not, we find in association with arthritis some local focus of infection which discharges a constant stream of toxins or pathogenic agents into the blood. The quantity can be so small that the person may remain totally unaware of what is going on, until the body finally reacts, and becomes seriously ill. As a rule, various changes take place in the blood and scientists such as Dr von Bremer, recently also Dr Isel, have found viruses in the blood as well. Nevertheless, no definitive and conclusive explanation has so far been presented despite all the research and theorising.

I have observed that patients suffering from rheumatoid arthritis usually have a family history of gout, arthritis or some other rheumatic disease. There would thus appear to be a definite predisposition to this condition, as it is the case with many other diseases. Not everyone with a dental abscess will be afflicted with rheumatoid arthritis. One person may come down with some kidney problem, another with a heart condition, while yet another one is likely to find that a circulatory disorder develops; only a fourth one may develop rheumatoid arthritis or some other ailment. And there may also be one who will escape unscathed. You see, it very much depends on the predisposition mentioned above, and even though the individuals concerned have the same life-style and diet, the disease is triggered either by some pathogenic agent, that is, microorganism, or by toxins.

The frightening thing about rheumatoid arthritis is that, without an apparent reason, the joints in any part of the body can become afflicted. The heart may be affected too. There are times when it seems that the ailment is improving because a loosening-up of the joints and great relief is felt. Then, suddenly, for some inexplicable reason, there is a relapse and the condition deteriorates. These relapses usually occur during the cold seasons, in late autumn, winter or early spring. A warm dry summer often encourages what appears to be a real improvement.

TREATMENT GIVEN BY ORTHODOX MEDICINE

Orthodox medicine has not so far been able to find any satisfactory cure, although the pharmacies are overflowing with 'remedies' for rheumatism. For the most part, the disease has been, and still is, treated with salicylic acid preparations. At first it was thought that this was at long last a specific for a hypothetical, supposed causative agent, but these hopes were soon shattered. Why? Because the duration of the disease was hardly shortened and heart complications began to appear as frequently as they did before – and all this, by the way, was openly admitted by orthodox doctors. The salicylic acid preparations merely palliate the pain and inflammation in the joints, but not without unpleasant side effects. Gastric troubles may follow, head noises, cases of dizziness that can take on such proportions that onlookers believe the patient to be drunk. These are additional disorders brought on by medication. Aspirin and similar salicylic preparations may be better tolerated, but they are not so effective as pure salicylic acid. Then, one day, Schottmueller introduced Pyramidon to combat rheumatic arthritis – and what happened? This drug had even worse effects on the general well-being of some patients. The formation of white blood cells (to be more exact, granulocytes – containing granules that become conspicuous when dyed) was prevented. This gave rise to agranulocytosis, from which some patients died. Sulphonamide drugs were indicated only for the primary infection, not for the already established rheumatoid arthritis.

CORTISONE

Then the great need for a cure seemed to have found its answer in the discovery of cortisone, a hormone secreted by the adrenal cortex. It was acclaimed as the wonder cure. Such enthusiasm about a new remedy is frequent, but when it does not justify the faith placed in it it is quickly forgotten. The reasoning behind the use of cortisone was a theory put forward by a Canadian scientist named Selye. He maintained that the cause of arthritis was to be found in the normal defence mechanism of the body and that cortisone prevents this mechanism from becoming active, in other words, it paralyses it. According to him, this should cure the disease.

When cortisone is administered, the pains and inflammation immediately disappear, but the patient is not really cured, because as soon as its action has been exhausted and if no further dose is given, the old symptoms return. So the duration of the illness is not at all affected by the drug. What is more, it is known from animal experiments – and autopsies on patients who died during treatment – that prolonged medication with cortisone tends to atrophy the adrenal cortex. In fact, cases have been known where the cortex had virtually wasted away completely. If the body is given a substance which it should produce itself, then the organ which normally has this function will degenerate because it has become superfluous. The same principle applies to the muscles. If they are not exercised they will grow weak and flabby, resulting in atrophy, wasting away. We have the same evidence of such a thing happening in the case of diabetes and treatment with insulin. The doctor will readily admit that insulin is a help but not a cure. Part of the pancreas, the part that actually produces insulin, begins to degenerate if too much of the medication is given. Orthodox medicine is aware of this fact and a conscientious doctor will prescribe the absolute minimum dose necessary. He does not want to discourage the pancreas from manufacturing its own insulin, or perhaps even cause the still active islets of the pancreas to degenerate as well. It is obvious that the treatment which produces results without the need for insulin is to be preferred at all times.

ACTH
The hormone product ACTH (adrenocorticotrophic hormone) has been on the market for some time now. It is a hormone produced by the pituitary gland and in some ways its effect is the same or similar to that of cortisone. In this case, however, the body is not given the adrenal hormone direct, that is, administered from outside, but the adrenal cortex is stimulated by a hormone to manufacture its own. Far from degenerating, it hypertrophies, or grows much larger in size. The effect of this medication is not as sudden as that of cortisone, for the adrenal cortex must first be activated by ACTH to produce a sufficiently high hormone level in the blood, which in turn is intended to ensure freedom from pain. When administration ceases, the harmful consequences experienced with cortisone will not occur, because ACTH preserves the function of the adrenal gland. Nevertheless, the question arises as to whether we have not merely carried the catastrophic effect of cell degeneration one step further. In this case degenerative changes take place in the pituitary gland, which normally produces ACTH for the body. Since the pituitary holds a key position in the body's hormone production (it manufactures a considerable number of different hormones), the hormone balance is disrupted and the resulting damage may be even more difficult to rectify than the arthritis itself. As far as hormone preparations are concerned, however spectacular their effects may be, one must always remember that only one side of the coin is seen at a time, and the other side may look quite different.

I once had the opportunity to discuss these points with a doctor who had lectured on this subject and he frankly admitted that he would not use these remedies for himself. Should the need arise, he would look for another, more conservative way of treating the disease. Of course, I do not deny that in some cases the use of the new medications may be justified, but let the doctor and patient alike consider very carefully what side effects they might produce and what the ultimate, rather than the immediate, effect might be. Careful analysis and observations have led me to conclude that all hormone and organ preparations should be viewed with the utmost caution before prescribing or taking them.

COMBINATION TREATMENT FOR ARTHRITIS

Very good results can be achieved in the treatment of rheumatoid arthritis by combining or applying the available therapies. First of all, the patient must change over to an absolutely natural diet, which is, of course, always indicated for cancer, arthritis or gout and all similar diseases. The conclusion about diet is supported by the fact that these diseases do not exist in less developed parts of the world, as I have seen for myself. It must be that our faulty eating habits and way of life in the West account for the problems we bring upon ourselves, or that they are at least contributory factors. Unfortunately, this opinion is not shared by many and even some doctors still do not seem to consider their patients' diet as a decisive factor for their improvement and cure. Not long ago a patient told me that her previous doctor had always taken good care of her but never once did he mention a change of diet. Rather, in his opinion diet did not play any part even in the treatment of cancer and the patient could eat anything he wished. Such an attitude and advice call into question the professional capacity of a doctor who is obviously behind the times. Surely nutritional therapy has yielded convincing proof of the importance of proper diet in treating most ailments and a doctor should not overlook the potential benefits, especially when it can contribute so much to his patient's welfare. The clear evidence should be enough to make him want to change his opinion. For my own part, I am firmly convinced that there is no illness in which a proper diet does not play a part, whether it concerns the laying of a good foundation from which to counteract the patient's sensitivity or the provision of healing factors. Diet should be given serious consideration even if it only assumes a supporting role on the way to recovery.

DIET

A diet of natural foods is of primary importance when treating rheumatoid arthritis. Follow the diet given under the heading 'Natural Food' (see pages 463–9). Only unadulterated, unrefined foods should be eaten, just as the Creator provided them in nature. In preparing them we should be guided by the same principle: food should be left in its natural state as far as possible. Cooked animal protein, such as meat, is detrimental according to my experience. For better results, adopt a predominantly vegetarian diet and include plenty of raw foods. Curds or cottage cheese, as animal-derived protein, are good for you. If you cannot abstain from meat altogether, it is permissible to eat a little beef or veal, but pork, sausages, and processed and canned meats should be completely out of bounds. Caution should be exercised as regards fats; they should be of vegetable origin, cold-pressed and unrefined. Keep off heated fats or fried food. Vegetable oils, such as cold-pressed olive, sunflower, poppy, or linseed oils, should be used in their unrefined state. Anyone suffering from rheumatoid arthritis should never have denatured white sugar on his table. For sweetening, honey and natural sweetness from grapes, sultanas, currants and raisins must take the place of refined white sugar. These dried fruits can be put through a mincer so that they can easily be added to foods for sweetening. Raw rose hip purée made without white sugar is an excellent substitute for the usual jams. Not only white sugar but also white flour and white flour products must be scrupulously avoided. On the other hand, wheat germ taken in limited quantities is an excellent addition to the diet. If vegetables are not eaten raw, care should be taken in their cooking. Never boil vegetables but simply steam them in a little water to preserve their minerals and vitamins. Raw salads are very good seasoned with whey concentrate (*Molkosan*) or with lemon juice and oil; never add salt and sugar.

If at all possible do not use table salt or sharp spices, but replace these by fresh culinary herbs and yeast extract, or use *Herbaforce*.

NATURAL REMEDIES

For internal use, *Nephrosolid* is an excellent remedy for the kidneys, as it increases the secretion and expulsion of urine. Nephrosolid contains *Solidago* (goldenrod) and other herb extracts. Another effective remedy I like to prescribe is *Imperarthritica*, also a fresh herb extract. It contains, among other important ingredients, *Petasites off.*, *Polygonum avic.*, *Betula* and *Viscum album*. To remedy circulatory disorders and venous stagnation, *Aesculaforce* is indicated. This herbal complex contains horse chestnut, melilot (sweet clover), witch hazel and arnica, all excellent for the veins. *Kelpasan* is a good mineral supplement and increases the haemoglobin content at the same time. *Echinaforce* will relieve inflammatory conditions. These remedies, in combination with *Petasites officinalis* and *Viscum album*, will make great improvement possible, the latter helping considerably to regenerate the affected tissues.

Should the breathing be restricted in any way, you will find *Usneasan* of great help. This remedy is prepared from larch moss and if used in conjunction with external applications of mucilaginous extracts such as *Wallwosan* or *Symphosan*, a fresh herb prep-

270

aration containing comfrey, you will obtain a great deal of relief. Furthermore, it will be to your advantage to alternate with a massage oil such as *Toxeucal*, made from camphor and various extracts, including eucalyptus and the fresh leaves of poison ivy (*Rhus toxicodendron*). Packs made up of *clay* and *pulped cabbage leaves* are also beneficial. To obtain the best results apply them in alternation. It has been found that an application of *grated carrots* also relieves the pain.

Biological injections will overcome the pain even faster. Homoeopathic remedies are injected subcutaneously and quickly take effect. *Formic acid 12x, Lachesis 10x* and *Urtica 6x* (stinging nettles), all have proved their worth in this respect. Mistletoe preparations, especially *Plenosol* (Dr Madaus), lend additional support to the curative action of these medicines. Start with the potency 0 and increase gradually to the stronger 1.

By following the above advice, rheumatoid arthritis can be successfully treated. You should find that most doctors who practise natural therapy will be prepared to give the appropriate homoeopathic injections.

FANGO (MUD) CURES
I remember some particularly severe cases where the patients followed all the advice given above, yet a fango treatment in Italy was still necessary to effect a cure. Where professors and doctors at Swiss clinics have been hard pressed to find some satisfactory treatment for their patients, a fango cure in conjunction with the natural remedies suggested in the previous section has proved a superb biological treatment – the best there is. Patients who could hardly move around anymore became quite capable of taking up their normal work once again. Should a fango cure in Abano or Montegrotto in Italy become necessary, the financial sacrifice it may require will no doubt seem worthwhile if the patient can regain his health and former efficiency.

If you combine a fango cure with the other three treatments already mentioned, you will not only make possible a cure of the disease, but will also ensure that it is permanent. Take the biological remedies and ampoules for injection with you so you can use them to a limited extent. When taking the fango cure, be careful not to force or overdo things. After four or five treatments take a day off.

For a change, take a bath in the hot springs of a grotto. These natural sauna baths are widely available in these Italian spas. It is

271

a good idea to sweat in the bath one day, and then to have a fango treatment the following day. This programme may prove to be rather strenuous for some patients, but it will be easier than having to put up with the dreadful consequences of arthritis when it is not treated naturally. The natural way is always the best way. As to the question of diet, as the suggested regime could be a little difficult to follow in Abano or Montegrotto, it may be advisable to take some crispbread, raw cane sugar, honey and raw carrots with you, or try to obtain them locally.

FURTHER ADVICE ON HOW TO GET WELL AGAIN

If you wish to regain your health, you will have to pay special attention to what is natural and follow the advice already given. This implies that you should beware of the many patent medicines that claim to be able to cure or improve your condition quickly. For a permanent cure, more is required than just a few injections. In fact, both the doctor and the patient need a lot of patience and perseverence. The doctor must pay close attention to the patient's reaction to the various treatments if rheumatoid arthritis is to be cured. Still, the important thing is that that relief is possible. If the result achieved is to be permanent, the patient must continue to follow a diet of natural foods and to take limited amounts of the remedies from time to time. The idea is to prevent a return of the same illness. If you have the financial means you might take a fango cure in Italy once a year; doing so will help combat an existing disposition to arthritis. This treatment, together with the other advice presented, if followed, will give the patient every chance to keep fit in the future.

The Living Cell

The cell is a tiny but perfectly designed and incredible unit of every living thing on earth. Like so many other things it is a miracle of Creation. Our body is a harmoniously cooperating organisation of single cells, similar to the many individual citizens in a country. The earth's population is now five billion, a tremendous number when you think about it, but relatively small in comparison with the total of about 100 trillion (100,000,000,000,000) cells that make up the body of an adult person. And this miracle, the human cell, is on average only 0.02 mm (1/1000 inch) in diameter. If you want to get some idea of this tiny structure, take a soft-boiled egg as a comparison. On the outside is the cell membrane (the shell), then we find the cell plasma (the white) surrounding and protecting the nucleus (the yolk), the most important, highly organised and complex part of this tiny unit – the control centre.

Cell Metabolism
The cell's metabolism is yet another miracle at work, one whose workings scientists rack their brains to puzzle out. Although we do have some knowledge of the internal processes, this represents only a fraction of what actually goes on in the cell. We know, for example, that the cell takes in proteins, sugar and salt solutions together with various minerals and that it releases some substances, in a sense, waste material. But why is it that one kind of cell selects this or that substance for itself, while another kind attracts different substances? In other words, what enables the cells to make this selection? No one has yet been able to discover the answer to this question.

Sick Cells
If an engine is not lubricated for any length of time, it will overheat. If we ignore the whining and grinding noises caused by dry bearings and do not replace the oil at once, the engine is bound to suffer damage. Similarly, a cell's efficiency will diminish if it lacks the required substances, or if it does not receive sufficient quantities. The cell will become sick if such a deficiency continues for some time so that it has to draw on and eventually exhaust its reserves. In the case of vitamin deficiency we speak of 'avitaminosis'. As soon as the deficiency is recognised and the required substances are provided, the individual cell will recover and with it the complex organisation of cells, the tissue, will be restored to health and begin to function properly again. For this reason the art, or rather the capacity, of a good doctor becomes evident in his ability to diagnose these deficiencies and choose the appropriate natural remedies. The damage will then be rectified.

The Degenerated Cell
A degenerated cell could be described as a criminal in the cellular 'state' or organisation, since it operates in a way similar to criminals in society. They ignore the law, do what they want and take what they like without any concern for those around them. Of course, it takes time for a person to sink so low mentally and morally that he becomes a cold-blooded criminal.

The same applies to a cancer cell, a cell that has degenerated into a malignant one. It is just like a criminal who lives at the

273

expense of others and without consideration ravishes and destroys whatever lies in his way. But, you may ask, what makes a healthy cell degenerate and become malignant? What complex series of errors and detrimental influences cause the degeneration? Careful observation and experience has already given us a good insight into the things that may contribute to the change, although we do not yet understand all the causes leading to the mutation that transforms a normal cell into a giant or malignant one.

KNOWN CAUSES

I am fully convinced that many causes work together and put such great stress on the healthy cells that they have to give in; the harmony of their natural life and function becomes so disrupted that they degenerate and become malignant.

1. Predisposition is often responsible for cell degeneration, that is, it may be due to the inherited genetic make-up. However, such a predisposition need not lead to cancer if one's life-style is sensible.

2. An inadequate diet, a constant companion of our modern way of living and eating, upsets the body's biological balance and so damages the entire cellular system.

a) Too much protein intake, and of a poor quality, plays a considerable part.
b) Fats have a bearing on the development of cancer. Animal fats and fats lacking in unsaturated fatty acids are especially detrimental.
c) Disturbances in the mineral metabolism caused by the consumption of refined foods have proved to be a contributory cause of cell degeneration.
d) Avitaminosis, as well as a deficiency of other vital substances, seem to be strongly implicated in the development of cancer, but research in this area is still inconclusive.
e) Metabolic disorders, for example chronic constipation and constant fermentations in the intestines as a result of dysbacteria, are also very damaging.

3. Lack of oxygen plays a decisive part in the development of cancer. Experience has shown that people who take plenty of exercise in fresh, clean air are less at risk than those who engage in mental work or have to work in closed rooms. It would therefore be advisable to walk more rather than go everywhere by car, to spend one's free time walking in the woods and meadows instead

of sitting in a pub or bar talking politics, or wasting one's time in front of the television set or in the pursuit of similar pleasures.

4. Toxic gases and radiation which pollute the air today are also carcinogenic, or cancer-producing, factors. So beware of them!

5. It has been proved beyond doubt that some chemical additives to our food are carcinogenic. Colourings, flavourings and preservatives are worse cell poisons than was previously thought, and it is for this reason that many government agencies have started to ban them. They follow the example of Germany in this respect, where the efforts of doctors, especially those engaged in research into vitamins and minerals, succeeded in persuading the Government to take such measures.

6. Certain medicines, such as those that are, unfortunately, still used all too frequently in chemotherapy, especially derivatives of tar, contribute to cell degeneration. This is of particular significance today, when people are accustomed to swallowing tablets for just about anything.

7. Poisons in the form of pesticides and herbicides are often used indiscriminately. These can stick to vegetables, for instance, and are taken into the body through carelessness or lack of forethought. The result can be extremely damaging since lead, arsenic and copper are much more toxic than is generally realised.

8. The biological balance in plants can be disturbed because of errors when using fertilisers. If such produce is eaten for any length of time, it can also upset the biological balance in the human body.

9. Tenseness and indurations disturb and slow down the metabolic processes and foster the development of cancer. It is therefore strongly recommended that regular exercise be taken for relaxation as a prophylactic therapy. Indurations, lumps and growths such as scars and warts should be carefully watched. Never scratch or irritate them.

10. One of the most serious factors in the development of cancer is stress, that is, worries and anxieties. The extent of its influence is, of course, closely linked to our mental attitude, whether we give into negative thinking rather than being positive and optimistic whenever we feel depressed. Worries and anxieties are detrimental to the liver and have been a contributory cause of cancer for thousands of people. There is nothing more harmful to the life of our cells than continuous or repeated mental stress. Indeed, it poisons the blood and lymph and undermines the very life of the cells to a greater extent than some of the other factors listed above, even when taken together.

The long list of detrimental influences on the health of our cells shows that determining the possibility of cancer is simply a question of calculation. Every one of the described factors adds a few more percentage points to the possibility of contracting the disease, and as soon as the total of 100 per cent is reached, the negative influences will pull down the scales, the cells will become damaged and the disease, which can bring such pain and sorrow, will strike.

Once a tumour has formed, surgical intervention helps to calm one's fears by removing it. However, the danger to the rest of the tissues can only be stopped if all contributory factors to the cancer are tackled. We should not be content with the surgeon's reassurance that he has been able to find and remove everything and thus feel absolutely safe. Hormone treatment and radiotherapy create added problems for the cellular system and will not save a patient who has undergone surgery from the need to completely change his dietary habits and life-style.

The patient's mental attitude towards the illness and all other vital matters must be put on a healthy basis. True, this may not always be easy for the convalescent, especially if members of his family lack the necessary understanding and do not support him. Nevertheless, he should make a serious effort since it will help to improve his condition and contribute significantly to his cure. At the same time, he will make life easier for himself and those around him. No doubt, this will be a blessing in itself.

The Spectre of Cancer
While the world's medical specialists argue about the causes of cancer, more and more victims die every year. Some researchers try to blame a virus for its development, considering the disease to be a localised one affecting certain groups of cells. Others are just as bold in defending their view that cancer is a disease affecting the whole organism.

It is possible that viruses do play some part in the disease, but the researchers who believe that cancer is a disease that affects the whole body may be closer to the truth than the others. The view that cancer is a disease brought about by civilisation finds strong support through the investigation of conditions in less developed parts of the world, where cancer is comparatively unknown. According to my observations, cancer has more than one cause, it is the culmination of a combination of many causes, in other words, it is a complex disease.

A Question Still Unanswered
Thousands of pages have been written about cancer, yet our critical questions remain practically unanswered. Histologists with their modern ultramicroscopes or electron microscopes have so far not been able to tell us why a healthy cell becomes a cancer cell. It is for this reason that the early diagnosis of cancer is so difficult. Public information and lectures often make cancer appear to be a simple and straightforward problem and, for example, women over forty are encouraged to visit the doctor for a regular check-up. The doctor keeps telling them that there is no reason to be anxious, that everything is in order – and the women lose their fear of cancer. Then, quite suddenly, and in spite of the doctor's reassurances, a woman notices a hard lump. She rushes to a specialist who asks, with a slight tone of reproach in his voice, 'Why did you not come to see me sooner?' When she answers that the family doctor has been checking her regularly for years the specialist is naturally embarrassed and worried. Indeed, cancer is a difficult problem even for a capable physician and his efforts to prolong a patient's life can often be in vain.

OTHER BAFFLING QUESTIONS
The conscientious doctor is sometimes baffled because a seemingly serious case takes an unexpected turn for the better. On the other hand, the opposite can also happen: the patient seems to be making fine progress but suddenly the picture changes and the illness takes such a rapid turn for the worse that no skill, no effort, is able to arrest it. Even the best surgeon, highly skilled in his profession, may suffer the tragedy inflicted by the merciless Angel of Death in that his best friend, sister, mother or even his own wife passes away prematurely. Or the scourge of cancer may take hold of the doctor himself and all the efforts of his colleagues, using the most up-to-date therapies, prove to be in vain.

All this is very sad and we are filled with sorrow. For how can one help the patient to escape such an end? It would be a great relief for all of us, would it not, if there were some natural remedy that could cure the disease. Sadly, though, even the most experienced specialist knows of no such remedy. True, there are some good medicines that may have brought relief for some patients, but unfortunately there is no specific remedy for cancer, one that cures it without fail. What is more, it seems that we will never find one. This, too, is a tragic prospect. Once again, patients, nurses, pharmacologists, as well as doctors, are confronted by a puzzle. Is

277

it not true that conscientious efforts are being made to find a cure, and endless hours and huge sums of money are being spent on research? Should it all be to no avail? Is it not true that those who seek will also find?

A plant may lack sufficient, or the right kind of, soil. Its fruits may be affected by a fungal disease. Insect pests may destroy some too. The site where the plants grow may not be the best one; perhaps they need plenty of light and sunshine but they grow in a dark and shady area, or they need a little sun but receive too much. If the orchard-keeper neglects the proper care and fertilising of his trees, the specialist to whom he turns for advice will not be able to overcome these deficiencies by using a single patent remedy. I think we will all understand this illustration without any difficulty, and by applying it to the factors contributing to cancer, we should also understand the difficulties of treating this disease. A remedy may be the best there is, yet it can only help towards effecting a cure. We can take a plant remedy that stimulates the liver, for example barberries from the Himalayas or the common butterbur, which have done much good in treating the disease, but the problem of cancer will not be solved by just one remedy alone. Perhaps it may alleviate the pain, arrest the growth of a tumour, even bring about an appreciable improvement to the patient's general condition. Other improvements may be noticeable, but none of the available remedies will actually be responsible for a complete cure. The reasons for this are explained in the sections below.

Is Cancer a Localised Disease or One Affecting the Whole System? It will first be interesting to consider some of the arguments put forward by doctors of the highest calibre about some of the basic questions concerning cancer during a recent court case in Germany. How difficult it must be for judges to reach the right decision in such cases, especially when the views of specialists contradict each other! How can judges possibly be expected to make sense of it all?

Professor Bauer from Heidelberg, a famous and respected expert in the field of cancer, maintained that cancer is a localised disease and can therefore be tackled by means of the scalpel and radiation, that is, by surgery and radiotherapy, with varying degrees of success. However, two other well-known surgeons, Dr Albrecht and Professor Zabel, expressed opposing views. In common with many others, they were of the opinion that cancer is a disease affecting the whole system and that with the surgical removal of a tumour the actual disease is only partially treated, let alone cured. The great number of deaths that occur during the first year after an operation, in spite of radiotherapy, seem to speak out strongly in favour of this second view. A further aspect may be added, for it is thought that certain materials leave the malignant tissues, enter the bloodstream and lymph and, of course, the cells. This has a detrimental, if not poisoning, effect. According to this opinion, we can conclude that it is not only migrating cancer cells but also these separate materials that can lead to metastases in the course of time. The American school of thought seems to support this opinion. However, the available literature is not clear on whether the detached and circulating materials are in fact the same as those viruses discovered first by Dr Nebel of Lausanne and later by Professor von Brehmer.

The claim that cancer is a communicable disease, under certain conditions, may no doubt be a new thought to many. As many people find this possibility alarming, the question is dealt with separately below (see pages 280–1).

THE COMPLEX NATURE OF THE CAUSES

In spite of all the new views about cancer, I am sure we are not mistaken in taking the cause to be a combination of factors, including nutrition, housing conditions, occupation, lack of oxygen and necessary exercise, as well as the mental state and attitude of the person. What is more, it can no longer be denied that an inherited predisposition contributes to cancer. The empirical fact that it is possible for therapies to be useless even if employed in the early stages of the disease, according to personal disposition and the reaction of the body, is a reason for sadness on the part of all therapists. No other illness presents more surprises to the doctor, even the specialist, than cancer. He may be successful in treating a severe case, but a seemingly mild one can suddenly take a turn for the worse against all expectations.

There is a practical lesson to be learned from this. It is absolutely necessary to take certain precautionary measures, particularly once you have reached the age of forty. You should be sure to avoid all carcinogenic influences. This means primarily tobacco, most chemical medicines, also colourings and flavourings in food and drinks. Another thing to avoid is constant or prolonged overtiredness. Mental and emotional stress and strain, worries and constant feelings of depression are equally dangerous. They should be combatted right away and every endeavour made to overcome them.

Anyone who has seen the suffering and pain of someone afflicted with cancer of the larynx or lungs will not find it too difficult to give up smoking for ever. If you suffer from rheumatism or arthritis and are sensitive to volcanic influences, you should keep away from radioactive treatments because the water of volcanic springs that are radioactive can also cause cancer.

All in all, do not be overanxious, yet still be sensible and careful. You do not want to do what is harmful while thinking you were doing yourself some good. Strong stimulations can destroy, whereas milder ones can be beneficial.

Is Cancer Communicable?

Even though it is said that in experiments it has been possible to transmit cancer from sick animals to healthy ones by infecting them with toxins from malignant tissues, there is absolutely no evidence that cancer is communicable in humans; it has also been proved that cancer can result if certain tissues are subjected to the influence of poisons over a period of time.

Nevertheless, it has been noted that when a marriage partner has died of cancer the other partner often falls victim to the insidious malady some time later. But this observation does not prove that the disease was transmitted to the partner; there is indeed another reason.

As a rule, both partners will have eaten the same food and lived in the same house and environment. Their work or occupation would often be similar, and the same is true of their philosophy of life, producing similar mental and emotional demands and stresses. In accordance with their physical predispositions, the existing bioclimatic conditions can also have the same effect on them. All these deliberations show that the cancer which killed one partner did not directly infect the other, but the same illness resulted from a combination of the same causes. Working together, these causes eventually led to cancer in the other partner as well.

Then there is the time spent in caring for the patient and the deep sympathy felt for his suffering. Both are a strain on the energy reserves, apart from the shattering experience of the loved one's eventual death, the resulting loss being difficult to bear. The feeling of loneliness after decades of companionship can be overwhelming. In fact, just as joy and happiness strengthen and help to overcome an illness, so constant sorrow and anxiety can contribute to producing an illness, turning it into infirmity that may end in death.

We must not forget that not everyone has the necessary inner strength to recover from losses and problems successfully, and this fact should be taken into account as another factor to be added to the total of all other causes.

If cancer really were communicable, it would no doubt claim many more victims than it does and would be far more dangerous than it already is.

Susceptibility to Cancer Despite a Healthy Life-Style

Vegetarians often claim that one cannot get cancer if one leads a natural life. So it is an understandable tragedy when someone with a healthy life-style and strictly vegetarian diet falls victim to cancer. But what explanation is there for the fact that vegetarians, advocates of natural remedies and treatments, even leading figures in this field, succumb to cancer? Unfortunately, this really does happen, even though they may try to keep it a secret. True enough, experience has proved that a diet too rich in protein, especially animal protein, can contribute to the development of cancer, whereas a healthy diet based on vegetables and fruit does reduce one's susceptibility to it.

ADDITIONAL PRECAUTIONS

It must be taken into consideration that vegetarians, perhaps even without realising it, can take into their system a number of carcinogenic substances. How? Mainly through pesticides and similar sprays, as well as colourings, flavourings and many other chemical food additives. Food that is natural and 100 per cent pure can only be guaranteed if you produce it yourself, and then by organic growing methods. Furthermore, it must be noted that the development of cancer is not solely dependent on diet. It is no doubt beneficial to our health, however, if we eat the right kind of food, because we are then more likely to avoid the substances that promote cancer.

However, it is easy to minimise the advantage gained from a healthy diet by ignoring other factors that are closely linked with a natural life-style. If you have to live and work inside all the time you are subject to a serious lack of oxygen, which must be remedied through plenty of exercise. It is also wrong to curtail the time allocated for rest and relaxation only because of being too conscientious and responsible. Why? Because doing so only produces a situation in which you live under constant stress, and this inevitably leads to tensions in the body, which in turn trigger mental and emotional ups and downs. Once physical tension has disturbed the mental balance the result can be cell irritation, and if this continues over the years it may also be a factor in the development of cancer. For this reason, true inner happiness and optimistic confidence are wonderful remedies, creating a different basis for life. Worries and anxieties, however, when added to overtiredness, can be even more dangerous in stimulating the development of cancer than can errors in diet.

This may well explain why some people who stick strictly to sound rules of nutrition nevertheless fall victim to cancer. No doubt you can now see that caring for our mental condition is just as important as adopting the right kind of diet. It is also true that the person who is able to maintain his mental balance finds it much easier to relax, slow down and keep calm, even though life may be stormy all around him. This ability will save much energy and help to avoid tension. If your duties are highly demanding, and you cannot reduce them, then make it a point to get plenty of oxygen, at least before going to bed; take a quiet walk and, what is even more important, do retire early. Is it not true that you get little done in the evening or night when your mind is tired? You will not be able to do as much as you want to, and you will have to make a far greater effort than you would in the morning after a good night's rest, when the problems we face seem much less overpowering and are easier to solve than the night before when vigour and efficiency levels were low.

So there are quite a few things we have to watch in our difficult and critical times if we want to protect our health. Happily, we can do justice to what we have to do if we use sound common sense and judgment and act circumspectly, even though we may have to make some sacrifices. Such precautions are all in the interest of good health.

Birthmarks and Cancer

I have noticed many times that we cannot be too careful with birthmarks. Take care not to scratch them; they are best left alone, for to try and get rid of them by means of remedies or surgery is not without danger. In fact, it can mean that cancer cells, which might be present, begin to spread. Probably the best time to do something about a mole (nevus), if you do want to remove it because it is too unsightly, is during childhood. Even then it is most important to choose a highly skilled surgeon who is fully aware of all the dangers involved in its removal.

Birthmarks may remain inactive for decades and then, quite

282

suddenly, at the age of fifty or over, they begin to play up. A Swiss immigrant in British Columbia, western Canada, told me recently about such a case. A friend of his who had a birthmark on his lower back finally had it removed. Eighteen months later he began to notice glandular swellings and other abnormalities all over his body. On further examination they were found to be metastases of a malignant kind.

Even a simple irritation of a birthmark, especially when the irritation is continuous or repeated, can pose a grave danger. Clothing can cause such an irritation or the habit of scratching the mark, perhaps even making it bleed. In time, this irritation can have serious consequences.

PRECAUTIONARY MEASURES

If you insist on having a birthmark removed surgically, go on a strict *liver diet* in preparation for the operation. The best diet is one that serves as nutritional therapy for cancer patients. Take *Petaforce* at the same time, since this remedy helps to prevent metastases. The point to remember is that you should not simply go to have the mark cut away without first preparing the body in a prophylactic sense. Nor is it advisable to have a little tissue cut out for examination (biopsy) unless the same precautionary measures have been carefully observed and the liver diet adhered to consistently for one or two months. In this case, too, it is necessary to take Petaforce as a precaution to avoid the formation of metastases. Following this advice could certainly save many a person from disaster, possibly even from death.

In lectures and medical literature doctors keep pointing out that it is important to begin treatment early whenever cancer is suspected. But what is meant by 'early'? There are many people who regularly visit their doctor, are carefully examined, and yet fail to prevent what is going on in the body which neither they nor the doctor can detect or foresee. Hence the question, 'What should you do to successfully prevent cancer?' Providing an answer to this question is not at all easy. In our modern times there are too many factors that disturb the normal cell in its biological balance, changing a normal cell into a cancerous one. Mutation, the process of a healthy cell changing into a sick or degenerated one, is still a mystery and all efforts to solve it have so far been unsuccessful.

No one can deny that the stresses of modern life are partly to blame for various diseases, whether it be vascular disorders or cancer. Neither can anyone deny that increased radioactivity contributes to cancer. Chemical sprays as well as chemical additives in food are also contributory factors, as discussed above, together with the refining of food items and the thoughtless consumption of these foods. In addition to the constant stress and strain, the increased mental tension of our times probably plays a great part in laying the foundation for the development of the disease. We know, for instance, that worries and anxieties are bad for the liver, and what is bad for the liver is also detrimental to the endocrine glands. The resulting effects also share the blame in the disease's development.

Therefore we must consider the contributory factors and then make a conscientious effort to avoid them. Of course, it goes without saying that it is essential to follow a natural rhythm, or way of life. Overdoing things, in other words extremes, should be avoided, as should everything that is not in harmony with nature; these things can only be detrimental to an already weakened constitution. Once we have come to understand that we must adopt a positive attitude and life-style in order to escape the tentacles of one of the worst illnesses of our times, a birthmark will not be the reason for putting ourselves in danger of dying from cancer.

Smokers' Cancer

The tobacco industry has all the power and money to prepare and mount an effective campaign to play down the warning sounded worldwide against smoking, especially the smoking of cigarettes. It sets out to silence all knowledge concerning the fact that smoking causes cancer. What is more, it is just possible that the tobacco industry may be successful in finding some scientists, well-known chemists and medical professors who will endeavour to prove the contrary. However, even though the American Medical Association might accept another ten million dollars from the tobacco industry – as it has happened before, to our disbelief – the damage to health is there for all to see. Much can be bought with money, but not necessarily good health.

Of course, there are other causes of cancer of the lips, tongue, larynx, bronchials and lungs, but this fact does not mean that smoking is less of a cause of cancer, or, more accurately, an irritation and causative factor. It is not the nicotine, which affects the coronary vessels, that is to blame for smokers' cancer, but the tar, or phenol to be more specific. This chemical irritant is able to make the cells degenerate, leading to cancer. It is true that not every smoker becomes a victim of cancer. The chemical cell irritation caused by the tar is not enough, as a sole cause, to trigger cancer. As stated earlier, a predisposition to the disease is necessary. Not every smoker can be sure whether he has this predisposition or not. But he can be quite certain of it if his parents suffered from cancer or arthritis.

HEALTHY HABITS

It is certainly unwise to expose oneself to the danger of cancer because of some so-called pleasure. Think of the terrible suffering cancer of the larynx or lungs can mean. If you have ever had to watch a victim of this tragic condition slowly dying in agony, no doubt you will muster the courage and consider it your urgent duty to warn others of the dangers. Honest records and statistics show that by far the greater percentage of the above-mentioned kinds of cancer occur in smokers and those who work with tar.

It is not difficult to admit that smoking does not quite agree with a young person to begin with. This is a fact. Still, the tiniest bit of inherent cowardice may cause the young person to overcome the natural aversion to smoking because he does not want to be different from his peers – he does not want to be an outsider. Nor does he fancy being teased; above all, he wants to appear grown up and so imitates the adults.

Instead of trying to overcome inhibitions and inferiority complexes by doing commendable work, some young people learn to smoke and drink, habits that are detrimental to their health. While acquiring a taste for these things they develop an internal insensitivity but this price is paid without much thought, since the end result helps to suppress their feeling of inferiority.

It is a strange thing that if something tastes bad and bitter or burns on the tongue, once one had become used to it, the palate even comes to like it. But should not exactly this reaction move us to embrace only good and healthy habits? Of course it should! And by the way, the craving to suck something can be satisfied in a completely harmless way. Simply keep some raisins in your pocket and eat them whenever you experience the desire for a cigarette. Raisins are stimulating because of the valuable grape sugar they contain. This is not only nourishing and strengthening but also much tastier than nicotine and tar products. If you are able to help someone give up the vice of smoking, you will be helping him not only to save a considerable amount of money but, what is more important, you may also save him from the cancer that might otherwise catch up with him in later years.

Deadly Dangers in the Water

My experiences in the tropics have often urged me to point out the dangers that await a traveller if he drinks unboiled water in tropical or subtropical regions. By doing so, it is possible to take in pathogenic agents and parasites that can actually put one's life in jeopardy.

Unfortunately, even in our temperate zones it has become a hazardous thing to drink water, as was evidenced in an article published as long ago as 19 April 1964, in the journal *Nationalzeitung* (No. 178), entitled 'Carcinogenic Substances in Water'. The article discussed the results of analytical tests of the water in Lake Constance and its catchment area. According to the author, the results indicated that the water analysed contained considerable amounts of carcinogenic substances. Even though the author did not sufficiently exploit the material, his presentation of the findings was enough to make us take note. We must remember that many toxins, besides the effluents from industries, can enter rivers and lakes without our realising it. For example, quite a number of poisonous sprays are used in agriculture, and deposits of leaded petrol and diesel oil accumulate on the roads. Rain and the water from melted snow take up these and many other substances, eventually washing them into the rivers and lakes. Tests have also shown that the groundwater in certain places already contains certain amounts of such pollutants, none of which are at all conducive to good health.

All these factors make carcinogenic agents accumulate in our system. Say someone is a smoker. The tar from the tobacco will give him a few per cent of carcinogenic substances; radioactivity in the air will add a few more per cent, so will sprays, especially if they contain DDT; then a few more per cent will be absorbed from chemical medicines, especially if derived from tar; a further amount will come from food additives, irradiated foods, as well as smoked meat and fish. If the carcinogenic substances from polluted water are added to these other tragic influences, it is quite possible that the total of 100 per cent cancer-producing substances will have accumulated in that person's body. This may be enough to form a tumour if an appropriate irritation in the body also takes place. Since cancer claims an increasing number of victims in our times, it is essential to identify the many causes that can lead to it.

Beware of Carcinogenic Substances

Now that it is generally known that certain substances are carcino-genic, many people are more careful about what they eat and drink. It has been found that all tar products have a carcinogenic effect. Some of these are medicines, for example headache and sleeping tablets, or analgesics, but so, too, are some artificial colourings, flavourings, preservatives and improvers that, unfortu-nately, are so often added to our food. Tar released in the process of smoking tobacco can also produce cancer. Sadly, people who have to live in towns and cities are unable to avoid inhaling air that is polluted with carcinogenic agents. It is also almost impossible to escape from increased radioactivity, which is present in our food, even in milk and water, and in ever-increasing quantities. How sensible and necessary it is, therefore, to keep away from any carcinogenic substances when we are able to.

To do this, however, we need to know and remember what they are at all times. We must not remain indifferent, telling ourselves this or that is not so bad after all. It is a fact that many little things add up to make one big one, and that the cumulative effect results in the disaster we are all trying to escape from!

SOME WARNING EXAMPLES

I could quote many examples to prove that there are a number of possibilities leading to cancer. Once a farmer from Emmental came to consult me about a large tumour he had. First I asked him what he himself thought might have caused the problem. Without much hesitation he told me that he had always tended to eat too much pork and smoked meat. As smoked meat is indeed carcinogenic because it contains tar, the patient was perhaps correct in his assumption. Moreover, many a gardener and farmer may not even realise that most of the sprays they use, especially those containing derivatives of tar, can cause cancer.

Years ago it was nothing short of a celebration if a person went to a fashionable coffee-house in order to enjoy some cake baked with 100 per cent natural ingredients. During the Second World War many food items were not available, or at least were in short supply. It was then that substitutes began to be introduced, and since it is often easier to use essences and the like, substitutes continued to be preferred. Using artificial products instead of natural ones has become more and more prevalent today. But few people stop to think that when they eat a cassata or any other ice-cream made with artificial colours and flavours, they are actually

287

ingesting carcinogenic substances. The chance of adding carcinogenic agents is ever-present wherever chemicals are mixed in food
to improve its flavour, aroma and colour. Today there are enough
dangers around that can lead to sickness that we do not even know
about. Knowing this fact should deter us from exposing ourselves
to damage by things we do know about and so could avoid.

It is unfortunate that so few people attach any importance to
leaving nature natural. Nevertheless, we should take care and do
everything in our power to eat and drink nothing but natural food
and drinks that will do us no harm.

Seven Basic Rules for the Prevention of Cancer
The following seven rules will give you an idea of some of the
effective precautionary measures you can take to prevent cancer
as far as you possibly can. You should endeavour to follow these
rules at all times.

RULE ONE
We live in restless, uneasy times, beset with many failures and
disappointments. Instead of putting the emphasis on the manifold
problems and difficulties confronting us, we should try our best to
keep calm and maintain our equilibrium. If we let worries and
anxieties dominate us, we should not be surprised if our health
begins to suffer; we will become agitated and our mental and
emotional life will be impaired, even come under stress. In such
circumstances is there any wonder that spasms occur and mental
tensions attack and damage our cellular system?

We must fight against depression in our outlook and attitude,
because constant mental and emotional pressures, given time, can
act like a physical cell poison. Depressive worries lead directly to
tension in the body and if the condition is allowed to continue, it
will contribute considerably to the development of cancer. So if
we do not want to suffer undue damage through worries and the
like, we must make a determined effort to shake off everything
that might upset our equilibrium, our inner calm and balance.
However, that does not mean we should become apathetic or
lethargic, for indifference is no remedy whatsoever. On the contrary, we must endeavour to go about our work with a happy
spirit and with bold determination try to find release from our
worries. If we do all that lies in our power to do, then we can
remain calm and take care that our spirit is filled with uplifting,
optimistic things and that we enjoy nature's precious gifts with joy

and gratitude. There are some people who give in to their worries and anxieties to such an extent that their depression makes them oblivious to the most beautiful scenery and glorious sunshine. It is to them that we especially recommend the precept 'Happiness means health'.

RULE TWO

We should make sure to always eat what nature offers, in as unadulterated or natural a state as possible. Proper nutrition is more important than you might think. It is a proven fact that devalued, refined foods containing artificial additives and residues of sprays, but lacking vital substances and other nutrients, help to prepare the groundwork for the development of cancer.

Our diet should always contain more alkaline foods than acid ones. A lack of minerals and unsaturated fatty acids can also contribute to the degeneration of cells. Furthermore, overeating and digestive upsets accompanied by fermentations and intestinal gases are basic causes of cancer. If you turn these remarks over in your mind, you will realise that it is up to yourself to make the necessary changes in your diet, always laying stress on a choice of wholesome, unadulterated natural food.

RULE THREE

We must not poison our body fluids and cells with chemicals. For this reason it will be clear why it is essential to avoid all medicines used in chemotherapy that are capable of disturbing the normal cell metabolism. Watch out especially for medicines based on tar. The compulsive consumption of tablets and narcotics is also responsible for upsetting the biological balance, physically as well as mentally. Smokers may delude themselves into thinking that nicotine is not really harmful and has no influence on cancer, but it is an established fact that the phenols – tar – contained in tobacco are carcinogenic. Why be foolishly deceived and suffer the tragic consequences?

RULE FOUR

No one but a person who cannot walk can imagine life without the use of his legs. The importance of our legs only begins to dawn on us when we see someone who cannot use them. And yet, time and again we commit the error of giving in to convenience; we take the car instead of walking. The way things are going it appears that before too long many people will use their feet and legs only to operate the accelerator! But this neglect is absolutely wrong; it robs the body of an essential source of strength. Walking and hiking help us to breathe deeply, so that we regularly inhale sufficient oxygen to keep the cells healthy and elastic. Cancer cells lack oxygen, and since lack of oxygen is one of the main causes leading to cell degeneration, we must never neglect the regular intake of oxygen. Engage regularly in walking and hiking!

RULE FIVE

Take great care that the cells do not receive any unnecessary physical irritation. The liver, too, should be paid constant attention and given more care than all the other organs. If the liver does not experience any functional upsets or failure, it is impossible for cancer to develop. The liver is the most important bulwark in the fight against cancer, and no cancerous cell degeneration is possible as long as this marvellous laboratory is working properly. We should therefore always make every effort to keep it working efficiently.

RULE SIX

Since the hazardous effects certain rays have on our body cells are known today, we should beware of them. Not only do radium and X-rays constitute a double-edged sword for the cells, but the ever-increasing radiation in the atmosphere plays an important part in cell degeneration. Volcanic areas with high radiation levels can trigger cancer, depending on the individual's predisposition and susceptibility. I have seen cases where lymphogranulomas developed within a few days, especially in women who had received treatment in hot volcanic springs and with fango (mud) packs. Cosmic rays, which together with the so-called earth rays can cause tensions, are also able to trigger cancer if someone is exposed to them regularly over a period of time. We should always be aware of these dangers and avoid them where possible.

RULE SEVEN

The endocrine glands play an important part in our body and should be cared for so as to keep them functioning normally. Maintaining the right balance will prevent unnecessary problems. Interestingly, there are some people who have such a favourable predisposition, despite the unbalanced and turbulent times we live in, that they experience no problems with the functioning of their glands, particularly the sex glands. However, not everyone is so fortunate and well-balanced; there are some people who push themselves too hard, while others suffer constantly from inhibitions. Both tendencies are responsible for unnatural conditions of irritation and are harmful to the cells. Excessive irritation and tension encourage cancerous degeneration of the cells if they occur repeatedly. In this case, harmony in one's emotional life is a necessary requirement if one wants to keep healthy.

FURTHER HINTS

If you make a determined effort to observe the seven rules given above and take care to put them into practice, you need have no fear of falling victim to cancer. Following this advice will benefit the general condition, even for those who may have inherited unfavourable tendencies and susceptibilities. It is true that it is not always easy today to lead a life that is in harmony with these rules, but when you consider the pain and trouble you can save yourself and those close to you, surely the effort would be worthwhile!

Even if someone already has cancer toxins in the blood, or perhaps even a tumour, he should not give up hope. A thorough change of life-style and diet can be a purposeful and decisive step towards a cure. Good natural remedies lend added support in this direction. *Petasites* preparations, for example *Petaforce*, have often reinforced the healing process.

It is, however, a different story if the liver is already affected. In this case, not only one battle but the whole fight is lost, and there is little point in continuing to bother the patient with diets and treatments. True, for some patients it has been possible to stabilise the condition even where the liver was affected, but where all other circumstances were favourable, although it must be said that such cases are rare exceptions.

PREVENTION IS EASIER AND BETTER THAN CURE

People whose parents have succumbed to cancer, even one parent, usually inherit a certain predisposition to the illness. Anyone falling into this category would be advised to be doubly careful and go over the seven rules at least once every three months. This review will help you to make the necessary changes while there is still time for it. Mind you attend to this early enough, so that you will not fall victim to a terminal illness.

Unfortunately, only a few people heed the warning and take preventative measures when they are young. And it is for their sakes, for those who are grateful for the right directives, that I consider it worthwhile giving the above advice. If you follow the recommendations, you will live to see that prevention and caring for your body will pay rich dividends. It is better, less expensive and less painful than first succumbing to sickness and then trying to combat it by means of costly and often useless therapies. If this principle is true of any illness, it is certainly so in the case of cancer.

Remedies for Cancer

Although there is no such thing as a specific remedy for cancer, and probably never will be, nature makes some helpful plants available to us. These plants are able to aid and exert a prophylactic effect. The plants described below represent just a sample of those that can be useful. Additional information can be found in my book *Cancer – Fate or Disease of Civilisation?*

BUTTERBUR

Known by the botanical name *Petasites officinalis*, butterbur has achieved wide recognition as a remedy. In the first place, its antispasmodic effect eases tension in the cells and reduces the patient's susceptibility to pain. Secondly, it has an anticarcinogenic effect. No wonder that some doctors claim to have noticed fewer cases of metastases after operations when the patient had been given a good *Petasites* preparation before and after surgery. As butterbur is a nonpoisonous plant, it can be taken in large amounts without any danger of side effects. Some cases are known where this simple plant, in conjunction with a change of life-style on the part of the patient, has produced remarkable results.

MISTLETOE

This peculiar parasitic plant likes to live on certain trees and is also known as *Viscum album*. It, too, has proved to be a good plant remedy for cancer, because of its effect of stimulating the cell metabolism. As this is generally very weak in cancer and arthritis patients, mistletoe preparations are beneficial for both diseases. Mistletoe can be given in the form of drops or by injection.

CELANDINE AND OTHER REMEDIES

Celandine, also known by its botanical name *Chelidonium*, is a further effective help, as are preparations made from *Podophyllum*, *Boldocynara*, *Lycopodium*, *barberry* and all other plants that stimulate the liver. Cancer patients always suffer from liver insufficiency, so it is understandable why plants that stimulate the activity of the liver can help to improve the patient's condition. Since there is usually a vitamin C deficiency as well, we recommend that the patient take *Bio-C-Lozenges*, in addition to a diet rich in vitamins.

ECHINACEA
This plant has proved its reliable effect on all kinds of inflammation and is therefore a good supportive remedy. It can be used internally and externally.

COMFREY (WALLWOSAN)
Comfrey (*Symphytum officinale*) is a fine pain-reliever in cases of cancer of the stomach and intestines. For this reason it is usually prescribed for diseases of these organs.

LACTIC ACID PREPARATIONS
In more recent times research has shown that lactic acid is also beneficial in caring for cancer patients and should be considered for this purpose. *Molkosan, sauerkraut juice and vegetable juices* taken alternately will improve the patient's condition and quench his thirst, however great it may be.

Bacteria and Viruses
These two types of micro-organism have been the subject of many books and lectures. There are even university institutes wholly devoted to research into them. So what do we know – and what can we do about them?

Bacteria
Bacteria are very tiny, but are discernible under a microscope. Even though they have been thoroughly researched, they are still as dangerous as ever. Just think of the bacteria that at one time caused such dreadful diseases as the bubonic plague, cholera, typhoid fever and tuberculosis. Improved sanitation has helped to eradicate the epidemics that in medieval times decimated entire towns and villages, so we have cause to thank hygiene, including effective sewage systems and clean drinking water, for stemming the tide.

In the past, tens of thousands used to die of tuberculosis. As recently as fifty years ago consumption, as it used to be called, was still considered more dangerous than cancer because men and women were carried off in the bloom of their youth. Happily, a change of life-style, healthier housing and living conditions, more nutritional food rich in calcium and vitamins, breathing oxygen-rich air and exposure to plenty of sunlight were found to be the means to almost eradicate tuberculosis. Moreover, the patients who were released from sanatoriums as cured would have developed an immunity to the disease. The bacteria would have been encapsulated and rendered ineffective and if the patients continued to observe certain guidelines they would be unlikely to suffer a return of the disease.

The important thing in protecting oneself against bacteria is, therefore, to strengthen the body's defences – the immune system. A deficiency in vital substances or nutrients, as well as unhealthy external conditions, can weaken this wonderful defence system or even destroy it. Expressed in military terms, this would mean creating a weak position in an otherwise well-protected and defended front line. The enemy would be able to penetrate where the defences were down – and so it is with the immune system in its fight against invading bacteria.

Viruses
For a long time the existence of viruses remained unknown, perhaps for the reason that they are much smaller than bacteria and invisible even under an ordinary microscope. However, since the invention of powerful ultramicroscopes and electron microscopes it has been possible to use more sophisticated methods of investigation and make viruses visible. We have therefore been able to learn more about what they do and the dangers they pose to man and beast. In the case of bacteria, specific medicines have been developed that retard and stop their multiplication and growth, in some cases actually destroying them. But viruses are much tougher and in no way affected by, say, antibiotics. Little has so far been achieved in finding a way to combat them successfully.

MY OWN EXPERIENCE
Some twenty years ago, one of my patients displayed certain symptoms which made me suspect a virus as being the cause of her illness. The woman, a Yugoslavian, complained about unnatural tiredness, accompanied by headaches, susceptibility to colds and catarrh, loss of appetite and intestinal trouble. It seemed as if everything in her body was upset. Her symptoms reminded me of a condition I had read about in a medical publication, for which

a virus was to blame. The fact that all known herbal and homoeo-pathic remedies had failed to bring her relief strengthened my suspicion that nothing but this specific virus could be responsible for her condition.

The syndrome observed in the patient matched the symptoms attributed to the cytomegalovirus. However, as I wanted to be absolutely certain I sent the lady to a hospital where the laboratory was headed by a virologist I knew personally. I explained to him that I suspected the cause of her problem to be the cytomegalovirus. He did not think so, however, especially as the symptoms were not so obvious to him that he could confirm my opinion there and then. Nevertheless, he agreed to do a blood test. To his great astonishment what I had suspected proved to be true.

I then asked him what he would recommend to help the patient, and he suggested building up and improving her general condition of health since there was no specific remedy to combat the virus.

TRIAL WITH NATURAL REMEDIES

I had no choice but to try out the remedies I knew and had available. To strengthen the immune system and regenerative mech-anism I prescribed *Echinacea*, a plant that builds up the body's own defences. I can speak from my own experience because when I visited the tropics *Echinacea* helped me to acquire resistance to malaria, which is one of the reasons why I decided on this remedy to fight the virus. Moreover, I put her on *Lachesis 10x*, a snake poison in homoeopathic dilution, in order to tackle the viral toxins. Thirdly, I indicated *bee pollen* and *royal jelly* to support the body with special nutrients. Besides taking these remedies, the patient was asked to change her diet to one made up of raw food, raw vegetable juices, natural brown rice and lactic acid products.

THE RESULT

Three months later the patient was feeling much better. After another hospital check-up, performed by the same virologist, he confirmed that the lady's condition had improved significantly, providing the basis for an encouraging prognosis. In answer to my question as to whether or not it was possible to get rid of the virus altogether, he told me that he did not think so. Then he used an interesting comparison to illustrate what was going on in the pati-ent's body.

295

A HELPFUL ILLUSTRATION

The virus, my virologist friend explained, could be seen as a villain who has been thrown out of the house itself but has stayed on the veranda. As soon as the circumstances in the house change – or the body's overall condition deteriorates again – the villain is there ready to slip into the house to cause havoc once more. This illustration reminded me of something that once happened in our own house. A family of sables climbed from the trees into the attic, where they created an awful racket. What could I do but have some of the trees near the roof cut down, and close up every hole through which they could possibly enter. A few years later, however, a creeping plant grew up the wall unnoticed, giving the sables the chance to climb in and become a nuisance yet again. Once more we had to block everything up, but this time we got rid of them for good because we made sure there were no openings left anywhere.

Perhaps this is an odd, not quite scientific, way to illustrate the problem we have with a virus, but it helped me to understand the researcher's point of view.

We have only one option in order to fight pathogenic agents, in this case viruses, for which there is no known antidote or remedy, and that is to support the body in defending itself, by helping to mobilise its defence forces, or mechanisms. Thus, if we want to take up the fight against viruses and win it, we must do all we can to back up the body's own regenerative power. The virologist in the Swiss hospital agreed with me. This is the only correct way to treat viral diseases.

LOSS OF IMMUNITY

We are no longer absolutely in the dark when it comes to treating cancer. There are some biological means that help to normalise the body's weakened defence system without causing undesirable side effects. It is now understood that cancer, the disease, is not restricted to a tumour, that is, a localised problem; rather, it is a chronic ailment affecting the body as a whole. For this reason measures must be taken to detoxify the body. How do we do this? First, we stimulate the liver, the organ whose role it is to filter out toxins. Then there is the need to regularise the intestinal flora. Next, the body must get plenty of oxygen. Finally, the patient requires a natural wholefood diet, with plenty of raw food, brown rice and lactic acid products. In this way we can fight cancer or do much to prevent it. At no time should we consider it an inevitable blow of fate.

With viruses the situation is similar, although less simple, because they usually attack the immune system. Where the body's resistance has been damaged by the sum total of pathogenic effects and an inherited weakness in the immune system, a viral attack is able to destroy what is left of the existing regenerative forces. In such a case, not just one battle but the whole war will have been lost.

AIDS – Worse than Cancer

Acquired Immune Deficiency Syndrome, AIDS for short, is the worst disease known to us that is caused by a virus. Hundreds of thousands of people, all over the world, have been gripped by shock and fear. So far, however, the orthodox medical profession has not found a remedy. Every victim is, in a sense, condemned to death. True, there is a waiting period of 2–5 years before resistance breaks down completely. Death is then caused, not by the destructive virulence of the virus, but by a lack, or loss, of the body's defences, a failure of the regenerative mechanisms, a disease the patient might easily have overcome under normal circumstances.

WHAT PROTECTION IS THERE?

If the media are right, hundreds of thousands of people in the United States and Europe alone have already fallen victim to AIDS. What can be done to prevent it? A widely read American newspaper gave the advice (with which I agree) to lead a morally clean life, rejecting all sexual excesses and other perversions of the body, mind and emotions. This disease has spread mainly, but not exclusively, among those who practise these things, having taken on epidemic proportions. Infection is said to be possible via the mucous membranes, primarily the sex organs. I do not like to write about things like these, I would rather talk about positive aspects of therapies and treatments that are intended to take care of our health and fitness. Still, I may be able to transmit a glimmer of hope, comfort and advice to the fearful.

A GLIMMER OF HOPE

I am aware that virological institutes are working frantically to find an antidote for the ultramicroscopic villain. It is hoped, and it would be good fortune if this hope could be fulfilled, that the search will be successful and that many people will thus be spared great suffering. But what can one do before medical science discovers a specific remedy?

Protection against the virus can only come from the help we give the body by leading a healthy life and by improving and strengthening its general condition.

For this reason the intake of food rich in vital substances, vitamins and minerals, is essential. The food of modern civilisation actually weakens the body, undermines the defences and hinders the system from deploying its forces and displaying its regenerative powers in the first place.

It is important to try and reduce the virus's chances of development as much as possible by eating, pure, alkaline food with a high vitamin content. Doing so, it is likely that the body's own regenerative forces will be built up. I read a newspaper report only recently which confirmed the assumption that a diet made up of such food can bring successful results. The case in question concerned a child born with the AIDS virus whom the doctors at the Robert-Koch-Institute had given two more years, at the most, to live. At the same time they told the mother that the baby's life could possibly be extended a little longer with the help of a vitamin treatment. According to the newspaper article, she followed this advice and every day gave the child two kiwi fruits, two grated apples with lemon juice, rusks and the juice of three oranges, in other words, pure, excess alkaline food with natural vitamins. Every two months she took her child for a check-up at the paediatric clinic. After some time the doctors were able to tell the happy mother that the last examination revealed a negative result – the AIDS virus no longer showed up. The child could be considered cured. Judging by this example, can we not draw the logical conclusion that every AIDS patient should live on only pure fresh food, that is, a diet of fruit and raw food? Besides the fruits mentioned in the article, the patient should also eat avocados, papaya, and perhaps bananas – fruits that are available all the year round.

A well-known tennis player came down with AIDS, and was diagnosed as such by the doctors of St Vincent hospital. This same person was completely cured by means of a special diet high in vitamins but low in protein, a protein-free fruit diet. Today he plays tennis with the same verve and vitality as he did before.

PLANT REMEDIES TO BACK UP TREATMENT

There are a number of plants that I have come to know for their efficacy in combatting viral diseases: *garlic, horseradish, bear's garlic (ramsons), butterbur (Petasites), lichen-acid-containing Usnea, and Echinacea, the purple coneflower.* I can vouch for the good results achieved with patients with viral infections who had taken these natural remedies, in addition to adopting a sensible and healthy life-style.

It would be worthwhile if doctors were to try these plants when treating their patients. *Echinacea,* in particular, contributed to keeping myself and my friends free from malaria in the tropics, and should therefore be included in any treatment given to those suffering the dreadful viral disease AIDS. Instead of sitting around waiting for the end to come, an experiment could be made involving a complete change of life-style and the indicated plant remedies. It may be that a cure is possible.

There is no doubt the AIDS disease has scared many, above all the young, making them rethink and modify their ethical views, especially their attitudes towards sexual morality. And I appeal whole-heartedly to doctors and dieticians to try everything in their power so that something positive rather than alarming will soon be reported by the media.

Remember, nature is bound to have a way, but it must be sought. And he who seeks can expect to find a solution.

Our Teeth

The importance to our health of having good teeth is still not sufficiently appreciated. It is the same with health in general. We begin to value it only when we have lost it and are sick. Many people think it is enough to know that there are doctors available if they need them, and they do not worry any further. They similarly rely on the dentist if something goes wrong with their teeth, and for this reason they do not give any thought to the importance of keeping their teeth healthy. In a figurative sense, we could call the teeth the front line defences of our body.

Healthy Teeth and their Defence Action

Metaphorical speech being the oldest and most effective way of explaining something, I would like to compare the teeth to armour-plated turrets. The hard outer tooth enamel could be called the armour-plating because the enamel is the toughest tissue of the body, built up of very hard calcium fluoride. The enamel possesses

299

a thick enough layer of calcium fluoride – in our illustration a strong armour-plating – to be able to do justice to all the demands made on it for the usual 60–80 or even more years of our life, provided we have inherited the proper basis for this from our parents, especially if our mother's mineral metabolism was efficient and her body had all the necessary minerals when she was carrying us.

Next to the armour-plating is the calcified tissue called dentine, which can be compared to porous limestone. The dentine is protected by the tooth enamel, the armour-plating mentioned above, and cannot be damaged or injured in any way as long as the enamel is intact.

The canals in the tooth leading to the root are the pulp canals. The larger central part is known as the pulp chamber, the spongy tissue of the tooth containing nerves and blood vessels. In our illustration these canals and chambers might represent crew quarters, from which it is seen to that all operations in the turret are properly directed.

In both the pulp canal and the pulp chamber there is also a breathing system, and a lymphatic and nervous system. The nerves could be compared to the crew manning and operating the test instruments, warning and listening devices, in short, all possible communication instruments and apparatus. Any unusual happenings, any attacks from outside, an unexpected bump, an excessive demand and the like are immediately reported to the central control, figuratively speaking, the headquarters. If a break-in or some other danger is imminent, a warning is sounded – pain sets in. The attackers in this case are bacteria. No doubt the Creator made the nerves, which transmit the feeling of pain, not to torture us but to make us aware that something is wrong in the body. We are then able to do something about the problem.

WHY WE NEED HEALTHY TEETH
We need healthy teeth to enable us to chew well, which is essential for proper digestion. Only if we make full use of our salivary glands will our food be properly assimilated and agree with us. There is a reason, then, why we have six large and many more small salivary glands, which secrete various alkaline substances that are of the utmost importance to the whole digestive process. If food particles are sufficiently insalivated, the later stages of digestion will be made much easier.

It is interesting to note that the teeth stay healthy if they are used correctly and given hard food to chew. This is exactly the opposite of what we know about other instruments, which usually wear out when used a lot. The pressure exerted when biting acts as a kind of stimulus for healthy teeth. The periodontal nerves transmit this stimulus to the blood vessels and more blood is supplied. The increased blood supply means better nutrition and guarantees constant regeneration of the tooth. Thus, anyone who eats hearty meals that force him to chew vigorously strengthens his teeth and keeps them healthy. On the other hand, if you get into the habit of eating primarily gruels, soup and soft food you miss the chance of forcing your teeth to be active and stimulated, laying the groundwork for later tooth decay. Apples are an excellent fruit to eat as they need chewing and their acidic juice also cleanses the teeth.

To keep physically healthy and fit, adopt a good and natural diet and take care that your teeth remain healthy and strong.

Dead Teeth

Unfortunately, it is possible to have dead teeth, and these could be likened to turrets without a crew. Their defences are gone and the enemies from outside are able to invade. No one is left to carry out repairs; no one is there to replace the damaged calcified tissue of the dentine or to take care of regenerating what becomes defective. Such a tooth may be repaired and closed up from outside, but if the dentist does not sterilise everything properly, bacteria may spread again inside the tooth and sooner or later cause its destruction. The only protection still left is the cementum around the root. Also surrounding the root is a network of nerves and blood vessels.

WHY CORRECT NUTRITION IS NECESSARY

Not only solid food but also wholefood is necessary to keep the teeth healthy, for the blood can only supply the nutrients and materials needed for regeneration and repair that it has available. If we do not take in enough calcium, even the best machinery ready to do the repair work cannot function because the necessary substances are lacking. A bricklayer will not be able to build a strong wall if he does not use enough lime or cement in his mortar. The same principle applies to our teeth. Deficiencies of calcium, vitamin D and fluoride, besides other vital substances, tend to prepare the way for weakness and degeneration.

Such degenerative symptoms, particularly dental caries and also degenerative effects apparent in the jawbone, are the consequences of our modern denatured food, our eating habits and life-style. People in less developed parts of the world, who have not yet been affected by modern ways but live a healthy natural life, generally possess fine teeth. There are indeed some primitive tribes, as we might describe them, who would provide a dentist with no work whatsoever. He could merely admire their beautiful teeth. For one thing, these people have inherited good teeth with the necessary armour-plating of excellent enamel.

So if you have children, see to it that they eat plenty of food rich in calcium and, in addition, give them a calcium preparation such as *Urticalcin*, the well-known nettle calcium supplement, as required. Should anything abnormal be noted, for instance oversensitivity to heat and cold, or perhaps painfulness when chewing, a visit to the dentist is called for. Any minor damage may then be quickly put right. Bacteria can easily invade once the protective cover or armour-plating, the tooth enamel, is broken, however small the crack may be. They cannot eat the enamel since it is too hard, but they enter the cracked protective surface and settle in the dentine, proliferate and ultimately destroy it. It is therefore of the utmost importance to act quickly. Do not wait until you get toothache, but visit your dentist regularly for a check-up and repair of minor damage, if necessary. Following this advice can help you to avoid the discomfort of a nerve treatment and dead teeth, which, after all, constitute a health hazard. The subject of caring for your teeth is discussed further in a later section (see pages 303–8).

THE CONSEQUENCES OF DEAD TEETH

As the expression indicates, a dead tooth is completely lifeless. Since it can no longer be regenerated, bacteria are able to form pus and abscesses. It may seem strange, however, that pain, or a toothache, is not always felt. An X-ray picture will disclose the presence of a granuloma full of bacteria at the root apex, or there may be an abscess full of pus. Still, even this unfortunate condition does not always cause pain. These abscesses or cysts scatter toxins, triggering headaches, dizziness, indisposition, rheumatic pains, neuralgias, neuritis and many other illnesses. The effect on some people is such that they never again feel quite well, and the slightest overexertion or change in the weather will make them feel indisposed. Good natural remedies and other medicines often give little relief, because the problems I have just described return again and again, making the person feel depressed. Of course, these symptoms may stem from a liver disorder. Conversely, the cysts may affect the liver if they happen to be in the teeth, tonsils or certain other parts of the body. When the dangerous abscesses are tackled by resection of the dental root, or the bad teeth are simply pulled out, the patient is suddenly freed from all his problems.

I have known patients who lived a healthy life and were never really ill, yet they were not really well either, because they did nothing about their dental abscesses. They would suffer from headaches, slight indisposition, excessive tiredness or pains somewhere in the body, but these would temporarily disappear with treatment. The condition always changed, however, when the abscesses were finally dealt with. These patients would suddenly feel better than they had done for years.

It is especially important for those of us who live in our so-called civilised society to take much better care of our teeth than we generally do. For this, of course, we need to have a good dentist. However, there are other things we need to do in order to care properly for our teeth. These requirements are dealt with below.

Care of the Teeth

THE DISADVANTAGES OF CIVILISATION

After considering the facts, it will be agreed that from the point of view of our health, care of the teeth is more important than any beauty or body care. Of course, when I was a little boy I am afraid I heartily disagreed with the idea of cleaning my teeth every day. It seemed enough of a restriction to my freedom to have to wash daily and keep blowing my nose. Why should I be bothered with even more work? Couldn't my teeth keep themselves clean? I wondered. Indeed, I thought they could, because I had heard of primitive tribes who live a natural life, close to nature, and they had beautiful teeth without ever having to brush them or give them special care. But eventually I learned that on account of our modern diet and way of living, we have lost many of the advantages that those primitive peoples still enjoyed. My parents told me that bacteria settle between the teeth, attack and destroy them. They get into every crack, multiply and eventually cause tooth decay. The questions remained, 'How do primitive people cope with bacteria? Why do their teeth remain healthy and beautiful? Are the bacteria unable to invade, multiply and cause decay, just as they do in civilised people?'

303

THE ADVANTAGES OF PRIMITIVE PEOPLES

Of course, primitive people in unspoilt areas of the world are exposed to the same tooth-destroying bacteria that affect people in the industrialised world, but the enamel of their teeth is harder and does not allow the bacteria to penetrate and lodge in crevices; that is why their teeth remain healthy and resistant. But why are the teeth of those people so excellent? The answer is simple: their food is unadulterated, natural, not like ours that has been changed, refined, denatured, bleached and adulterated – to our detriment. Our faulty nutrition impairs healthy resistance, not only in the teeth but also in the bones, indeed the entire organism; we have become soft.

Solid, unrefined food as originally produced by nature enables those primitive peoples to use their teeth for the purpose originally intended by our Creator. They use their teeth in such a way that the function of chewing is properly exercised, and the teeth are cleaned at the same time. Wholewheat bread and bread or cakes made with whole corn require vigorous chewing, and so does all the rest of the hard food that makes up their diet. Thorough chewing guarantees a maximum health benefit from the outside, while healthy nutrients make for internal health, vigour and resistance.

A NATURAL DIET AND DENTAL HYGIENE

A healthy, unrefined diet will supply sufficient calcium, fluoride and other important elements to keep the dentine and enamel in perfect condition. Primitive people have such beautiful teeth because their crude diet supplies all the elements they need to preserve their teeth in a healthy condition, whereas we, with our denatured food, suffer from all sorts of deficiencies. Beautiful teeth do not depend on being Chinese, African or Indian or whether you are white, yellow, black or brown; they depend on a natural diet. The proof of this is found among North American blacks who have been living in that modern, industrialised society for some generations. It is only since they left their native lands and adopted the diet and customs of their new environment that their teeth have begun to show signs of deterioration. Now dentists have plenty of work among the blacks of Chicago or Virginia. Their healthy resistance has disappeared and those who turn their backs on natural foods have to care for and brush their teeth just as much as anyone else. Anyone who adopts the life-style and eating habits of our modern 'civilised' society becomes prone to disease, including, of course, bad teeth.

Should we clean our teeth? Certainly we should, for we no longer possess natural resistance to tooth decay and therefore have to assist nature mechanically to remove all food particles, plaque and undesirable bacteria from the surface and crevices of the teeth.

To ensure healthy teeth, we should adopt a natural diet. This is the first decisive step. It is essential to have a wholesome diet of natural foods and also plenty of exercise in the open air and sunshine. The teeth will then be able to do their work for an entire lifetime. As regards proper nutrition, it is important to choose wholegrain or wholemeal (wholewheat) bread that contains rye in addition to wheat, since rye is rich in fluoride which is necessary for the development of strong tooth enamel. Among some tried and tested breads are 'Walliser Roggenbrot' (100 per cent rye bread made in Switzerland), Vogel's wholegrain flake bread, Risopan crispbread and 'Waerlandbrot'. Other similar breads may also be available in your locality.

However, because our bodies have become degenerated through the introduction of modern foods, we must, as a second step, go in for special tooth care. Even if we occasionally eat some black rye or wholegrain bread, this will not make our teeth any healthier. True, there are still some people who have good teeth, even among Europeans, but if an analysis is made of their diet it will be found that it is based on wholefoods and that they follow a natural way of life. In the mountain areas of the Swiss canton Valais the people still eat a famous dark rye bread, and this is no doubt one reason why they seem to have excellent teeth. Vigorous chewing gives the jaw muscles plenty of exercise, and this kind of natural massage assures better blood circulation. There must be other countries, too, where in some areas the population lives primarily on natural food and has good teeth as a result.

When I was a young man in my late teens I too had bad teeth as the result of an unnatural diet. I then changed my eating habits and within three years my dentist assured me that my teeth showed definite signs of hardening. At the end of six years, he congratulated me on my change of diet and said that my teeth were in excellent condition, with hard and healthy dentine. Now, in my old age, I still have the same good teeth I had in my youth. So, to safeguard the teeth, all refined foods should be avoided. To start with, white sugar and flour should definitely be left out of your diet. Every school and every dentist's waiting room should display comical educational posters, acting as constant reminders of the two enemies of strong teeth, white sugar and white flour, and the cartoons on these posters should become as popular as Mickey Mouse. Such vivid warnings would make our schoolchildren constantly aware of the agents responsible for bad teeth. Who knows, maybe they would even contribute to banning the culprits from our tables!

BASIC RULES FOR CARE OF THE TEETH

A few rules for care of the teeth might be useful to everyone. First of all, the teeth should be cleaned every day with a good and simple cleansing agent. It can be a toothpaste that does not contain any strong chemicals, for example *Rosemary Toothpaste*, or it can be ashes or some other natural material. Every small sign of decay should be given immediate attention so that you will be spared the problem of dead teeth. Small defects when neglected may result in having to kill the nerve, and years ago that was often the practice.

A tooth without a nerve is a dead tooth and, in a manner of speaking, becomes a foreign body in the mouth. Such a tooth must be watched carefully, for it may precipitate the formation of granulomas, ideal nesting grounds for germs. A little thing like that can endanger a person's general health because the bacteria and metabolic toxins discharged into the bloodstream can cause various ailments, although the teeth themselves may not be painful at all. Nothing seems to be wrong with the teeth, yet the person may suffer from rheumatic fever and does not know why. Arthritis may develop, possibly leading to rheumatoid arthritis and other serious ailments, all stemming from granulomas or abscesses. Some of the other problems attributed to them include cardiac pains and troubles, palpitations when walking upstairs or uphill, kidney and liver dysfunctions, as well as other organic upsets – all without our knowing what the cause might be.

American doctors are generally credited with the discovery of these problems emanating from germ-ridden dead teeth. The sad thing was that in the case of articular rheumatism, rheumatic fever, some dentists short-sightedly extracted not only the dead teeth with their abscesses, but also all the good ones. This, of course, was wrong, although many doctors worldwide followed this method. The error was later recognised, but not before a lot of damage had been done.

An acquaintance of mine, a railway employee, was forced to have all his excellent teeth extracted because a doctor had decided that they were the cause of his heart trouble. He was unwilling to have this done, but gave in because he was afraid the insurance company would refuse to continue his policy. Unfortunately, the removal of his teeth did not cure his heart problem. A nature cure did eventually succeed in doing so, but, alas, nature treatments, however effective, could not bring back his extracted teeth.

DENTAL TREATMENT

Never deceive yourself into thinking that a small dental defect will eventually correct itself. Visit your dentist right away. Have your teeth checked regularly and have the dentist look out especially for any dead teeth.

A capable dentist, at the first sign of articular rheumatism or heart trouble, for example, will X-ray the teeth to see if an abscess may be the cause of the trouble. The effective treatment of this type of inflammation requires professional knowledge and skill. If you have waited too long, so that you need large fillings, be careful as to the material used. Some people experience unpleasant side-effects when certain amalgams are used to fill a cavity, chief among which are mercury and silver. Depending on the individual's constitution and potential resistance, these amalgams can trigger heart trouble, a dazed state or headaches, making him unable to perform mental work efficiently. These symptoms persist until the amalgam fillings are removed. Once that is done, the problems that may have been plaguing a person for years usually disappear. Some material resembling the tooth substance should be used to fill the pulp canals, wherever possible. Gold crowns have often proved their worth, too, but they are not suitable for everyone, especially those sensitive to metals. The reaction in this case may be a mild form of heart trouble. Remove the gold and the problem goes too. If such a sensitivity to metals exists, the dentist cannot use them for your fillings, particularly silver, since its effect is worse than that of gold. However, the degree of sensitivity will vary from one person to another, depending on the individual's constitution, especially the lymphatic system.

When fitting a crown, a good dentist will take great care to see that it fits well. It must come well up into the neck of the tooth, leaving no space, as this would become a breeding ground for micro-organisms. Neither should a crown be too long, as this might cause irritation and inflammation. The solution to these problems depends upon the dentist's skill. A loose crown can lead to suppurative conditions and an abscess formation which, when prematurely closed in, can cause the most dreadful pain imaginable because of the gases that are produced that have no way out. Under such painful circumstances the taking of anodyne drugs will be unavoidable. A further consequence of incorrect treatment could be the infiltration of bacterial toxins into the system, a situation that is not only bad for health but can endanger one's life. The heart may be affected; it may even stop beating momentarily. Great skill and experience in natural treatment methods would then be required to eradicate such an infiltration.

It should be quite clear from this explanation that it is foolish to take such problems lightly and to neglect seeking treatment at the earliest opportunity, even if you think you are too busy and have no time for it straight away. On the other hand, it is also important to consult an extremely experienced dentist because his knowledge will be indispensable in recognising the problem and subsequently providing the proper treatment.

Periodontal Disease (Periodontitis)
Despite any amount of skill and experience, it is extremely hard for a good dentist to treat the ever-increasing number of cases of periodontal disease with more than limited success. This disease, characterised by chronic gingivitis (gum inflammation) and the gums becoming detached from the tooth surface, presents a difficult problem for dentist and patient alike. In fact, the teeth may become loose and fall out (periodontitis).

Massaging the diseased gums with *Echinaforce*, in alternation with *rhatany tincture* or a *herbal water containing rhatany and myrrh*, is a partial solution to the problem. In addition to cleaning the teeth, the necessary daily dental hygiene and massaging of the gums, take *Urticalcin*, in order to supply the body with additional calcium, and adopt a diet rich in vitamins and minerals.

Periodontitis is definitely not an infectious disease; it is the result of a deficiency, an avitaminosis, and this, of course, can arise quite easily if we live on modern refined foods. It is quite a different story among the American Indians and Africans, for example, who have not abandoned their traditional natural diet. Gingivitis and periodontitis are unknown among them.

Improvement can often be noticed when the patient changes his diet to a natural one, eating plenty of raw foods and avoiding products made with white flour and white sugar. However, patience will be necessary, since it will take time for the benefits of a change in diet to manifest themselves. Still, even though you might have to wait several months before the problem disappears, you will be all the more grateful and happy in the end. Alternatively, if you do not see fit to change your diet to a natural one, you can, in time, expect to face bigger problems, in spite of your dentist's efforts. The disease can spread to the jaw and cause you to lose all your teeth.

Beautiful Hair – a Natural Adornment

Visitors to oriental countries cannot help but notice the many, mainly young, Buddhist monks clad in orange robes and with their heads shaved. They are to be seen everywhere. Without even thinking you will compare them to the ordinary people with their beautiful dark hair. You will be convinced that hair is indeed an adornment. We in the West like blond, brown and black hair; even auburn or red hair can be very appealing. Women with auburn hair were considered especially beautiful in ancient Greece. But when we compare the thick bluish-black hair of the Indians in the Americas and India, and other peoples, it is not easy to say whether it is because of mere admiration or a little envy that we consider their bountiful hair so desirable. The inhabitants of those lands do not yet see any need to spend money on preserving their beautiful locks. Baldness is a peculiarity predominant among white people. It must be an acquired characteristic, for baldness simply cannot have been the Creator's original purpose; it is presumably a consequence of civilisation.

The Structure of the Hair

The anatomic structure of the hair, like so many other things in the body, is a technical miracle. Although the hair has no feeling, it is not dead matter either. Perhaps it could best be compared to a plant with a bulb-shaped root. The hair root, or bulb, is embedded in the skin, about 3–5 mm deep ($\frac{1}{8}$–$\frac{1}{5}$ inch), and is connected by blood vessels from which it receives the nutrients necessary for the hair to grow. The daily rate of growth is about $\frac{1}{4}$–$\frac{1}{2}$ mm. A tightly knit network of lymphatics envelops the hair roots. The salty lymph is thought to act as an electrolyte in the electrical function of hair. Strong electric charges in hair cause visible sparks when combing it in the dark. The hair of very excited or ecstatic people lights up in the dark and when photographed the effect is seen as a kind of halo. Great mental disturbance and agitation is observable in the hair, when viewed under a microscope, as notches of variable depths. So it is possible, for example, to discover if someone has had a nervous breakdown the previous year.

A medical book I once read described hair as a 'barometer of the soul'. In fact, extreme shock can make one's hair turn grey in a short time. Some people who were buried under rubble when conscious and could only be freed some days later, emerged grey-haired. When I visited a hospital in Guatemala I also observed Indian children whose long black hair showed strains of white, in this case caused by vitamin deficiencies. Their bodies lost the ability to produce black pigment the moment the deficiency disease had started, and the colour of the hair remained white as long as the disease lasted. Only after recovery did the colour return to its original black.

We can see, then, that the hair not only mirrors what goes on in our mind but also our physical condition. For instance, during pregnancy some women's hair becomes very oily due to increased activity of the sebaceous glands. But once the child is born the function of the glands returns to normal. This again goes to show that the condition of the hair is closely linked with one's physical condition. The same principle applies in the case of animals. A shiny coat in dogs and horses is a sign of good health, but if it is dull or rough looking, it is high time for the vet to look for the underlying problem in the animal's system.

A healthy hair is strong, being able to support a weight of about 80 g (just under 3 oz) without snapping. A diseased hair, however, will tear when a weight of 30–40 g (about 1½ oz) is suspended from it. The healthy pigtail of a Chinese or Indian woman is able to support about 2½–3 tons before it snaps. Of course, the resistance of a single hair depends also upon its relative thickness. People who live close to nature have thicker and stronger hair than those who do not. Generally speaking, the more refined our food and life-style, the finer will be our hair.

When a hair is pulled out, the root, held fast in the dermis, is able to manufacture another hair shaft. However, eczema and other diseases affecting the scalp can make this part degenerate and die, so that the affected areas become bald. Typhoid fever is usually responsible for the loss of all hair, but the hair bulb does not actually die and the hair has been known to grow back even more luxuriantly after recovery, when the capillary vessels and lymphatics have returned to their normal function.

Hair Colour
The colour of the hair is manufactured near the hair roots, where an inner layer of cells contains pigments of various colours. That

is why there are so many shades of hair, from blond to red or black. Hair colour is part of an individual's genetic make-up. True, the hairdresser can use chemicals to change your natural shade to one that is completely different. Nevertheless, the original colour will return at the roots as the hair continues to grow. So, if your hair is dyed or bleached and you do not wish it to be known, you will have to see your hairdresser regularly for a touch-up. It has become the fashion to change one's hair colour according to whim, but this may not always be appreciated by the passport control at international borders, for example, unless you have the entry 'hair colour' altered accordingly. Irrespective of the modern extremes and changes, the natural variety of hair colours and characteristics is just as lovely as the charming variety of shape and colour seen in butterflies, birds, fish and other marine creatures, not forgetting the beauty of flowers.

Turning grey seems to be somehow connected with the activity of the sex glands. The hormone production of these glands diminishes with advancing age and the hair seems to go grey at the same rate. As already mentioned, however, dramatic mental and emotional shock, as well as continual stress and worries, can also be responsible for premature greying. It is often noticeable at the same time that the activity of the gonads is weakened. It could be genetic that some people turn grey in the bloom of youth. Unfortunately, however, grey hair does not usually suit the person's youthful looks. It is different with a face wrinkled as a result of rich experience and a hard life; silver-grey hair in such a person often seems a fitting crown.

Care of the Hair
Natural beauty calls for care if it is to remain, and this principle applies to our hair too. The best care we can give it is a natural way of life with plenty of exercise in the open air and a sensible diet. Remember, the hair is a reflection of our general condition of health.

Since hair contains silica, iron, copper, arsenic, manganese and sulphur, it stands to reason that plants in which these elements are found prove to be excellent for its care. Naturally blond people will find that washing their hair with *camomile* and then applying *onion hair tonic* is a superb treatment. Dark-haired people achieve better results with *birch* or *nettle* lotions. If you rinse your hair with diluted *Molkosan* (3 tablespoons to 1 litre/1¾ pints of water), it will retain its natural brilliance.

For care of the scalp, and to combat hair loss, massage it with *Bioforce Cream*, preferably a day before washing it. This natural cream contains lanolin, genuine St John's wort oil and the extracts of fresh plants. If fungal disease has caused a loss of hair, dab the affected areas with diluted Molkosan and, after drying, dust with *Urticalcin* powder. This treatment usually helps to get rid of the infection in a short time.

Excessively oily hair is often a problem for young people around the age of puberty. In the case of girls, this is generally due to a temporary disruption of the ovarian function. In order to help, the cause must be treated; *warm underwear* is recommended and *warm herbal sitz baths* are necessary, taken every night until relief is achieved. Some older men try to keep their hair by using expensive tonics, but these preparations often benefit the manufacturers and advertisers more than those who would like to see an end to their bald pate. Really, all is in vain, because once the hair bulbs have gone, no new hair can grow.

Most people look after their hair in one way or another, even though they may not have grasped the idea that the basic care and treatment has to be from inside the body itself. In other words, by eliminating any existing internal deficiencies, the appearance of the hair will improve. I often hear from patients who have taken silica and a biological calcium preparation who tell me, 'My hair is beautiful again.' They are elated and surprised at the same time.

External care will no doubt benefit your hair to some extent, and so will a good hair tonic. However, if you do not see to it that you put your 'internal house', your body, in order, and do not take in sufficient calcium and silica, all external treatments will be of little use. And it is really quite easy to do something about it. The usual problem is lack of calcium and silica, but if a woman's hair is too greasy, her hormone production is poor. Then it is important to treat the hormone glands, perhaps by taking a good homoeopathic preparation such as *Ovarium 3x* and regular *sitz baths* in order to assure good circulation. If the stagnation is bad, *Aesculaforce* will help rectify the trouble. Proceeding in this way, there will be an indirect beneficial influence on the hair. Moreover, if you follow this treatment you will not merely benefit your hair; the general condition of your health will improve, since many other body functions depend on the proper functioning of the glands.

HAIR AND SCALP LOTIONS AND HAIR RESTORERS

There are all kinds of hair and scalp lotions advertised and no doubt some of them may be quite good. However, there is one remedy that is always available and does not cost much; it is also the best possible hair tonic and restorer. It is the common *onion*. Onions contain sulphur and this natural sulphur is an excellent skin lotion. If you have any hair or scalp problems, take half a raw onion and rub it well into the scalp before washing your hair. This treatment is very effective and will stimulate hair growth. If you do not feel like using raw onions, use an *onion hair lotion*. For better results use a hair nutrient as well, *lanolin*, which contains vitamin F. In its natural state pure lanolin (*Adeps lanae*) is too thick and sticky, so that it has to be processed or at least mixed with oil. *Bioforce Cream* is such a simple preparation. Incidentally, lanolin (wool fat) is not obtained from sheep's meat but from sheep's wool. It is certainly biologically appropriate if we use the things nature provides for certain purposes. Since lanolin serves to keep the sheep's wool, hair and skin in good condition, it can be of service for our hair and skin too. My own successful experiences of using lanolin have proved this assumption to be true. Of course, *nettles*, in the form of an infusion or a fresh plant extract, provide us with an excellent hair tonic, especially in the case of skin eruptions on the scalp. Many people recommend *birch leaves* too, but the best tonic of all, I believe, is the onion.

So if you wish to have a healthy scalp and beautiful hair, there are plenty of remedies from which to choose. The ones I have just mentioned will no doubt give good results.

The Skin

The Functions of the Skin

Not everyone is aware of the fact that the skin is an organ just as vital as the kidneys, stomach and intestines, and even as essential as the liver. A person would die in a few hours without the function of his skin, and that is much quicker than if his stomach and intestines were to be taken out. One third of the blood in the human body is to be found in the capillary vessels in the skin. In an adult the skin covers an area of approximately 2 square metres (21 square feet), and it is therefore one of the largest organs of the body. One square centimetre (0.155 square inch) contains about three million cells and a number of tiny structures whose functions are essential to good health. We do not feel the cold as acutely as heat and therefore feel less pain when exposed to severe cold than to extreme heat. This is because every square centimetre of our skin contains two or three structures that register cold sensations and about six times as many that register heat. Depending on the area of the body, there are about 10–20 hairs to every square centimetre, also 12–15 sebaceous glands and 90–120 sweat glands, in accordance with the texture of the skin, whether it has fine or large pores. If all the fine capillaries were to be connected together, they would extend to about 1 km (⅝ mile), and the even finer nerves would be four times as long.

If we touch a piece of material with our fingertips, trying to find out whether it is pure silk or linen, twenty-five tiny structures cooperate to help us test the fabric. We could catch a finger in the door and feel nothing at all if it were not for the 200 sensation structures per square centimetre of skin that communicate the injury to the brain via the sensory nerves. Scalding, burning and a Baunscheidt (stimulation) treatment can cause the formation of large blisters filled with fluid, with the top layer of skin becoming separated from the one beneath it.

The outermost layer is called epidermis and consists of cells. The deep inner layer, the corium or dermis, is much thicker and consists of fibrous tissue. The epidermis has more than twenty cell layers that contain no blood vessels, which is why the skin does not bleed when it is rubbed off, nor produces any sensation of pain. However, when the dermis, which lies under the epidermis, is touched or brought into contact with water, there is an immediate reaction. When engaged in physical work, handling earth, sand, lye and the like, soapy water rubs off several layers of the epidermis when the hands are subsequently washed. But on the following day there will already be the same number of layers as before, because the epidermis is continually replaced from underneath. Once this function is disturbed, we get hard and horny skin or abnormal flaking, with loose scales of dry, dead skin, as is so often the case with the scalp. If you wear the same underwear for too long, the offensive smell is due mainly to millions of dead skin cells and dried sweat.

THE SEBACEOUS GLANDS
Our skin is like living leather, with a built-in automatic lubrication system in the sebaceous glands that becomes active in accordance with the skin's needs. Dry skin (lacking oil) is extremely sensitive, making one much more susceptible to colds and infections, and also to radiation damage. When washing with soap, not only is

the dirt removed but sebum is dissolved at the same time. This means that the skin is deprived of the necessary oil and its protective function is diminished. For this reason it is especially important in the winter to use a good skin oil after washing with soap. Experience has shown that *St John's wort oil* is the best skin care oil known to us; it is truly excellent for the skin and especially for the capillaries and nerves embedded in it. However, since it is rather greasy it should be mixed with essential oils from plants, which provide the added bonus of enhancing the soothing effect of the St John's wort oil. We have produced such an excellent mixture with our orangy-red-coloured *Skin Oil*. It would be a good idea to keep a bottle in your bathroom on account of its importance in skin care and as a massage oil.

If there is an insufficient secretion of the sebaceous glands, causing the skin to be rough and chapped, the application of a cream containing lanolin is indicated. *Bioforce Cream* is a natural and effective remedial cream that is soon able to revitalise the skin. This tried and tested cream contains lanolin as a base, as well as arnica, sanicle and other medicinal herbs that have proved their worth in skin care. Bioforce Cream is also recommended as a protection against sunburn, with the best results being obtained if it is applied to the skin the day before exposure to the sun.

THE EFFECTS OF SUNLIGHT

Sunlight of a certain wavelength is especially intense in the mountains and by the sea, changing white tyrosine to a brown colour. This pigment, which tans the skin so beautifully, is on the one hand a protection against burns and on the other, a stimulus for the manufacture of antibodies for various infectious diseases, especially tuberculosis and diseases of the throat and chest.

As individuals it seems that we are still not well enough informed about the importance of sunlight for our well-being. Otherwise we would find out just how much or how little can benefit our health. If we were to put our children on a natural diet rich in calcium and let them spend more time in the open air and sunlight, rickets and scrofula (tuberculosis of the lymphatic glands) would be unknown. The ultraviolet rays change ergosterol, which is present in the human body, into vitamin D. And it is generally known that a deficiency in calcium and vitamin D is mainly responsible for rickets and lymphatic problems.

Beauty and well-being are highly dependent upon the general

315

tone and buoyancy of the body, and both are significantly increased by exposure to sunlight.

With regular exposure to sunlight, the way we look and feel will both improve, giving us a better physical appearance than we had before. It has been found that exposing the skin to sunlight increases, in a manner of speaking, the voltage of the nerve system so that the whole body will experience greater vitality. The skin is like an antenna that absorbs and emits rays. For this reason some people appear to refresh us and others sap our strength; when in the presence of the latter if feels as if all our energy were being drained, tiring us very quickly.

It is interesting to note that sunlight on the skin also heightens the efficiency of our sensory organs. We are able to hear and see better when we let the sun recharge us.

THE SWEAT GLANDS
The manifold functions of the sweat glands have only gradually come to be recognised. The body has about two million sweat glands, each one being about 5 mm (about ⅕ inch) long. Without perspiring, they evaporate 1–1.5 litres (1.7–2.6 pints) of water during the course of a day. If exudation is increased by means of a steam bath, a sauna bath or by living in the tropics, the body is able to give produce up to ten times this quantity of water.

If it were possible to combine all the sweat pores into one single tube, its diameter would be about 25–30 cm (10–12 inches). The size of such a tube makes it easy to understand why so much water is able to escape. Taste a drop of sweat and you will see that it is salty; on litmus paper its reaction is acid. In fact, sweat contains sodium salts, potassium, sulphuric acid, iron, phosphorus, lactic acid and as much urea as one kidney excretes, for which reason the skin could be called the 'third kidney'. The skin can exude arsenic and other poisons, possibly resulting in eczema and other skin eruptions. This shows the wisdom of treating skin problems internally as well as externally. Indeed, it explains why sweat treatments have cured many an illness.

The sweat glands are the units of a temperature control system that makes life in the tropics more bearable. By evaporating water through the sweat glands it is possible to lose heat of up to 500 calories. Keep the functions of the skin in good working order and you will be observing one of the most important rules for good health.

DETRIMENTAL INFLUENCES

When I visited Mesopotamia (between the Euphrates and Tigris rivers) I went to a small museum at the edge of the ruined city of ancient Babylon. There I saw vessels that had been used by women of those bygone times for the storage of oils and creams. According to ancient records, the women even used plants as a basis for the preparation of cosmetics and aromatic oils, as it is still the practice in those areas among Arab and Bedouin women. On another visit, this time to the Indians of the Amazon region, I became acquainted with a plant from which a fatty red dye is obtained. The natives use this extract to paint the body and face and it adheres to the skin for weeks, not even soap being strong enough to remove it.

Beauty culture is almost as old as the human race. The desire to look attractive and to improve one's looks is somehow inborn and it is especially women who take full advantage of the possibilities. However, although cosmetics can be beneficial to the skin and its functions they can also be detrimental, as, for example, are all creams and other preparations that block the pores and impair or stop the exudation of sweat, thus making the skin flaccid and tired looking. Frequent powdering also has the same effect. This explains why some women with tired skin certainly do not look their best without their make-up and can give you quite a shock if you see them first thing in the morning. Without make-up a forty-year-old woman who has been accustomed to applying non-biological cosmetics for many years may look like a seventy-year-old grandmother.

The skin is, and should be, the expression of one's good health, so if you want to help nature a little by caring for your skin, use nothing but biological cosmetics, especially those of natural plant origin, since they stimulate and support the skin's natural functions. Other cosmetics are little more than paint, a veritable deception.

WHEN THE FUNCTIONS OF THE SKIN ARE IMPAIRED

It is understandable that the indigenous peoples of, for example, Africa, South America and the South Sea islands enjoy a better skin function than people who have to wear thick clothing all the time; the native people in hot climates often walk around wearing very little clothing, if any, and their bodies are in constant contact with the air, sunlight and often with muddy water, thus promoting a more efficient skin function. Since in colder regions of the earth it would be impossible to do this, the people living in northern

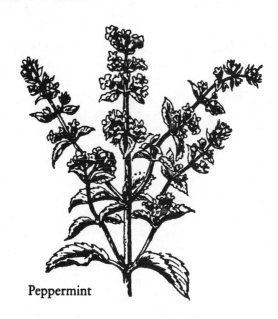

Peppermint

Europe must have followed a healthy instinctive desire to stimulate their bodies by taking regular saunas and improving the effect even further by cooling down afterwards in cold water or by rolling in the snow, for these customs also keep the functions of the skin in good order and, in turn, benefit the whole body. For the same reason some people with a healthy instinct like to go hiking or swimming. They practise such a sport on a reasonable scale, and if they ski it is done in a sensible way, climbing up the mountain slope instead of using a ski-lift. Other people find greater pleasure and advantage in massaging the body or having it massaged regularly. They use an effective oil that stimulates the functions of the skin, keeping it healthy and in top condition.

Impaired skin functions can have extremely detrimental consequences. When you do not perspire enough you should frequently drink an infusion of *elder flowers, peppermint* and *lovage;* you can take them either in alternation or as a mixed herb tea. In addition, it is recommended to take a weekly *sauna* over an extended period.

Certain parts of the body can sweat excessively, for example the hands, feet and armpits. Is there anything one can do about this condition? Yes there is; you can stimulate the kidneys with a good *kidney tea* containing *Solidago* (goldenrod), and *Nephrosolid kidney drops.* The skin, the so-called 'third kidney', will be relieved as soon as the kidneys themselves have been activated. Additionally, in accordance with the method of the ancient Chinese, take *sage tea* or *Salvia drops* (made from fresh sage) regularly. If the perspiration, especially under the arms, has an unpleasant smell, the best external remedy is *Hamamelis Soap*, which contains witch hazel and thyme, and is an excellent means of supporting the treatment with sage drops or tea. Daily washing with Hamamelis Soap followed by the application of *Bioforce Cream* has also proved successful in cases of feet that sweat excessively.

Dry, scaly skin that is flaking off can be effectively treated by the external application of *St John's wort oil*, in alternation with *Symphytum Cream* or *Symphosan*, which contain comfrey and other herbs. At the same time, take *Violaforce*, a tincture made from heartsease (wild pansy). If the condition is caused by dry psoriasis, you will also have to dab the affected area with *Molkosan* every day. Callouses, causing skin that is as hard as a lizard's, are the result of a disease of the endocrine glands, often connected with avitaminosis (a disease caused by vitamin deficiency), and will require special treatment of the underlying cause.

Sensible Skin Care

It is important that the skin care you practise protects and benefits the skin rather than damages it. The reason why I raise this point is the great number of cosmetics on the market and the persuasive advertising used to sell them. Unfortunately, only very few of this host of products really are kind to the skin. You see, the term 'skin care' only applies correctly to products that protect the skin, are good for it, keep it healthy, indeed, even heal and rejuvenate it. Only skin that functions properly can remain healthy and reflect freshness, perhaps even youthfulness. This requires, first and foremost, good circulation, for this alone guarantees adequate nourishment of the skin.

The second factor to consider is the importance of stimulating the skin's ability to breathe, or at least ensuring that this is not impaired. Cosmetics that block the pores prevent the skin from breathing properly. Such products include powder, certain other cosmetics and many creams containing fat, filling materials and stabilisers which the skin is unable to absorb. If the skin is not treated in the right way, it will begin to look withered and will age prematurely.

In addition to physical treatment to stimulate the circulation and regenerate the skin, there are some first-class plants that can be used for this purpose. *St John's wort* (*Hypericum*) is most frequently indicated and widely used. Its oil-soluble ingredients promote good circulation in the skin because even the finest capillaries will be activated. Plants that contain mucilage, for example, comfrey and some mosses, rejuvenate the skin and, in time, can even soften wrinkles, since the skin tissue will recover its youthful tone. It is therefore most beneficial in the care of your face if you soak some cotton wool with *Symphosan* and dab your face with it after washing, or regularly apply *Symphytum Cream*. Should you suffer from eczema and dry skin, wash the affected areas with an infusion of heartsease (wild pansy) every day.

Badly functioning sebaceous glands tend to dry the skin and require the use of a cream made from plant oils, lanolin and vitamin F. Whatever cream you decide on, it should supply the skin with the substances it lacks. Creams with a vaseline base are not truly satisfactory because vaseline is difficult to saponify and the skin cannot absorb it. *Bioforce Cream*, on the other hand, is excellent for dry, even cracked and chapped skin. I would advise that any rich skin cream be applied sparingly; remember, too, that the skin absorbs oil or fat more quickly in cold weather than in warm weather.

Non-greasy creams based on something other than plant mucilage generally contain ingredients that block the pores. The skin suffers and loses its smoothness if the treatment continues for some time. Oiling the skin, especially after a bath and washing with soap, is to be recommended, since soap removes the natural oil produced by the sebaceous glands. A good oil that stimulates the skin is indispensable in winter and whenever engaging in water sports.

It is imperative that the perfumes added to skin oils and creams be only from natural essential oils. Perfumes derived from chemicals can harm the skin. Also remember that the skin derives no benefit whatsoever from being covered with thick layers of all kinds of cosmetics. Healthy skin only needs a little help when greater demands are put on it through exposure to the sun, water, cold and wind. The wisdom expressed in the saying 'You can have too much of a good thing' applies to the care of your skin and cosmetics too.

SKIN BLEMISHES

No one likes to have skin blemishes, yet it is not uncommon for young people to have a problem with spots, especially at the age of puberty. A spotty face can even create an inferiority complex if all lotions and creams fail to help. This is another reason why the problem of impure skin should be tackled at the roots. The recommendation to be careful about what one eats and adopt an appropriate diet is not always received with appreciation, but it is necessary, since the trouble is basically the result of ingesting the wrong food.

If you suffer from spots it is of the utmost importance to reduce your intake of fats by half or three-quarters. What is more, take great care to avoid heated fats and oils, animal fats being especially detrimental. Cakes, biscuits, pastries, and all other sweets should be left out of the diet altogether or at least drastically reduced. Eggs, particularly boiled eggs, omelettes and other egg dishes are like poison for impure skin. Only fresh, soft white cheeses such as cottage cheese or quark are digestible, but no other kind of cheese. Raw vegetables, natural brown rice, potatoes boiled in their skins, cottage cheese and horseradish are nutritive and remedial and contain plenty of essential vitamins and minerals. Hot spices tend to make things worse. Some external remedies that have proved very effective are *Echinaforce* and *Molkosan;* one day apply Echinaforce to the affected area, the next day use Molkosan, and continue in daily alternation. Apply a little *Bioforce Cream* to any patches of dry skin. For internal treatment take *Violaforce*, a tincture made from heartsease (wild pansy), and also Echinaforce.

Avoid squeezing spots and blackheads, unless you apply Molkosan to disinfect them right away. Otherwise you will only spread the bacteria, which usually settle in the inflamed skin pores. In other words, if you want to prevent the condition from getting worse you have to be very careful. Also, do not handle or work with turpentine, floor wax, paints and modern detergents; if you have to use them, make sure to wear rubber gloves for protection. *Symphosan* helps to improve and regenerate skin that has large pores and looks withered. Its content of plant mucilage is responsible for this action. And another thing, it is not always advisable to wash with soap. Cleansing the skin with oil and then wiping it with alcohol is often more beneficial for impure skin. Finally, I cannot emphasise strongly enough how important it is to improve your general health by adopting a natural way of life. Your skin will then derive great benefits too.

SHOULD OILS BE USED FOR SKIN CARE?
It is true that nature itself sees to it that our skin receives the oil it needs, and for this purpose we have been given the marvellous

sebaceous glands, which work automatically. I have noticed that people in less developed parts of the world tend to have much oilier skin than we have and they never have to worry about dry skin. Unfortunately, the sebaceous glands of people living in industrialised societies work less efficiently and there is a very good reason for this. The fact that we go against, rather than cooperate with, nature – through our unnatural way of life, our food, clothing and general living conditions, and doing our work shut inside closed rooms that are often overheated in cold weather – discourages the proper functioning of the skin and the sebaceous glands.

To remedy this situation we must give our skin all the help it needs in the form of a good oil. It is advisable to always lubricate the body well before going for a swim, whether in a cool freshwater lake or river or in the sea. Doing this will help the body to retain its warmth and you will not shiver or feel chilled even if the water is cold. I am writing this from personal experience, although I must admit that I have a good basal metabolic rate and circulation, so I do not chill easily. The oil treatment is especially recommended for sensitive people, even more so for the prevention of chills after stepping out of the water.

On the other hand, it is not necessary and does not benefit the skin in any way to smear so much oil on the body so that it looks all greasy. Oil should be used sparingly and massaged well into the skin. Avoid oils that are scented with synthetic perfumes, which make the bathers smell even from a distance. Pure *olive oil* mixed with a little *lemon oil* is a good and inexpensive skin lotion for bathing. If you want to buy a ready-made oil, look for a skin oil that is based on *St John's wort oil*, because this is a most excellent skin-food on account of the lipoids it contains. It is important, when shopping, to ask for a skin oil that is made from natural, red St John's wort oil; reject any oil that is artificially coloured.

Care of the skin requires not only the use of oil but involves common sense when exposing the body to the sun, light and air. An efficient skin function is the basis for proper glandular function and for general well-being.

WRINKLES AND SKIN WITH LARGE PORES

As a rule, smooth skin is a sign of youthfulness and good health and it is not surprising that women in particular make a great effort to maintain this desirable condition for as long as they possibly can. But it is not simply a matter of giving nature a helping hand by applying plenty of powder, make-up and creams. In fact, the liberal use of such products may achieve just the opposite of what is desired. The real answer lies in taking care in one's youth, living in a natural way and not worrying too much or constantly giving in to anxieties, for we know that stressful problems are wearisome and undermine the body's reserves and well-being. They do indeed age us prematurely and foster the formation of wrinkles. Of course, constant tiredness on account of overwork or pursuing pleasures night after night can also harm one's health and impair one's youthful looks. It is understandable why so many people want to cover up these flaws in their faces by using all kinds of cosmetics.

What is less understandable is why some girls plaster their young and radiant faces with make-up. Make-up is supposed to hide what is ugly, but what could be more beautiful than glowing health, smooth and youthful skin, red cheeks and lips as nature coloured them.

The skin cannot breathe naturally if the pores are blocked with cosmetics. In consequence it degenerates; the pores become larger. It is just as unsightly when the skin begins to slacken early, developing more wrinkles than would be expected as a result of the normal ageing process.

NATURAL BEAUTY CARE

Much time is often wasted in efforts to improve one's looks cosmetically. Yet how much easier it would be to keep the body healthy and, in particular, to take good care of the sex glands right from the start. Their efficiency contributes to maintaining youthfulness longer. For this, sunlight, deep-breathing and exercise are important. Anyone who spends most of his time in heated rooms, rarely moves around in the open air, never goes for walks or hikes or practises some other sport in moderation, should not be surprised if he becomes like a hothouse plant and grows old before his time. Remember, exercise in the open air, perhaps gardening or walking, has much to do with keeping young and fit. Regular showers, alternating between hot and cold water, are also beneficial since they promote good circulation. Recommended, too, are good plant remedies for effective external application, such as *Symphosan* tincture or *Symphytum Cream*, and *Violaforce*. These two remedies, applied in alternation, help to reduce the size of the pores and rejuvenate the skin.

For a reliable skin care programme rub in Symphosan, a tried and tested comfrey preparation, every morning after washing.

Afterwards, as a protection against strong sunlight or biting wind, apply *Bioforce Cream,* which contains lanolin, but it is not necessary to do this daily. Then, before going to bed, soak a cotton pad with *Violaforce* and dab over the whole face. In order to help the sebaceous glands, use a natural skin oil, or the lanolin cream already mentioned, two or three times a week. This treatment may be sufficient for everyday use, provided you are not too exposed to cold and sunshine. It is quite a simple treatment and you will derive great benefit if you take care of your skin like this for a few months. It will look much younger and the pores may even return to normal.

Impetigo

Young people often suffer from pustules all over the face and on the back. The condition may be attributable to a disturbance in the internal hormone secretions and especially associated with the sex glands. At the same time, an external bacterial infection – mainly staphylococci or streptococci – may also be diagnosed. This unpleasant condition usually provokes inhibitions and the sufferer tries to get rid of the disfiguring infection as quickly as possible. So he keeps squeezing the pustules and spots, only to spread the infection with his fingernails. The bacteria keep on spreading, the affected areas and spots growing larger and more inflamed. In time, the lesions secrete a fluid which, when dry, develops into yellowish crusty sores, of a rather unsightly appearance. In the past mercury ointments were used to combat this condition, but in modern times penicillin or sulphonamide creams have become more popular, both of them giving better results than those with a mercury or tar base.

Biological Treatment

This unpleasant condition can also be treated with biological remedies, an excellent one being *Molkosan.* Used externally, this natural, concentrated, whey product, containing 15 per cent lactic acid, will give good results. Soak a cotton pad with it and dab the affected areas. Repeat the application after about five minutes, this time using *Echinaforce* instead. Molkosan kills the bacteria and Echinaforce prevents infection. When a pustule comes to a head and you feel like squeezing it open, do so only with sterilised cotton wool. Immediately afterwards, apply Molkosan and Echinaforce as indicated above. Do not use soap for washing, but cleanse the skin with 45 per cent *alcohol* to which a few drops of *arnica tincture* have been added. When you suffer from pustules your skin is rarely dry, but if it should be, apply *Bioforce Cream* once a week.

Internal treatment is also necessary and you should adopt an appropriate diet. My book *The Liver, the Regulator of Your Health* contains guidelines for such a diet. In addition, you should take Echinaforce regularly. And if you want to reduce the formation of pus, take *Hepar sulph. 10x*. On the other hand, if you want to stimulate it in order to promote faster cleansing, take the same remedy in the fourth potency (4x). In order to activate the glands, it is also advisable to take at least one *Kelpasan* tablet daily.

Reliable Remedies for Fungal Infections (Mycosis)

No matter where mycosis occurs, it is difficult to eradicate. However, as with all skin conditions, *whey* has proved to be of excellent value even for mycotic diseases, that is, fungal skin diseases. But since not everyone is able to go to a dairy in the country and obtain fresh whey, many patients like to use the concentrated whey as available in *Molkosan*.

A patient told me once that she had suffered from this troublesome problem for years despite all her efforts to get rid of it. The fungus had settled under her breasts and on her arms, causing frequent soreness, and for more than twelve years she had used all kinds of remedies without success. Then she learned about Molkosan and an African plant remedy, *Spilanthes*, which complements and reinforces the healing effect of Molkosan. After applying these two remedies in alternation for about two weeks, she was pleased to note great improvement. The skin had been rehabilitated and was clear once again.

It goes without saying that such a splendid result makes one glad, if only because of the great patience the sufferer must have had in order to endure the unpleasant problem and its bothersome effects in spite of years of treatment. Think of the discouragement and disappointment first of all, then the great relief when the stubborn fungus disappeared in a relatively short space of time, restoring the skin to normal.

Diseases of the Nails

It is one of nature's wonders that the body is able to use silica and other minerals to provide the toes and fingers with tough horny plates. By diseases of the nails I do not mean deformities of the nails and diseases of the nail roots caused by the use of nail polish and manicures etc. The nails and hair are usually an indication of the person's general condition of health. As a rule, those who suffer from metabolic disorders have neither strong nails nor healthy-looking hair. The nails and hair become brittle and lose their natural structure when there is a deficiency of minerals and trace elements. In such cases, the only worthwhile thing to do is to treat the basic cause of the problem.

Athlete's foot and nail mycosis are stubborn infections. It is easy to acquire the fungus from infected scales of skin dropped on the floor of changing rooms in public swimming baths, or through contact with persons who suffer from the infection. If you want to treat these infections successfully you will have to cut the nails to the quick, perhaps even using a nail file. Apply *Bioforce Cream* during the day and, before you go to bed, tie some absorbent cotton soaked in *Molkosan* round the affected areas, leaving it on all night. The following night *Spilanthes* should be used instead of Molkosan. Continue using these two remedies in alternation for quite some time. I remember one doctor from Berlin telling me once quite excitedly that in his many years of medical practice he had never known an effective remedy for athlete's foot and nail mycosis until, by chance, he came across Molkosan whey concentrate when he was standing in for another doctor elsewhere. The good results in combatting these infections may be due to the effect of concentrated lactic acid together with lactic enzymes and nutritive salts.

A simple inflammation of the cuticle can be treated successfully with *Bioforce Cream, Molkosan* and *Echinaforce*. For the treatment of more serious cases of inflammation, for example onychia, use *horseradish tincture* instead of Molkosan. Finally, eating food that is rich in calcium and silica is an excellent way to strengthen the nails, as is the supplementary intake of *Urticalcin* and *Galeopsis*.

The Feet – our Faithful Servants
Only when we look upon our feet as faithful servants will we show enough appreciation to pay them proper attention and give them the good care they deserve. Do you realise what an important function the feet have to fulfil through an entire lifetime? They carry the body, irrespective of its weight, and take us wherever we wish to go. Yet looking at the changing fashion in footwear, especially as indulged in by the ladies, we begin to see the discrepancy existing between the unfair treatment of our feet and the

constant care they need and deserve. We must not close our eyes to this fact.

When I was young I often heard adults use the term 'flat-footed Indian' when they were describing someone who had really bad flat feet. Later on in life I had the opportunity to visit the Indians personally and, to my enlightenment, I saw for myself that such a description of their feet was completely out of place. True, there are Indians called Blackfeet, but I never saw one Indian with flat feet, a sad and frequent occurrence among many other people. People in less developed societies, as long as they stick to their traditional habits and walk barefoot most of the time, have strong and healthy feet that make others living in a more industrialised society truly envious.

Is it not true that our poor feet spend much time imprisoned in often unsuitable shoes? No wonder they are often just as degenerated as our teeth! It is indeed important that we give appropriate care and attention to our feet in return for their lifelong faithful service.

The Structure of the Feet and the Need for Proper Care

The bones of the feet are of a very simple design, but the structure and arrangement of the muscles is a technical masterpiece. The muscles are designed for walking on uneven ground, that is, natural ground. If they are not exercised they degenerate and the shape of the foot will change. The foot will lose its efficiency and especially the long muscles, the long flexors of the toes, will become slack. Changes in the natural structure of the feet will lead to deformities such as flat feet, splay feet, club feet, and whatever other names they are known by.

It was for a good reason that Priessnitz, Sebastian Kneipp, Rickli and other nature cure teachers recommended again and again that we walk barefoot as much as possible, particularly in the summer. It is good to walk on dew-wet grass early in the morning. This is refreshing and strengthens the foot muscles, while walking on uneven natural ground provides the feet with an invigorating massage. These recommendations are explained in greater detail on pages 332–4. However, there are many other ways in which we can care for our feet. These are the subject of the following sections.

Care of the Feet

What long and faithful service is rendered by our feet! We take it for granted that they will support the whole weight of our body and take us wherever we want to go every day of our life. Nevertheless, as a rule we neglect the daily foot bath that they so urgently need and deserve. For the feet perform not only a mechanical but also an eliminative function, although this may generally be ignored. Everyone knows about perspiration of the feet and although it can become offensive and unpleasant when excessive, so that we would like to get rid of it, it does have a purpose. Suppressing this perspiration can have extremely serious consequences. Granted, it is most disconcerting when others become aware of the strong odour, and cases have even been known where smelly feet led to a divorce. Excessive sweating of the feet should really be looked upon as being the action of a safety valve of the body; when it reaches the point where it becomes embarrassing the sufferer should do something about stimulating the kidneys and the skin by natural means. For if you try to suppress foot sweat, the toxins will remain in the system and cause havoc, leading to various ailments. The types of problem that might arise from such action, together with some suggested alternatives for dealing with excessive foot sweat, are discussed on pages 330–31.

Above all, it is most important to look after our feet and wash them daily. Since the feet are excretory organs and the sweat rids the body of toxins, it is even more important to wash your feet every day than it is to wash your face. This cleansing is very important to one's general well-being. Although there are incidents mentioned in the Bible where 'washing of the feet' had a symbolic meaning (for example humility), we should never overlook the intrinsic therapeutic value either. The washing of feet in the Middle East is almost a ritual because most people wear sandals and recognise the hygienic and health reasons for doing so. We should do it for the same reasons. To convince yourself, try washing your feet every day for one month and you will notice how your general feeling of well-being improves.

At the end of the day, if you feel tired and perhaps have a headache, try a *herbal foot bath* and see how it will soothe you. Add to the bath wild thyme, juniper needles or any other aromatic herbs and your feet will feel refreshed and invigorated. To increase the effect, after the foot bath apply a good oil that stimulates skin function; *St John's wort oil* or *olive oil* can be used for this. Even if done only once a week, this oil treatment is most beneficial. Another soothing foot oil is *Juniperosan*.

Daily care of the feet takes only a few minutes but it pays dividends in good health and saves medical bills. Try to do it on a regular basis. Further guidelines for proper foot care are given immediately below.

The importance to our health and well-being of caring for the feet will be clear from the preceding sections. Other interesting points will also be explored in the following pages. However, this section sets out to provide some useful guidelines on caring for the feet in general, as discussed above, as well as dealing with specific problems that may be experienced.

1. To start with, go and buy yourself shoes that are sensible and fit the foot rather than the fashion.
2. In the second place, take note of the following three points:
   (a) Wash your feet daily; afterwards knead and massage the muscles, then rub the feet with a little foot oil, such as *Juniperosan*.
   (b) If you suffer from rheumatism, arthritis or an ailment that causes water to accumulate in the feet, it is useful to add a tablespoon of *herbal sea salt* to a foot bath. This bath should last 15–30 minutes, at a constant temperature of 37°C (98.6°F).
   (c) Sore feet should be bathed in an infusion of *mallow* or *sanicle*.
3. Never try to suppress foot perspiration by means of strong substances. The result could be damaging to internal organs. The correct approach is to stimulate the kidneys for better elimination of wastes. Bathe the feet in an infusion of *sage* and afterwards rub them with a little *Juniperosan*. This amounts to a pleasant foot care regime and can get rid of foot perspiration in a natural way, given time.
4. For eczema and athlete's foot a foot bath with an infusion of *wild pansy (heartsease)* or *cranesbill* is recommended. After the bath dab *Molkosan* on the affected areas and as soon as it has dried, apply *Bioforce Cream*.
5. Blue areas, which are caused by dilated capillaries, should be treated like varicose veins. Take *Aesculaforce* orally and apply it externally as well.
6. For cold feet take *foot baths*, alternating between hot and cold water. Prepare the warm bath with an infusion of thyme, immerse your feet for three minutes, then place them in cold water for three seconds. Repeat this sequence for a total of about twenty minutes.

Make sure the temperature of the warm water remains constant by adding fresh hot water whenever necessary.

7. A burning sensation in the feet, as often experienced by older people, should be treated in the same way as item 6. The burning is caused by strictured vessels, and remedies that act to dilate them again must also be taken internally.

If you have ever had any trouble with your feet you will keenly appreciate that healthy ones are a real blessing. It is always recommended that they be given preventative care, for our general condition of well-being often depends on the state of the feet. Also remember that cold feet are bad for the kidneys and, in the case of women, the pelvic organs.

Dealing with Excessive Foot Sweat

Is it a good thing to get rid of foot sweat? Or is perspiration a natural process through which the body disposes of toxins tnat it could not otherwise eliminate? This second assumption seems to be correct, or else so many unpleasant consequences could not have resulted when sufferers tried to suppress perspiration of the feet.

Just recently I received a letter from a woman in Zurich telling me that while her husband was doing military service his foot sweat was suppressed and as a result he developed a skin disease. Foot sweat is often suppressed by people in military service, but this is no cure; rather, it can be detrimental in as far as the effects will be either a skin disorder or some other problem. For example, I have never found a person suffering from any form of lung trouble to be plagued by excessively sweaty feet. Specialists in lung diseases with whom I have discussed this phenomenon have confirmed my observation. Hence the logical conclusion that the direct and deliberate suppression of foot perspiration or some other excretory body function, can mark the beginning of lung problems or may be connected with them. If you want to get rid of the troubles incurred there will be no other way but once again to induce the feet to sweat. You may wonder how this can be done. Well, the suggestion below is simple enough, but carrying it out successfully is quite another matter.

A doctor in Berlin once helped himself by sprinkling carbide powder on the insoles of his shoes. The moisture exuding from the feet generates heat through its contact with the carbide, which serves to draw out yet more moisture. In this way foot sweat is induced artificially. It was reported that the doctor used this method to cure several cases, including patients with lung diseases that had previously failed to respond to any other treatment.

The thing to remember is that it is fundamentally wrong to try to suppress foot sweat. If the odour becomes too unpleasant, bathe the feet frequently; wash them with a herbal infusion and afterwards oil them with a good, aromatic skin oil, for example *Juniperosan*, that is easily absorbed. Also, change your socks and stockings frequently. These measures will do no harm and can only be beneficial. Remember, the natural functions of the body should never be suppressed because through them the system is able to work properly.

High Heels or None at All?

The question of heels does not arise in areas of the world where people walk barefoot. In temperate and cold regions, however, the question is a valid one. It is interesting, however, that when travelling through South America you will see many more high-heeled shoes worn by women than is common among modern women in more northern regions. In fact, I had the impression that South America might have been the birthplace of high-heeled shoes. On one occasion I was watching an Indian girl from the slums of Lima. As soon as she was out of sight of her shack she quickly took off her shabby footwear, hid it under a bush and put on a pair of fashionable high-heeled shoes. She then proceeded to swagger along the street like a queen!

In rural areas where there are only dirt roads, high heels are, of course, most uncomfortable. The natural uneven ground, meadows and fields call for sensible shoes or going barefoot. So if someone leaves a lonely farmstead and goes to live in the city, the temptation to follow modern fashion trends is often too great; high-heeled shoes are worn, even though they may make walking rather awkward and difficult, indeed even painful. And if a woman is so used to wearing high heels that she cannot do without them, her feet will no longer be normal and healthy. Her tendons will have become so deformed that it will be difficult and painful for her even to stand on her bare feet.

FOOD FOR THOUGHT

I am often surprised to see young girls strutting along in high-heeled shoes, or else in slipper-like shoes with thin soles and no heels at all. Both extremes are harmful and inappropriate; both force the body into an unnatural position, causing it to tire more quickly and suffer damage. The blood can become congested, leading to varicose veins.

There is a natural reason why walking barefoot does not cause any problems. You simply would not walk for long along a hard and even road surface, but over meadows, fields and forest ground, all of which are uneven surfaces that support the arch of the foot, for movement acts like a massage. Judging from the standpoint of zone therapy, you will happily realise that the whole body benefits as a result. It is for this reason that walking barefoot in warm weather when you are on holiday or when working in the garden is an effective and invigorating natural treatment.

In contrast, when you have to walk on surfaced pavements and roads, a heel of 2–2½cm (about 1 inch) is just right. This height will provide the position for the foot that tends to tire the legs and body the least. Additionally, an arch support may be the answer for feet that ache or tire easily. There is usually no need for special insoles because there are carefully made shoes with a built-in support on the market.

If you stop to think that the feet have to carry your whole body weight day after day, you will agree that they most certainly deserve comfortable, well-constructed shoes in addition to daily attention. All this is surely part of a proper health programme.

Walking Barefoot

Walking barefoot is increasingly becoming a thing of the past. In fact, nowadays many people associate it with poverty or eccentricity – they look down on it. Just try it and dare to go for a long walk without your shoes and watch how many glances of surprise, pity and even contempt you will attract. What does this indicate? That the onlookers have all but forgotten or never learned the benefits of walking barefoot. They know nothing of the peculiar, mysterious power it can convey, or else they would not react the way they do.

Of course, there are many whose feet are untrained and would not be capable of walking barefoot over stones. But if you go for an early morning walk on dewy grass you will soon notice that going barefoot makes you feel really good, generating new strength when you have been feeling tired and worn out. It is like recharging one's batteries, so to speak, recharging your run-down nerves with energy. It seems as if Mother Earth is giving off energy that improves the glandular functions. That is why I consider it rather strange that, although overtired and worn-out, we do not take full advantage of this simple regenerative treatment, which is able to stimulate our endocrine glands to increase their activity.

Whenever we are in the garden, woods and forest, fields and meadows, we should make full use of the opportunity to take off our shoes and socks or stockings and walk barefoot, especially in the summer when the ground is warm. Take care, however, to walk only on natural ground, for the more unspoilt the ground the greater will be the benefit derived from its magnetic field. Never believe that walking barefoot on asphalt, concrete or any other artificial surface will do the same good. No, it is better to wear your shoes on this kind of surface, because you will not stand to gain anything by it, rather the opposite. Also, do not cool down your body even further by going barefoot when it is cold or wet. In certain mountain or rural areas the children can often be seen going without shoes throughout the entire summer, even when it is cold and raining. Their parents follow the custom of putting away their children's shoes and socks at the beginning of spring, only bringing them out again when the winter has set in. But even during the summer months a rainy spell can cool the atmosphere so much that bare feet will no longer benefit the health. It should be clear that it would be much better to be reasonable and sensible as regards the wearing of shoes in inclement weather.

On the other hand, if walking barefoot is done sensibly, it cannot be recommended highly enough as a remedy for all those who are worn-out and overworked, and who suffer from glandular insufficiency and other problems. If you feel tense because of stress and overwork, why not try it and see how you will obtain soothing relief.

The ancient Greeks were not as weak as the people of our modern age, yet they seem to have understood the revitalising benefits coming from the ground, or else they would not have passed on to us the old legend of Gaea, the energising Mother Earth. The legend tells of the giant Antaeus, son of Gaea, who was invincible as long as he touched his mother, the earth. When wrestling with him his adversary was able to defeat him only because he noticed that Antaeus regained new strength every time he touched the ground, but that his strength diminished as soon as he was lifted in the air. Granted, this is only a legend, but the story must have been based on certain observations of natural phenomena, for it is a fact that the earth holds wonderful regenerative powers capable of imparting energy to our bodies. A simple test is all that is needed to prove this assertion. Even though it has not yet been possible to discover and prove scientifically the actual cause of this elemental force, our experience of it cannot easily be refuted.

WALKING AND EXERCISING ON DEWY GRASS IN THE MORNING

Not everyone may find it easy to get up early in the morning and walk, run or do their exercises on the still dewy grass. Perhaps you live in a town with narrow streets and would find it inconvenient to go outside and seek out a green meadow before breakfast in order to do a little morning exercise. Still, it would be a most refreshing activity for all the many town dwellers who are normally locked up in their rooms and offices, before actually having to surrender to the hustle and bustle of a busy day.

How much to be envied are those who still live close to nature, who in the early morning carry out their natural exercise by making hay or doing general farm and garden work. Even though they may not realise it, these people are conditioning their bodies all the while. To them it is nothing but their work, part of their daily routine. It would be a first-class restorative to take a holiday on a farm and get up early and join these people in their early morning chores so as to regenerate our bodies which have been wearied and worn out during the working year. Think, too, of the opportunity you would have of learning from nature, helping you to adopt a more optimistic view of life.

Early morning exercises require deep-breathing, and this will help to drive out the remaining traces of weariness from our bodies, enabling us to start the day's work refreshed, even more so if we are able to walk on dewy grass. Sebastian Kneipp was one who called attention to the effects of dew, and it is beneficial to our health if we make use of nature's gifts. Civilisation has robbed us of much of our freedom by forcing us to live in cramped houses and towns, but nature teaches us little things that can make up for this loss to some extent. Observing these lessons can help us to maintain a reasonable physical balance while having to accept the hustle and bustle of everyday life.

Periostitis

'Just a minor cut on the foot, a little torn skin. Such a thing is bound to happen when working in the garden or fields. I'll let the wound bleed freely and will be able to forget all about it.' So I thought when I injured my left foot some time ago. Over the years such injuries had often happened and no further trouble had resulted. I naturally thought that it would be the same this time.

Within two days, however, the foot became inflamed and the first signs of blood poisoning could be detected. Two clay poultices made the symptoms disappear; but instead of continuing the treatment as I should have done, I did nothing further, being too busy to look after myself. From time to time, especially at night, I noticed a dull pain which seemed to go deeper and deeper. After about ten days it became so bad one night that I could hardly bear it. Because of neglecting to treat the infection, inflammation of the membrane covering the bone (periostitis) had evidently set in. Clay poultices no longer helped, or to be more specific, I could no longer tolerate the poultices. Soaking the foot in a herbal bath did nothing towards relieving the pain either.

After two terrible nights I decided to apply the *Baunscheidt (revulsion) treatment* (see pages 438–9) and after about two hours the pain had completely disappeared. The inflammation had been drawn to the surface and the cause of the pain eliminated. How much more simple is such a treatment than the allopathic method involving pain-killing drugs and surgery. Had I undergone allopathic treatment it would have meant weeks or even months in bed. Only someone who has experienced relief from pain through natural and reliable means can appreciate how wonderful it is to draw from nature's storehouse the wide variety of remedies and treatments available to us.

Strained Ligaments and Sinews, Sprained Ankles

There is a way to alleviate the pain and restore to normal any sprains and strained ligaments in the quickest possible time. This is what you must do.

Beat until stiff the whites of 3–5 eggs. Add a strong substance that will increase the rate of the blood and lymph circulation to a maximum. If you live in a southern region, use *eucalyptus* or *camphor leaves* but before adding them to the egg whites put them through a mincer two or three times until they are transformed into a paste. Dried leaves should be ground to a powder, or crushed in a mortar. Or maybe you have some eucalyptus or camphor leaves already in powder form. If you have camphor powder available, use 20–30g (about 1 oz). At any rate, add the leaf powder or camphor powder to the stiff egg whites, mixing the ingredients thoroughly. If neither camphor nor eucalyptus powder is on hand, use finely chopped *pine buds or needles* (from any coniferous tree) for the paste and mix with the egg whites. Spread the mixture on the painful area, then dress with wide strips of cloth and bind loosely with an elastic bandage. As the egg whites harden the paste will provide a firm and strong dressing. If necessary, renew the dressing after two days. After that, massage the affected part with *comfrey tincture* (*Wallwosan*), followed by the application of *raw cabbage poultices. Pulped raw potatoes, curds* or similar ingredients can also be used for the poultices.

This treatment will relieve the pain after only a short time, perhaps within a few days, and it is therefore better than suffering pain and not being able to walk for 4–6 weeks or even 2–3 months.

Massaging the injured part with light movements directed towards the heart will speed up the healing process.

Finally, warmth is necessary in the case of all bruises and internal injuries of ligaments and muscles. So see to it that the affected parts of the body are kept warm at all times.

Back Problems
After some great physical strain or effort, particularly at the end of a day of heavy housework or gardening, people often complain about their aching back. Yet the cause of the pain is not necessarily connected with general tiredness caused by the work. Many other causes can be responsible for backache and if it keeps returning it is advisable to look for the true source of the problem.

If the pain is relatively high up, causing a feeling of contraction, the person may actually be suffering from kidney trouble. Should the pain be felt a little lower down it may be the symptom of prostate (in the case of men) or bladder trouble. Backache can also stem from a degeneration of the bones, for example in a case of 'arthritis deformans'. A change in the position of the uterus can also trigger backache, and even muscular rheumatism may be interpreted as backache, as can sciatica when it starts higher up.

Backache being a nuisance, the sufferer seeks to get rid of it quickly. For this purpose use a good warming ointment. Apply *Symphosan* for a change. It is also beneficial to place some moist, hot *hay flowers* or *camomile*, tied in a cloth, on the painful area. Should this treatment not alleviate the pain and improve the condition, it is advisable to consult a doctor in order to identify the real cause of the pain, which can then be treated accordingly.

Hernias (Ruptures)

The peritoneum is so well designed that it does not easily become ruptured, even if it is subjected to exceptional strain once in a while. The healthy body is equipped with such good reserves of strength that one really wonders how it is possible for the abdominal wall to rupture in so many different ways. Observations show that some people inherit a tendency to ruptures, while with others a post-operative scar serves to weaken the abdomen. Once a weakness exists, it only needs a degree of pressure or a violent bout of coughing for a hernia to result. Thus, a hernia is not only caused by lifting heavy weights.

When the peritoneum is torn, the intestine can protrude through the front wall of the abdominal cavity. If the intestine is not pushed back in at once, flatulence can make it impossible for it to be returned to its normal position. The result is a so-called strangulated hernia, which requires immediate surgery. However, if the hernia is not strangulated, it is possible that a well-fitting truss can retain it in place, thus giving some relief.

Preventative Measures

It is always useful to know what you can do to prevent certain problems from arising and this also applies to preventative measures after surgery. For example, it is advisable to massage the abdomen regularly with *Symphosan*. This will help to strengthen the stomach muscles and prevent unwanted deposits of fat. At the same time, if every week you take two *sitz baths* in an infusion of *oak bark*, the effect of the regular massage will be enhanced. Keep-fit exercises also strengthen the abdominal muscles and the entire front wall. But be careful not to overdo the exercises. Be sensible, too, when practising a sport, whether it be rowing, skiing or whatever. A sensible approach guarantees good exercise that will strengthen, but not strain, the abdominal muscles and wall. Incidentally, if you practise some physical exercise regularly and sensibly, you will be much less prone to hernias in the first place than if you only sit around and do mental work.

For internal treatment, herbs that contain silica, such as *horsetail* and, especially, *Galeopsis*, are excellent. And to not forget to take *Urticalcin*, a biological calcium preparation.

337

A Selection of Medicinal Herbs

Only some of the more important herbs are considered in the following pages, since a detailed description of the extensive domain of the plant world would demand far greater attention than could ever be given in this limited space.

How a Good Herbal Remedy Is Developed

Establishing the Therapeutic Effects

To establish the effects of a natural plant medicine one must first of all be capable of observing accurately and interpreting correctly. In every age there have been people endowed with intuitive insight which enabled them, by personal experience and observation of others, to determine what plants are most suitable for curing a given condition or illness.

The effect of various substances on the human organism can be observed with greater accuracy after two or three days of fasting. Needless to say, one would only experiment with plants and substances known to be nonpoisonous. After taking one plant or another, it is possible to judge the relative merits – how it affects the bowels, the kidney, the stomach or the appetite, or whether it stimulates the functions of the body in some other way. If the body is in good condition, certain important effects can be easily perceived. In homoeopathy this is the so-called 'proving' of remedies on healthy people.

A doctor or other health practitioner can observe the effects of a remedy on the patient himself. If the patient reports that a particular remedy has other effects on him than those already known, the doctor will naturally take note of such observations. If other patients experience the same effect, then the doctor will realise that the medicine has a novel, so far unknown, reaction. A new remedy, or a new application of one, will have been discovered!

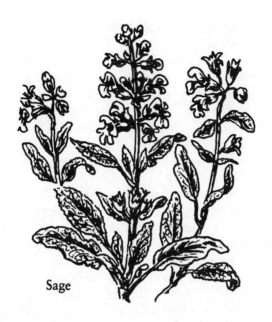

Sage

Combining Remedies

The purpose of combining remedies is to enhance the effect of one through the addition of another.

If a calcium deficiency is to be treated, it will be necessary to make sure that there is not a deficiency of silica at the same time. If there is, the patient must take both minerals. Supposing he also suffers from night sweats and at the same time wants to get rid of a bad cough; for the first, *sage (Salvia)* would be needed and for the second, extract of *pine buds* or *lance-leaf plantain (also known as ribwort, or Plantago lanceolata)* would be the indicated remedy.

It will be clear, therefore, that in order to cure different illnesses, the doctor can choose a suitable combination of remedies, but he must be careful that the individual remedies are compatible. There are some that vitalise the body, while others have a relaxing effect. As a rule, a knowledge of pharmacology is required to be able to choose and combine remedies correctly. Still, even in former times, when physicians were not so well trained and informed as they are today, they hit upon remedies by accurate observation and careful analysis of their findings. They were successful in discovering effective combinations, with one remedy increasing the effect of another, so that the action of the combined ingredients was greatly improved. However, if the combined remedies do not complement one another, not being compatible, the total effect can be reduced rather than enhanced.

The importance and effectiveness of combining different substances is illustrated in the case of vitamins. For example, an easily assimilated calcium preparation is not necessarily absorbed into the system if there is a deficiency of vitamin D, or if the two are not taken together. The body cannot absorb the calcium if there is a lack of vitamin D and, conversely, the vitamin D will not benefit the body if there is a lack of calcium. One complements the other.

In the body we find a similar interdependence of functions. Hydrochloric acid and the digestive enzyme pepsin work in close association with each other in the stomach. Pepsin can break down the food proteins only if the gastric environment is kept acid through the presence of hydrochloric acid in the right concentration; otherwise pepsin is completely ineffective. There are many associations like these, and if we are to produce medicines that fulfil their intended purpose, we must find out more about them.

To combine just any kind of herb or extract with another, hoping that eventually one may be lucky and suddenly invent something outstanding, is clearly the wrong thing to do. There are certain herbs and other natural remedies which, when combined, tend to harm rather than benefit the system. To ascertain the overall effects and be able to combine them correctly requires the gift and powers of accurate observation and a certain amount of intuition, a flair that comes from experience and training. Moreover, it is not always possible to judge the material components alone, for there are many substances and factors which have yet to be discovered but nevertheless play a part in the total effect. For this reason it is necessary to reckon with unknown as well as known factors.

Consider, for example, certain combinations of remedies that were used in the Middle Ages and are still as effective today as they were then. This is undoubtedly because of their rich content of vitamins and enzymes. Even though such factors were unknown when these remedies were originated, the skilled observers became aware of their effects and a new remedy was found and from then on employed in curing sickness. Practical experience in such circumstances is just as valuable, if not more so, than scientific knowledge of the exact chemical composition.

Unknown Factors
Very often an alkaloid or some other chemical substance in a plant is believed to produce a certain effect. If the alkaloid is extracted and administered, the symptomatic effects may be the same or similar, but the lasting effect will probably be different. The chemist is unable to explain this, because his analytical procedures are not sufficiently refined for him to be able to pinpoint those substances which are commonly termed 'unknown factors' and which are responsible for the overall effect produced by the plant. It is therefore essential that all natural remedies be taken as an organic whole, in the same form as nature produces them. Those who merely consider the so-called 'active substance' in a herbal preparation demonstrate a superficial understanding of the subject.

For example, if we extract arnicin from the arnica plant, it will never have the same effect on the heart and blood vessels as the extract that has been made from the whole arnica root. The same principle applies to carrot juice. By using just the isolated carotene as a provitamin, it is impossible to obtain the same medicinal effect as it would by drinking the pure and natural juice. Pure lactic acid as found in sauerkraut also differs in its action from the whole sauerkraut, because the acid is associated with other substances in the fermented cabbage and these possess their own curative properties. Some of these intrinsic properties are still unknown.

These few examples show that the things nature provides in their unadulterated and complete state represent the best source of our remedies. Nature is and will remain the most reliable pharmacy. Anyone gifted with an awareness of what nature has to offer will not be disappointed in his search, whether he be a medical researcher or just eager to learn. Nature will be his willing teacher and will unlock the secrets of its marvellous healing powers.

How Herbal Remedies Can Be Used
Every plant contains various minerals, vitamins, ferments, enzymes, oils, resins and mucilage. All these components in their natural proportions have a specific effect on the body.

Tea (Infusion)
In many places it is still customary to make a herbal tea or infusion in order to treat health problems. In fact, this is the oldest form of preparing herbal remedies. Unfortunately, however, an infusion only utilises the water-soluble properties of a plant.

341

Tincture
The preparation of a tincture using alcohol as a base, as opposed
to water in the case of an infusion, is more advisable, since in
addition to the water-soluble substances, those soluble in alcohol,
such as resins, oils and other specific active ingredients (for example
arnicin and petasin), will be extracted. What is more, an alcoholic
tincture keeps well and can also be diluted, that is, to obtain
homoeopathic potencies. The body is able to assimilate substances
contained in an alcoholic solution better than those dissolved in
water. In times gone by, only dried plants were used in the preparation of tinctures but today fresh plant extracts are preferred,
since they contain a higher concentration of the active ingredients.

The Spagyric Process
Many years ago Dr Zimpel developed the spagyric process in
which plants are fermented by means of yeast fermentation. The
carbohydrates ferment and are changed into alcohol. During this
process certain medicinal properties are released and are also
changed. New enzymes develop and these enhance the overall effect
in the case of some plants, whereas in others, for example plants
containing mucilage, the effect is diminished. This fermentation
process, like any other method, has its advantages and disadvantages. In more recent times, Dr Strahtmeier has again started to
use the fermentation process, with good results.

Lactic Fermentation
Lactic fermentation has been used for centuries in China, Korea
and Japan. In those countries it is employed to prepare medicinal
herbs and to change vegetables into hearty condiments and what
are known as *kimchi*, spicy pickled dishes similar to sauerkraut.
Although the lactic fermentation of various vegetables has the great
advantage of activating a plant's beneficial properties, this method
of preparing food has not yet found the popularity it deserves. The
remedial effects of plants used in the treatment and prevention of
diabetes, arthritis, rheumatism and cancer could be even more
beneficial if they were prepared in this way. That is why *Molkosan*
and vegetable juices should not be regarded merely as food, but
also as remedies. It appears that the importance of preparations
containing lactic acid will increase as radiation levels increase in
our modern environment.

Powder and Tablets

The whole, dried plant can also be made into a powder, which in turn can be used to produce tablets. The advantage of a powder and tablets is the fact that they retain all the plant's substances, including the ashes. On the negative side, sensitive ingredients are lost in the drying process, although the minerals, oils and resins remain fully effective. Remedies taken in powder and tablet form are ideal for use as laxatives and to stop diarrhoea, as well as to aid the digestion and eliminate worms. Papaya preparations are a good example in this respect.

Fresh Plant Trituration

In this method of preparing plant remedies, freshly cut or harvested plants are triturated with lactose, grape sugar or some other basic medium. Experience has shown this method to be one of the most effective. Unfortunately, as the process is slow and intricate, it is rarely used. Trituration has proved its worth in the manufacture of *Urticalcin*, since it allows the natural calcium to be prepared in such a way that the body can easily absorb it.

Oil Extracts (Preparations Made with Oil)

Oil is used in the preparation of *St John's wort oil* and other body oils, since it dissolves resins and other oil-soluble substances, which the skin will absorb for the benefit of the whole body. For example, the red dye of St John's wort is oil-soluble and much more effective in the form of an oil than as a tincture.

Crushed Fresh Plants for Poultices

Applying fresh crushed plants to an affected area is also a reliable form of treatment and has become more popular in recent times. Many people have either heard of or experienced cures effected by applying cabbage leaf poultices. If followed correctly, this method does a lot of good, avoiding the need for expensive medication. Besides cabbage leaves, many other medicinal plants and herbs can be used for poultices, so that their active ingredients will be absorbed via the skin. *Rumex alpinus* (giant dock) is an excellent medicinal plant. When crushed and applied to the back of the neck overnight, it will alleviate headaches and nervous tension. In the tropics, crushed greater plantain (*Plantago major*) is used for the treatment of ulcers and boils with good results. Crushed *Echinacea* leaves are marvellous for inflammations, and crushed comfrey leaves relieve arthritic pain.

343

The above examples show that medicinal plants can be used in a variety of ways to obtain reliable results. Plants are indeed the link between inorganic minerals and the human and animal body. Since the body is only able to absorb and assimilate minerals in the finest form possible, it is of great benefit that plants were designed to do the preliminary work of processing the minerals. They absorb these inorganic substances from the ground, processing them in such a way that our body is able to assimilate them.

Alpine Plants and Lowland Plants – Which Are of Greater Value?

Observations and Practical Experience
The above question does not have a simple answer. There are many aspects that have to be taken into consideration. For instance, I first noticed that strawberries grown in my garden in Teufen (about 900 m/3,000 feet above sea level) had less sugar content that the same variety grown in the Engadine (about 1,500 m/5,000 feet above sea level). I wondered if this could be attributed to the humus in the soil of the Engadine moors or to the intensive sunlight there. Interestingly, I also noticed that the sugar content of the lowland strawberries increased if the summer was a warm and dry one. I had to conclude from this observation that warmth and sunlight are mainly responsible for sweetness. Feeding also plays an important part; our strawberries are given a sufficient quantity of organic lime, which would account for their being sweeter than if the soil was not fed at all. So then, various factors must be weighed up before we can come to the right conclusion. By the way, carrots also do better in the Engadine than in Teufen, being sweeter and better flavoured. For this we must not only thank the strong, warm sunshine but also the higher elevation of the Engadine, its excellent climatic condition, and the richness of the soil.

Not every high elevation has the same merits. The southern Alps enjoy many more hours of sunshine than the northern range. For this reason plants do much better in the more southern areas than in the northern regions. In some of the latter areas they have only stunted growth before dying. Naturally, medicinal plants are also affected by these regional and climatic differences. For example, *Solidago* that has been grown in the higher Engadine has a better and stronger effect on the kidneys than that grown in the lower region of Teufen and, interestingly, that grown in Teufen is still better than any grown in the districts below an altitude of 500 m (1,500 feet).

Scientific Experiments
Some time ago, Professor Flueck delivered an interesting lecture to members of the Swiss Association of Apothecaries dealing with exactly these observations and the many factors that combine to produce active substances in plants. The lecture was based on the results of experiments in which various medicinal herbs had been grown at different altitudes but in identical soils. The experiments enabled Professor Flueck to prove beyond doubt that the therapeutic value of the plants does not depend solely upon the altitude at which they grow. In order to accurately identify the other factors involved, the experiments were fully controlled; the same plant was grown at different altitudes but in the same kind of soil in every case.

Better growth and content of active substances was achieved with the plants grown in sheltered mountain valleys, exposed to sunshine but protected from the winds, than with those grown at higher altitudes with equal exposure to the sun but unprotected from the winds. For this reason certain plants were found to do better at middle elevations than at higher altitudes. Others produce a higher content of medicinal properties if grown in the shade, or at least semi-shade, but these are usually exceptions to the rule.

So if an alpine herb proves to be more effective than others, having a higher content of active substances, it cannot always be attributed to altitude alone. Rather, it depends upon the kind of plant, its hours of exposure to sunshine, the temperature of the atmosphere and the degree of protection from severe winds. It is therefore not at all surprising that plants growing in mountain valleys protected from the winds tend to contain more active ingredients than those growing at lower altitudes.

However, Professor Flueck's experiments led to the astonishing observation that plants grown in the middle altitudes had a higher content of nutrients than those grown at high elevations. In view of my own experience, having been successful in growing mountain plants, his findings made me wonder. However, further investigation gave me the solution to the mystery: it was the species, or variety, of plant rather than the elevation at which it grew that really mattered.

Alpine Plants
The alpine plant is usually richer in its constituents and medicinal value than its lowland relative. I have proved this for myself through analysis. For example, the lowland yarrow contains less

essential oil and is less aromatic than the highland yarrow from
the Engadine, the Lower Engadine to be exact. Mind you, it may
be true that the soil and the abundant sunshine and warm atmosphere, also the greater intensity of ultraviolet rays, exert an influence on the quality of the plant.

The conclusions drawn from Professor Flueck's experiments
were arrived at with little, if any, consideration of the influence of
ultraviolet radiation and this would lead one to believe that these
rays are not so important in plant life, at least as far as their
principal active elements are concerned. However, there are other
constituents to be reckoned with, even though they are not generally considered 'active substances'. These elements, especially the
trace elements, seem to depend upon ultraviolet light to a far
greater extent than the more common principal substances,
although little is known about the relationship between trace
elements, ultraviolet radiation and mountain climate, as Professor
Flueck admitted. To obtain scientifically acceptable evidence in this
matter would involve costly experiments. In any case, what really
matters are the results of our practical experience with herbs and
herb extracts. For instance, we know it to be true that St John's
wort grown at alpine altitudes is richer in active substances and
more efficacious than the same plant grown in the lowlands or at
an intermediate elevation. The tincture obtained from the former
is a much darker shade of red than that prepared from the lowland
plant. Hence we must conclude that the medicinal dye content is
greater. The plant itself looks different from the ordinary lowland
Hypericum perforatum; it is shorter and more compact. And since
it is indigenous to the alpine regions it is distinguished by the name
Hypericum alpinum. You will see, then, that it is the alpine plant
which is richer in medicinal value and content; the variety of plant
is the clue to the mystery's solution.

What is true about St John's wort also applies to goldenrod.
The alpine variety is small and bushy and instead of one flower
stem, like the lowland kind, it has 12–15 arising from its small
rootstock. The alpine variety of *Solidago* is more aromatic and
stronger, contains more essential oil, and its diuretic effect is far
stronger than that of its lowland cousin.

Other Noteworthy Influences
It is quite obvious that experiments made with some lowland
plants, *Belladonna* for instance, are less conclusive as regards the
influence of mountain climate and than those made with plants

that are actually native to higher elevations. The condition of the soil has to be considered too, because the bacterial flora of lowland soil has usually been damaged by artificial fertilisers and cannot offer the same favourable basis for growth as the naturally fertilised ground of mountain valleys, the humus of which is brought down to the valleys every spring by the avalanche snow from where the ecology has not been interfered with. This kind of soil is ideal for promoting exceptionally good growth of plants, their medicinal content being the best possible because the mountain valleys provide the perfect biological conditions for these plants. Additionally, the sheltered valleys offer another advantage in as far as the plants are less exposed to strong winds than on mountain heights. That is why they thrive in these alpine valleys, and are especially aromatic and effective as raw materials for fresh plant preparations.

Scientific research is no doubt of great interest to the therapist and can tell him a lot. But when it comes to assessing the medicinal value of a herbal preparation, there is no substitute for practical experience with actual patients. A pure remedy, made from the whole plant, contains a complex of active elements, some of which are known and others unknown. For this reason, it is the practical treatment of a patient that really matters in determining whether a preparation is effective or not. This is why the medical researcher needs the cooperation of the herbal therapist in order to develop the best remedies from nature's bountiful storehouse for the benefit of the sick. After all, is this not the real purpose of all medical research? At least, that is what it should be!

Angelica (*Angelica archangelica*)

When the black death, the plague, raged in the Middle Ages, terrified people scoured the woods and marshes for medicinal herbs. They dug up angelica by the running streams and in damp clearings, for they felt certain that this plant would help them. Next to a plant called butterbur (in German, 'plague root'), angelica was considered the most important remedy for combatting the plague. Contemporary descriptions of those dreadful times contain the most remarkable stories of the reliable help these remedies must have given. The old chronicles report that anyone who kept a piece of angelica root in his mouth all through the day would be preserved from the plague. Be that as it may, the strong aromatic taste of this root is due to an essential oil and the valerian, malic and angelic acids it contains.

347

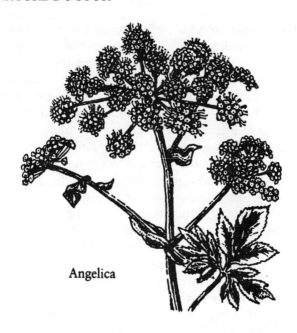

Angelica

The fresh plant extract has a marvellous effect on the digestion, helping to overcome loss of appetite, irritation of the stomach lining and also stomach cramps. For these complaints, take ten drops in a little water three times a day, half an hour before meals. Moreover, it is excellent for bronchial and deep-seated catarrh if a few drops are taken with a little honey once an hour.

The seeds of angelica are also used. For example, a liqueur can be made from them. And here is the recipe for the genuine angelica liqueur known as 'Vespétro':

Angelica seeds (or chopped angelica root, if you are unable to obtain the seeds) 60g (2 oz)
Fennel seeds 8g (¼ oz)
Anise seeds 8g (¼ oz)
Coriander seeds 6g (⅕ oz)

Grind all the seeds together in a mill or crush in a mortar, put in a bottle and add 200 g (8 fl. oz) of pure alcohol. After eight days strain the mixture through muslin or cotton wool and mix it with a solution of 1–1.5 litres (2½ pints) of water to which 500 g (1lb) sugar (preferably grape sugar) has been added. And there you have it!

There is no better or more pleasant remedy for digestive upsets or flatulence. Let us imagine a monastery in the Middle Ages. There the monks would enjoy a glass of this golden drink before appearing for duty in the morning. Late in the evening a guest arriving with an upset or chilled stomach would be given a glass of 'Vespé-tro', and just a small sip would have a quicker and better effect than any of today's chemical liquids or tablets.

Bear's Garlic/Ramsons (Allium ursinum)

This outstanding medicinal plant has been wrongfully neglected for a long time and in quite a few books on herbalism it has not even been mentioned. Even in some of the best books only garlic is listed. *Allium ursinum*, with its distinct pungent smell, is generally called bear's garlic or ramsons. Its leaves resemble those of the lily of the valley and, as both plants grow in the shade of the woods, one is often mistaken for the other. Bear's garlic thrives in damp but healthy ground and is sometimes found so plentifully along the sides of streams and brooks that it could actually be cut with a scythe.

The considerable sulphur content of bear's garlic acts on the skin, the bones and the bronchial tubes, especially when there is an abundant secretion of phlegm.

Intestinal flatulence, with a burning sensation in the abdomen and an irritation of the bladder, accompanied by a strong urge to urinate, will be alleviated by means of bear's garlic. So, too, will chronic intestinal catarrh, when the mucous lining of the stomach and intestines has become very sensitive. Best of all, however, is the effect that bear's garlic has on hardening of the arteries. In this respect it can considerably lengthen the lives of older people. Bear's garlic juice or bear's garlic tonic can help prevent a stroke, and if a person has already suffered a stroke, this simple plant can restore him to health better than some of the most expensive proprietary medicines. Elderly people who have high blood pressure and are in danger of a stroke can ward it off with four plant remedies: *bear's garlic (Allium ursinum), mistletoe (Viscum album), hawthorn (Crataegus oxyacantha)* and *Arnica (Arnica montana)*. So why risk falling victim to paralysis when simple natural remedies exist that will prevent a stroke and at the same time strengthen the heart and the vascular system, giving new life to the body?

To benefit fully from bear's garlic it may be eaten fresh and uncooked as a salad or mixed with other vegetables. Steamed with a little oil, it is similar to spinach and, although not as beneficial as when eaten raw, it is still better than ordinary vegetables.

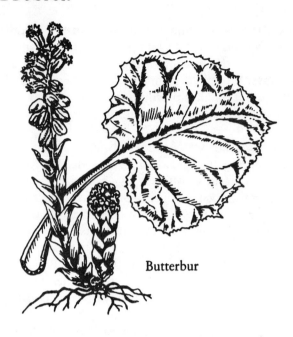

Butterbur

Taken as a wine or tonic, or an extract in the form of drops, it has also proved invaluable. If you do not wish to go to the bother of gathering the leaves yourself to use as a vegetable, you can take advantage of the fresh plant extract, in which all the goodness of the plant is preserved.

Butterbur (*petasites officinalis [hybridus]*)
During the past few years butterbur, or *Petasites*, has proved itself as a valuable remedy, one that has achieved quite astonishing results. Since it is a strong remedy, the mother tincture is not usually tolerated by the average patient and it has to be potentised to 1x or 2x, or even higher. If the patient, for example one suffering from a tumour or cancerous growth, notices a very strong reaction, he will have to take the remedy in a weaker potency. Let me add that this reaction is a sign of having made the right choice, that the remedy is appropriate. All that is left to do is to ascertain the potency that is tolerated by the patient. To find the individual tolerance, it will be necessary to ignore the usual directions; instead, add one drop of *Petasites* to a glass of water (200 ml/7 fl. oz) and take frequent sips during the day. After 8–10 days the body will have become used to that particular strength and the dose can be increased, using one drop to 100 ml (3.5 fl. oz) of water. Continue taking this dilution for eight days, then add one

350

drop to 50 ml. In time, the body will tolerate *Petasites* in even stronger doses.

This remedy attacks tumours, growths and all other pathological cell changes very forcibly. In cases of diseases of the respiratory tract, for example the lungs, *Petasites* should be given highly diluted. Recently, I spoke to a professor of medicine in Germany with whom I had left samples of the tincture for experimental purposes, and he confirmed that *Petasites* is a 'strong' medicine. He said that doses of only one drop gave rise to severe reactions in sensitive patients. It must be added that *Petasites* is quite harmless and nonpoisonous, so that strong reactions need not be any cause for alarm. Doctors who complain that our natural remedies are not potent enough to produce a satisfactory therapeutic reaction should try some of them to find out for themselves that fresh plant extracts can be as spectacular in their effects as many chemotherapeutic drugs, with the added advantage of their being harmless and nontoxic. This fact proves that nature holds many hidden powers which could be utilised for the benefit of the sick.

Not long ago I received a letter describing the treatment of an animal with *Petasites*. A terrier had developed a growth on one of her nipples, but this remedy soon reduced it in size.

Petasites is one of the best, if not *the* best, natural remedies, often giving better results than one hopes and expects in cases of tumours, especially those of suspected cancer or actual cancer. If it is taken together with *Viscum album*, the reliable fresh plant extract from mistletoe, or in the form of a combination remedy made up of these two remedies, it is possible to experience satisfactory results even in cases where chemotherapy has no more to offer.

So when the doctor says that he has done everything possible, and that there is no hope left for an improvement in a patient's condition, remember *Petasites* and *Viscum album*. These two remedies, together with an appropriate diet containing plenty of fruit juices and vegetable juices, can often achieve an improvement in the patient's general well-being. At any rate, this treatment can definitely reduce sensitivity to pain and make life easier.

Latest Research Findings
The medicinal use of *Petasites* goes back to the Middle Ages, or even earlier. The more we study the plant the more impressed we become with its good effects on a whole range of complaints, and the therapeutic spectrum of its active substances.

Petasites has a wide range of applications as an analgesic (a pain-relieving drug) and excellent results have been reported in connection with its use for headaches, migraines, menstrual cramps, toothache, painful wounds and many other aches and pains. It is at its most effective when taken in tablet form as *Petadolor*. This remedy provides temporary or complete relief from pain, and has also been known to cure the underlying problem.

Considering the fact that many people swallow chemical analgesics almost without thinking and become dependent upon them, it is understandable that doctors and patients alike appreciate the availability of a nontoxic and nonaddictive pain-killer.

A real-life experience proves that *Petadolor* is absolutely harmless. A patient from the Swiss canton of Graubuenden who felt tired of life swallowed some eighty Petadolor tablets hoping to put an end to his suffering. However, afterwards he must have had second thoughts because he contacted his family doctor. The doctor telephoned me, as the manufacturer of Petadolor, in order to find out about the remedy's ingredients and toxicity. I reassured him that the remedy is completely nontoxic and gave him the name and address of a pharmacologist who had conducted many experiments with it. The phamacologist subsequently confirmed that Petadolor is harmless. In fact, the doctor did not even have to pump out the patient's stomach, even though an overdose had been taken. Later on, he telephoned again, reporting that the patient felt none the worse except that he had passed a large amount of water and in a short time had lost a lot of weight. But despite his experience he felt very well indeed and no longer intended to commit suicide. Incidentally, the doctor went on to suggest that the remedy might be used for the treatment of dropsy and obesity.

Petadolor is not as fast-acting as many chemical medicines, but its harmlessness no doubt offsets this small disadvantage. In approximately 50 per cent of patients who take it the pain-killing effect is relatively fast, but in 30 per cent it is slower, taking about an hour to counteract menstrual cramps and migraine. In approximately 10 per cent of patients, especially cancer patients, it begins to work only after about three days, but then the effect is stronger than that of morphine. About 10 per cent of all patients respond very little or not at all to the remedy. It may be, however, that in time a greater concentration of the active substances will bring relief to these people too.

Since Petadolor is able to ease cramps and spasms, it helps to calm and tone the nerves. Faster results are obtained when Petadolor tablets are dissolved on the tongue, because in this way the active elements are dissolved by the saliva and absorbed via the mucous membrane.

Curing an Addiction to Chemical Analgesics
In recent years there has been a frightening increase in the number of people becoming addicted to pain-killing drugs. It is therefore welcome news indeed that *Petadolor*, if taken regularly, can cure the habit comparatively easily. Thousands of people can now obtain great relief through this simple herbal remedy. Taking one tablet every hour can break the addition within a few weeks. Petadolor can even relieve in a relatively short time severe cases of migraine headaches that are accompanied by the typical vomiting of bile. Some patients had suffered from such attacks for years before taking Petadolor. However, it must be said that the normal dose of two tablets three times a day is not sufficient for this purpose. In severe cases the tablets should be taken every hour, or even every half hour, and allowed to dissolve on the tongue.

Welcome Help for Painful Menstruation
It is a relief for women and girls to know that *Petadolor* can help most cases of dysmenorrhoea, the pains and cramps associated with difficult menstruation. I have received testimonials from women who have been helped by this simple natural remedy, where stronger chemical medicines had previously failed. Hence Petadolor should be kept in every medicine chest and travel bag, every hotel and factory reception desk and the staff room or sick bay of every store. In one Basel store Petadolor was given to about forty saleswomen for headaches and menstrual pains, and they all expressed their appreciation for this natural remedy that has no side effects whatsoever.

An Effective Remedy for Asthma
Of all the available plant remedies for asthma the various butterbur preparations stand out as being the most effective. These are *Petastites officinalis extract, Petadolor tablets* and, for exceptionally stubborn conditions, *Petaforce capsules*. All these preparations are made from 100 per cent plant extract and are reliable antispasmodics. A senior consultant at a Kneipp sanatorium once related the case of an asthma attack that would have killed the patient if it had not been for the doctor's help. The strongest chemical medicine, which the doctor had reluctantly administered before, was

353

not as effective as the *Petasites* preparations he then gave the patient. Moreover, it is gratifying to know that *Petasites* not only provides effective short-term relief but in time will bring about a cure.

The effect is not always the same with every patient, since there are various kinds of asthma (see pages 96–8). To back up the treatment, it is often necessary to prescribe a biological calcium preparation, for example *Urticalcin*. One asthmatic told us that such a treatment with *Asthmasan* had practically rid him of his problem, even though he used to suffer from almost unsupportable attacks every time there was an atmospheric depression, or föhn, in the air.

Treating Cancer with Petaforce

Petasites in a high concentration has been given to cancer patients for some years now and the good results achieved have induced researchers to continue their tests. It is not impossible that desperate cancer patients who face an uncertain future will eventually be helped by means of *Petasites*, and this possibility gives us reassurance and hope. Much store has been placed on certain potential cancer remedies that have been publicised widely in the press, causing a sensation, but almost as suddenly as they appeared so they disappeared. However, observations relating to the use of *Petasites* extracts have consistently shown for decades that the plant has a certain influence on the general development of cancer. Of course, only time will tell how far this plant can help to solve the problem of cancer.

Encouraging results have already been recorded. For example, the senior consultant of one large hospital told me that he gave *Petasites* extract to all patients after surgery, with the result that no metastases occurred (the cancer did not spread) and the patients' condition remained stable. Another example concerns a sixty-year-old patient who was taken to hospital suffering from a ramified malignant growth in an advanced state. The doctors held out no hope and informed the lady's son that they did not expect her to live much longer. Nevertheless, the patient was put on *Petasites* extract and, to the great astonishment of the doctors, she was discharged from hospital a few weeks later.

Cases like this last one give grounds for the hope that *Petasites* contains active substances that can be of great help in the treatment of cancer, and no doctor should ignore its potential. Experience has shown that *Petasites* definitely alleviates the unbearable pain suffered by cancer patients in the advanced stage of the illness, when even morphine injectons begin to fail. Every cancer patient should be given *Petaforce*, a *Petasites*-based preparation, in addition to the doctor's usual therapy. Our own results justify the assertion that Petaforce can be of great benefit to cancer patients: it reduces the danger of metastasis, considerably improves the patient's condition and prospects of a cure, and makes the existing pain more endurable. Moreover, Petaforce is a harmless, nontoxic plant remedy without any side effects, for which reason doctors and patients should not hesitate to make full use of its medicinal properties.

Notable doctors continue to use Petaforce and to obtain promising results from their experiments. It is hoped that, together with a special regime, it will eventually play an essential part in solving the difficult problem of cancer. There is another specific observation to back up this hope. As a rule, a turn for the better is noticed on the third day of treatment with Petaforce; the patient's condition improves and pain becomes less severe. Satisfactory results have even been obtained in cases of cancer of the liver, which usually leaves little hope for the patient.

Comfrey (*Symphytum officinale*)

Comfrey grows, for the most part unnoticed, near farmyards, in ditches and by river banks. Because of its excellent medicinal effects it should be lifted from its obscurity and used more widely. Even in ancient times it was employed to heal wounds and broken bones, especially fractures of the leg. It is for good reason, then, that people gave it common names such as 'knitback', 'bruisewort' and 'healing herb'. Considering its good services in cases of fractures alone, it deserves more attention than it usually receives. Comfrey, especially when taken in a homoeopathic form, promotes the healing process and speeds up the formation of new bone cells, which is probably due to the fact that it contains 0.8–1.0 per cent allantoin. This substance is known to encourage granulation and the formation of epithelial cells. Comfrey also contains choline and other, still unknown, elements.

Symphytum growing in the wild has a strong effect on the central nervous system and should be taken only in small amounts. There are about twenty varieties of comfrey, some of which are cultivated for fodder. One is *Symphytum asperum* or *asperrimum*, which is mainly grown in the Caucasus area, while *Symphytum peregrinum* is a Ukrainian variety. *Symphytum orientale* can be found in an

355

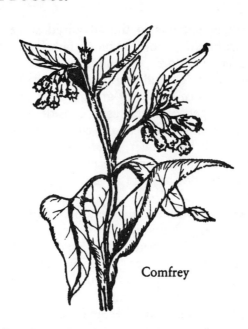

Comfrey

area covering Armenia and running all the way to the north of Iran. These three varieties are valuable because of their leaves. While animals avoid the leaves of common comfrey, or *Symphytum officinale*, they enjoy these three kinds; pigs especially like them. The leaves of these three varieties of *Symphytum*, as well as of Siberian comfrey, are said to contain vitamin B_{12}. The curative mucilage is present in the leaves, but in larger amounts in the roots. In the United States the leaves are even used in salads.

Comfrey is a fine remedy for an injured periosteum (the connective tissue covering the bones), for festering wounds, wounds which refuse to heal, and leg ulcers. There is hardly a better remedy to be found for the external treatment of gout, in which case the raw root should be grated and applied to the affected part as a poultice. If fresh roots are not available, use the tincture (*Wallwosan*) instead. The tincture also provides effective relief from neuralgic pains, for instance troublesome facial neuralgia. In both cases, *Symphytum 3x* is a good supportive remedy if taken internally.

Wallwosan should be rubbed very lightly into the affected parts, because gouty conditions, injuries to the periosteum and periostitis react unfavourably to forcible massage. After applying the tincture it is beneficial to follow up the treatment with *packs of clay, cabbage, giant dock (sorrel),* or *goldenrod*.

Wallwosan should be taken internally not only in cases of frac-

356

tures, gout and neuralgic pain, but also for all sorts of injuries, as well as before and after an operation. Once the bandages, stitches or clips have been removed, the fresh scars can be treated with Wallwosan. Apply the tincture lightly and the healing process will be speeded up.

Additionally, healing can be accelerated and unpleasant post-operative conditions avoided by drinking *vegetable water*, chiefly that from *boiled potatoes* and *leeks*. The *raw juices* of the *cabbage* family are excellent and have a curative effect. The idea is to make use of all these available means in order to derive their combined benefit. It is to your advantage to let comfrey help you, and to increase its effect by using all other available remedies as well.

Symphosan – a Tried and Tested Remedy

Symphosan consists of a mucilaginous tincture prepared from the fresh, raw *Symphytum officinale*, a hairy boraginaceous plant, and various other fresh plant tinctures.

Years of experience have shown that Symphosan, when taken orally, is excellent for treating inflammations of the stomach and intestinal linings. However, even more important is its external use. Applied as an ointment, it will alleviate gout and pains in the joints which manifest themselves when degenerative changes in them begin to occur and a grating noise can be noticed when flexing the joints.

It is important to adopt a strict natural diet as well, for the cure must come, in the first place, from within the body. Gratifying results can be achieved with this treatment if the patient is willing to follow it faithfully. There is no reason for arthritis sufferers to lose hope if they use Symphosan and plan a well-regulated diet. In this way, the degenerative progress of arthritis or gout can be arrested, as has been proved in long-standing cases where all other therapies had failed.

Inflammation of the nerves (neuritis) may also be treated success-fully with Symphosan. In fact, wherever there are painful parts in the body, or wherever there is any sensitivity to pressure which manifests itself in the peripheral nerves, Symphosan can be rec-ommended as a simple, natural and efficacious remedy.

It is extraordinary what a regenerating influence Symphosan has on the skin. Wrinkles, crow's feet and other signs of premature aging will be regenerated by its continuous use. As far as age allows, it is possible to have a firm, youthfully fresh skin. Sympho-san is therefore a valuable cosmetic and should not be missing

357

from the dressing table. It does more than improve the appearance, it promotes good health, and true beauty is identified with health. If Symphosan is used for cosmetic purposes, it should be alternated with a good skin oil.

Abrasions, cuts and injuries which take a long time to heal will respond favourably to Symphosan and heal more quickly. It relieves pain and is anti-inflammatory, and also helpful for haematomas, that is, blood blisters and swellings filled with effused blood.

Use Symphosan externally and take *Aesculaforce* orally for good results in cases of phlebitis. Leg ulcers respond to a local application of Symphosan. First, dab the affected part, but if it stings too much, just dab the surrounding area until the pain subsides, for this too has an alleviating effect.

SYMPHOSAN'S SEVEN INGREDIENTS

To obtain a therapeutically balanced preparation, the fresh plant extract of *Hypericum perforatum (St John's wort)* is added to the pure product of *Symphytum officinale (comfrey)*. St John's wort is well known and proven as a remedy for the blood and for wounds, and as such, helps to intensify the effect of Symphytum.

Hamamelis (witch hazel) is, in the experience of the North American Indians, one of the important wound-healing remedies. It has gained a deserved place in modern medicine too.

Sanicle is another tried and proven country remedy, especially indicated for badly healing wounds, cuts and grazes. It has been used by people in the country for centuries. Unfortunately, it is quite rare in many areas.

Solidago virgaurea, also known as *goldenrod* and *woundwort*, has also been used to treat wounds since time immemorial. It is anti-inflammatory and speeds up the healing process. Its content of essential oils, tannins and saponins may be responsible for these valuable effects.

Arnica, which may be found anywhere in Switzerland up to a height of about 2800 m (8,500 feet), has been recognised as an aid to healing wounds for thousands of years and is acclaimed as such in the oldest herbal records. Contusions with extravasation of the blood into the adjoining tissues are also cured by means of an extract from the root. Arnica will encourage proper capillary circulation, which makes it an important ingredient that enhances the effectiveness of the other plant remedies.

Besides these six ingredients making up Symphosan, there is yet one more. It is *houseleek (Sempervivum tectorum)*, a plant that

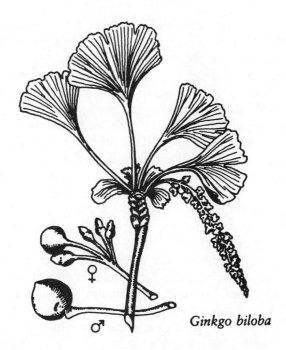

Ginkgo biloba

used to be found growing on the roofs of old houses in Switzerland, especially on thatched ones. It may not have been a good thing for the roofs, but the householders certainly knew how to take advantage of the fresh plant to treat inflamed eyes, burns, scalds, ulcers or sores and wounds, for which it is a cooling and healing medicine.

All these outstanding herbs are combined to make Symphosan a truly remarkable remedy that should be kept in every medicine chest and rucksack.

Maidenhair Tree (*Ginkgo biloba*)

I first came across the tree called *Ginkgo biloba* some years ago, while on a visit to the Far East. There were some very fine specimens near Nagasaki, Japan – the city destroyed by an atom bomb. The trees had fortunately survived. Now *Ginkgo biloba* is also grown in Europe's temperate zone, its leaves containing the same active substances as those grown in Asia. In fact, I planted a maidenhair tree, as it is also called, in my garden ten years ago, and it is doing well.

As a result of our modern life-style and environmental disruptions, vascular diseases have increased considerably; in this context it seemed appropriate for me to take a closer look at the *Ginkgo biloba* tree. My contact with Dr Wilmar Schwabe and his research team enabled me to gain a thorough knowledge of the medicinal effects of this extremely valuable plant, and it is noteworthy that preparations made from it have caused no side effects whatsoever. In cases where the brain does not receive sufficient blood, the tincture made from the leaves has proved to be efficacious. Also, a deficient supply of oxygen to the brain can be remedied quite rapidly, which is very important after a stroke. Blood viscosity, that is, its consistency and rate of flow, will improve in a short time. This makes it possible to eliminate the symptoms of a defective circulation, such as headaches, buzzing in the ears, problems with hearing and sight, depression, and a state of fear and panic.

Some people over the age of seventy have registered a notable improvement in health after only 4–6 weeks when they have taken a double dose of the tincture three times a day (the normal dose is 15–20 drops three times a day). Relief is even more certain when a low-protein diet, but one that is rich in vital substances, vitamins and minerals is also followed. Although scientists believe that ginkgo flavone compounds are responsible for this plant's diverse effects, other yet undiscovered substances in the plant must also be given some credit for these benefits.

It is possible to normalise high blood pressure after just a few weeks of taking *Ginkgo biloba*, probably because the blood's viscosity will be favourably affected. We do not know of any other plant remedy that is as beneficial for the brain, central nervous system and vascular system. Moreover, it is interesting to note that the tincture produces a welcome secondary effect, the stimulation of the kidneys and pancreas. Improved blood circulation and supply of oxygen ensure that the cells of the central nervous system are better nourished, hence more efficient. Furthermore, the circulation in the skin, therefore the functioning of the finest capillaries, will be promoted. When *Hypericum* is taken at the same time, ten drops on an empty stomach every morning before breakfast, this will influence the circulation even more. Anyone over the age of fifty would do well to take *Ginkgo* drops for a few months, since various body functions can thus be improved. For when there is better blood circulation, the entire body will benefit from a general cleansing process. The use of this remedy in daily alternation with *Vinca minor* has also given very good results.

Vascular constriction caused by nicotine can also be favourably influenced – but one has to stop smoking. Circulatory disturbances in the arms and legs, even diabetic vascular damage, will diminish.

In cases of varicose veins, the regular taking of *Ginkgo* drops will counteract the formation of blood clots (thrombosis). Everyone who is reasonably sensible and natural in his approach to nutrition and life-style will be able to achieve a veritable regeneration and rejuvenation when taking a course of these drops.

I have received many encouraging letters from patients who have found *Ginkgo biloba* to be an excellent remedy for a variety of complaints. In February 1986, one lady wrote:

'I have been taking this remedy since October 1985. For years I kept getting a pain behind my left eye and when out walking I would involuntarily swerve to the left, often bumping into people. I even feared I had a brain tumour, but neither the eye specialist nor X-rays discovered anything like that. Tests of the throat, nose, ears and sinus were all negative. One doctor said that vascular and circulatory problems were to blame and prescribed *Ginkgo biloba*, "the best remedy there is," he added. And that reminded me of your article in *Gesundheits-Nachrichten (Health News)*, where you recommended *Ginkgo biloba* for the same complaints.'

A nursery-school teacher recently told me that her eyesight had deteriorated so that she could no longer read even when wearing her glasses. Several months earlier she had started taking *Ginkgo biloba* regularly, about thirty drops every morning and night. When she tried her old pair of glasses again she was amazed that her sight had actually improved. I asked myself why this might be so and came to the conclusion that *Ginkgo biloba* had had a regenerative effect on her eyes because it promotes good blood circulation even to the capillaries, thus also improving the supply of oxygen. In fact, I would be glad to hear from anyone whose eyesight had improved after taking *Ginkgo biloba* for some time. Incidentally, it stimulates other sensory functions too, for example the hearing.

Another patient said: 'I began to notice an improvement in my circulation after taking 15–20 drops daily for about a month. The feeling of heaviness in my left foot and leg has almost gone and the migraine headaches are now less frequent.'

A further effect is highlighted in the following letter:

'A little while ago I began to drink *Ginkgo* tea and I must say that its effect is outstanding. Blood supply to the head has improved. Every night my nostrils seemed to be blocked, but now this is better. What is even more important, I'm not as forgetful as I used to be, and if I do forget something I find it easier to recall what it was. Another thing, before I began to take *Ginkgo biloba* my right arm tended to go numb while I was asleep and I had to shake and massage it several times to get the circulation going again. Now I no longer suffer from this.'

I might add here that *Ginkgo biloba* tincture, made from the fresh leaves is stronger and more convenient to use than the tea prepared from an infusion of dried leaves.

A lady in Bremen, Germany, had a similar experience to the one recounted above:

'I have been suffering from insufficient blood supply to the brain since my youth. It has caused me a great deal of anxiety, even an inferiority complex and lots of tears. As soon as I learned about *Ginkgo biloba* I went to get it from our local pharmacy, which stocks your remedies. That was three weeks ago, and I already notice that I can think better and more clearly and my memory, indeed my general health, has improved. I feel happy again.'

Ginkgo biloba is also indicated in cases of concussion. As soon as the patient feels better and has recovered, the remedy should be taken to stimulate blood supply to the brain. Pain and complications in the legs caused by menstrual problems can be eased if *Ginkgo biloba* is taken in alternation with *Vinca minor*. It is recommended to take the first remedy early in the morning one day and the second one the next day, and so forth. Doing so will improve the circulation right down to the finest capillaries.

Horsetail/Shave Grass (*Equisetum arvense*)
Horsetail, or shave grass, is to be found as a rampant weed growing chiefly in damp clay and sandy soil, on railroad tracks, untilled ground, on meadows and alongside paths in the fields. In former times this silica-containing plant was used to clean tinware in some areas of Europe. There are more than twenty varieties in Switzerland, although only *Equisetum arvense* is used for medicinal purposes. Some varieties are even poisonous, for example *Equisetum heleocharis* which contains a toxic alkaloid called equisetin. This variety is larger than the common horsetail and, like *Equisetum palustre*, a marsh plant, it should never be used as a medicinal herb. In the remote past shave grass grew considerably taller, attaining the height of a tree, as has been proved by fossilised specimens dug up from the earth.

Today we must content ourselves with the small, rather delicate plant. It has a finely wrought structure and it stands like a tender young fir, pliant yet tough. A flood can knock it to the ground and drag it from its roots, but the little horsetail takes root anew and stands erect. What gives it this toughness and resilience? If we

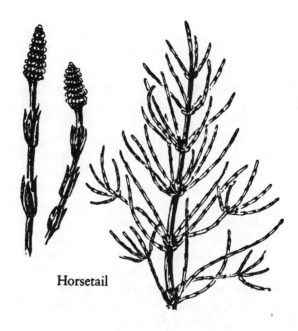

Horsetail

analyse its ash constituents, we will find that it contains 60–65 per cent silica and 15 per cent calcium, with the balance of 20 per cent being made up of other minerals.

From this analysis it is evident that silica, as the predominant element, is mainly responsible for its curative effect. *Horsetail tea* has a diuretic effect, stimulating the kidneys; it also helps to cure haemoptysis (the spitting or coughing up of blood), whether it comes from the lungs or the stomach. There is only one other remedy that can compete with horsetail in alleviating this condition and that is tormentil extract. Silica is of great importance in the regeneration of the tissue, as is calcium. Diseases of the respiratory tract (the lungs, bronchial tubes and pleura) and the glandular system likewise depend upon silica for help. Hence an infusion of horsetail or an extract from the fresh plant will be most beneficial. There is only one other plant so far known that contains more silica than horsetail and that is the hemp nettle (*Galeopsis dubia*), with 72 per cent. These silica-containing plants are also very good for the skin and shave grass baths are frequently recommended for the treatment of various skin diseases.

Lady's Mantle (*Alchemilla vulgaris*)

Was this plant given its name because its leaves are shaped like a cloak, or because it can ward off women's illnesses in particular, and so protect them from harm? Perhaps both attributes have influenced the choice of this name. At any rate, let us look at this herb more closely. To do so we must leave the flat lowlands and climb up into the hills, not too high, though, for lady's mantle grows at about 550–640 m (1,800–2,100 feet). Its true home, however, is the alpine meadows of Switzerland, where in close proximity we also find silvery lady's mantle (*Alchemilla alpina*), a plant which looks a little more attractive but is less demanding as regards nutrient intake since it grows in poor stony soil. The less conspicuous common lady's mantle (*Alchemilla vulgaris*) favours rich soil and it can be seen growing alongside the proud monkshood (*Aconitum napellus*) in hollow places where the earth contains the humus and nitrogen in which these two plants delight. You can also come across it near alpine dairies, where it proliferates together with the giant dock (*Rumus alpinus*). It grows very large in these places because of the rich soil.

The healing potential of lady's mantle is of particular benefit to women and has also proved its worth in cases where the connective tissues lack sufficient strength, causing a tendency to hernia. It should be pointed out, however, that such constitutional problems require that an infusion made from the plant should be taken regularly for at least a year.

The freshly pulped leaves of lady's mantle help wounds to heal quickly when applied externally. If you sustain a scratch or a cut while walking or hiking in the mountains, there are plenty of effective remedies all around. A few flowers of St John's wort rubbed between the fingers and placed on the cut (or crushed arnica root), with pulped lady's mantle bound on top, will make an inexpensive curative dressing. A word of caution is needed here: pick the plants only where they are clean and never from the wayside or near an alpine dairy.

Formerly, good ointments used to be made from the fresh leaves of lady's mantle and also its root. These ointments and creams were used to dress wounds and treat mild ruptures. A tea made with lady's mantle will also stop children's diarrhoea without any side effects.

Lily of the Valley (*Convallaria majalis*)

This woodland plant with elegant sword-shaped leaves and delicate white flower bells not only brings joy to our hearts in the spring when we come across it on our walks, but also strengthens and stimulates this organ, albeit that few people are aware of it. As long ago as the Middle Ages, lily of the valley was held in high esteem as a heart medicine. Later, however, when the more potent digitalis, or foxglove, was discovered, lily of the valley fell into disuse. An English doctor, by the name of Withering, found digitalis in the tea mixture of an old woman herbalist who used it to cure dropsy. This happened in the year 1785 and digitalis has been used ever since.

However, in recent times, we are beginning to realise that we have wrongfully neglected lily of the valley and that the plant that produces the most dramatic effect is not necessarily the best one. After many years of using digitalis as a heart medicine we have come to know some of its side effects. For example, we know now that digitalis is cumulative, which means that it remains in the heart muscle for quite some time and so prolonged treatment may seriously damage the heart. Lily of the valley, however, does not pose the same danger, since within four hours the glycoside, the active substance, is broken down by the body, although its medicinal effect continues for much longer.

Convallaria – the Latin name for lily of the valley – is best used in the form of a standardised fresh plant extract, together with *Scilla maritima* (sea onion or squill). It strengthens the heart muscles and extends its favourable effect to the blood vessels. If the patient is given the same dose as would be given with digitalis, its action will be more gentle and produce no side effects such as are engendered by accumulation. Digitalis sometimes proves ineffective in cases of a weak heart resulting from influenza, pneumonia or other lung and infectious diseases, whereas lily of the valley invariably does the job more effectively. This plant can, and should, be used as a pre-operative heart tonic and it will also have a salutary effect if used after an operation. Those who engage in competitive sports, where a strain is often placed on the heart, will find *Convallaria* a real help. I have also had excellent results when using it to treat heart complications which occurred during or after kidney diseases and have found it most reliable in the treatment of arteriosclerotic conditions, high blood pressure and symptoms characteristic of degenerative and premature aging processes.

There is no doubt that lily of the valley is a remedy to be used

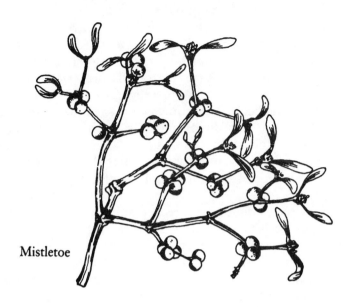

Mistletoe

for all kinds of heart trouble. In addition, the unpleasant heart symptoms accompanying hyperthyroidism will be alleviated by taking it, in which case digitalis would not be indicated at all. *Convascillan* is an excellent heart remedy combining lily of the valley with sea onion or squill. The latter plant is described on pages 380–81.

Mistletoe (*Viscum album*)
Each December, as the festive season approaches, shop windows and market places are decorated with the famous mistletoe branches with yellow-green stems and white berries. How many people realise, however, that this plant contains within it such wonderful curative powers? Mistletoe, known also by the Latin name of *Viscum album*, is not only used in the observance of an ancient custom, but is also important in the treatment of prematurely aged arteries. The fresh extract of mistletoe is one of the best remedies for the loss of elasticity in the arteries, a hardening of the arteries accompanied by high blood pressure. Combined with bear's garlic and hawthorn it will safely arrest, perhaps even cure, the progress of this tragic accompaniment of old age. These herbs, together with garlic and passionflower, are contained in *Arterioforce* capsules. Also, when combined with the Indian drug *Rauwolfia serpentina*, mistletoe becomes a high-blood pressure medicine beyond

compare. Centuries of experience with mistletoe and the latest results of research on *Rauwolfia* have enabled us to produce the outstanding combination remedy called *Rauwolfavena*.

However, for the treatment to be effective it is important that the levels of salt and protein in the diet be drastically reduced. The importance of mistletoe as a remedy can be illustrated by the quantity used in Germany alone, where 170–190 tons are processed every year.

Mistletoe extract is, of course, used to treat more complaints than just high blood pressure. It is indicated for headaches that are accompanied by dizziness, for spells of vertigo where there is a tendency to fall backwards, for people suffering from agoraphobia and a wavering gait and for those who experience attacks of 'pins and needles' in the limbs and who suffer from constant cold feet. *Viscum album*, used in conjunction with the indicated heart remedies, is beneficial for sudden attacks of palpitations coupled with vascular spasms, difficult breathing and nightly attacks of asthma. For treatment take 5–10 drops, 3–5 times daily.

Moreover, in the search of an effective herbal remedy for cancer, mistletoe and butterbur have given good results so far. For this reason, no one suffering from malignant growths should forget to take mistletoe. The fresh plant extract, as well as homoeopathic injections, have proved invaluable in this respect.

Finally, it is a matter of record that people who have suffered for years from pains in the joints because of chronic arthritis or arthrosis have been cured by homoeopathic mistletoe injections.

Mugwort (*Artemisia vulgaris*)

Pliny, writing in ancient Rome, as well as Gmelin in modern times, noted that *Artemisia* derived its name from the ancient practice of lining the shoes with the leaves to prevent tiredness. It is also said that Roman soldiers put mugwort in their sandals in order to ease their march into Helvetia.

People who have spent their holidays in the canton of Tessin, Switzerland, must be familiar with mugwort, for it is one of the toughest and most widespread weeds in that district. It is easily recognised because it reaches a height of almost 2 m (5–6 feet). Anyone not well acquainted with the various members of the *Artemisia* family might mistake mugwort for wormwood, as it resembles the latter in taste and smell.

The claim that mugwort relieves tired legs can be proved quite simply. After a long walk, bathe your feet in an infusion of mugwort and discover for yourself its soothing effect.

Apart from an essential oil and bitter substances, the herb also contains inulin, a substance similar to a carbohydrate but one that is tolerated by diabetics, unlike ordinary starch and carbohydrates. This makes it possible for the body to receive natural sugar-like substances without the need to engage the pancreas (the islets of Langerhans) in their digestion. Diabetics should take advantage of mugwort. The finely chopped leaves can be used in salads as an additional flavouring. In former days mugwort was also well known as an ingredient for stuffing geese and ducks. In fact, this is still the custom in some areas.

In cases of chronic diarrhoea, stomach or intestinal catarrh, and the widespread problem of intestinal worms, mugwort is an ideal remedy. Moreover, the fresh plant extract is one of the few effective medicines for the treatment of hystero-epilepsy, a form of falling sickness which appears to be connected with ovarian dysfunction. Mugwort is also an ingredient in *Dr Zimpel's epilepsy medicine*, which is closely based on the formulae developed by Paracelsus.

Mugwort is a diuretic and also encourages the menstrual flow when it has for some reason become retarded. Five drops of the fresh plant extract in a glass of water, sipped throughout the day, will suffice for this purpose.

Nettles (*Urtica dioica, Urtica urens*)

In the spring, when the snow has melted and the warm wind thaws the ground, life once again begins to stir in Mother Nature's womb. On sunny slopes, steep paths and even on disused refuse heaps, the green, finely serrated leaves of the nettle appear. Hardly anyone notices it, but it quietly grows while using its juices to produce a medicine that can bring health to many, and even save lives. If only people knew about the benefits of this plant and used it. Many a sufferer of tuberculosis would not have died had he but gone out of his way to gather nettles and avail himself of their goodness. How many children might have had their waxen looks changed and their red cheeks restored, if only their parents had realised what wonderful medicinal value the despised nettle has to offer! Much hard-earned money would not clink unnecessarily into the pharmacist's till, if young nettles were used as a restorative every spring.

No other plant can equal the nettle as a remedy for anaemia,

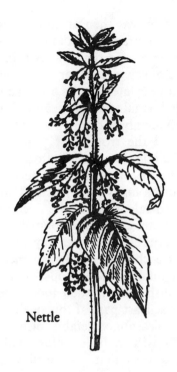

Nettle

chlorosis, rickets, scrofula, respiratory diseases and, especially, lymphatic problems.

It is most appropriate that nature has given this plant the protection of stinging exterior. Without it, we would probably never have the opportunity to benefit from its healing power. Animals, with their instinctive knowledge of what is good for them, would not leave us even one leaf.

The stinging nettle is rich in calcium, phosphorus, iron and other important minerals. It also belongs to the small category of plants that contain vitamin D. We already know that this vitamin is important in the development of the bones as well as for the assimilation of calcium. That is why eating raw nettles, either pulped or in the form of nettle juice, has a quick and reliable effect on rickets.

Many years ago I gave a lecture in Winterthur and mentioned that the stinging nettle was a wonderful help to those suffering from tuberculosis or weak lungs. A year later, I again delivered a lecture in that same hall. This time, a man from the audience stood up and announced in front of everybody that he had heard me describe the marvellous healing powers of the stinging nettle the previous year. His wife was then at home ill with tuberculosis of the lungs. Since her doctors could hold out no real hope of a cure, he began giving his wife food that was rich in calcium. Every day he gave her the juice of raw nettles, or added finely chopped nettles to her soup. Now, a year later, to the astonishment of her doctors, this man's wife had regained her health. I myself was just as surprised as the 300 members of my audience. I do admit that the daily nettle hunt and the trouble of putting them through the mincer to extract the juice is quite an effort. However, it is worthwhile considering that it can help a sick person to regain health.

Young nettles can be finely chopped and sprinkled on soup as a garnish or added to salads. Since the juice is not very tasty it is better to mix it in with whichever soup you prefer – vegetable, potato or oatmeal. A tablespoon per day for an adult and a half to one teaspoon for a child has sufficient medicinal properties to take effect. For an infant, 5–10 drops of the extract each day, added to different dishes of mashed foods should suffice. If you want to profit from at least part of this healthy remedy and at the same time enjoy a pleasant vegetable dish, you can also steam young nettles in oil with a little onion. This will give you an excellent spinach-like dish that goes well with mashed or sauté potatoes, besides being tasty. So make it a point to search out the places where you can gather nettles; only pick the young shoots and you will be able to have nettles on your menu for months.

Perhaps some of my readers feel that they have no time to look for and prepare these wild plants and would prefer to buy the juice ready-made. Of course they can do this; but no prepared medicine – even an extract from fresh plants – can have as good an effect as the extracted juice from a plant freshly gathered or the fresh plant used by itself.

The calcium complex *Urticalcin* contains *Urtica*, which is the Latin name for nettles. As the name implies, Urticalcin is a compound containing various kinds or combinations of calcium, with the addition of fresh nettles. The way in which homoeopathy makes use of nettles will be explained in the section on 'Homoeopathic remedies' (see page 397).

Oats (*Avena sativa*)
It is common knowledge that horses derive their strength largely from eating oats. They are nourishing for people too. Whenever we have an upset stomach we most likely take oatmeal gruel or porridge, for this will usually correct the trouble. As a food oats

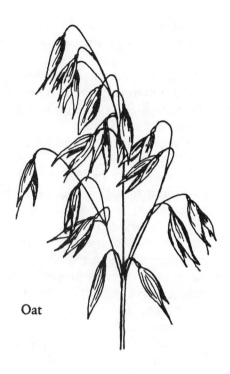

Oat

are good for man and beast, but that is not all: oats are also a wonderful remedy. Even in its earliest stages, when the oat plant is just a tall grass, it has remarkable healing powers. Few people realise that when the ears are just beginning to form, when it is juicy and breaking into flower, this green grass is at its richest in avenin, which is unsurpassed as a nutrient for the cells of the nervous system.

You can prepare a perfect nerve food at home simply by putting the flowering oats through a mincer, or by chopping them up in some other way. Cover the green mash with warm water and let it stand for about two minutes. Then strain and sweeten with honey, unrefined sugar, grape sugar or grape concentrate. The green oats can also be put through the mincer together with raisins or currants, then covered with warm water and strained as before. In this way they will be sweetened during preparation.

When the green oat plant is about 40–50 cm (15–20 inches) high it is usable for this oat drink, and is most potent during the flowering period. As long as the grains are juicy the oats can be used for this tonic.

The resulting oat drink is a wonderful tonic which, if taken

371

regularly over a period of time, will calm and regenerate the nervous system, giving it new energy. Its use is also recommended for diabetics.

Even after the oats have been harvested the straw can be used to make an infusion, although it is not as potent as the juice from the green oats. Still, it will be found quite effective in cases of catarrh, coughs and febrile conditions. A decoction of oat straw added to the bath water is especially good for children whose skin function needs stimulating.

There are still other uses for oats, for even the grains make an excellent tea. If you cannot find gleanings in the field, use the oat grain together with the husk, as fed to horses. Sweeten the tea as you would the oat drink described above. It has a tonic effect, and if taken when the mucous membranes of the stomach or intestines are inflamed, it is a superb soothing remedy.

Homoeopathy employs the freshly pressed juice from the green oats for its outstanding nerve remedy *Avena sativa*, which is the Latin name for the oat plant. This remedy is particularly useful for children and sensitive people. The same extract, together with the extract of Korean ginseng, is used to make the reliable nerve tonic for adults called *Ginsavena*.

Papaya (*Carica papaya*)

Every time I see papaya fruits on display in a shop I remember the time I spent in Lagunas, on the Marañon river. It was there that I acquired the habit of looking for a papaya plant after every meal. I would break off a leaf and eat some of it to aid the digestion and as a prophylactic, even if it was only a piece the size of a large coin. It may even be possible that my regular chewing of papaya leaves may have seen to it that the many kinds of parasites did not really bother me on my repeated travels in the tropics, even though I may have swallowed them with my food. True, I was always very careful, but even so, dangerous amoebas, hookworms, oxyurias, ascarids, whipworms and many other parasites, are rampant in the tropics and multiply rapidly, laying millions of eggs. There are some that draw blood from the intestinal linings; others cause inflammation, even abscesses and ulcers. They penetrate the liver and as a direct or indirect consequence thousands of victims die, often literally wasting away.

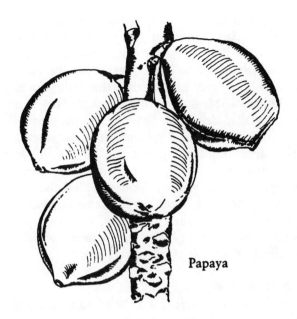

Papaya

A *Superb Remedy*

It is interesting to note that wherever there are dangers to our health nature provides a local means of resistance or remedy. Papaya thrives in hot and humid tropical regions. I came across some marvellous specimens in Lagunas, where the trees grew to about 3–4 m (about 10–13 feet), the trunk to a diameter of about 20–25 cm (8–10 inches), bearing 20–25 fruits, which hang on the trunk between the axils of the large leaves. The ripe yellow fruits hang more towards the bottom of the tree; further up they are still green and unripe. They look like melons, are hollow inside and full of small, black, moist, round seeds. The active substance of papaya is to be found mainly in the unripe fruits and in the skin of the ripe ones, but this skin is usually peeled off and thrown away. The fruit pulp is yellow or pinkish, with an unusual taste, which it may take a while to become accustomed to.

As I suggested above, the fruit aids the digestion, so make it a habit to eat a slice after meals if you are visiting the tropics. The strong taste is less noticeable when papaya is mixed in a fruit salad together with pineapple, bananas and mangoes. It also helps to add a little lemon juice. Incidentally, papaya and pineapple mixed together in a blender make a tasty and refreshing drink.

Although a certain German pharmaceutical company mentions the use of only ripe papaya in their product, the real medicinal

373

effect is not obtained from ripe fruits. The curative properties, especially papain, are found in the unripe fruit, the seeds and leaves. Papain can be obtained by scratching the skin of unripe fruits. Immediately, a white juice oozes from the incision, similar to latex in a rubber tree. Left to dry, this milky juice becomes a yellowish rubbery substance – raw papain. This is an excellent remedy, employed to deal with two specific problems. First of all, it kills – or rather, digests – all intestinal parasites that usually settle in the large and small intestines. So if you eat a piece of papaya leaf after every meal, as I used to do, you will not be plagued by troublesome worms. You can also chew and swallow a teaspoonful of the black seeds for the same purpose. This simple preventative measure, if taken regularly, will keep you free from infections too. The second type of problem for which papaya has proved an effective remedy is described below.

Help for the Pancreas
Papaya stimulates the pancreas and helps to digest protein. If you happen to indulge in too much protein, eat some papaya and you will find that the feeling of fullness and listlessness disappears in a matter of minutes. No wonder, then, that *Papayasan*, which is made from papaya leaves and the juice of unripe fruits, is such a helpful natural product. In fact, Papayasan has proved to be an excellent remedy for a range of pancreatic problems, including fatty stools caused by insufficiency of the pancreas, even typical pancreatitis. Papayasan should preferably be taken in conjunction with *Kelpasan* because of the latter's potassium iodide content. Diabetics will benefit from Papayasan too, since it is a great aid in digesting fat and protein. Anyone who suffers from diabetes should take two Papayasan tablets after every meal and will be delighted at the effect of this natural remedy.

If you intend to travel to a subtropical or tropical region, even if only for a short visit or vacation, do not forget to take some Papayasan with you. Remember, two tablets after every meal can save you from a lot of trouble. It is much better to pay a little attention to your body and care for your health than fall victim to amoebic dysentery or some stubborn worm infection and the bothersome consequences.

Pimpernel Root (*Pimpinella saxifraga*)
In the Middle Ages, women must have often sat talking and exchanged advice on all sorts of subjects. The medical practitioner

often lived miles away from a hamlet or fortified castle and there were no telephones to summon him or her. Sometimes it might have happened that some young noblewoman was unable to give her new-born baby sufficient milk and, often within the walls of the castle itself, some wise old woman would be found to give advice. Later, a young girl would be hustled through the gates and over the drawbridge with orders to find some pimpernel roots somewhere outside. Having been well washed, these roots would be placed in the noblewoman's bosom and within 6–8 hours there would be so much milk that the pimpernel roots would have to be quickly removed and thrown away.

Thus, old stories and records tell us of the wonderful effect produced by the little pimpernel. Today we have other remedies that may be easier to come by and apply (for example *Ricinus communis 3x*) but wherever the pimpernel may be found, it should prove to be as great a help as it was in days of old. Nursing mothers might try to discover whether its effect is as good as the old records say it is.

Today, the pimpernel's main attribute is the wonderful effect it has on the vocal cords in cases of catarrh and sore throats. Pimpernel roots, chewed throughout the day, will have a much better effect than all the expensive patent medicines with their fancy packaging and labels that promise miracles. There is only one drawback, pimpernel roots are far from palatable, even though they are not so bad that one would want to reject them altogether. In the wintertime, when catarrh is so prevalent, one can come to appreciate the pimpernel's great benefits.

If hoarseness is allied to the catarrh, chew pimpernel roots with rowan berries; both remedies can usually be bought in a dry state at a pharmacy or herbalist. For extremely bad cases, *fresh pine bud syrup (Santasapina Cough Syrup)* is another excellent remedy.

Formerly, pimpernel root was recommended in cases of calculus and skin eruptions. That our forefathers prized pimpernel as one of the means of protecting themselves against contagious diseases can be seen from the old saying:

To be healthy and fit, eat garlic and pimpernel,
You can then hope to live to an old age as well!

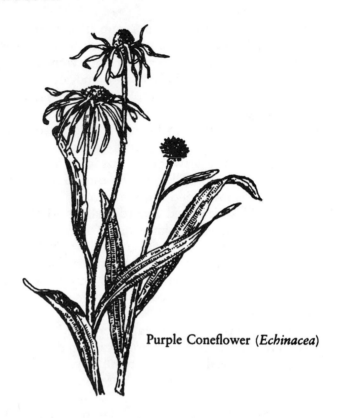

Purple Coneflower (*Echinacea*)

Purple Coneflower (*Echinacea purpurea* and *angustifolia*)

My Introduction to Echinacea

It was in the 1950s when I met Black Eagle, the chief of the Sioux Indians. Besides his tribal tongue, he spoke very good English, so we were able to talk about our mutual appreciation and love of plants, their curative powers and practical uses for various ailments and emergencies. I found even his philosophy of life to be very similar to my own. He too looked at nature as a creation of the great Artist of the Universe.

We both shared the same views regarding man's responsibility towards nature, which involved not only thinking of what we can get out of it but rather doing all we can to protect and preserve it. Because of the many things we had in common, a close bond of friendship developed between us and one day he embraced me affectionately and professed his feelings of brotherly love towards me. It was a most interesting experience, not least because of the different tribal customs he introduced me to. Being over ninety years old at the time, he was able to relate many experiences he had had with the white man. More than once I had to interrupt, expressing my deepest sympathy and sadness at all the injury and suffering the people of my own skin colour had inflicted upon him and his people.

Black Eagle's ideas about illness and disease were of great interest to me, and in this respect we discussed the importance of medicinal herbs as well as nutrition, or proper diet. He believed that the white man's customs and habits had overtaxed the regenerative powers our Creator, or nature, had implanted in us and that he often had only himself to blame for the resulting diseases.

A Sacred Plant

It was from Black Eagle that I learned about the curative effects of various plants growing in South Dakota, the home of his tribe. One plant in particular enjoyed his special appreciation. Considered as sacred, this medicinal herb had been a life-saver on many occasions. His ancestors, he said, used it to cure cases of blood poisoning.

Even snake poison could be made ineffective with it. When someone was bitten by a poisonous snake, he told me, another person would suck the bite until blood began to flow. Of course, the attendant would spit the poison out. Next, the leaves and roots of the plant were chewed up, preferably by the unfortunate victim himself. The juice was swallowed but the masticated plant was applied to the bite and bandaged. This treatment was repeated at least twice, and then repeated again on the second and third day. By the fourth day, the effect of the poison would have disappeared and the victim would be out of danger.

These Indians used to do the same thing to treat injuries. Again, the masticated plant would be placed on the affected part, and a serious situation would never arise provided this plant was on hand and was applied immediately. Certain arrow poisons could be neutralised by the same method. And if one wanted to prevent susceptibility to colds and catarrh in bad and blustery weather, he only had to chew the leaves or roots of the plant. The ingested juice would build up resistance to everything we now call infectious diseases.

The Two Varieties of Echinacea

Then Black Eagle showed me this highly prized plant, or plants to be more exact. I discovered that it was the coneflower, *Echinacea angustifolia* and *Echinacea purpurea*. One of the two varieties, *Echinacea angustifolia*, has a tap root, and I still remember how deep I had to dig to get it out. The other variety has a rootstock and does not penetrate quite so deep into the earth.

The chief explained that both plants were equal in their effect. But having heard so many marvellous things about what this plant could do I began to think it was almost too good to be true. Still, I took some seeds back home with me and began to grow *Echinacea* in the Swiss lowlands as well as at an elevation of 1,600 m (4,500 feet); that was in Teufen and in Brail (in the Engadine), where I used to have a house with a large garden. At first, the plants were quite sensitive to the cold in the mountains, but I persevered for ten years until they became acclimatised and began to produce flowers.

Blood Poisoning Cured

One day I was cutting grass on a steep meadow when I hit my foot with the scythe. It was careless of me, but I did not immediately disinfect the cut, only bandaged it with a handkerchief and carried on with my work. Because of this negligence, it was not surprising when blood poisoning set in. Well now, I thought, this is a chance to put our herb to the test and see whether the Indians were right. I proceeded exactly the way Black Eagle had taught me. Already a long blue line was visible on the leg and higher up, in the groin, there was a swollen lymph node. So I covered the whole leg with a dressing of crushed *Echinacea* leaves. Furthermore, I chewed some and swallowed the juice. In fact, I ate the whole plant. Now came the surprise, for within quite a short time the inflammation and infection were gone. This experience convinced me that everything I had been told about *Echinacea* was true.

Protection against Malaria

Some time after the above experience, I travelled to the Amazon region and visited a jungle where malaria was rampant. I was accompanied on this study tour by a colleague who had been working with me in Peru, a man who was well acclimatised to South America.

I took the risk of travelling without malaria drugs, but I did take *Echinacea* tincture daily, about forty drops every morning and evening. During the first few days we put up a mosquito net, but in the native huts the mosquitoes were able to slip through the chinks in the bamboo floor. We even killed some blood-filled insects under the net.

My colleague had no confidence in *Echinacea* and declined to take any. Like myself, he must have been bitten hundreds of times. The area we visited around the Upper Marañon was notorious and feared for malaria. Although I was bitten all over, I was astonished that I did not once come down with a fever attack, whereas my colleague returned home with a bad case of the disease. Unfortunately, he had not taken any remedy. He believed that his sixteen years in Peru had made him immune to malaria. However, the area where he had been living, at our farm in Tarapoto, was malaria-free, unlike the Amazon region we visited on this occasion.

Thirty years later, a medical check-up brought to light that I had once had a malaria infection, which could only have been during this visit to the Marañon. As I had never suffered so much as a bout of fever or any other symptom of the disease, I came to the obvious conclusion that *Echinacea* may well help to prevent malaria.

Reinforcing the Immune System
Researchers have been taking a keen interest in *Echinacea*, with the aim of isolating its medicinal properties. First they tried, without success, to find the substances that prevent the growth and development of pathogenic organisms, since it was thought that this is what happens.

It was much later, however, when they discovered that the effect of *Echinacea* is not attributable to some antibiotic property, but to its ability to reinforce the body's own defence mechanism. Medical science began to realise then that here was a very remarkable plant indeed. After all, the immune system is one of the most important things in our body. Without its proper functioning, without a good defence mechanism, we could not survive. We are constantly subjected to the attacks of millions of germs. However, these agents can multiply and cause damage in the human body only if they find the breeding ground necessary for their survival and if the defence system is weak.

The immune system is weakened by our modern, unnatural way of life. It is therefore understandable that a herbal remedy such as *Echinacea* is gaining in stature.

SCIENTIFIC EVIDENCE
Scientific research has confirmed that *Echinacea* improves and builds up immunity, even though it has not been possible, to date, to isolate a specific substance that is responsible for its remedial effect. I myself am convinced that no such active substances will ever be discovered because it is not some specific chemical that can be credited with the medicinal effect, but the complex of vital substances contained in the plant as a whole. It is the same with all other medicinal herbs; it is the entirety of substance – all the active and supporting substances in the plant – that achieves the desirable results. This is especially true in the case of a herb whose properties stimulate the immune system, since it acts not just on a single organ but on the body as a unit.

I have been able to prove for myself that *Echinacea* activates the immune system, and that it is therefore a great aid to the body's resistance to micro-organisms. Time and again I have seen those with a weak lymphatic system and who suffer constant attacks of colds and catarrh, particularly children, overcome this suscepti-bility when put on regular medication with *Echinacea* preparations such as *Echinaforce*. Many parents have told me that their children have become more resistant to infectious diseases; the same is true of sensitive adults. Because of my practical experience, I maintain that *Echinacea* builds up the body's own defences, above all, the efficiency of the phagocytes.

Scientists have discovered that *Echinacea* is able to render the hyaluronidase (an enzyme) produced by bacteria ineffective, pre-venting their proliferation. This helps us to understand why *Echin-acea* neutralises snake poison, which also contains hyaluronidase.

Without doubt, *Echinaforce* can be used with confidence for every case of infection or infectious disease. It supports the body in every part where its defence mechanism needs to be improved, increasing overall resistance.

Sea Onion or Squill (*Scilla, Urginea maritima*)

Along the shores of the Mediterranean, more specifically the blue waters of Greece by the Peloponnesian peninsula, an extraordinary plant is found. It shoots up out of the dry ground on a stem more than a metre (3 feet) high and is crowned with a dense spike of small white flowers. The stem has no leaves and if you dig down for its root, you will come upon a large bulb which, on average, is about 15 cm (6 inches) in diameter and over 1 kg (2 pounds) in weight. This is the genuine sea onion or squill that flourishes in the dry ground and the fragrant sea air and is known to the botanists as *Scilla maritima*. The plant contains an essential oil, scillitin, or scillin, besides other important substances, and was used as an internal as well as external remedy even by the ancient inhabitants of the Mediterranean region. They praised its medicinal effects in the treatment of various heart troubles, oedematic congestion, and breathing difficulties. They also used it to aid those who suffered from extreme cold in the hands and feet, whose urine was pale and watery, whose pulse was light or rapid, or whose upper air passages were affected with catarrh. It was found especially helpful in treating the kind of heart trouble that is accompanied by difficulty in dispersing water and expelling phlegm caused by catarrh, and by itching of the skin. More recent observations, based on the experience of those ancient herbalists, have confirmed the efficacy of fresh squill extract in curing the range of symptoms just described.

This natural plant remedy can be of great help in treating these problems. Large doses are unnecessary. In fact, to achieve good results no more than five drops of 3x potency (1/1000 dilution of the mother tincture) need be taken at one time.

A combination of lily of the valley and sea onion produces a very good remedy, *Convascillan*. Where once it was necessary to give strophanthin – a virtual whip for the heart – it is now possible to provide help with this gentle and reliable *Convallaria* complex, which supports rather than drives the heart. The effect of Convascillan is also long-lasting, another point in its favour.

Wild Fruits and Berries

Barberry (*Berberis vulgaris*)

Roaming through the valleys of the Swiss cantons of Valais and Graubuenden, bright with the autumn sun and a riot of colours, the happy wanderer will find not only hedgerow after hedgerow of wild rose hips, but also many bushes replete with sprays of barberries. Of course, barberries grow in other areas too, but wherever they are, most people go past the wild fruits without realising that they have wonderful healing powers. The clusters of these red oblong berries are a delight to the eye and, together with autumn flowers and leaves, make a beautiful bouquet. Still, few people are aware that these berries can be eaten and are, in fact, one of the best nerve tonics available. No other wild berries are as rich in vitamin C and many people suffering from 'nerves' could, on their walks in the country, benefit enormously by picking some and chewing them slowly before swallowing them. A general check-up of the population would no doubt prove that many people nowadays need such a tonic.

A raw barberry conserve, made from well-ripened berries, is rich in vitamin C (ascorbic acid) and other vitamins. However, if copper vessels or utensils are used to cook and strain the conserve, the copper acts as a catalytic agent and destroys most of the vitamin C.

Since the vitamin content is mostly lost in cooking, the barberries should be processed raw in order to obtain a nutritious and remedial conserve that keeps well. Thorough tests have shown that the best way to produce barberry conserve is as follows. Put the freshly picked and fully ripe barberries through the mincer. Then squeeze the pulp through a sieve. The pips and skins will remain in the sieve and you will have the clean purée and juice. Add 100 g (3 oz) of raw cane sugar to 500 g (1lb) of barberry purée and stir well. When the sugar has dissolved, add 200 g (7 oz) of honey and finally 200–250 g (7–8 oz) of thick grape sugar syrup. Stir the

382

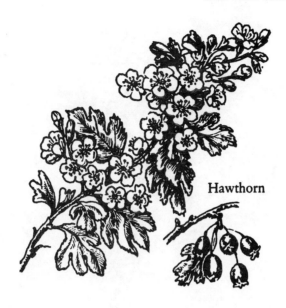

Hawthorn

mixture until well blended. If the mixture is too thin, add a little more raw cane sugar. Then, pour into glass jars as you would with jam.

On a commercial scale, this conserve is made by condensing grape sugar under a vacuum and then slowly adding the raw purée. Experimental research has established the excellence of this natural remedy in the treatment of bad nerves. It also has a wonderful effect on the kidneys and on any scorbutic tendency, such as bleeding gums.

Hawthorn (*Crataegus oxyacantha*)
The splendid remedy, *Crataegisan*, is made from the dark red berries, haws, to be found hanging in small bunches from the thorny hawthorn shrubs by the wayside or in the meadows every autumn. When I was a child, my friends and I called them 'mealy berries'. We children did not know anything about them, except that they were good to eat (their pulpy inside is not unlike cooked sweet potato) and of course we ate them because there was probably nothing else at that particular moment. Certainly we did not need those berries when we were young, for *Crataegus* is a heart remedy, and is particularly valuable in cases of weak heart muscles.

When arteriosclerosis, high blood pressure and, especially, a hardened and constricted coronary artery are diagnosed, there is

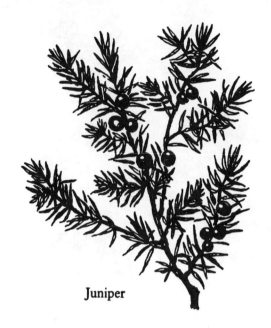

Juniper

no doubt that *Crataegus* is the best, the most harmless and the most reliable remedy that can be taken. *Arnica*, mixed in the right proportion with *Crataegus*, makes up a compound remedy that has benefited many elderly people, even to the extent of lengthening their lives.

Crataegisan is a successful remedy for angina pectoris, when heart cramps occur. These cramps are usually accompanied by stabbing pains in the region of the heart resulting in difficult breathing and a weak, irregular pulse. In this case, where immediate relief is necessary, take 5–10 drops every half hour. When the pains subside and the cramps have eased, 15–20 drops taken three times a day will suffice.

For cardiac dilatation, the main treatment should consist of *heart hormones* and *Crataegus* taken at the same time.

Juniper Berries (*Fructus juniperi*)
People who like sauerkraut will be familiar with juniper berries because they are often added for flavouring. But then what do we do? We pick them out and leave them on the side of the plate. Occasionally they are mentioned in a cookery book as a spice, and it may also be remembered by some that grandfather often used to chew them first thing in the morning. Besides that, juniper

berries have been more or less forgotten. Old herbals say that the eagle lives to an old age because it feeds on juniper berries. They contain a delicate essential oil and much sugar, yet they do not taste sweet because their bitter constituents override the sweet ones.

Sufferers from gout and rheumatism find that juniper berries are an excellent remedy because they help to increase the elimination of uric acid by way of the urine. Be careful how you use them, however; too much may irritate the kidneys, and this is easily done if you take the juice or extract. If someone suffers from nephritis or similar kidney conditions, he should take juniper only in homoeopathic doses, *Juniperus communis 1x* or *2x*.

For cases of asthma, and particularly the excessive mucous catarrh that may result from the disease, juniper extract is most beneficial and its use should be alternated with that of barberries and rowan berries.

Oedematous conditions (excessive accumulation of fluid in the body) and acute inflammation of the bladder (cystitis) will respond to juniper in the form of an infusion, essence or extract.

Eat juniper berries every morning before breakfast, one berry the first day, two the second day, and so forth until you reach twenty and then go back, reducing the amount day by day to just one. This is very good for stimulating the appetite and strengthening the stomach and will benefit the glands.

Moreover, if you tie some juniper needles in a muslin bag, and place this under the hot tap when you run a bath, you will have a good remedy for rheumatism and gout.

Rose Hips (*Rosa canina*)

Not only are the modest but beautiful flowers of the wild rose, so unjustly called *Rosa canina* or 'dog rose', a pleasure to behold, but the fruit too is delightful as it splashes its bright red across the autumn landscape. Where the hips have not been harvested they look, in winter, like little red gnomes with white caps of snow, and many a hungry bird has enjoyed these nutritious berries when everything else has been buried under the ice.

As a food, rose hips are excellent for many reasons. The fully ripe hips contain natural fruit sugar and taste as sweet as any jam. They are nourishing because of their many mineral salts, such as calcium, silica, magnesium and phosphorus. Incidentally, phosphorus is good for the brain and no doubt our little feathered friends have to use theirs, dashing about in the winter weather,

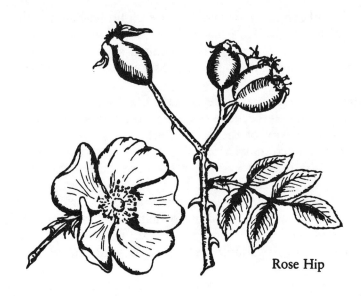

Rose Hip

and who knows whether the phosphorus in rose hips is responsible for their feathers being always so bright and shiny. On the other hand, silica may contribute to the beauty of their feather coats. Our little friends must owe their peace and contentedness, in spite of their lively acrobatics, to the vitamin C in rose hips, since this vitamin has a calming effect on the nerves.

Now you know why rose hip products are also valuable for us humans. Nature always shows us the way, while science can only try to give us an explanation of the reasons.

Rose hips are one of the best sources of vitamin C. Rose hip pulp is not only a tasty, slightly tart conserve but a medicine, a nerve food, conforming to the old principle, 'Let food be your medicine and medicine your food.' It is important, however, to remember that rose hips should not be boiled as heat destroys much of their remedial properties. Eat a slice of bread thickly spread with raw pulp every day and you will be taking your daily requirement of vitamin C. If a conserve is made from the pulp and sweetened with grape sugar or other fruit sugars as described below, you will have the added advantage of getting the best kinds of sugar, ones that are easy to assimilate, and you will be providing yourself with food of a high calorific value.

Rose Hip Conserve

Gather the ripe berries of the wild rose, the hips, and spread them out to mellow in a dry shady place. Make sure they are not piled up on top of each other in the box or basket, otherwise they will go mouldy, rather than overripe. When they are nice and soft, put them through a mincer to obtain a thick red purée. Use a wooden spoon to rub the mash through a sieve in order to separate the little seeds. A red paste will come through the sieve and can be scraped off with a knife or spoon. This paste, rich in vitamin C, should now be mixed with half the quantity of honey or grape sugar (the consistency of honey). That is all there is to it! Although uncooked, the mixture will keep well, preferably in the refrigerator. It is wholesome and delicious. A teaspoonful a day will provide the daily requirement of vitamin C and can help a hard-working person more than any of the commercially manufactured vitamin C tablets.

Rose Hip Tea

Having made the conserve, you will have the seeds, skin and some pulp left over. These can be dried and used for making tea, especially in winter. Rose hip tea is most beneficial. It has a delicate flavour and can be served with lemon or milk, according to taste. It is rich in silica and, perhaps for this reason, is an excellent kidney remedy. Seriously ill people who cannot take any other herbal infusion are quite safe with rose hip tea.

Rowan Berries (*Fructus sorbi*)

In the autumn, the rowan tree (European mountain ash) produces beautiful red berries. If you spread these berries out in a shady place and dry them, you will have a reliable remedy for hoarseness. Just chew them and the problem will quickly disappear. Also, some people in rural areas still make jam from the ripe berries.

Sea Buckthorn (*Hippophae rhamnoides*)

There is hardly another shrub with edible berries that is so widely distributed as sea buckthorn. It can be found growing from the north of Portugal to the Pyrenees, across the Alps, then south in the Balkans, over in Turkey, and to the east in central Russia, Mongolia, Korea and Japan. If all the berries could be gathered and processed, they would be more than enough to cater for the vitamin C requirement of all humankind.

Once our bodies have become deficient in vitamin C, we are

much more liable to succumb to infectious diseases. That is why we should see to it that the deficiency is rectified, especially in springtime. Although barberrry and rose hip purées no doubt play an important part in correcting vitamin C deficiencies, sea buckthorn berries are no less valuable in terms of their extremely high content of vitamin C. During the time of year when a wide selection of fresh vegetables are difficult to obtain, or very expensive, and fruits have lost part of their vitamin content because of long storage, the need for vitamins is even greater and many people like to tide themselves over the vitamin-poor period by eating *Bio-Buckthorn-Conserve*.

Vitamin C has to be taken daily since the body can store only minute quantities. It is found in the endocrine glands, the supra-renal and pituitary glands, and there is no doubt that it is essential to the normal functioning of these important glands.

As a rule, cancer patients show a definite lack of this vitamin. It is therefore recommended that people with a predisposition to cancer and those who are victims already, increase their intake of foods that are rich in vitamin C.

To ensure good health, the daily intake of vitamin C should not be less than 50 mg, and it is better if it can be obtained from such natural sources as sea buckthorn, raspberries, lemon juice and rose hip and barberry purée.

Sea buckthorn has even more to offer us than its high vitamin content. Its berries also contain other vitamins, for example, water-soluble vitamin B, fat-soluble provitamin A and even vitamin E. These natural, biological vitamins are vital for keeping the body healthy, fit and efficient. Various acids, such as malic and tartaric acids, have also been identified in these berries. The sea buckthorn berry seeds can also be used to produce an oil of which the dietary value is unquestionable.

If you suffer from constant infections and bleeding of the gums and mucous membranes, you would do well to take sea buckthorn products as a dietary supplement. Sea buckthorn berries being rich in many vitamins and trace elements, it is obvious that the products based on them are recommended for children and adults alike as food supplements and a tonic.

In Switzerland, sea buckthorn grows abundantly in the upper Inn valley and in Ticino, especially in the Maggia valley. When ripe, the orange-coloured berries nestling between olive-green leaves are quite conspicuous, and in the wintertime birds can be seen enjoying them to the full. We use sea buckthorn extract as one of the ingredients in our vitamin preparation called *Bio-C-Lozenges*.

A Brief Guide to Selected Homoeopathic Remedies

The subject of homoeopathic remedies is so vast that the examples given below represent only a small selection of what would otherwise fill several volumes.

Aconitum napellus (Aconite, Monkshood)

The erect and splendid aconite, with its hood-like, blue-purple flowers, can be as poisonous as it is medicinal. This beautiful plant is known by many names, for example monkshood, friar's cap, wolfbane and mousebane, and is native to the Swiss Alps. There you will find it on the alpine meadows, where the ground is rich, in damp hollows between low shrubs and in thinning woods right up to the highest elevation where the conifers grow.

Every part of the plant is highly poisonous. The whole plant, including the subsidiary tuber, which is developed from the root for the following year's growth, is used to make a tincture for homoeopathic purposes. If this tincture was to be taken pure, it would result in certain death caused by cardiac paralysis and damage to the spinal cord. But diluted a thousand or one hundred thousand times, aconite becomes one of the best and most reliable homoeopathic medicines.

Aconitum is the best first aid in cases of inflammations that tend to become febrile. In infectious diseases, especially when the skin is hot and dry, *Aconitum* in the third and fourth decimal potency (3x or 4x) has a rapid and highly beneficial effect. It diverts the toxins from the blood and the tissues to the skin and encourages perspiration. A rush of blood to the head (hot flushes), such as many women experience during the change of life, is best dealt with by *Aconitum 10x*; for even better results this should be taken together with *Ovarium 3x*. It is helpful to take *Aconitum 4x* in alternation with *Belladonna 4x* at the onset of an acute illness when fever, a feeling of unrest, hot flushes, palpitations, uneasiness and a state of anxiety are present. When perspiration breaks out and the patient has calmed down, the treatment with *Aconitum* can be stopped and only *Belladonna 4x* or some other indicated remedy need be taken.

Homoeopathic *Aconitum* and *Belladonna* should be in everyone's medicine chest, for they are more frequently used than any other remedy for first aid. However, we do not recommend *Aconitum* tincture as it is dangerous, even though some doctors prescribe it for neuralgia caused by a cold, for gout and for rheumatism. There are other, safer remedies available that are just as effective. *Aconitum* is a mydriatic, that is, it dilates the pupil if it is put in the eye. *Belladonna* has the same property due to its atropine content. To achieve the best results, *Aconitum* should be given in the fourth decimal potency (4x), for stronger persons perhaps in the third (3x); five drops in a glass of water taken at hourly intervals will be enough.

Atropa belladonna (Belladonna, Deadly Nightshade)
This attractive plant with its thick stems or branches and leaves is somewhat similar to the tobacco plant. However, its axillary flowers, dull brown to dark purple in colour, indicate that it is neither the tobacco plant nor the ground-cherry (Chinese lantern), but belladonna, the medicinal as well as deadly nightshade.

The ripe, shiny black berries often entice children to pick and eat them – with fatal results. Many a child has had to pay with his young life because of being tempted. On the other hand, in considering this plant we cannot overlook its many benefits, even though we are aware of its poisonous properties. As is true of people, plants can have good and bad characteristics, and this is the case with belladonna. It is known to have killed people, but it is also famed as a life-saver.

Belladonna is partly responsible for the rediscovery of the homoeopathic principle of similarity. Dr Hahnemann once found himself completely at a loss as to what remedy to prescribe for a sick woman, until an unconscious child was carried in to him. The child's face was suffused by a bluish-red colour and Hahnemann realised immediately what had happened when the father showed him the pretty black berries he had snatched from the child's hands – belladonna poisoning! By chance, the physician noticed that there was an extraordinary similarity in the appearance of the women and the child; both had a bluish-red flush on the face. The causes were different but the results were the same. The doctor suddenly realised what he must do, the significance of which has only become fully recognised and appreciated in our time: '*Similia similibus curantur*', the ancient Hippocratic teaching and principle of similarity.

As soon as Hahnemann had given the child something to make it vomit, he went out with the father, broke off a branch of the belladonna with flowers and fruit, and squeezed the whole thing into some water. By diluting it to about 4x he prepared the yellowish-green liquid into a medicine, which he then gave to the sick woman. Noting her reaction, the doctor followed this up with a second dose, and a few more, until the woman was finally out of danger. Thus, the child's belladonna poisoning saved the woman's life and at the same time brought about a deeper understanding and knowledge of another law of nature.

Belladonna can always be given with success where a condition is the result of poisoning, whether from an internal or external cause, and where it manifests itself in the nervous system and the brain, for example through headaches, a rush of blood to the head accompanied by a racing pulse, delirium and where every movement of the body, even a simple movement of the eyes, aggravates the condition. *Belladonna 4x* is indicated when an illness reaches a sudden crisis; when the patient is sensitive to light and his pupils are dilated; when the mucous membranes are dry, hot and inflamed – and when any one of these symptoms is accompanied by a high temperature. For the intellectually alert, the vivacious person, young people who have to concentrate mentally and draw heavily on their brains, or for those who lead an intellectual life, *Belladonna 4x* is a wonder medicine.

Belladonna 4x is a quick and reliable help in cases of infectious diseases such as measles, scarlet fever, whooping cough, conjunctivitis, whitlows and even pneumonia, especially in its early stages.

It is important to keep *Belladonna* in your medicine chest; if used at once when needed, many a serious problem can be avoided. The remedy works if there is a threat of meningitis. If grandfather exhibits a suspiciously red face, the same remedy will avert an imminent apoplectic fit. Auntie may be troubled by sudden neuralgic pains, a brother or sister may come home from work with stomach, intestinal, liver, bladder or biliary cramps, or the cramps may be somewhere else in the abdomen – they will all find relief from five drops of *Belladonna* taken in a small glass of water. This first aid rarely fails. Cramps that develop suddenly, beginning in the anus, are relieved within a few minutes by *Belladonna*. It has even been effective in cases of bed-wetting.

With respect to dosage, the potency used generally is 4x. Typical *Belladonna* cases should not receive potencies below 6x.

Coccus cacti (Cochineal)

This is a marvellous remedy for whooping cough and when combined with *Drosera* (sundew) its effect is astonishingly fast. *Coccus cacti* (cochineal) is one of the ingredients in *Thydroca*, the reliable whooping cough drops. If these drops are used at once, possibly prior to the onset of the characteristic symptoms, as a prophylactic, the whoop may be aborted.

It is strange that *Drosera* is a carnivorous plant and *Coccus cacti* itself has little to do with plants. To obtain the raw material for this whooping cough remedy one must travel far: to Algeria, the Canary Islands, or to Central America where cactus plants abound in desert areas and stony wastelands. The search goes on to locate a genus of cactus called *Opuntia coccinellifera* and on it one will find a small insect about 3 mm long, which feeds on the juicy flesh of its host. The insect has a broad shell and leaves behind a red stain when it is squashed on a piece of white paper. Do not be shocked to learn that this is the female cochineal insect, the raw material for the wonderful homoeopathic whooping cough remedy called *Coccus cacti*.

In addition to its beneficial effect on whooping cough, students and supporters of Dr Rademacher have found that *Coccus cacti* has an excellent effect on the kidneys. Observations made at a Vienna clinic confirm that all kinds of spasmodic blockages, respiratory blockages and pneumo-tubercular coughs also benefit from it. In the great Homoeopathic Repertory by the well-known American authority Kent, *Coccus cacti* is recommended for diseases of the central nervous system.

Physicians in earlier times used this remedy in material doses, that is, the mother tincture, for severe kidney disorders, but homoeopathy generally employs the medium potencies 4x–6x.

Guaiacum officinale (Guaiac, Resin of Lignum vitae)

In Paracelsus' time, merchants brought home a sort of wood that was said to contain a medicinal resin. This wood was extraordinary because it sank in water, obviously being heavier than water, and this made it different from any other wood known at the time. It was found in the West Indies and South America and, when heated, a resin flowed from it that became a remedy for consumption.

Today, *Guaiacum 1x* is one of the best medicines for pharyngitis. Five drops on a little sugar, taken every one or two hours, will almost certainly stop the symptoms in a short time. In fact, after two or three doses the patient will notice that the soreness has already begun to ease. *Guaiacum* acts as a specific in such cases, and bad-smelling sputum or perspiration is usually a sure indication for its use, at a medium potency, three times a day. Stabbing, tearing pains in the joints, with gouty deposits in them, have also been relieved by means of this remedy. *Guaiacum* is therefore an important ingredient in several ointments and embrocations. Used together with *Lachesis*, *Guaiacum* will bring quick relief for those who suffer from tonsillitis.

Kalium iodatum (Potassium Iodide)

This is one of the remedies that is greatly misused by orthodox medicine, insofar as it is given in large material doses. Professor Bier has promoted the success of potassium iodide and has proved that it is one of the best expectorants for catarrh and will even arrest the development of catarrh if used in the strengths 4x and even 6x.

Those who are predisposed to rheumatism and chesty colds will find *Kali iodatum 4x* an excellent and speedy means of help, even for bronchial and pulmonary catarrh. Even chronic cases respond favourably to the remedy. *Kali iodatum* is indicated for post-pneumonia treatment, in cases where phlegm is still present and seems to sit deep in the chest, threatening to develop into consumption. The best results are obtained when it is alternated with *raw pine bud syrup* or *Imperatoria (imperial masterwort)*.

As a final observation, the main effect of kelp can no doubt be ascribed to its content of *Kalium iodatum*.

Lachesis

Do not be shocked, dear readers, when I tell you that this remedy is made from snake poison, taken from a viper (*Lachesis muta*, or bushmaster) whose bite, if unattended, leads to certain death. However, when homoeopathically potentised, in this case diluted a billion times, *Lachesis* is a valuable medicine.

We owe the discovery of this remarkable remedy to Dr Constantin Hering. It has no doubt saved many more lives than have ever been lost through the bite of the bushmaster. Blood poisoning, septicaemia, chronic ulcers, boils, carbuncles, smallpox, scarlet fever, severe cases of measles and other diseases just as serious, can be safely and reliably treated with *Lachesis*. Whenever a disorder is accompanied by a bluish appearance of the skin, you can be sure that *Lachesis 12x* will help.

Lachesis 12x is a superb remedy for problems occurring in the left side of the pelvis, especially women's complaints.

After a serious illness, when all sorts of toxins are circulating in the bloodstream and the body is fighting to eliminate them, *Lachesis* can be of great service.

Where typhoid fever is concerned, *Lachesis* is one of the most useful and reliable medicines. After a stroke, especially in cases where the left side is paralysed, *Lachesis* as well as *Arnica* are often given with good results.

In cases of pulmonary abscesses, gangrene of the lung or very bad tonsillitis and other serious throat diseases, this remedy can help where all others seem to have failed. I have often seen tonsillitis completely disappear after an injection of *Lachesis 10x*, without any ill effects.

This remedy should be kept in every home, for whenever a serious illness threatens to induce blood poisoning, there is no better medicine available. The safest potencies to use are 10x or 12x.

Daphne mezereum (Daphne, Spurge Laurel)
The last muddy streaks of snow are still lying on the upland meadows and under the rhododendrons when the bright red blossoms of the daphne already catch our eye. The homoeopathic remedy *Mezereum* is prepared from the bark of this attractive but poisonous plant.

It is a wonderful remedy for shingles, facial erysipelas and vesicular eruptions, those itching little blisters on a red background that become worse when scratched.

For deep-seated varicose ulcers this remedy is second to none.

Mezereum is indicated for dry mucous membranes accompanied by dry and irritating cough and a feeling of constriction across the chest, which occurs especially during the night, as well as intense thirst with burning pains in the throat and a raw nasal discharge. Even in acute cases the remedy must not be given in potencies below 3x.

Sepia officinalis (Sepia)

Let me describe the merits of this wonderful homoeopathic remedy, one that is not recognised by the orthodox section of the medical profession, and you will no doubt become quite enthusiastic about it. First, however, do not turn your nose up when I tell you that *Sepia* is obtained from cuttlefish 'ink'. If you have ever visited the Mediterranean or other southern seas you must have come across those curious creatures with their tentacles and know that they eject a dark brown ink-like fluid. In former times painters used this ink from the cuttlefish but today the chemical industry produces a dye known as sepia.

Did you know that *Sepia* is one of the best medicines for women's problems? Frail women who tire easily after only a short walk or who perspire excessively, causing them to smell unpleasant and feel listless, have their best friend in *Sepia*, a remedy that benefits the whole body. In the United States they call it the washer-woman's medicine. It helps the overworked, the tired, the sad, and those who complain of backaches.

Chronic skin eruptions that itch and burn, little blisters around the joints, the desire to sleep during the daytime and insomnia during the night, vertigo, a poor memory and similar conditions can all be alleviated and cured if *Sepia* is taken for a certain period of time.

The potency required depends upon the sensitivity of the person; robust people can use a lower potency (4x), while those with a more delicate constitution may require higher potencies (6x–12x) for the best results.

Tarentula cubensis

It is hardly believable that the poison of the hairy Cuban tarantula should possess such remarkable curative powers when homoeopathically diluted, but it does. Boils, felons (whitlows), or any other infection of the fingers or under the nails are cured by *Tarentula cubensis* as if by a miracle. In most cases the affected parts are characterised by a bluish colour and cause severe, burning pains, particularly during the night. For small abscesses on the hands and feet, as well as whitlows, there is no better medicine. *Tarentula* is without a par among homoeopathic medicines in the treatment of furunculosis (the recurrent appearance of furuncles and boils). To produce immediate results, use the injection method.

As a word of caution, *Tarentula cubensis* should only be used in high potencies (8x–12x). It is also important not to confuse *Tarentula cubensis* with *Tarentula hispanica* (Spanish tarantula).

Urtica dioica, Urtica urens (Stinging Nettle)

The fresh plant extract from the stinging nettle (see pages 368–70) is known in homoeopathy as *Urtica mother tincture*. In addition to glycosides, tannic acids and formic acid, it also contains a good quantity of silica (40 per cent of the ash constituents), the same proportion of calcium, as well as phosphorus, iron, sodium and a little sulphur.

Urtica is a most reliable remedy for arthritic ailments, inflamed joints of a gouty nature, diminished urine with increased sedimentation and bladder irritation.

In such cases, exudation through the skin becomes acrid and is accompanied by an unpleasant odour. This is the result of an insufficient kidney function and may in time lead to a skin eruption that itches and burns, especially at night. For these symptoms, take ten drops of *Urtica* mother tincture in a glass of water, sipping it during the day. In addition to *Urtica*, the kidneys can be further assisted with *Solidago* or *Nephrosolid*. Take sips of both remedies, alternating one with the other.

Four Biochemical Remedies

Calcarea fluorica (Calcium Fluoride)

If your teeth hurt when you eat, if they feel a bit loose, or if the enamel becomes brittle and chips off easily so that bacteria can enter through the crevices, causing tooth decay, then it is high time for you to remember *Calcarea fluorica*, a biochemical remedy to counteract mineral deficiency. At the same time, *silica* (see page 401) should also be taken because it is equally important for the construction of the teeth and bones.

Incidentally, it is not surprising that the mountain peasants of the Swiss canton of Valais possess such beautiful teeth, because the famous whole rye bread they consume is a rich source of calcium fluoride.

This mineral is important for the connective tissues and for this reason should be taken before and after operations so that granulation, such as scar formation, can take place more quickly and without interruption. It has also been suggested that a deficiency of calcium fluoride in the system must play some part in the tendency to hernias.

Always remember that nature will be able to rectify problems as long as the necessary raw materials are present. This principle should be observed in our diet and if it is, the body will respond, but if our diet is deficient, we must see to it that the necessary materials are supplied.

Recently, interesting observations have been made concerning the effect of this mineral on hard swellings of the tendons and ligaments, dilations of the tendon sheaths (known as 'ganglia') and even glandular tumours and hard cyst formation. It is gratifying to know that, besides other treatments, such a simple natural medicine as *Calcarea fluorica* will benefit these conditions. It would, of course, be unreasonable to expect too much from any given remedy, because we must remember that disease is hardly ever attributable to the deficiency of a single cell salt. Others, too, may be lacking and need to be replaced.

It has been found that cataracts of the eyes are usually associated with a deficiency of *Calcarea fluorica*, and their treatment should include taking this mineral in alternation with *Kali chloricum* (potassium chlorate). Sclerotic deposits on the eardrum, which may give rise to deafness and 'head noises', as well as painful whitlows and itching, and eczematous diseases of the skin are also relieved by taking this remedy for a period of time. *Calcarea fluorica* should be taken together with *Millefolium* (yarrow) or *Aesculaforce* to improve the elasticity of the walls of the veins in all cases of haemorrhoids (piles), varicose veins and phlebitis (inflammation of the veins).

Babies with teething problems will respond to *Calcarea fluorica*, taken in alternation with *Calcarea phosphorica* (calcium phosphate). I should also mention that mothers can more quickly regain their figure after the birth of their babies and prevent a pendulous abdomen, which is caused by a relaxation of the abdominal muscles and ligaments, if they take *Calcarea fluorica* or the calcium complex *Urticalcin* regularly during pregnancy.

Calcarea fluorica is generally given in the potency 12x, but for some rare cases it may be 6x. The normal dose is two tablets (0.125 g each), three times daily.

Natrum muriaticum (Cooking or Table Salt, Sodium Chloride)

The type of person most likely to benefit from *Natrum muriaticum* can be described as follows: puffy face, with watery-looking skin; thin, in spite of having a good appetite; feels the cold acutely especially along the spine and back, as well as in the hands and feet; easily exhausted by mental and physical work; cannot stand the heat of the sun; inclined to headaches and migraines; easily agitated and upset. If one tries to comfort such people they become bad tempered or angry. Their bowels function badly and the stool is dry, hard and crumbly. In the case of women these symptoms are accentuated during and after their periods, which are always irregular. A typical aversion to bread can often be noted. There either seems to be a great yearning for salt or a definite aversion to it. Those who have a number of these characteristics will find *Natrum muriaticum* an excellent and quite harmless remedy.

It has an immediate effect on infants and small children when there are disturbances of the bowels or liver, and it is a splendid worm remedy if taken regularly for a long time.

Patients with Graves' disease (exophthalmic goitre) will find speedy relief by taking *Natrum muriaticum*. In cases of vasomotor disorders, palpitations with a feeling of faintness, and an irregular pulse (such as every third stroke out of rhythm) the medication has a very good effect. Skin eruptions with light-coloured watery secretions, eczema, acne and skin blemishes, especially when accompanied by dry mucous membranes, also respond to treatment with *Natrum muriaticum*.

In cases of constipation, the potency 3x is indicated. All other disorders will benefit from a medium potency, such as 6x, or better still, a higher one, from 12x to 30x. Highly strung persons always respond better to higher potencies.

Natrum sulphuricum (Glauber's Salt, Sodium Sulphate)

The German chemist J. R. Glauber discovered this salt in 1658 and it still bears his name today. Although it is water-soluble, it is absorbed with difficulty by the intestines and, if its curative powers are to be utilised, it has to be taken in biochemical trituration and attenuated to the sixth decimal potency. Only then is *Natrum sulphuricum* fully absorbed, benefiting the body without any side effects.

One of its important merits is that it increases the secretion of bile into the duodenum, thus aiding the digestion generally and that of fats in particular. Its action also extends to the blood. In cases of haemophilia, a disease characterised by loss or impairment of the clotting ability of blood, so that even a minor cut or injury can put the patient at risk of bleeding to death if the right action is not taken, *Natrum sulphuricum* will improve the condition. Naturally, it must be taken over a long period of time; moreover, its effectiveness is enhanced when *Millefolium* (yarrow) is taken at the same time.

Diabetics will find *Natrum sulphuricum* a great help if taken in conjunction with the fresh plant extract of *tormentil*. Other indications include liver problems, especially after recovery from jaundice, an inflamed bile duct or an inflammation of the small intestine.

For 'early-morning diarrhoea' with flatulence, it is a specific, but should be alternated with doses of *clay water* (healing earth). Metabolic disturbances, having their origin in a liver dysfunction, are remarkably improved by *Natrum sulphuricum 6x*, two tablets taken three times daily – a simple remedy that gives fast relief! Also in cases of obesity, mild cases of dropsy, certain kinds of asthma, chronic malaria, and the well-known spring rashes from which many adolescents suffer, *Natrum sulphuricum 6x* brings prompt relief.

Nursing mothers should not take this remedy because it reduces the flow of milk. On the other hand, at the time of weaning it has been found to be of great help. People who are always pale or whose eyes are slightly yellowish instead of white and tend to feel depressed and moody should take this remedy from time to time.

Terra Silicea purificata (Silica)

This fine remedy is valued in biochemistry as much as it is in homoeopathy, and I will try to describe its most important uses as briefly as possible.

Silicea is used for suppuration of every kind, but only when it has established itself properly or is already dispersing. In the early stage *Hepar sulph*. *4x* should be given to encourage the elimination of pus. The healing process should then be left for *Silicea 12x* to accomplish. In northern lands, silica is used by the peasants for every sort of suppuration, especially for boils. For inflammation of the bones, necrosis of the bones, tonsillar abscesses, dental fistulas, indeed for any sort of fistula, silica is a slow but sure remedy.

Silica is the right remedy to use for felons (whitlows), problems with the hair roots and the disrupted growth of hair and nails.

Give silica to lymphatic-scrofulous children with swollen glands; there is no better remedy than this for improving the child's whole constitution. As a rule these children are thin, or else puffy with a swollen stomach, and have a poor appetite and little stamina, as well as an uncertain state of mind.

Those who suffer from lung problems and scrofula should take silica together with a homoeopathic calcium preparation. Silica is very good for the skin and the connective tissues, and is successful in the treatment of excessive hand and foot perspiration that has an unpleasant odour and causes the skin between the fingers and toes to become sore. Problems arising from suppressed foot sweat can also be dealt with satisfactorily by silica, but it is probable that the sweat will be re-established after having been wrongly suppressed in the first place. This is something to be welcomed. In fact, never do anything drastic to suppress foot sweat, unless you also stimulate the function of the skin and kidneys so that elimination is increased through these two escape routes. In that case, the foot sweat will eventually disappear without any harmful consequences.

People who always feel cold and shivery, even when they are active, might try taking silica. After several weeks it will improve the basal metabolism, and their vitality and joy of living will gradually return.

Hard lumps in the breast, perhaps even malignant ones, will benefit from the continued use of silica. Wounds that refuse to heal will improve if it is sprinkled over their surfaces. This external method of treatment has proved its value for leg ulcers (*Silicea* for external use, *Hypericum perforatum* and *Aesculaforce* to be taken internally). Apart from its medicinal value, if silica is taken over a long period of time, it will improve the condition of the hair and promote a clear complexion.

Silicea is sometimes prescribed in the 6x potency, but usually it is 12x. Some physicians use 30x with good results. Take two tablets two or three times daily.

If you wish to use *Silicea* as a powder, simply crush the tablets.

Modern man and woman,
Living under constant stress,
Must go back to Nature
And relearn how to live
In harmony with its peace and tranquillity.

Seasonings

Culinary Herbs Are Medicines

Culinary herbs could be such a rich blessing if only we were sensible enough to plant and cultivate them in our own garden. Moreover, if we realised that these herbs not only make our food tastier but also have real medicinal value, we would not hesitate to avail ourselves of their curative properties by adding them daily to our food. Seasoning that is good for health means using herbs, but it is sad to say that the importance of fresh herbs for our well-being is still too little appreciated. All of us should know each herb and its value as a flavouring and as a medicine, however small or ordinary it may be. To help you acquire this invaluable knowledge, let us consider some of these herbs more closely.

Parsley

Parsley is, of course, well known but often only used to garnish a dish. But did you know that it is a good remedy for the kidneys? Bearing this in mind, why not add it, finely chopped, to soups, sauces and dressings, to cottage cheese, and sprinkle it on salads, potatoes and other dishes? It will enhance the taste of your meals and provide you with vitamins A and C, as well as traces of vitamin B_{12}, which is important for the formation of red blood corpuscles.

Celery, Celeriac

Celery (leaf-stalks) and celeriac (the turnip-like root) are good vegetables for people suffering from rheumatism and gout, and for those who want to do something about preventing these two diseases. If you use the roots, stalks and leaves to season your food on a regular basis, it is most unlikely that you will ever suffer from renal gravel or stones. Celery is also a notable remedy for dropsy.

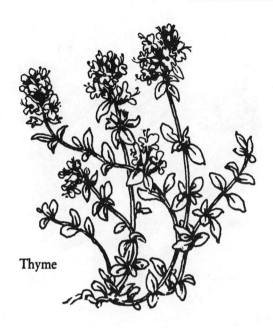

Thyme

Marjoram

This herb originally came from North Africa, where it is still valued as a mild but reliable nerve tonic. Marjoram increases the amount of water eliminated by the body and is therefore used to ease bladder trouble. It also stimulates the bowel movement, helping to regulate it.

Thyme

Thyme is very popular because of its fine aroma and flavour. What is more, it has an antiseptic property and is able to regenerate mouth bacteria.

Rosemary

Isabella, Queen of Hungary, had much to do with rosemary's reputation as a rejuvenating tonic. This simple but beautiful shrub with its little leaves and flowers is known everywhere as a sweet herb and a remedy and is used in herbal medicine because of its beneficial effect on the vasomotor nerves and the heart nerves. This aromatic herb should be used much more widely for culinary purposes, to enable us to benefit from its goodness. In fact, famous

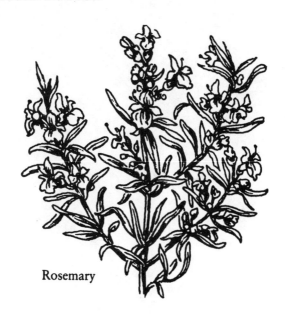

Rosemary

chefs have been adding rosemary to sauces and gravies, roast meat and saltwater fish for a long time. Vegetarians, too, should not forget to use plenty of this herb.

If you add rosemary to old wine you will get a good heart tonic, which will benefit anyone suffering from low blood pressure or who is always pale and weak, as well as older persons. A glass of rosemary wine is a good pick-me-up for convalescents recovering from a bout of flu or similar infectious disease; it will speed up their recovery.

Savory
In the Middle Ages, savory, or bean herb (*Satureja hortensis* in Latin), grew in every monastery garden and still today it is prized as a kitchen herb. It was used for seasoning and as a remedy, and Abbess Hildegard of Bingen, Germany, a reputable medieval herbalist and recognised as such even in modern times, recommended savory as a valuable herb.

The common name 'bean herb' tells us something about its culinary use; indeed, some cooks maintain that there is no better flavouring for beans. Moreover, if you season vegetables with savory, you will not suffer wind as an after effect. Many good cooks also flavour meat dishes and chicken with aromatic savory.

Anyone suffering from low blood pressure would do well to use savory in addition to hyssop in the preparation of food. This herb was also highly valued in the Middle Ages because it was thought to stimulate the gonads.

Lemon Balm

Lemon balm is often grown in kitchen gardens, its pleasant aroma not only attracting humans but also bees which feed on its nectar. It makes a fine tea, and if your nerves are frayed and need calming, a cup at bedtime, sweetened with honey for an even better effect, will help you sleep since it is mildly soporific. Many women like to drink the tea because it is good for menstrual problems and cramps. In days gone by, balm tea was recommended for tobacco poisoning. And in the seventeenth century the Carmelite monks in Paris prepared an excellent 'balm spirit' that soon became famous. The ingredients were lemon balm, betony leaves, lemon peel, a little coriander, cloves and cinnamon.

Although you may know lemon balm mainly for its use as a tea, it can also be added to food for flavouring. It may also be true that few people know of another application of balm; the fresh leaves can be crushed and gently rubbed on bee or wasp stings. This has a soothing and healing effect, similar to that obtained by applying crushed ivy leaves.

Basil

This plant has been cultivated since ancient times. It is probably native to India, where it was known as *Arjaka* in ancient Sanskrit. The aromatic herb is a good source of food for bees, but is also valued as a kitchen herb and a remedy. In ancient Egypt basil served as a medicine for snakebites, scorpion stings and eye troubles. The crushed leaves were also applied to painful parts in cases of rheumatism. Basil's remedial effects are due to its content of rhymol, eugenol and camphor. Pliny recommended basil tea as a remedy for nerves, headaches and fainting spells. The Greeks used basil not only to prepare aromatic baths to strengthen the nerves, but also for flavouring must (the juice pressed from grapes before it has fermented), wine and liqueurs. Basil is used in northern Germany to season the famous Hamburg eel soup and in the preparation of gherkins (pickled cucumbers). In Italy, particularly in the south, it is found in practically every garden because it is used widely for seasoning – and food to which is has been added is always very tasty.

Lovage

Lovage can reach a height of over 2 m (6 feet) and is used in the same way as celery and celeriac (see page 404). It is probably native to Asia, where it is used to make highly flavoured sauces. The plant is known for its diuretic effect, which is no doubt due to an essential oil. Lovage stimulates the appetite and makes a good soothing remedy for flatulence and digestive problems in the intestines.

Chervil

This herb, called *Anthriscus cerefolium* in Latin, is much appreciated as a medicinal plant in Bern canton, Switzerland. The smell of chervil is strong, somewhat sweet, aromatic and slightly reminiscent of anise. Chervil's effects are digestive, dispersing, blood-thinning and diuretic. You can prepare an excellent herbal tea in the spring by adding it to dandelion and yarrow. This combination is particularly indicated for the treatment of scrofula, dropsy and a tendency to eczema.

Caraway, Anise, Coriander, Fennel and Dill

The seeds of these five plants have a warming effect and are good for the stomach and intestines, especially in cases of chills and inflammations, as well as other upsets.

An infusion of fennel and anise is also appreciated for its good effect when small children suffer from stomach and bowel problems of any kind. Nursing mothers will find dill helpful in stimulating lactation.

Leek and Other Varieties of Allium

A number of the *Allium* varieties – there are about 250 in all – serve as vegetables, spice plants and remedies. They contain garlic oil, its chief component being allyl sulphide, which is responsible for their characteristic smell. All varieties of *Allium*, for example leeks, are good for the blood vessels, keeping them elastic and preventing premature aging. If you eat plenty of chives, garlic, and, in the spring, bear's garlic (ramsons) – all of which are from the *Allium* family – intestinal worms will be eliminated.

Chives

Of all varieties of *Allium*, chives (*Allium schoenoprasum*) are probably used the most widely. Chives are found all over Europe, East Asia, the Orient, and from the Caucasus right up to Siberia.

Add finely chopped chives to salads, gruels, cottage cheese, potatoes and vegetables for flavouring and to enrich the nutritional content. If you have no garden, you can grow chives in a pot on a window sill or balcony. During the winter months, move it to another light area of the kitchen.

Bear's Garlic (Ramsons)
Bear's garlic also belongs to the *Allium* family and is called *Allium ursinum*. Use it for seasoning or as a steamed vegetable. Mix finely chopped bear's garlic with other salads or serve it on its own.

As a hot dish, steam it together with spinach in a little oil, but even without the spinach bear's garlic is very tasty. As a spring treatment, bear's garlic is the best remedy for cleansing the blood, gallbladder and liver of wastes that have accumulated during the winter months. For those suffering from arteriosclerosis (hardening of the arteries) with high blood pressure, bear's garlic is a remedy and food at the same time. They should eat it regularly every day, finely chopped and added to salads.

Garlic (*Allium sativum*)
Today, tourists visiting the great pyramids of Egypt, seated unsteadily on the back of a camel or in a sleek automobile, are probably unaware that the overseers of the pharaohs were not only responsible for the construction of these great architectural masterpieces but they faced the additional problem of feeding a great army of workmen. Herodotus, the Greek historian, wrote that during the time of the building of the Cheops pyramid 1,600 silver talents (about 3.5 million pounds sterling) worth of garlic, onions and radishes were purchased to keep up the workers' strength. The Egyptians considered garlic and onions as sacred plants, to which they attributed all manner of magical powers able to ward off evil spirits and the effects of their wicked deeds. The Greeks and Romans also used garlic as a medicine and for seasoning. From the Bible we learn about the prominence the Jews gave to it, and their constant use of garlic for thousands of years is perhaps partly responsible for the endurance and tenacity of this people. The Semitic people seem to suffer much less than others from hardening of the arteries and poor functioning of the lymphatic glands. The Turks and Russians make much use of garlic to season their food and their older people are less likely to suffer from high blood pressure because they eat it regularly.

Many people, however, do not like the pungent smell of garlic.

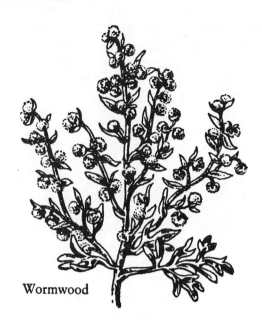

Wormwood

Yet there is a simple remedy to dispel it quickly; just eat some fresh raw parsley at the same time. You can make a tasty sandwich by slicing a garlic clove onto a slice of buttered bread and adding a little *Herbaforce*.

Like all foods that have a penetrating smell and a strong taste, garlic should be taken in small amounts only, otherwise it could be harmful, especially to the kidneys. Garlic as well as onions contain a sulphurous essential oil that is probably responsible for its effectiveness as a vermifuge, an agent that causes the expulsion of intestinal worms. Garlic milk is excellent for this purpose, as described below. Crushed garlic can also be added to a wormwood infusion instead of milk, to be drunk or used as an enema in the same way as garlic milk.

Half a clove of garlic, placed between the gums and cheek, will often soothe a headache. Earache and headaches often respond to a garlic or onion poultice applied to the back of the neck.

Garlic Milk
This is an effective remedy for eliminating intestinal worms, as well as for sciatic pains. If taken over a prolonged period of time it will also cure sweaty feet.

A garage mechanic who had suffered from sciatica for a consider-

410

able time, and for whom the doctor could not offer any help, was advised to drink garlic milk daily. He took the advice and within a few days the pain was greatly relieved. At the end of a fortnight it had disappeared completely.

Garlic milk may be prepared cooked or uncooked. In the raw state, uncooked, it is more potent. Cooking lessens the smell somewhat and the effect is still quite satisfactory.

To make garlic milk use a garlic press, obtainable from hardware stores, to crush the garlic. Add the pulp to uncooked milk (two raw cloves to 100 ml/3.5 fl. oz) and drink it. If you prefer, you can boil the garlic in the milk.

For the maximum effect one should drink 200 ml (half a pint) of this mixture daily. The same mixture can also be used for enemas.

Of course, not everyone reacts in the same way and not every remedy produces the same results in every person, but in the case of a bad sciatica attack, it is well worth giving this simple remedy a try. According to the individual, one of three different therapies should produce results: formic acid treatment, adjustment by a chiropractor, or garlic milk.

Onion (*Allium cepa*)

Although onions are healthy and can be used for seasoning in many ways, they do not agree with everyone, especially people whose digestion is not too good and who tend to suffer from intestinal fermentation and flatulence. Such problems can be exacerbated when onions are eaten.

Raw onions have a mild diuretic effect. They are rich in vitamin C, and if eaten regularly and in small quantities they are good for the nerves. In cases of congestion, a headache, earache, toothache and inflammation of the eyes, especially after a chill or cold, an onion compress on the back of the neck can relieve the pain and often disperse it entirely. For this purpose, wrap the finely chopped onion in gauze.

When a person is feverish, with a congested, burning head, an onion compress applied to the soles of the feet will be very helpful, and if the heart is affected, a compress on the calves of the legs will give quick relief, or at least act as an auxiliary to another remedial treatment. For gout and diabetes, as well as for hardening of the arteries, onions as a food are a vital part of the treatment.

A sulphurous essential oil is responsible for the onion's good

411

effect on the skin and scalp, especially in cases of dandruff and loss of hair.

In homoeopathy *Allium cepa* is the best remedy for a running cold. It is often enough just to leave half an onion on the bedside table so that the odour can be inhaled through the night. Every morning and evening cut the dried part away. If this does not effect a cure, it will still bring great relief and help towards a speedy recovery.

For colic and wind in the umbilical region, and for infants and small children who have bladder cramps along with reddish, smarting urine, *Allium cepa* is a harmless and reliable remedy. If you do not have extract of *Allium cepa* in your medicine chest, cut a thin slice of onion, dip it into a glass of warm water for a few seconds then remove it and take a sip of the water every hour. You will be astonished at the prompt relief this will bring.

Shallot (*Allium ascalonicum*)
In addition to the common onion, the small, flavoursome shallot, also called scallion, is widely used for flavouring. Its botanical name is derived from the name of the ancient Philistine town Ascalon on the Mediterranean coast, which has been rebuilt in modern times.

The shallot is native to Palestine, where the crusaders came across it and brought it back to Europe. With regard to its use in cooking and as a remedy, it can be used in a similar way to the common onion and the leek.

Cress
Some of the cress varieties used for food are garden cress (*Lepidium sativum*), watercress (*Nasturtium officinale*), nasturtium (*Tropaeolum majus*) and alpine cress (*Hutchinsia alpina*). In all, about 90 different varieties are known in the temperate zones of the earth. Some are used for flavouring, and most of them have a medicinal effect, although varying in strength.

According to recent research, cress (like horseradish) contains a kind of penicillin and is a great help in improving mouth and intestinal bacteria. Having a modest content of iodine, cress is a dietary remedy for thyroid problems. It is recommended as a remedy for scrofula, and when taken regularly it will reduce an inherent tendency to skin eruptions. At the same time cress is good for kidney problems; in particular, it helps to prevent the formation of kidney stones.

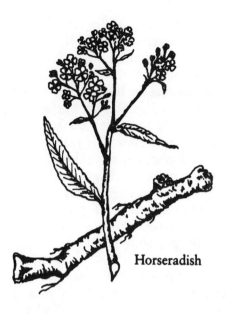

Horseradish

Cress on its own makes a wholesome salad, but it should also be added to other salads. In fact, it is very important that we avail ourselves of its medicinal values by eating it regularly. If you are in the habit of preparing vegetable juices daily for the sake of their vitamins, always add a little cress. The popular seasoning salt *Trocomare* contains various cresses among its ingredients which largely account for its fine aroma and taste.

Horseradish (*Armoracia rusticana*)

Since horseradish is one of the healthiest seasonings there is, it should be used much more in the kitchen. It is rich in vitamin C and is the best known dietary remedy for scurvy, only raw sauerkraut being equally effective. Horseradish has a regenerative effect in cases of dysbacteria and helps to overcome functional disorders of the pancreas. It is a good seasoning agent for diabetics, being curative at the same time. If you use it as a seasoning in the spring, in small amounts but regularly, it will help in the fight against 'spring fever'.

It has recently been discovered that horseradish contains a considerable amount of antibiotic substances, including a kind of penicillin, which explains why horseradish syrup (see below) is so effective in cases of throat diseases. Also because of its antibiotic properties horseradish tincture is of great benefit when treating

413

wounds that are not healing well or are forming proud flesh. Even when other remedies have proved ineffective, horseradish tincture will not only bring relief surprisingly quickly, but will actually cause the wound to heal.

For home use, tincture of horseradish may be prepared in the following manner. Grate some fresh horseradish, mix it well with pure alcohol and let it stand for an hour or so. Then filter it through some gauze or muslin. The resulting tincture can be used on wounds, cuts and grazes as an antiseptic. Although it may sting somewhat, it will be most effective and the pain and soreness will quickly disappear.

Grated horseradish can be used in place of onions when these, applied as a poultice, have not succeeded in stopping, for example, a bad headache. Simply apply the grated horseradish to the back of the neck.

Horseradish being one of the spice plants that have a reliable medicinal effect, it should be grown in your garden, if you have one. It will then always be available. Add horseradish to carrot salad and the latter will be less sweet and more palatable; many men, especially, prefer it in this way. The flavour of cottage or curd cheese is also improved by horseradish, and the same is true of salad dressings.

Always mix a little grated horseradish into your salads. In addition to making the salad taste better, horseradish will reduce any tendency to colds and chills.

For older people, horseradish, as well as garlic, is a most excellent medicine. Both regenerate the blood vessels, especially the arteries, and reduce the blood pressure. If you are over the age of forty, you should give these two remedies serious consideration. They serve an important purpose, act in a regenerative way, and are stimulating.

However, you must be careful not to use too much horseradish, since it is very strong. The Chinese make a horseradish relish that, if eaten without your knowing what it is, will take you by surprise as the pungent flavour goes up your nose, indeed, it seems, even to your brain, causing temporary discomfort. The sensation is severe and definite, as with any other strong stimulation, but do not forget that the effect is also one of cleansing.

Horseradish Syrup
If the symptom of catarrh refuses to disappear, try horseradish syrup. This remedy is also indicated for the treatment of weak lungs

and other bronchial and respiratory problems, since horseradish contains an antibiotic substance similar to penicillin.

Prepare the syrup by adding honey to the grated horseradish. Mix well and press through muslin. The residue should be cooked with a little water and raw (unrefined) cane sugar, pressed out again, and then added to the syrup. This provides a strong medicinal mixture.

Black or Spanish Radish (*Raphanus sativus*)

The black or Spanish radish is the best possible liver medicine you can have right in your home. But you should not eat too much of it, or else it will be harmful. Taken frequently in small quantities, it can help liver patients to prevent bilious colic and many kinds of digestive problems.

Radish Syrup

Finely grated radish, sprinkled with raw cane sugar in order to make a syrup, provides a good medicine for chronic bronchial catarrh. To save on the amount of sugar used, first press the grated radish through muslin and then add sufficient sugar to form a thick syrup. Made in this way it should keep for weeks and you can take some every day. This is also an inexpensive and reliable help in the treatment of persistent whooping cough. For those who do not want to take the time to make the syrup, or who are unable to obtain black radishes, radish syrup prepared in much the same way can be bought.

In cases of gallbladder trouble, ten drops of raw radish essence (*Raphanus-Perkolat*) in a tablespoon of water, taken three times a day, are sufficient to give relief. You may use this radish essence for whooping cough and bronchial catarrh in conjunction with the syrup. Add ten drops to a glass of water, sweeten with honey and sip throughout the day.

Salt as a Medicine

Salt is a remedy for many ailments, but not in the form in which it is usually ingested. Bathing in sea water is recommended for glandular disturbances, which so often result in obesity. The thyroid also benefits from sea-bathing, and anyone who suffers from goitre or similar thyroid problems (hypothyroidism and hyperthyroidism) will obtain good results from it too. If you live in a landlocked area and do not have access to the sea, you can use dry or moist salt packs at home to draw away water from the tissues. For this reason, anyone suffering from oedema, swellings of a dropsical nature, will find salt packs an answer to his problem.

Gargling with salt water is an excellent substitute for the more expensive antiseptics and herbal mouthwashes sold over-the-counter – the effect is just as good.

In cases of catarrh or inflammation of the mucosa, tepid salt water should be sniffed up the nostrils, which should then be rinsed with clear water. This simple treatment, when practised regularly, will reduce any susceptibility to respiratory ailments, that is, catarrh and sore throats. Naturally, if you do live by the sea, it would be better to use sea water, provided that it is uncontaminated. Use cooking salt instead, if that is all you have available.

Salt has a good effect when used externally and it is also beneficial when taken orally. However, for internal use common cooking salt, iodised or fluorinated salt should not be used if at all possible, only sea salt or herbal salt, which are much better. The trace elements found in sea salt and herbal salt benefit the endocrine glands and normalise both hypofunction and hyperfunction. Obesity is often the result of insufficient glandular function, and in such cases ordinary salt will aggravate the condition by increasing the body weight still more. On the other hand, a herbal salt containing seaweed has the opposite effect. In fact, if *Herbamare* seasoning salt is used regularly, quite a few pounds of excess weight will be lost in a natural way.

Salt is an excellent preservative, even for fresh plant extracts, and does not reduce their therapeutic value. *Trocomare* herbal seasoning salt contains eight different fresh herbs with an antibacterial effect. If you are susceptible to, or are exposed to, infectious diseases, Trocomare will prove invaluable as a prophylactic and will also have a favourable influence on any existing problems.

Salt is widely used in homoeopathy too (see page 399), where it is known by the name *Natrum muriaticum*.

Various Diets and Treatments

Serious Vitamin Deficiency in the Spring

In the past, the consequences of vitamin deficiencies through the winter months and into the spring used to be much more drastic than they are today. The problem was little understood and therefore left without any real solution. People in remote areas often suffered greatly during these months because of an acute lack of food rich in vitamins. Many old people would die in the winter or spring because their strength was at an all-time low for this very reason.

Even today at this time of the year there is a general susceptibility to colds, bronchial catarrh and infectious conditions of the mucous membranes; these are always a result of a deficiency of vitamin A and other substances. By taking food rich in vitamin A you can, as a rule, avoid inflammation of the eyes, eyelids and cornea, and the nuisance known as 'night-blindness'. A lack of vitamin A in the body is responsible for the stubborn failure of wounds to heal properly.

It is good to know that the varieties of pepper, as well as tomatoes, contain plenty of vitamin A; unfortunately, however, in winter they are not always widely available or are relatively expensive. It is therefore more than welcome that carrots are usually on the market – and somewhat cheaper. Their vitamin A content is, of course, well known. So make it a point to eat fresh carrot salad every day, or to drink fresh carrot juice. Commercially prepared carrot juice with lactic acid is also recommended, and is appreciated by those who have little time to prepare the juice themselves. Health food stores stock concentrated carrot juice, such as *Biocarottin*. This is a good supplement to overcome vitamin deficiency. A word of caution is needed, however, for people who suffer from high blood pressure; try to eat more salads rather than depending on juices alone, since the regular intake of carrot juice can raise the blood pressure.

THE NATURE DOCTOR

Further Observations

In a series of experiments some animals were given food that did not contain vitamin A, resulting in the development of gravel and stones in the kidneys. To eliminate the stones, they were then given food rich in vitamin A. The experiments were indeed successful and the elimination was confirmed by means of X-ray pictures. This is a clear warning to us never to go without food that is rich in vitamin A.

Other symptoms of vitamin A deficiency are bleeding gums, which are more frequently seen in the spring, and blue-red spots in the skin, which occur when blood seeps into the tissues as a result of leaking blood vessels caused by the deficiency. These undesirable blue-red spots show up mainly in the legs, where they can eventually turn into ulcers. Vitamin A deficiency can also lead to a loss of appetite and the limbs feeling as heavy as lead. In some cases frequent nose bleeds are experienced or existing piles begin to bleed slightly; these symptoms are often accompanied by cardiac insufficiency.

Scurvy used to make itself known with similar symptoms, posing great problems to ships' crews for a long time, until the importance of vitamin C was discovered. Sauerkraut then came to the rescue. The great seafarer James Cook used it successfully to keep his crews free from scurvy, and others later followed his example. Instead of sauerkraut you can eat white cabbage salad, flavoured with a little lemon juice; the effect is the same.

Way back in the Middle Ages a physician by the name of Carier discovered that an extract made from pine and fir buds or shoots was a good remedy for scurvy. Later research proved that the buds or shoots of coniferous trees have the highest content of vitamin C. You have here the reason why pine bud syrup, when prepared with the raw juice, as in *Santasapina Cough Syrup*, has a twofold effect: in cases of catarrh it soothes the mucous membranes and it also improves the general health of the patient because of the pine buds' vitamin C content.

Nearly all wild fruits are rich in vitamin C and contain valuable fruit sugar. Barberries, rose hips and sea buckthorn berries are marketed in the form of tasty conserves that keep well. Your vitamin C requirements in the winter and spring months will therefore be met if you take these purées. An especially effective addition to them are combinations such as *Bio-Sanddorsan;* this contains sea buckthorn as well as rose hip purée, both of which valuable for your health and also very tasty. Children like to eat Bio-

418

Sanddorsan as a sandwich spread. It is an advantage when something that is necessary can also be made palatable, especially as far as sweet-toothed children are concerned, because then they will happily take in the thing that benefits their health. I once overheard a child say, with sad face, that things that were tasty were bad for you, but things that were supposed to be good for you had a nasty taste. I have never forgotten this remark and since then have tried hard to produce health foods that taste good at the same time. This is possible by using well-thought-out combinations, such as the one I achieved in *Bio-Sanddorsan*. Another easy way to avail oneself of vitamins is by taking *Bio-C-Lozenges*, made from fruit extracts such as acerola cherries, sea buckthorn, rose hips, passionfruit, lemons and blackcurrants.

It is not only wild fruits and berries that are good for us in the spring, there are also a number of wild vegetables that sprout in the milder regions where there is no snow, or where it has melted. To name but a few, we can find dandelion shoots, watercress, nettle shoots, bear's garlic (ramsons) – and many others that can be used for salads. These plants often seem more like weeds and we might pass them by without a glance. It would be much better if we were to make use of them and their appreciable content of natural vitamins.

Internal Cleansing in the Spring

As soon as the warm rays of the sun hit the windows in the spring conscientious housewives are usually gripped by a peculiar restlessness that urges them to declare war on every trace of dust, dirt and disorder in the home. Similarly, such a challenge to spring-clean confronts each and everyone of us and we get the overpowering feeling that our bodies need cleansing, in order to rid them of all accumulated wastes. Then a certain 'spring fever' or fatigue seems to gradually reduce, or slow down, our enthusiasm. Even though we may have had enough exercise during the winter to keep our bodies in trim through movement and deep-breathing, we still feel that somehow our reserves of energy are at a low ebb. Of course that is quite true since the food that was stored in the autumn will have been losing more and more of its vitamins and other vital substances. Another problem are the many days without any sunshine, so that our body is even less able to utilise the vitamins properly. Heavy winter clothing, especially thick waterproof coats, hinders the normal breathing and perspiration of the skin and in this way contributes to impaired body functions.

419

What You Can Do

There are a number of things you can do to combat 'spring fever' successfully. First of all, practise more physical and breathing exercises. Even vigorous walking or hiking will help you to exhale a substantial amount of accumulated wastes. It may make you sweat a little, and that is good because it stimulates the skin and helps it to exude toxins. Only be careful not to catch a cold; as soon as you arrive home, change your damp underwear.

You can do even better than that by sweating properly in a steam bath, either taking a sweat bath at home or a sauna. This will make the skin eliminate toxins faster than anything else. But beware of overdoing it; be reasonable and watch your heart. This treatment can be made easier and safer if you take a natural heart tonic.

At any rate, you can see that there are some wonderful possibilities for assisting the body to eliminate wastes and toxins by excreting them through the skin as much as possible. So do not forget to treat your body to this kind of beneficial 'spring-cleaning'.

FOOD RICH IN VITAMINS AND MINERALS

The fact that 'spring fever' is partly a result of a deficiency in vitamins and important minerals should impel us to include in our diet plenty of early spring and wild salad greens and fresh vegetables. Then there are certain flowers and leaves that make superb herbal teas. For example, the bright yellow flowers of coltsfoot are a means of eliminating any phlegm and catarrh that may still linger on after the winter has passed. An infusion of various new leaf shoots is a rich source of minerals; as soon as the raspberry plants, blackberry branches and blackthorn and hawthorn bushes put forth tender new shoots, busy yourself with gathering them to prepare a wonderful spring tea from these fresh leaves. Do the same with young strawberry leaves and the tender shoots of the birch tree. Not only does such an infusion supply you with certain nutritive salts, but it also stimulates the kidneys to function more efficiently – an important aspect of any spring-cleaning treatment.

When the stinging nettles have grown large enough, gather some young shoots every day and add them, finely chopped, to your salads. They are delicious when lightly steamed as a vegetable, tasting something like spinach – which, incidentally, can also be used – or make them into a salad if you prefer. A little finely chopped bear's garlic (ramsons) will enrich any salad and a number of people enjoy bear's garlic leaves lightly steamed as a vegetable.

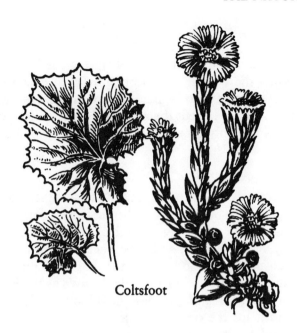

Coltsfoot

Remember, however, bear's garlic has a piquant flavour and it is better to use it fresh according to the principle 'You can have too much of a good thing.' Of course, this guideline applies to all strong flavourings and seasonings. Another spring vegetable is the radish, of which there are several varieties. Use them wisely in accordance with the same principle, for a little is good for the liver, but too much can harm it.

Many people in the country know of another wild salad herb that stimulates the liver – young dandelion leaves. When these are fresh and tender they should be eaten as a salad every day. If we want to avail ourselves of their benefits even during the warmer season of the year, when the plants are already fully grown, bearing flowers and seeds, there is still a way to enjoy dandelion salad. Here is how. On a mild spring day, when the soil is sufficiently moist, lay out a dandelion bed by making deep grooves into which you plant a row of dandelion roots. Lay the roots in such a way that they appear to be like a long rope in the groove. Cover them with garden peat and soil. When the shoots push through the earth, cut them immediately. This method will give you tender dandelion shoots right into the autumn months. Their effect on the liver is marvellous. During our cleansing treatment in the spring we must do all we can to stimulate the liver. Only by doing so can we be sure of success in fortifying one of the body's most important organs.

Many people are of the opinion that a 'spring cure' has fulfilled its purpose when the bowels are thoroughly cleansed. And, it is true, the intestines do have to be paid due attention. Nevertheless, strong laxatives will not benefit them as much as they deserve. Any treatment should not only cleanse or purify, but also build up and heal.

A WELL-BALANCED PROGRAMME TO IMPROVE THE METABOLISM

In order to improve the body's metabolism it is necessary to stimulate the bowels as well as the liver, gallbladder and kidneys. The normal activity of these organs can be achieved by a treatment that helps to cleanse the blood and which has been put together according to an Oriental 'cure' or formula. Known as the Rasayana Programme, it cleanses and purifies the blood, normalises the metabolism and helps the organs to function properly. This programme is outlined in detail in the next section.

It is important to point out that no drastic or extreme measures should be taken in any such treatment. Years ago, some people in the country would use arum, a strong plant, to cleanse the lungs in the spring, but their view was based on the principle 'the more the better'. However, this is not true, nor is it sensible, for much harm can come from it. Rather, be reasonable in following a spring-cleansing programme. Consider your general health and take sufficient time to allow your body to gradually adjust to the change. If you are sensible in carrying out the treatment, and follow it through successfully, the result will be better health and increased efficiency and vigour. The care and effort required will certainly be worthwhile.

Programmes to Purify the Blood

In the past it used to be the custom in the country to carry out a programme of cleansing the blood every spring. People would gather fresh leaves from blackberry and raspberry bushes, strawberry plants and ribwort (ribgrass), coltsfoot flowers and, where possible, cowslip. They would pour boiling water over these young green shoots and flowers and drink the infusion in the morning and evening. Honey was added to sweeten it.

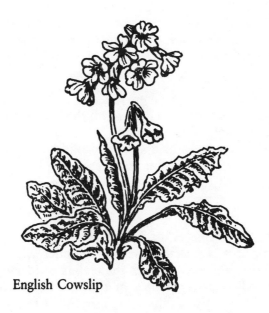

English Cowslip

This 'spring tea' is still recognised for its pleasant effect on our well-being. Those who take it regularly are convinced that it purifies the system, purging it of the winter's metabolic wastes and infusing the new energies of spring. Some medical practitioners may turn up their noses, discarding the idea of blood-cleansing as being erroneous and unscientific, but there is no doubt that such herbal cleansing stimulates the body's mechanisms and in this way achieves an overall cleansing effect.

According to the views held in ancient India, the blood and the circulatory system can and should be purified from time to time. *Rasa* is the ancient Indian word for the blood or body fluids, and *Rasayana Kalpa* is the name used for a blood-cleansing programme following the model and method of the ancient Indians.

In fact, the programme consists of four remedies, one each to stimulate the intestines, liver, kidneys and stomach:

1. *Rasayana No. 1* is a herb tablet that stimulates and cleanses the intestines.
2. *Rasayana No. 2,* is also a herb tablet; it contains curcuma root (Indian saffron) and serves to stimulate the liver.
3. A special *kidney tea* stimulates the kidneys and the excretion of wastes through the urine.
4. *Arabiaforce,* an Arabian plant essence, improves, regulates and

423

balances the function of the stomach lining and the mucous membranes of the intestines. This remedy is made according to an old herbal recipe that was brought to Europe by Paracelsus. The herbal ingredients come from the Near and Far East.

These four remedies taken together serve to 'spring-clean' the body and are of special benefit to all those who suffer from constipation and sluggish metabolism.

For even better results and to consolidate them, take the above-mentioned 'spring tea' after completing the Rasayana Programme. Your body will respond to this good care, and will enjoy greater vitality and energy.

Kelp and 'Spring Fever' or Fatigue

Since kelp is a seaweed some may wonder what this plant from the cool ocean has to do with the feeling of laziness or listlessness experienced by many people at the onset of spring. Well, many things in life are astonishing, not least the fact that this ocean plant can help to replenish the body's deficiency of minerals and vitamins that causes this unwelcome and bothersome feeling.

Kelp, a species of seaweed from the Pacific Ocean, is rich in minerals and for this reason has been successfully used to reduce obesity and treat thyroid problems, as well as to combat 'spring fever'. Its successful application for both purposes has been confirmed by an increasing number of people. Kelp is always at our service with its rich content of important trace elements and it is therefore the simplest, and possibly the best and least expensive, remedy to combat 'spring fever'. The easiest way to go about it is to take one *Kelpasan* tablet after each meal. If you suffer from Graves' disease (exophthalmic goitre) or hyperthyroidism, it is important to take kelp only in homoeopathic potency (1x–6x) because the effect of the remedy depends on the appropriate dilution being used.

Water and its Therapeutic Effects

Several years have passed since I visited the headwaters of the Amazon river, but I still remember watching the natives bathe in the dirty waters of a tributary of the Marañón. In other tropical areas I often saw the same thing happen, natives enjoying themselves in the muddy water, in some cases the water being absolutely black, while other streams appeared more yellow or red. The Indians and, especially, their children would romp about in these dirty rivers without any fear of becoming sick as a result. At any rate, they always seemed very happy and seemed to enjoy their dip. In spite of the obviously good effect a swim seemed to have on them, I never mustered enough courage to go in the water myself.

However, one day I felt exceptionally tired and worn out and decided to derive some benefit from the refreshing water. After all, the temperature was 40°C (105°F) in the shade and took a lot out of me after a while, especially as it was combined with extremely high humidity. I had to keep reminding myself of the need to breathe deeply in order to cope a little better with the unbearable atmosphere. All I wanted was a refreshing bath to bolster my spirits. Even so, I still did not have the courage to jump in the river, but it occurred to me that I could ask a native woman to go and fetch me some water in a large earthenware jug. I stood on a bamboo footbridge between two huts and as she brought the water I poured it over my head, letting it run down all over me. The Indian woman was kind enough to keep bringing one jug of water after another, and it was not long before I felt quite refreshed, even though the water was not as cool or as clean as I would have wished it to be.

The Mystery Solved
Much later I took a bath in a mud pond in the north of Scandinavia. When I stepped out of the muddy water I felt completely refreshed and began to think about the effect a little more closely. It suddenly crossed my mind that we apply clay-water compresses because they are better than simple water packs. And then there are mud baths and fango mud packs; these too are judged to be more effective than simple water packs. Then it dawned on me that the muddy, that is, dirty, water was not that bad after all; I realised that it can still have a therapeutic effect in spite of its uninviting appearance, provided, of course, that the muddiness is nothing but natural dirt accounted for by clay or some other kind of earth.

On a later visit to the southwest of the United States I came across a river that looked red, quite appropriately called Red River. The puzzling question was 'How do this and similar rivers get their strange colour?' The answer is quite simple: there is either red or yellow clay dissolved in the water, thus colouring the water accordingly, or they contain marshy soil and are black as a result.

I can well imagine that Sebastian Kneipp would have been over-joyed if he could have seen such coloured river water. His natural instinct and intuition would have encouraged him to immediately investigate the medical effects of these waters. In fact, some time later an analytical chemist proved to me, by means of an apparatus which measured the electric tension in the water, that water carries energy that is transmitted to the human body. We filled a bath tub and then used the apparatus to measure the electric field in it. After the bath had been used we measured this once more and found that the electric field had decreased, thus proving that the energy had been transmitted to the person in the water.

The Origin of Water's Therapeutic Effects
Not every kind of water has the same electric field, nor does it have the same therapeutic effect. The result depends upon the 'ballast' substances contained in the water, such as clay or black mud, which are responsible for the electric charge. Minerals dissolved in the water can also add medicinal properties. These substances are usually picked up by the water as it flows from its source deep in the earth and on its way passes over mineral deposits. It is these substances that account for the remedial effects of water when used for bathing and drinking. Any colouring matter, which we at first consider to be impurities or dirt, will have been added to the spring water as it flowed over deposits of clay and minerals. Thus the therapeutic value, as well as the content of minerals and its energy or power, is produced in a natural way, and that is of importance to us.

When I was visiting the South Sea islands I had similar opportunities to see the natives bathe in dirty, muddy waters. But please do not misunderstand my meaning, for I am not referring here to dirt resulting from the unhygienic environment I also saw there – human excrement or pollutants, or bacteriological dirt from other sources that can be channelled into the water. I am not talking about this kind of real pollution, but rather the natural process of earth and minerals being absorbed by the water, changing its clear colour. Naturally, coloured water is not necessarily unsuitable for bathing, although one has to be extra careful in the tropics because of the abundance of parasites that pollute the streams. Just think of the dangerous schistosomes, liver flukes and micro-organisms galore, which transmit all kinds of dangerous diseases.

You have to be even more careful with drinking water. There are some wonderful mineral waters available, but some water also contains poisonous minerals, some of which I came across in North, Central and South America. It can happen that a stream may come from a mineral spring in which is dissolved arsenic, copper or other heavy minerals that make the water poisonous and dangerous to drink. For this reason it is not possible to drink water from just any spring or source as one is able to do, for example, in Switzerland. It is often possible to recognise such dangerous springs by the discoloration of the rocks and stones, which turn yellow, greenish or other colours. Sometimes crystals can be found in the riverbed which taste sharp and burn the tongue.

The same rule applies to water for internal or external use as applies to plants: many plants are curative whereas others are harmful or can only be taken in a diluted form. It is true that nature has much to offer that is beneficial, but we must also keep our eyes open and make sure that we use only the things that are truly good for our health. There is no point in being careless and ignorant and so causing ourselves harm. Remember, always make sure to use only the things that are helpful and safe.

It is common knowledge that not all mineral waters have the same effect and it would be foolish to ignore the fact that the mineral content of a certain water may be beneficial in the case of one particular illness but may not be so for some other physical disorder. Similarly, not everyone is helped by the same thing. For example, strong people are more resistant, whereas those who are sensitive and weak always have to remember that although a mild stimulation can be good, anything stronger may be harmful. Hence, be careful. Volcanic areas with strongly radioactive springs can do much harm to sensitive people, and may even have a paralysing effect and endanger their glandular functions. If you become aware of an adverse reaction when staying in such places or taking the waters, it will be better to avoid them. On the other hand, do not forget that people of a stronger disposition and nature may benefit from a stay in volcanic areas. What may harm a weak person can possibly cure a stronger one. The simple rule is 'Know your own limitations and weaknesses.'

The Therapeutic Value of the Sea
People who do not live by the sea dream of the beach and surf, especially when they sit down to plan their holidays. They long to see the play of the waves, how they break on the immovable rocks, roll and foam and then fizzle out on the golden sands. The waves approach the beach, powerful and inexorable, run up on it and disappear, yet in spite of their awesome power they instil a feeling

of being soothed. We never tire of watching them; we are just happy and content to admire their endless movement.

Sea Air

In the morning and evening we feel the urge to stretch our legs and go for a walk along the beach. Some holiday-makers may still be tucked up in bed when we are already up and about, enjoying every minute of the exhilarating experience. The bracing sea air is tangy, salty, high in iodine, and its effect on us is instant. Old and lingering catarrh is loosened. Whatever else is left over from the colds and chills of the previous winter is on its way out because we breathe deeply on our regular walks along the beach.

Let me tell you, sea air is indeed a remedy for our respiratory organs and the endocrine glands; it cleanses and stimulates them marvellously. It has been said before that the thyroid in particular is stimulated by sea air and also by sea water and seaweeds, especially on account of their iodine content. However, if you suffer from Graves' disease (exophthalmic goitre) or hyperthyroidism, you must be careful to limit your exposure to these stimulants; in other words, if the sea air or bathing in the sea increases your pulse rate or causes a faster heartbeat, you should spend only short periods on the beach every day. Given time, the body will become accustomed to the impact of the marine atmosphere and you may gradually increase your exposure to a few hours daily. The more the disturbing symptoms diminish, the longer you can permit yourself the pleasure of spending time on the beach. So if you take care to do what is sensible and reasonable and not extreme, the therapeutic effect and cure will be much faster.

Sea-Bathing

Bathing in the sea has different effects on people. Salt water has an osmotic effect in as much as it draws water from the body. As a result, those people who always have some excess fluid in the legs will feel considerably better after bathing in the sea. Sea water will do the same for them as sea salt packs would do. If you tend to obesity, sea-bathing will usually help you to lose weight, even though you may not eat less. Excess weight and fat can be reduced because the sea stimulates the thyroid and gonads, thus benefiting the entire metabolism. All this is good for the figure and slimness may thus be within reach for some people. Sea air and sea-bathing are beneficial in cases of circulatory disorders, and diabetics will find sea-bathing good for them when they swim a lot and walk along the beach and over sand dunes. When stress and tension threaten your health do something about it quickly: take a holiday by the sea – there is no better remedy. However, while you are away from your work and duties, put them completely out of your mind and do not let the telephone interrupt your treatment. So, no telephone in your hotel room! 'Switching off' is absolutely essential during your holiday if you are to benefit fully from the 'cure' the sea can give you.

And there is one other rule you must observe: go to bed early during your stay by the sea. That means that you must cut out any kind of night life and remember instead that the early morning hours are the best. In fact, after an early and restful night it is easier to wake up, then go for a walk along the beach, feeling fully refreshed and fit. Remember, early to bed and early to rise, makes a man (and woman) healthy and gloriously hungry for breakfast! What better ingredients could you have for this meal than a delicious fruit muesli, wholegrain or wholewheat (wholemeal) bread with honey, and fruit-cereal coffee (*Bambu Coffee Substitute*)!

If you are able to organise your days by the sea properly, you can expect to benefit as much from them as you would from a holiday in the mountains. If we provide the body with all its needs, we will reap the desired health benefits irrespective of where we spend our holidays. However, just lazing around in the sun and heat is of no benefit anywhere. Instead, move around and exercise in the unpolluted air, breathe deeply and get plenty of rest during the night. If you eat healthy natural food at the same time, you will return to your duties after the holiday feeling rested, refreshed and optimistic.

Alternating Hot and Cold Water Therapies
Alternating hot and cold water applications are excellent for poor circulation and a fine aid to removing any congestion.

Apply hot water or herbal packs for about three minutes, then replace by a cold water pack, but leave this on for no longer than half a minute. Repeat the hot pack, followed by the cold, and continue in the same way for 20–30 minutes. The same principle applies to water-treading. Tread your feet in hot water for three minutes, then half a minute in cold water, and so forth. If you take alternating hot and cold baths, you must stay in the cold water only the same number of seconds as you were in the hot for minutes. This rule also applies to alternating hot and cold foot and arm baths. These applications should never make you feel chilled, but always warm and comfortable.

Steam Baths at Home

Steam baths are useful for dispersing congestions, making the urine flow again when retention occurs (older men often suffer from this difficulty) and relieving cystitis (inflammation of the bladder) and similar conditions of the bladder, as well as prostate problems.

These baths are easy enough to prepare at home. First make a steaming hot infusion of hay flowers (using the stalks, leaves, blossoms, seed and the hay itself), camomile, wild thyme or similar aromatic herbs. When this is ready, pour it into a large vessel, place a narrow plank or board over it, on which you can sit. Keep the steam and heat from escaping by covering yourself from head to toe with towels or sheets.

If you find sitting on the board to be uncomfortable, you might use some sort of wicker chair instead. If you do not have one, it may be possible to cut a hole out of the seat of an ordinary chair so that the steam can rise from underneath. In any event, you must keep your body warm and well wrapped in towels.

Keep adding more hot herbal infusion or hot water so that the steam continues to rise. It will be even more efficient it you can keep the infusion on a hot plate.

Such a steam bath is very effective, inexpensive to construct, and serves an excellent purpose.

Sitz Baths and their Medicinal Value

Sitz baths (in which only the hips and buttocks are immersed, hence their other name, hip baths) are part and parcel of good health care and, at the same time, complement effective beauty care. If you take regular hip baths, the circulation will be stimulated, which, in turn, will benefit the abdominal organs and health in general. Such regular care and attention is especially good for the ovaries, since they are easily affected by cold and congestions. Sitz baths increase the blood circulation and eliminate congestions, stagnation, irritations and any initial stages of inflammation of the ovaries and Fallopian tubes. Deformations and infertility can thus often be prevented.

Of what use are the best natural remedies if they do not reach the affected parts of the body because of congestion or circulatory disorders? We all know that life and healing forces are contained in the blood and that it is therefore important for the blood to

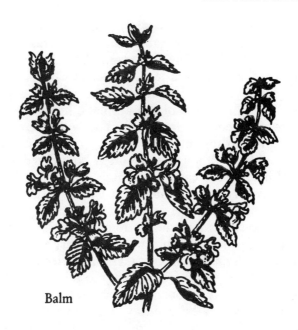

Balm

reach the ailing parts of the body. The best remedies for this purpose are water therapies, and for women, hip baths, or sitz baths, are the most indicated. Did you know that external symptoms such as oily skin, blackheads, dandruff, skin eruptions and itchy skin can be the result of poor functioning of the abdominal organs? One basic requirement of a thorough health and body care programme for modern women is the treatment and care of these organs.

A woman's mental and emotional balance and attitude are highly dependent on the good working order of the abdominal organs, especially the ovaries. Keep-fit exercises, walking and regular sitz baths help to provide the proper circulation a woman needs. Taking into account that her general well-being has much to do with the conscientious care of her health, surely any woman will want to see to it that this care is just another important part of her daily routine.

The addition of herbs in the form of infusions is highly recommended. For those who are nervous and tense, add lemon balm to the bath water; those who tend to feel tired and easily chilled will find thyme a good help; dry and flaking skin benefits from an infusion of wild pansy (heartsease); while comfrey is good for rough skin with large pores. Another way to treat rough skin is to apply Symphosan (comfrey tincture) after every bath. If the skin is sensitive or sore, it is advisable to add an infusion of mallow (cheese plant) or sanicle. Oily skin responds well to herbal sea salt.

Hay flowers (hayseed) and juniper needles can also be added to a hip bath. Or if you can obtain some eucalyptus leaves, they too are a good addition. Some of the aromatic herbs are stimulating while others have sedative properties. You will have to make your choice according to the intended effect. Even oat straw can be a beneficial addition, although it is often considered useless as a medicine. Whatever the case, a hip bath is more efficacious when a herbal infusion is added than if just water is used. It would be a pity to take so much time and trouble preparing a sitz bath if full use of the herbs as remedies were not made at the same time.

One or two hip baths should be taken every week. In cases of illness and necessity they can be taken more frequently. The time spent in the bath may vary from twenty to thirty minutes, and the water must be kept at a constant temperature of 37°C (98.6°F), which is accomplished by pouring off some of the water and replacing it with hot water. It is recommended that a hip bath be taken in the evening before going to bed, because you should not step out into the cold air afterwards or sit around in the house to cool off. A warm room is essential for such a bath, as a cold room absorbs too much body heat. Additionally, it is advisable to wrap up well with warm towels for extra warmth. A reduction in body temperature or even beginning to feel chilly is detrimental when taking a bath.

The best vessel to use for a sitz bath is, of course, one specially designed for that purpose; it will enable you to run off cooling water and add hot water, in order to maintain the required temperature. Lacking that, an ordinary bathtub will do, but you will have to keep a bucket of very hot water by the side of it. Use this hot water to top up the bath after removing some of the cooling water; to do this you will need a jar and another bucket for disposal. If all you have is a bathtub, you can take such a 'half bath' with the water reaching no higher than the navel. If you have an ordinary bathtub and a small hip bath, you can simply put a plank across the tub and stand the hip bath on it. You will need another plank or board as a foot rest. A hand shower attachment will make it quite easy to add more hot water, while the cooling water can be left to run out into the unplugged bathtub underneath. The advantage of this arrangement is obvious; at the end of your bath the water can be emptied straight into the tub.

Regular sitz baths are beneficial to your health, will preserve your youthfulness and, of course, have a great influence on your mental and emotional disposition and attitude.

The Schlenz Method (Baths of Increasing Temperature)

I once met the old high school teacher Rudolf Schlenz in Innsbruck and shortly afterwards discussed the Schlenz method with his son, Dr J. Schlenz. My conversations with these two men conveyed to me some of the spirit of the late Maria Schlenz, who had developed this type of hot water therapy.

Mrs Schlenz was neither a medical doctor nor a naturopath, but a simple housewife and mother. She had, however, an appreciation for nature and a gift for observation. In caring for her children she realised that they were too delicate to benefit from Kneipp's cold water treatment, so she thought of giving them hot water treatments instead. Some doctors had given baths of increasing temperature (*Überwärmungsbäder* in German) with good results even before she began to use them and continued to do so after the introduction of her method, but orthodox medicine in her native country paid no attention to her experience.

Later on, I made the acquaintance of Dr Devrient in Berlin, who was so enthusiastic about the Schlenz method that he published a book explaining these baths, as well as sauna baths, as used in practice. He made reference to the practical experiences with these baths recorded by his colleagues Dr Wilhelm Winsch and Dr Walenski. Whenever Dr Devrient stood in for another colleague, Dr Keller-Hoerschelmann, he came into contact with Swiss folk medicine. He himself was an ardent advocate of natural therapy methods and holistic medicine. It was obvious, then, that he also approved of hydrotherapy and, of course, the Schlenz method. Professor Lampert employed the same method with great success; in fact, it is known that he cured over a hundred cases of typhoid fever during World War II, without losing a single one of his patients.

Some time later I learned about the regenerative and curative effects of hot water treatments as used in Japan. The temperature of their baths surpasses that of blood temperature, and it is interesting to note that rheumatism and cancer are seldom heard of where these hot water baths are taken regularly. Some researchers even claim that swollen tissue can be rehabilitated if the water is kept 2–3 degrees Celsius above normal body temperature (39–40°C/102–104°F). And when the temperature is raised 4–5 degrees higher, that is, up to 41–42 °C (105.8–107.6 °F), tumours are changed and in time dissolved, according to these researchers.

It is possible that these claims are somewhat exaggerated; nevertheless, experience has shown that 'baths of increasing temperature' make a positive contribution in the treatment of tumours, especially when the effect is heightened by the use of appropriate herbs. Many a malignant ailment can be prevented by their use, and the prevention of frightening diseases such as cancer has become a great necessity in our time. *The Nature Doctor* has already given some good advice regarding the prevention of cancer (see pages 288–92) and here we add the further recommendation that you take a prolonged bath or Schlenz bath once a week. Its prophylactic effect can help to maintain your health. However, you should not simply be satisfied with knowing these things without acting upon the knowledge. That would be of little use to you. You should rouse yourself and apply the recommended treatment on a regular basis.

Schlenz Baths at Home
Before you decide to try out a Schlenz bath in your home, you should first get to know the exact method as used in a recognised Schlenz bath centre, to enable you to become familiar with all the relevant details. The bathtub used for Schlenz baths is generally longer than an ordinary one and should preferably be made of wood. But in modern homes this is rarely the case, so that a conventional enamelled or plastic bathtub will have to do. It is also necessary to remember that the head will have to be immersed, too, so that you will have to bend your legs a little in a shorter tub.

Since the head is submerged as well as the rest of the body the warmth will be equally distributed over the entire body and congestions towards the head will be avoided. A Schlenz bath will therefore give no trouble at all, even though you may not be able to stand an ordinary hot bath. Keep the mouth and nose just out of the water so that you can breathe. On the other hand, as this position is uncomfortable and difficult to maintain for any length of time, attach a belt at the top end of the bathtub, or a strong cloth, for use as a support for the head. Rest the head on this support under the water, leaving only the mouth and nose above it. To begin with, keep the water temperature at 36–37 °C (97–98 °F), that is, blood temperature; but be careful not to let the temperature drop. For this reason, it is important to have some

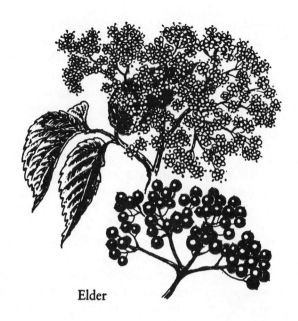

Elder

hot water ready to add as necessary, letting the temperature rise to at least 38 °C (100.4 °F). Before taking the bath, drink one or two cups of hot herbal tea – lemon balm, peppermint, elder or goldenrod. Add a few drops of *Crataegisan* if your heart is a little weak.

Increasing the body temperature by several degrees induces a kind of artificial fever, which is able to burn up a lot of wastes, just as with a natural fever. In this regard, we cannot help remembering a statement made by Parmenides, the father of metaphysics: 'Give me the power to induce fever and I shall cure every illness.'

Indeed, more healing can be done through increasing the body temperature than is generally thought possible. By raising the temperature to 40 or 41 °C (104–105.8 °F), disease-causing agents that are sensitive to heat will be destroyed. Regular Schlenz baths will have an effect on sensitive tumour cells or tissue, since they do not tolerate heat very well. Those who suffer from metabolic and circulatory disorders will benefit from a weekly Schlenz bath, as will anyone who has problems with the skin function and lymphatic glands, or who suffers from skin eruptions and eczema. In the case of all these disorders and ailments, regular Schlenz baths can lead to a complete cure.

When you first start, a Schlenz bath should last only half an hour. In time, you can increase the duration to two hours. In cases

435

of obesity it is advisable to add sea salt, brine or a good bath salt to the bath water, in addition to the herbs. An attendant should use a tough brush to vigorously brush down the patient's entire body once or twice during the bath. This has the same effect as an underwater massage and stimulates the capillaries. It removes congestions, and any unpleasant feeling of constriction will disappear.

When the time for the bath is up, sit upright, apply a little *Po-Ho-Oil* under your nose and inhale slowly, deeply and vigorously; then stand up, wrap yourself in a warm bath towel and go straight into a warmed bed without drying yourself. You will continue to perspire while you are there. Maria Schlenz, by the way, used hand-knitted wool blankets to keep the heat in. Your head and wet hair should be wrapped up warmly so that no part of the body can cool down.

A Schlenz bath taken at home has the advantage that you can go straight to bed and sleep. As soon as the body has stopped perspiring, wash it down with lukewarm water and apply *St John's wort oil* or some other body oil that contains this oil. Afterwards you will feel relaxed and pleasantly tired and will go soundly to sleep.

A few Schlenz baths can dispense with the need for costly hydrotherapy treatment at a spa. Then there is the added advantage of being able to prepare Schlenz baths right in your own home. If you wait until evening for the bath, you can still do some urgent work during the day, and you will feel fresh and energetic the following morning, after a good night's sleep.

In cases where the initial symptoms of poliomyelitis are present, the fresh hormone treatment recommended by *The Nature Doctor* (see page 53–4) should be followed up by a Schlenz bath. This can help you to prevent paralysis. Schlenz baths are of equal benefit to those who suffer from multiple sclerosis. They help to prevent the sad complications of this illness, which can make life almost unbearable. In view of the many benefits a course of treatment with Schlenz baths can give, this method deserves to be much better known and utilised than it actually is.

Kuhne's Cold Water Treatment
Louis Kuhne had an astute mind and understanding of natural healing and was able to use water most effectively for what is called 'stimulation' or 'irritation' therapy. He perfected his method to such an extent that his handbook came to be translated into

many languages, circulating in all parts of the earth. Unfortunately, he had no direct successor and no society or clinic took up his ideas with a view to spreading the Kuhne method, as was the case with the cures developed by Priessnitz, Sebastian Kneipp and other hydrotherapists.

Cold Water Friction Treatment
Especially valuable and important is a cold water massage Kuhne developed. A simplified form of this treatment can be undertaken in your own home. First, take a large container and fill it three-quarters full with cold water. Then put a board over the container to cover half of it. Sit on the board, having taken off the clothes covering the lower part of the body. Take a brush with a long handle, wrap a cloth around the brush, dip it in the cold water and rub round about the genitals. The cold reaction must only affect one part of the body and for this reason your hand should not be put in the cold water but remain dry all the time. Because of the cold reaction it is essential to maintain a constant body temperature by wrapping yourself in warm cloths or towels during the treatment, as is done during a steam bath.

The Kuhne treatment is best done at night, for it ensures more restful sleep because it draws the blood from the head to the abdomen, with the effect that it is much easier to switch off from distracting thoughts. If you find it difficult to go to sleep, you should try this method. Five minutes are often enough to draw the blood away from the head to the centre of the body, resulting in hyperaemia, increased blood flow. In accordance with the body's reaction and the purpose intended, the treatment has to be carried on for 10–15 minutes. However, always remember that you must not allow yourself to become chilled; the body should remain nice and warm for the effect to be beneficial. If you think that you could catch a cold because you keep dipping the brush in cold water and going over the same area again and again, you are actually mistaken. This part of the body has an abundance of blood vessels and is therefore less sensitive to the cold. When massaging, do avoid the region of the bladder because it is more sensitive. If your body does not respond to the cold water friction by making you feel warm, and you are quite sure that it does not, it would appear that the Kuhne method is not for you.

However, if your body responds well to cold water applications, the Kuhne method will give you the desired results. These cold water friction or massage treatments relieve headaches, congestions in the head, leaden fatigue, stomach upsets, loss of appetite and many other complaints. Frigidity as well as an exceptionally strong sexual drive can be treated successfully, so that in time it is possible to experience normal function of the sex organs. After a few weeks, cases of depression and melancholy can be improved and they may even be cured if the treatment is continued over an extended period.

Following the instructions given, you can practise these cold water massages at home and as long as the necessary care is taken, you will do no harm whatsoever. On the contrary, you will have reason to be astonished at the excellent results.

Revulsion by Means of Stimulation (Irritation) Therapies

It is the Chinese who seem to have a great deal of experience in the field of stimulation (irritation) therapy. On my visits to the Far East I was able to witness their mastery of this kind of therapy. I even watched them treat and cure gangrene by means of it. There was an old monk in a Buddhist monastery who gave this kind of treatment. One European patient told me in confidence about the excellent result in his own case.

Of course, the modern treatment is much milder than the old-fashioned methods. In the old days a white-hot iron was passed quickly over the affected area in order to induce stimulation or revulsion. Nowadays pungent roots containing mainly mustard oil, are used instead. First, hot compresses are applied to the area to be cured, then the grated roots are rubbed in, bandaged with cotton to keep warm and left to act for 4–5 hours. The active substances contained in the root pulp induce powerful stimulation, making the blood circulate vigorously in the area. The body responds by sending a great detachment of leucocytes and lymphocytes to the spot, so that an artificially induced inflammation breaks out. The purpose is to rally all available forces in the body. Congested blood vessels, tiny thromboses, toxins and metabolic wastes are dislodged and excreted. If the treatment is done properly, it is possible to cure old and even chronic disorders.

Some years ago I had the opportunity to give such a treatment with complete success. One day an old man from the Jura mountains came to see me about his leg, which the doctors were intending to amputate. The stimulating treatment I gave him opened up an ulcer on his leg that had been a long-standing problem. You should have seen the quantity of blood and pus that burst forth! And then the pain subsided all at once. Needless to say, after this thorough cleansing action the wound began to heal and the old watchmaker's leg was soon as good as new.

The Baunscheidt Method

The Baunscheidt method is similar to the Chinese treatment just described. However, Baunscheidt did not take it from the Chinese but developed his treatment based on his own experience and conclusions. This method achieves a simulation or irritation of the skin by means of an apparatus known in German as *Lebenswecker* (life reviver). After pricking the skin, *Baunscheidt oil* is rubbed in, the area is covered with cotton wool and the ingredients are left to work overnight. The following day the treatment is continued with the application of a lanolin cream (*Bioforce Cream*).

This therapy has given good results in the treatment of chronic ailments, even multiple sclerosis. The application is made on the left and right side along the patient's spine. However, it is not advisable to undertake a Baunscheidt revulsion treatment on the off-chance that it might work, but without being really familiar with it. If you want to use this method it is absolutely essential that you know the correct way of applying it. The same rule applies to any stimulation therapy and it is better to let a physiotherapist or biologically oriented doctor with the necessary experience give the treatment. The needles have to be used with great care and only on the muscles; never touch the glands or periosteum, which must not be irritated.

Stimulation therapies can be used successfully in cases where medicines fail to give results because the circulation in the affected parts is insufficient and the remedies do not reach them. The stimulation provided by these therapies is then an alternative and welcome means of assistance.

The Medicinal Value of Clay

From time immemorial clay has been used to cure many ailments. Yet this old remedy has often been rejected by those who could have benefited from it. Nevertheless, clay has never been totally forgotten and today it is once more finding favour. Among other things, it is particularly recommended as a treatment for tumours where external application is possible.

Also, there is an interesting account in the Bible of how Christ used clay to cure a blind man (John 9:11). Even though it may have been a symbolic act, we should not lose sight of the fact that earth or clay was used and that the Teacher of Nazareth surely knew of the healing elements of nature and respected them.

People who live closer to nature in less developed parts of the world treat many illnesses with clay, and veterinary surgeons make use of it too. Beauty specialists recommend it for face packs and athletes use it for strains and sprains. Clay applications have proved their worth for centuries. A combination of clay and herbs is especially recommended. Instead of using simple herb poultices, the herbal properties are combined with those of clay. Usually the clay is mixed into a paste, to which the hot herbal infusion is added to form a poultice. The poultice is then applied to the affected part of the body and the double action of the clay and herbs results in a more potent effect.

If you want to get the best out of a treatment with clay, you must be certain that you understand how it works. There are those who use clay where linseed or fenugreek seed should be applied, and this is quite wrong. For instance, clay should not be placed on a boil to collect the pus and draw it to a head. Hot linseed or fenugreek compresses will do this job far better, for the action of clay disperses, it never draws together or gathers.

Directions for the Use of Clay

According to the time of the year, clay poultices may be used either hot or cold. Those who are sensitive to the cold may prefer a hot poultice; a bag of hot herbs can be placed on top of the clay to help retain its heat. With a cold clay pack you can reduce the feeling of cold by a hot herb bag used in the same way.

For a small clay poultice, a tablespoon of clay, mixed with a herbal infusion to make a thin paste, will suffice. Spread the paste evenly, about 3–5 mm (⅛–⅕ inch) thick, onto a piece of gauze or linen and place on the affected part. In cases of inflammation, especially inflammation of a nerve (neuritis), *St John's wort oil* mixed with clay can work wonders and has the added advantage of keeping the poultice soft and easy to remove. Otherwise its removal can be unpleasant for those with sensitive skin as clay becomes hard and brittle as it dries. It is recommended that the poultice be applied at night and left on until the morning.

There are certain instances, usually in cases of chronic ailments, where it is advantageous to apply *clay and cabbage poultices* alternately. Since we know that clay disperses and cabbage draws together, the alternating actions will produce effects similar to those of a counter-irritation. This is often desirable in chronic rheumatic and arthritic conditions.

Taken internally, clay has a remarkable effect on diarrhoea and inflammation of the intestinal mucosa. Whatever medication is taken for these problems, it should be added to clay water.

Everyone could profit physically from an intestinal cleansing twice a year and the best clay to use for this purpose is the white, sand-free kind, although yellow clay is suitable too. Such a course of treatment should last a week at a time.

What Herbs to Use

For applying to tumours an infusion made from *horsetail* (shave grass) or *oak bark* produces good results when mixed with clay. Inflammation of the nerves is best treated with a mixture of *lemon balm* and clay; and for rheumatic problems, an infusion of *eucalyptus leaves,* needle-like *juniper leaves,* or *wild thyme* with clay is recommended. Never boil aromatic herbs and leaves; merely pour boiling water over them and allow them to steep in the hot liquid (infusion). Non-aromatic herbs can be boiled a little. When ready, strain and mix the liquid with clay to make a paste. If you infuse the herbs in a small cloth bag, this will be useful for laying on top of the clay-herb poultice when it is in position. As previously explained, this will help to retain the heat.

Herb Poultices

Herbs that favourably influence the function of organs when taken as teas, tinctures and extracts will also benefit us if we apply them as poultices, as practical experience will prove. Kidney herbs such as *Solidago (goldenrod), birch leaves* and *horsetail,* can be crushed or minced and applied raw to the region over the kidneys. This external application will enhance the effect of the same remedies taken internally.

The application of fresh plants will benefit the circulatory and lymphatic systems and ease stagnation in the vascular system. In fact, fresh plant therapy is easy. For example, *crushed sorrel, giant dock* and *rhubarb leaf* poultices applied to congestions, bruises, swellings and the like, have an excellent effect. They will dissipate the trouble much better than expensive commercial plasters and ointments. Various leaves found in the garden and fields are suitable, but care must be taken not to employ the leaves of poisonous plants. The leaves of *Rhus toxicodendron* (poison ivy) can cause a severe rash. *Belladonna* and other poisonous plants must not be

441

used either. In fact, poisonous plants, it must be remembered, are safe only in the hands of a professional phytotherapist. Other leaf poultices, for example ones made with *cabbage leaves*, can be applied without having to fear any complications. They are helpful in treating numerous ailments, and if there should be a strong reaction, simply reduce the time the poultices are allowed to remain on the affected area.

These poultices are easily prepared and always beneficial.

Cabbage Leaf and Other Herb Poultices
The curative properties of *cabbage leaves* are becoming more widely known now, even though the use of crushed medicinal plants on diseased parts of the body is by no means a new idea. Dr Blanc has written a booklet on the subject and many people have benefited from this inexpensive treatment. Many years ago I started to apply crushed *St John's wort* leaves and flowers in the case of inflammations of the nerves, with wonderful results. Whenever I used to get blisters from walking barefoot in the mountains in search of herbs, I always found some *goldenrod*, bruised it and put it, raw and fresh, on the sore spot, covered it with a leaf of lady's mantle and bandaged everything with a handkerchief. This enabled me to carry on walking and go about my business. The blisters did not bother me anymore and soon began to heal. In the case of kidney trouble it is a good thing to crush or mince fresh *birch leaves and goldenrod* and apply the raw pulp over the kidney area. Wrap them round with warm towels and place a hot water bottle on top for added warmth.

Cabbage leaf poultices or packs are excellent for the treatment of tumours. In the case of cancerous growths, their effect is very good when alternated with clay poultices. It sometimes happens that the condition or pain becomes aggravated at first, but after a while improvement usually follows. Cabbage pulp can cause a strong reaction; it can increase the secretion of urine, cause blisters, or simply dry out on the skin. Tests on myself and the testimonies of patients have always proved the effectiveness of these poultices.

Cabbage leaves are usually available in your kitchen, so why not try a pack when you suffer bruising, notice a growth or experience some internal inflammation? Apply the crushed leaves, in addition to taking the necessary oral medicine. Many chronic ailments can be successfully treated with *cabbage* and *clay packs* applied in alternation; one day apply the pulped leaves, next day the clay packs. In this way it is often possible to avoid the surgeon's knife.

Good results are also achieved with *onions* and *raw horseradish*. Some skin diseases clear up when a paste made up of *bran* and an infusion of *marigold* or *horsetail* is applied. Or you can soak some *wheat*, put it through a mincer, then mix it with marigold or horsetail to make a soothing and curative paste.

THE EFFECTIVENESS OF CABBAGE POULTICES – TESTIMONIALS

In many cases the orthodox doctor goes to no end of trouble to help a patient, but unfortunately, without success. Then, when a simple natural remedy like cabbage leaves produces a cure, we are astonished at how natural active forces, without depending upon laboriously collected human knowledge, can bring about almost miraculous results.

The case of a 62-year-old patient, who suffered considerably, serves as a good example. An infection, aggravated by eating sprayed cherries, resulted in the development of a fungus the size of a small coin on the lady's tongue. The doctor removed it with cautery (silver nitrate) and found it necessary to prescribe, in addition, eight days of radium treatment. After three weeks the patient left the hospital with a paralysed tongue.

Five weeks later, a large swelling appeared on her neck. It seemed that another operation would be necessary to remove it. Discouraged by the prospect of more surgery, the patient kept postponing it. Eight weeks later the pain had become almost unbearable but now an operation was considered out of the question. Instead, she received forty-three radiation treatments. Afterwards, the patient felt weak and thought death was inevitable.

At this point the doctors had given up all hope of curing her. The wound would not heal and constantly exuded pus. After nine weeks the patient asked to return home from the hospital and her family and relatives continued treating her with much care and devotion. Every ten minutes the dressing on the wound had to be changed and a special ointment applied. But despite all this kind attention the pain could not be relieved.

An acquaintance of hers who had read of cabbage poultices in my monthly magazine *Health News (Gesundheits-Nachrichten)* recommended this treatment and – lo and behold – within four days of trying it, the pus was discharging freely and the terrible pain receded. In spite of suffering from chronic constipation and headaches resulting from it, the patient felt much better and was delighted to be on the mend after a year and a half of illness. It is hard to believe that cabbage can achieve such success, but if this patient had not taken advantage of the treatment her condition would probably have greatly deteriorated instead of improving as it did.

The marvellous effect of cabbage leaves is truly remarkable and no doctor or medical practitioner who has the well-being of his patients at heart should ignore this lowly plant.

Here is another example, taken at random from the many testimonials I have received. A worried mother wrote asking for advice on how to deal with her child's swollen neck glands. Having followed the prescribed treatment, this is what she wrote:

'The trouble was soon put right by the remedies and cabbage poultices. Cabbage, in general, seems to be a marvellous thing. It seemed our thirteen-year-old son, who is 175 cm [5'9"] tall and whose voice has already broken, would not be able to get rid of a cold before having to go back to school the following Monday. He then complained of a really bad headache and yesterday afternoon, of a pain in and above his right eye. I was afraid of sinus trouble, so I put a cabbage poultice on his head just above the eyes and left it on for two hours. Monday came and off he went to school, returning in the evening still cheerful. The pain had completely gone.'

It is quite peculiar that the humble cabbage should have such outstanding healing powers and can give unexpected relief without any harmful side effects. What explanation is there? Well, cabbage not only supplies curative elements to the tissues but also eliminates toxins and other harmful substances from these same affected areas. This kind of remedy fills an important place, especially where nothing else seems to be effective.

The Potato as a Remedy

Raw, grated potatoes, mixed with a little milk, are an ideal remedy for the following conditions: slow-healing wounds or cuts, wounds that form proud flesh, infections or inflammations that secrete putrid matter, swellings, bruises, articular rheumatism and inflammation of muscles and of the periosteum.

Potatoes boiled in their skins, mashed when they are still hot and mixed with a little raw milk, can be applied as a poultice, like a clay pack. If you have a poor reaction to cold applications, use warm poultices. Those who benefit from cold packs, on the other hand, should use raw potatoes, grated or pulped.

A remarkable effect can be obtained by alternating three applications on three consecutive days. On the first day, apply a *potato*

444

poultice; on the second day, a *cabbage poultice*; and on the third day, a *clay poultice* made with a *horsetail infusion* and a little *St John's wort oil*. If you continue to apply these poultices for some time, even a severe swelling will yield.

Old potatoes should have their sprouts carefully removed because they contain a poisonous substance called solanin. These sprouts should neither be fed to animals nor used as food or as a remedy. If you prepare juice from fresh potatoes, or from old ones after removing the sprouts very carefully, do not be afraid that the juice could harm you. On the contrary, raw potato juice is well known as a remedy and has helped to cure many a gastric problem.

Raw potato juice is especially good for inflammation of the gastric lining (gastritis). For stomach ulcers drink the juice diluted with warm water first thing in the morning, before breakfast. The juice of one small potato will do. If you find it difficult to drink potato juice because of its not too pleasant taste, add it to a warm oat gruel or soup that has already been cooked. Potato juice, *Gastronol* and a mild, fibre-free diet will cure the most stubborn gastric ulcers, if attention is given to proper mastication and thorough insalivation of the food one eats.

Potato juice is highly alkaline and is a very effective antidote for uric acid conditions such as rheumatism and arthritis. Just remember that care must be taken to remove any solanin-containing sprouts before preparing it.

Papain – its Origin and Uses
In the lush woodlands of Florida there are found not only thousands of cabbage palms and many other tropical plants, but also a great number of wild papayas. The Indians living there have always enjoyed the juicy fruit because it is delicious and healthy. They also made use of the plant in cooking. Since time immemorial those primitive tribes have known that papaya leaves, stems and fruit contain a substance that breaks down protein. So, whenever the hunters happened to kill an old animal the cook would wrap the tough meat in papaya leaves and leave it overnight. On the following day it would be tender enough to be roasted over a fire. The substance which tenderises meat, called papain, causes a kind of predigestion process, one might say.

The handsome papaya plant resembles a small palm and has big leaves similar to those of a fig tree. It grows mostly in the Western hemisphere and is found in Central America, Guatemala and San Salvador, the islands of the Caribbean, in Brazil, even in the jungle, as well as in Florida. If you could visit the sites in the Brazilian jungle where trees are cut for timber or the area is cleared for other purposes, you would be able to make a very interesting observation that almost borders on the miraculous. In the dense forests there are no papayas to be seen anywhere, but shortly after the trees have been felled, papaya plants begin to sprout here and there. I met some Swiss settlers in the area who told me of their surprise at finding papayas growing where not one single plant could be seen in an area of 100–200 square kilometres (about 40–80 square miles) before it was cleared.

Where do these plants suddenly spring from? The answer escaped me for quite a while, but I found it in the end, and it is actually very simple. You see, birds like papaya too and when they find the fruit growing in clearings they swoop down and pick at them, seeds and all. Off they fly again and on the way their droppings, together with the undigested seeds, fall back onto the jungle floor where they remain dormant for ten, twenty, or perhaps even a hundred years or more, the reason being that the dense forest shuts out all sunlight from the earth, and without light they cannot sprout. However, as soon as a clearing is cut in the jungle the sunlight warms the earth, the seeds begin to germinate and within a year, because their growth is very fast indeed, you have a plant the height of a man.

The Indians enjoy eating plenty of papaya where they grow, and the white settlers have noticed this habit and copied it. Eating papaya after a meal makes for better digestion. Food rich in protein will cause no problems if you eat papaya, since papain breaks down protein. Being a good observer, you will soon discover that all those who eat papaya remain free from intestinal worms. In fact, all worms disappear when papaya is taken over a period of time. The seeds are especially effective as a remedy and it is recommended to chew some of them every time you eat the fruit. What is the reason for this desirable effect? Research has shown that papain simply digests the parasites made of protein; it not only helps to digest cheese, meat, eggs, and other protein foods in the digestive tract, but also any intestinal worms that may have settled there. It dissolves their protein organisms and destroys them in a simple and harmless way. Papaya could not be better described than as a simple food and an excellent vermicide. Even amoebas are destroyed by the papain in papaya seed as long as they are still in the intestines and have not settled elsewhere.

Because the ripe papaya fruit is perishable it cannot be transported over long distances. However, it was discovered that the unripe fruit, the stems and the leaves contain more papain than the ripe fruit – and this solved the problem of shipping. Obviously unripe fruits can be transported far more easily. Furthermore, the use of the milky juice which contains the most papain suggested itself. Preparations made with this juice aid the digestion and are useful remedies for the elimination of worms – a widespread problem in many areas of the world.

Papayasan contains papain in combination with the ingredients of the whole plant. It can therefore act in the same way as the whole plant provided by nature and taking it is the equivalent of eating the unripe fruit with its rich papain content.

Every doctor, nature practitioner and pharmacist, as well as every caring mother, will no doubt be glad to know that there is at last a worm medicine that is absolutely safe. According to the third edition of Professor Eichholz's *Pharmakologie (Pharmacology)*, even experts regard the usual worm medicines as risky and far from harmless, for he writes: 'The toxicity of all anthelmintic medicines should prompt the prescriber to consider whether it is preferable to tolerate the presence of parasites, rather than to take the risk of poisoning the patient.' If this is of concern to pharmacologists and pharmacists, how much more should it make the patient think. However, with a papaya preparation no one need fear, for it is beneficial to the digestion, assisting in the assimilation of proteins, and is absolutely harmless – even for pregnant women and people with weak constitutions.

In the short time Papayasan has been available it has helped many hundreds of people, and in the future it will aid thousands more who want to be free from the harm and danger of intestinal worms without any risk of side effects.

Worms are by no means to be taken lightly, whether it is *Oxyuris vermicularis*, the little threadworm that causes an itching irritation in the anus and can be found by the thousands in the large intestine; the ascaris or roundworm inhabiting the small intestine; the *Trichocephalus dispar* (whipworm), or any other intestinal parasites. They are all extremely harmful and can lead to severe disturbances in the composition of the blood, and cause conditions such as eosinophilia, anaemia, chlorosis and liver disorders. The chief factors responsible for these and other serious conditions are no doubt the metabolic toxins secreted by the worms.

The botanical enzymes of Papayasan break down protein and hence dissolve the cuticle of roundworms, threadworms and whip-

447

worms, and with the help of intestinal ferments will completely digest them.

The Therapeutic Effects of Milk

Milk has always been regarded as a remedy, not only as a food. Everyone knows that milk is an excellent source of minerals. It contains magnesium, manganese and many other minerals, including calcium in a form that can be easily assimilated. These minerals are found in a concentrated form in sour whey, the watery liquid that separates from the curd when milk is made into cheese. At the same time, they are improved and enriched through the process of lactic fermentation. The concentrated lactic acid with the milk enzymes, such as contained in *Molkosan*, has antiseptic properties, making Molkosan a good remedy for sore throats, catarrh and even laryngitis.The numerous applications of this valuable remedy are described in greater detail below.

Just as sour whey is a remedy, so is milk on its own and curds or soft skimmed milk cheese. They are each good for certain illnesses. For example, an inflammation of the gallbladder can be quite painful, but a compress of cold, unboiled milk will relieve the pain immediately. The actual inflammation will often subside after a short while and pass faster than with any other medication. Heartburn caused by indigestion, an overacid stomach, is easily neutralised by drinking unboiled milk, and this natural remedy is to be preferred to aluminium silicates. Milk, given in the form of injections, has also been effective in revulsion or stimulation therapies. Soft skimmed milk cheese (quark) has been used in poultices for grazes, bruises and benign swellings for longer than anyone can remember. The application never fails to give good results.

Molkosan (Whey Concentrate)

Although curd packs and several other milk applications are well enough known, whey, the serum of the milk, is the form most frequently used in caring for the sick. Both sweet and sour whey contains most of the milk's mineral nutrients, while cheese, which separates from the whey, is valued chiefly on account of its high protein and fat content. Enzymes, especially rennet used in the manufacture of cheese, doubtlessly play an important part in the therapeutic effects of whey. Milk itself is a wholefood, which implies that it contains all the necessary elements to sustain life. Among these elements are protein, fat, sugar, minerals and trace elements. So whey, the by-product of cheese manufacture, still has considerable nutritional value, actually much more than it was once thought to have. It is, therefore, of little wonder that in former times royalty and the famous from France and other countries made special journeys to Switzerland to take the world-renowned Swiss Whey Cures. Usually the visitors were afflicted with metabolic problems such as obesity, circulatory congestions, intestinal complaints, pancreatic insufficiency and flatulence. Whey cures also rectified conditions of dysbacteria, a complaint that is even more widespread today. Artificial preservatives and food additives, pesticide sprays etc., all contribute to the harm done to the body, which will have to put up a fight against them and their consequences.

Molkosan has helped a great deal in this struggle. If you want to assist the digestion, add a teaspoon or tablespoon of Molkosan to a glass of mineral water and drink this at mealtimes. Of course, you do not have to take mineral water, ordinary water will do just as well.

Molkosan regulates the secretion of gastric acid; it reduces an excess of acid and increases its quantity when there is a lack of it. Molkosan also benefits diabetics because the lactic ferments stimulate the pancreas. Thus, it is without a doubt one of the best drinks these patients could wish for.

Regular use of Molkosan will lower the blood sugar level and, at the same time, reduce the quantity of sugar in the urine. Of course, an appropriate natural diet must be observed too. A little patience is necessary, but after several weeks a positive change for the better will be noticed.

Having an efficient pancreas is important to obese people, as this gland influences the fat metabolism. Regular use of Molkosan will slowly reduce excess weight, especially if *kelp tablets* are taken at the same time. This does not mean, however, that people who are underweight will have to avoid taking whey concentrate, for it regulates the metabolism rather than having a specific catabolic effect. So both underweight and overweight persons will benefit. In short, Molkosan makes for better assimilation of food.

Molkosan can be applied externally with the same success as when it is used internally. It has proved to be more valuable in the treatment of pimples, eczema and cradle cap than many more expensive preparations. For the most part, eczema can be treated by dabbing on undiluted whey concentrate. In cases of skin impurities and blemishes fine results are achieved if Molkosan is

449

both taken internally and applied externally. Where athlete's foot and nail mould have not yet yielded to any other remedy, Molkosan will give quick and reliable relief. Just soak some absorbent cotton in it, bind this on the affected part and leave it on overnight. Dr Devrient of Berlin has confirmed that no other remedy for mycotic diseases is quicker and more reliable than Molkosan whey concentrate. When used to clean minor wounds, scratches and cuts, it is a first-class antiseptic.

For incipient tonsillitis or during the course of this disease, painting the throat with whey concentrate is most helpful. In fact, if it is done in the early stages, it may well prevent the disease altogether, especially when *Lachesis 10x* is taken at the same time.

Many years ago, I drew attention to my experience in the treatment of internal and external carcinomas with whey concentrate. Frequently, the mere swabbing of external cancerous growths and skin cancer has proved very effective. I vividly remember one special case of a cancerous tumour on the calf of the leg. When the surgeon had removed it he told the nurse in attendance that he felt doubtful about the wound ever healing. Still, we swabbed it with Molkosan and, to the surgeon's astonishment, it did heal very well and fast. Other successful cures have been achieved by giving whey concentrate orally and externally and I am happy to say that Dr Kuhl, having made his own experiments, now acknowledges the importance of lactic acid in the treatment of cancer.

Of course, I do not wish to say that such lactic acid preparations are a panacea, a cure-all, but they have certainly brought the treatment of cancer a step further along the road. Because Molkosan has a fairly high percentage of natural lactic acid, it is of immense value in a cancer diet. As a drink, diluted with mineral water, it is both prophylactic and curative in its effect. Dr Kuhl also recommends *raw sauerkraut* for this purpose, because of its lactic acid content.

It is, indeed, a great pleasure to see how the experiences and observations we began to report on in our magazine and books many years ago are now being confirmed as facts.

Once you are familiar with the many good effects of whey concentrate you will appreciate it and stop wondering why, in the past, even high-ranking personages did not consider it beneath their dignity to take 'whey cures' for the benefit of their health.

The Curative Effects of Wheat Germ Oil

In my discussion on wheat and wholegrain bread (see pages 516–9) I highlight the merits of wholegrain products and how the various cereals grown in different parts of the earth are a useful source of food that does not perish easily. It was only a few decades ago when researchers discovered that wheat germ is, in fact, an excellent remedy; this equally applies, of course, to wheat germ oil. Since more and more people are rejecting the use of chemical medicines, physicians, naturopaths and physiotherapists are ever more compelled to turn their attention to remedies that are made from basic materials as nature provides them. Many competent and skilled researchers have been studying the oils contained in cereal germs, and have found that the remedial effects of wheat germ oil are remarkable.

Wheat Germ Oil and its Two Important Elements

Wheat germ oil is high in polyunsaturated fatty acids and these play an important part in the development and maintenance of healthy body cells, as well as in the protein metabolism. They also contribute to the therapeutic solution of the problem of cancer. Polyunsaturated fatty acids, also known as essential fatty acids, promote internal oil oxygenation and, generally speaking, benefit the entire metabolism.

In the second place, wheat germ oil is important because of its valuable vitamin E content, which has also been called the fertility vitamin. Expectant and nursing mothers should take wheat germ oil regularly. Experience has shown that vitamin E is useful in helping to overcome a tendency to premature birth and miscarriage, since a deficiency in this vitamin is often found to be the cause. An extended course of wheat germ oil can help to prevent these unfortunate occurrences.

Furthermore, wheat germ oil can serve as a real help for menopausal problems and scanty, irregular or painful periods, if it is taken for some time. Weak sexual impulses, even impotence, can also be improved or cured if wheat germ oil is taken regularly. Yet this oil is not a stimulant drug, as is the case with preparations made from the African yohimbe tree bark; rather, it strengthens and normalises the functions of the organs in an absolutely natural way. It simply supplies the body with enough vitamin E to keep it functioning normally. For sexual weakness we recommend *A. Vogel's Wheat Germ Oil* or *capsules*; to increase the effect, take *Kelpasan* at the same time.

Heart Trouble and Circulatory Disorders

Wheat germ oil has proved such a good tonic for the heart that its use for this purpose deserves a special mention. The oil is always beneficial for circulatory disturbances in the heart, myocardial insufficiency or disorders, as well as stricture of the coronary vessels and other degenerative heart conditions.

Many people suffer from peripheral circulatory disorders and their consequences, others from circulatory disturbances in the brain, causing a weak memory, fainting spells, vertigo and related complaints. For all these conditions wheat germ oil is a superb remedy, especially when taken in conjunction with *Aesculaforce* and *Ginkgo biloba*, both of which are proven fresh plant preparations. We are certainly glad to have these preparations and wheat germ oil as a welcome natural remedy for many conditions.

Normalising Body Weight – Obesity and Leanness

Wheat germ oil improves the activity of the sex glands and is therefore an excellent help in the fight against obesity. If the treatment is supplemented by the intake of *Kelpasan*, a seaweed preparation, the thyroid and other endocrine glands will also be stimulated. The body weight will be regulated and the general condition of health improved without having to follow a strict diet. Furthermore, it is most gratifying to know that skinny people can normalise their weight with the help of wheat germ oil.

Incidentally, it is marvellous that sufferers from liver and gallbladder disorders can take wheat germ oil very well. My book *The Liver, the Regulator of Your Health* describes a practical liver diet which will benefit such people, especially if it is supplemented by wheat germ oil.

Hypertrophy of the Prostate

For this condition, an enlarged prostate, wheat germ oil has proved most effective, with even better results being achieved when it is taken together with *Sabal serrulata*, which is obtained from a palm that grows in Florida. Experience has shown that this plant remedy causes the enlargement to recede. If wheat germ oil is taken at the same time, its stimulating effect will give the success which *Sabal* alone could not produce. There are, of course, other good remedies for this complaint, and physical therapies are often necessary for a complete cure, but in the initial stages *Sabal* or *Prostasan* together with wheat germ oil capsules will suffice.

Dosage and Duration of Treatment
The normal dosage for adults is one tablespoon of wheat germ oil in the morning, at noon and in the evening. For children it is sufficient to give one teaspoonful three times daily. Wheat germ oil has a strengthening effect and is especially recommended when children and adolescents suffer from tiredness as a result of studying. As a tonic or prophylactic, adults should take one teaspoonful daily. Alternatively, you can take wheat germ oil in soup or in your breakfast muesli.

The duration of the treatment depends entirely upon the individual's needs. Generally speaking, if a vitamin or mineral deficiency is to be rectified, it is necessary to take the medication for several months. When the deficiency has been overcome, it is recommended to continue the treatment by taking half the dosage only, then a quarter, and then slowly phasing it out altogether.

After recovery, if you replace the former deficient diet by one made up of wholefoods, you will be able to manage without having to take any more concentrated vitamin products. However, if you continue to follow the denatured diet of the majority of people today, one including white flour and refined sugar, you will need to supplement it with vitamin preparations. Only in this way will it be possible to avoid a relapse. For this purpose, wheat germ oil is strongly indicated.

A. Vogel's wheat germ oil is a 100 per cent Swiss product and has the advantage of being cold-pressed in modern oil presses. That is why its content of the two main components – vitamin E and polyunsaturated fatty acids – is so high. According to absolutely reliable and objective analysis, it meets with the highest demands of both doctors and consumers.

Vitaforce
Besides the carefully manufactured wheat germ oil, there is also available a fortifying and body-building tonic called *Vitaforce*. This product is especially appreciated by those who have a sensitive liver and wish to use a good food supplement. It is a natural product, whose carefully balanced combination of ingredients is the result of exhaustive research, containing mainly sea buckthorn juice, orange juice, wheat germ and malt extracts, honey, bee pollen and the effective ingredients of a tropical fruit called durian (*Durio zibethinus*). The combination is a concentrated food supplement ideal for fortifying and maintaining the muscle tone and the functions of the sex glands. The effective ingredients of Vitaforce make

it an excellent tonic for all those who work hard, and particularly those who use up more energy than most, such as athletes. The tonic compensates for the high loss of energy.

Honey – its Specific Therapeutic Effect

It is interesting to study how that little wonder, the bee, makes its honey. We marvel, too, at the bee's body and how this small and delicate structure is able to manufacture a substance that would need such cumbersome machinery if done by humans. Then we marvel at the diligent industry of the bee as we watch its flight over the flowering countryside – but these aspects are not what I wish to speak about right now. Our interest, at the moment, lies in the remedial value of honey, which has earned a high mark for itself in natural medicine.

In the ancient world honey was well known and appreciated for its healing properties but as time went on that knowledge fell into oblivion. The rediscovery and scientific explanation of the value of honey, however, has enabled it once more to assume its rightful place among natural remedies.

A doctor wrote in a medical journal about having successfully used honey in the treatment of diphtheria. A 25 per cent addition of honey to another remedy was found to act as an antiseptic and prevented the diphtheria bacilli from propagating.

This experiment is without doubt proof of the fact that honey deserves attention as a folk medicine of long-standing. It is certainly no coincidence that years ago honey was prescribed as a remedy for exactly this disease. In those days, unlike today, there were no effective treatments for diphtheria, and honey, together with other remedies, no doubt was beneficial to the patients and may have helped to save many lives.

As regards natural remedies in general, I am sure that scientific research would find many an old piece of folk wisdom to be true. The Bible's recommendation, 'My son, eat honey, for it is good', is clearly well founded. Honey is indeed good for us because it has healing properties.

Dr Müller asserts that potential carriers of the diphtheria bacillus can render themselves much less dangerous to other people by the systematic consumption of honey. 'Carriers' are those who harbour the micro-organism of a disease but are not necessarily affected by it themselves, although they constitute a potential source of infection for others. Any remedy that eliminates this danger is most welcome.

The effectiveness of honey places it on the list of tried and proven remedial foods and our confidence in it is fully justified, even though there may be some people who cannot take it and have to forgo its goodness.

The Medicinal Value of Honey
There is no doubt that honey and its medicinal value were known as far back as biblical times, as it is mentioned in a number of ancient records. Honey is the best form of carbohydrate and is easily absorbed by the body. What is more, experience has shown that honey increases the medicinal effect of natural remedies that are good for the respiratory organs. If you want to take advantage of this fact, simply add the indicated number of drops of a given remedy to a teaspoon of honey or to warm water sweetened with honey. Sipping this honey water together with the remedies will enhance their effect; for example, in cases of catarrh or disorders of the bronchial tubes or lungs, the prescribed medicines will have a much faster and stronger effect if taken with honey. It is for this reason that the pine bud syrup *Santasapina* contains honey.

Honey Salve – a Healer
Mix a teaspoon of honey with 20–30 drops of *Echinaforce* tincture and you will have a splendid healing salve for grazes, minor wounds and cuts, boils, and even scabs and crusts.

For wounds that are refusing to heal properly, mix some honey with 10 per cent *horseradish*; the horseradish can be finely grated, or use the fresh juice or tincture. Apply this reliable natural remedy to the affected part, and you will be surprised at the good result. This mixture is an excellent remedy for whitlows, nail mould and similar stubborn conditions that suppurate and take a long time to heal.

Treating Arthritis and Gout with Honey Packs
If you suffer from arthritis or gout you will find the external application of honey a great relief. Add one teaspoon of *comfrey tincture* or *Symphosan* to four tablespoons of honey, mix thoroughly in a cup, then heat the mixture in a double saucepan (bain-marie). Fold a cloth three or four times, soak it in the hot honey mixture and apply to the parts where the pain is worst – the hands, elbows, knees and feet. This treatment is best given in the evening, so that you can leave the pack on overnight. In order to retain the heat for longer, place on top of the pack a bag of

cherry stones that have been heated on the stove; a bag of hot hay flowers or camomile will serve the same purpose. Then wrap a warm cloth around everything.

Some patients have been helped by this treatment to the extent that they were once again able to walk or move their hands without feeling any pain. It is worthwhile repeating these honey packs for several weeks until you find relief. If you do not have any herbs at your disposal, honey packs can be made without them. The effect will still be very beneficial, even though it might take longer.

The Wonder Jelly for Queen Bees – Royal Jelly

An Unsolved Mystery

Not everyone knows that a worker bee's busy life is over after twenty-eight working days. Or did you know that the egg cells that normally produce worker bees can, when fed with a special substance develop into queens? There is something mysterious about this wonder of nature. For one thing, the queens are considerably bigger than the other bees, and, what is more, they live sixty times longer. A very special nutritive fluid is collected by the workers for those cells which ultimately produce queens. Although this phenomenon has been the subject of extensive scientific investigation, the understanding of its exact nature still eludes the researchers and only some of the jelly's constituents have been isolated. The ancients perhaps knew more about it than we do, as we frequently find references to 'ambrosia', 'nectar' and other wonder foods in their writings and it is not unreasonable to assume that they were referring to what is now called 'royal jelly'.

Unfortunately, no reference as to how this ambrosia was obtained is to be found, so our assumption must remain speculative. There is no doubt, however, that royal jelly possesses biological qualities of the highest order, for it enables the queen to lay as many as 2,000 eggs daily, and this with a single fertilisation. This is, indeed, a marvellous biological achievement, which stands unrivalled in nature.

Royal Jelly Makes the Headlines

Scientific and popular periodicals have devoted much space to the subject of royal jelly. True, this promotion no doubt has something to do with cleverly disguised advertising, since every manufacturer believes his product to be the best on the market. On the other hand, these efforts demonstrate that today's world needs a biologically safe natural tonic, as opposed to a chemical or synthetic one. No one really knows how the bees manufacture the natural compound. All we can say is that the Creator gave them the necessary instinct to make this complex substance from the raw materials they have available in nature. What they produce proves the truth of the concept that 'Food should be medicine and medicines should be food.'

Some years ago the newspapers reported that the Pope had recovered from a severe illness after his personal physician, Dr Galeazzi, had prescribed royal jelly as a tonic for him. It also was reported that Dr Paul Niehans, an eminent endocrinologist and specialist in live-cell therapy, was of the opinion that royal jelly vitalises the glandular system in a similar way to an injection of fresh endocrine cells. These observations are a strong enough indication that it is indeed appropriate to pay much more attention to royal jelly in the future.

As long ago as in April 1956, at the Second International Biogenetic Congress held in Baden-Baden, Germany, under the chairmanship of Dr Galeazzi, many of the papers presented dealt with the research findings in connection with royal jelly.

Then there were the articles written by Professor Belvefer of Paris, who had been conducting research on royal jelly for decades. It is amazing to read his references to the findings made by a number of researchers, for example the fact that the queen bee is able to lay 300,000–450,000 eggs a year as a result of her feeding on this remarkable nutritive complex. This feat cannot be matched by any other creature on earth.

Further reports explained that royal jelly not only vitalises and rejuvenates through its effect on the endocrine glands, but also successfully combats whooping cough and asthma, especially in children. It has been found that children with a weak constitution soon pick up and have better appetites when given royal jelly. Benefits can also be obtained in cases of bronchitis, migraine, stomach and gallbladder troubles, digestive disorders, bad nerves and the peculiar kind of fatigue resulting from weak functioning of the endocrine glands. These and many other health problems can be improved considerably, if not cured, by taking royal jelly regularly. Moreover, it is maintained that people with a predisposition to cancer will benefit from a regular intake of royal jelly. It is also good for the skin when taken orally and when used for massage. For the latter, dilute some royal jelly with honey and water and massage the solution into the skin.

A Question of Cost
Many people have questioned the cost of royal jelly, since there is no uniformity of price. In the United States it can cost five, six or even ten times as much as it does in Europe, but the price tags on European products can also vary considerably. It is unfortunate that such products are not always honestly priced and, as a consequence, a good natural remedy can become discredited.

Our own *Gelée Royale* is marketed in 10 g (0.353 oz) jars and this quantity gives about a month's treatment. It is also available in the form of ampoules, called *Apiforce*.

Pollen
Every time sensational articles about pollen appeared in newspapers and magazines, the questions would be asked. 'What actually is pollen? Is it a product of the food industry or of nature?'

According to the biblical account of the Creation, pollen existed long before man. The earth had to be thoughtfully prepared for man's existence. For this reason, the plant world had to be made first, then came the animals and finally, man. So pollen existed even before the bees started flying from flower to flower. Pollen contains the male gametes of plants, which are essential to their propagation. Perhaps the wind carried these reproductive cells; otherwise the plants could not have been fertilised or pollinated before the arrival of insects. Today, bees are especially responsible for pollination, together with the wind. We have probably watched these busy insects in their constant activity many times. When bees visit individual flowers with their untiring zeal in gathering nectar, they collect something else at the same time. Their little legs touch the pollen, which in turn sticks to them in tiny grains, making the bees look as if they were wearing tiny yellow pants.

Since beekeepers are usually good observers, it occurred to them to make an experiment of collecting this pollen and feeding it to the bees during inclement weather. The result was that after 8–10 generations the bees that had been given this pollen food had grown bigger, stronger and healthier. They even built larger honeycomb cells. Their tongues had grown longer in relation to their overall size, and this was also an advantage, for these bees were able to obtain the nectar from flowers that ordinary bees were unable to reach.

So the beekeepers were prompted to look at pollen more closely. Experiments were made with mice, giving them a supplement of pollen. This resulted in several benefits. It was noticed that the mice became less susceptible to disease, their fertility increased visibly, their coats became shiny and healthy, and they remained free from skin diseases. The rodents' vitality increased noticeably, and they lived longer. These findings led to a further examination of pollen. An analysis showed pollen to be rich in vitamins and to contain nearly all the minerals and trace elements vital to man and beast.

Tiredness and Low Blood Pressure
Experiments have shown that pollen has a strong action on the human sex glands and, through them, on all the endocrine glands. People who always feel tired and weary are able to get rid of this tiredness by taking a teaspoon of pollen in the morning with their breakfast.

Pollen is excellent for low blood pressure, especially when taken together with seaweed, that is, *kelp*. If one drinks carrot juice in addition, which can be in the condensed form of *Biocarottin*, the unpleasant symptoms of low blood pressure, for example fainting and weakness, will usually be rectified after a short time. People who suffer from low blood pressure are often subject to sexual weakness, too, and therefore a deficiency in the sex glands. As a rule, taking pollen in combination with seaweed preparations can remedy this condition.

High Blood Pressure, Exophthalmic Goitre, Metabolic Disorders
If the blood pressure is too high, it is not advisable to take pollen. A necessary precaution would be, first of all, to bring down the pressure by eating a natural diet of whole rice, soft white cheese (cottage cheese or quark) and salads. This diet is described in detail on pages 128–9. Only when the blood pressure has been normalised can a person start taking pollen.

Those who have exophthalmic goitre, that is to say, a hyperfunction of the thyroid, should take pollen only after the functional disorder has been eliminated.

On the other hand, metabolic disorders such as constipation and diarrhoea can benefit from treatment with pollen.

Mental Strain
Those who do taxing mental work find bee pollen to be an extremely simple and natural energy food. With its help they are able to stand up to the intensity of their work for longer and feel less tired. In today's hustle and bustle of everyday life pollen is a

welcome food supplement, providing the help needed when great demands are made on one's mental capacity.

Not all the active substances of pollen have yet been discovered, but those that have been isolated, as experience has shown, are cause enough to recommend this natural product to everyone who lives a modern life.

Bee pollen, being very rich in vitamins and containing almost all known minerals and trace elements, has become a popular energy booster. Since nature provides us with this wonderful tonic food, we should prefer it to artificial or chemical products every time.

The Curative Properties of Chicken and Chicken Fat

The following story confirms the efficacy of an old natural remedy. A French-Swiss woman tried to lift a heavy pot of boiling water from the fire and, in doing so, slipped. She sustained scalds and second- and third-degree burns over a considerable area of her body, including the neck and chest. According to the doctor, her life was in danger. Fortunately, her husband remembered his mother's treatment for burns and scalds. She always used raw chicken fat. So, as fast as he could, he got some fresh chicken fat and proceeded to spread it liberally over the parts of the body that had been scalded. Before long, the burning pain was relieved and his wife calmed down, being able to sleep that same night. Within a few days the pain had completely gone and new skin was beginning to form over the scalded areas.

As I have already mentioned, fresh chicken fat is an old natural remedy and, next to *St John's wort oil*, one of the best treatments there is for severe burns and scalds.

And here is another experience with chicken fat which is just as interesting. In a lonely farmstead a young man hurt himself badly while felling a tree. The axe went right into his knee and cracked the knee cap. He dragged himself to the house with difficulty. There was no doctor for miles around and, of course, there was no such thing as a telephone. His father could not think what to do. Meanwhile, the boy's leg had become very swollen and discoloured. The lymph glands in the groin became swollen and painful. Blood poisoning had already set in. His mother then remembered that her grandmother had always used chicken fat in cases of blood poisoning. So she killed several chickens and spread the raw fat on the whole leg as thickly as possible.

The doctor, whom the family finally succeeded in contacting, could only come the following morning. As an experienced travelling country doctor, he did not consider the chicken fat treatment strange and appeared well satisfied with the young man's condition. He took the patient with him to the hospital for surgical treatment and in a short time the leg was completely healed. The mother was convinced that she had saved her boy's life by rubbing on the fat as soon as the blood poisoning became evident.

Some doctors may smile or scoff when reading about such simple natural remedies. However, they should not forget that these remedies have been known and used for hundreds of years and have outlasted many a modern chemical drug. These natural treatments are always near at hand and invariably provide help when other remedies fail. They will continue to do so long after many of the present-day products of the pharmaceutical industry have been discarded and forgotten.

Chicken as a Styptic

No less interesting is the story I heard from a Berlin doctor who was attached to the famous hospital 'Charité'. A person suffering from haemophilia had to have a minor operation and the doctors were worried about stopping the bleeding. A peasant who was a patient in the hospital happened to hear of their anxiety and when one of the doctors was making his rounds, he told him in his blunt rustic way that he knew of something that would stop the bleeding and was better than all the strong-smelling ointments in the hospital.

The doctor, who had formerly been a country practitioner for many years and had often obtained valuable information from his patients, did not ignore such words but asked, 'Well, what would you say was good for stopping bleeding?'

'Chicken would help, Doc, but it must be put on absolutely fresh and warm,' replied the peasant, and the conversation ended there.

However, the doctor did obtain a chicken before the operation, although perhaps more out of curiosity as to what would happen if he actually used it. After collodion treatment and everything else had failed to stop the bleeding, as a last resort, he cut a piece from the chicken and laid it while still warm on the patient's small incision, which was still bleeding. As if by magic, before the unbelieving eyes of the other doctors, the bleeding stopped.

Red Slug Syrup (*Arion rufus*)

When suffering from a serious condition, and everything else has been tried without success, red slug syrup, however unattractive it may sound, should be given a chance. Extraordinary results have been achieved with this syrup in the treatment of diseases where bacteria or bacilli play a part, for example ulcers, gastric ulcers and pulmonary infections.

Its preparation is quite simple. Place a layer of the large red forest slugs (*Arion rufus*) in a jar, cover with a layer of sugar, then add further layers of slugs and sugar until the jar is full. The minimum quantity of sugar should be about the same weight as the slugs, although you can use a little more.

After a short time the sugar begins to dissolve the slugs. On the second day, strain everything through a sieve. Then add a third part of alcohol, that is, one-third of the whole weight of the mixture. The remedy is then ready. (The residue in the strainer is of no further use and can be disposed of.) A tablespoon, or in serious cases a liqueur glass of the syrup, should be taken every morning before breakfast. The curative effect of this syrup is so extraordinary that even doctors who have experimented with it are simply amazed.

Although the preparation and perhaps even the mere idea of slug syrup may seem repugnant, such feelings can be disregarded when grave necessity arises. Farmers, who are less fussy about such things, are often pleased to avail themselves of this remedy. One young farmer who had stomach ulcers and was spitting blood had found no relief from chemical and natural remedies. He consented to take the slug syrup, this repulsive-sounding remedy, with the result that he recovered and today is once more able to look after the family farm.

Another report tells of a man who was suffering from some form of lung disease. The doctors had despaired of curing him. He too tried the slug syrup and is now quite well again. Many other successful examples prove that it is better to take a remedy, the thought of which may be repugnant, than to accept defeat in matters of health and perhaps even die as a result of neglect.

Of course, if you do not know what the syrup is made of you will not worry, for it does not have an unpleasant taste at all.

I would like to make one final observation. Cases of chronic bronchial catarrh can also be treated successfully with slug syrup, even if it has not responded to other medicines. Remember, however, when you buy the ready-made syrup, to make sure it is actually made from slugs.

Questions of Nutrition

Natural Wholefood

It is certainly difficult for a housewife to feed her family along scientific lines, for even an expert in the field of nutrition would find it a problem. In fact, what should you eat so that the body obtains all the nutrients, minerals, vitamins and trace elements for it to be adequately nourished? Who can dare to say that he knows what our individual requirements really are? Is it not true to say that every year, every decade, new discoveries are made in the field of nutrition? In fifty or a hundred years from now, if we could look back at the things we now think of as necessities for our bodies, we would probably be surprised at our ignorance of the elements which make up a healthy diet.

How much simpler it would be if man could accept the idea that a wise Creator has provided everything that is necessary including our food, in nature. If we look upon our food as something prepared for us by Him, for our well-being, then we will know we have at our disposal all the known and unknown nutritive elements we need. Being in their right proportions, they will contribute all that our bodies require. Primitive peoples are more sensible than we are in this respect. They take their food just as it grows and prepare it very simply, thus preserving its nutritive value. Does that not give our ailing society cause to think on these things?

New drugs are being discovered every day, yet we do not see a decline in the overall incidence of disease. On the contrary, certain diseases are becoming more prevalent, especially those that are connected with the metabolism of the cells and the central nervous system. Among the most notable are cancer and multiple sclerosis. Yet those two diseases are practically unknown among the natives of various so-called 'uncivilised' areas of the world. It is noteworthy, then, that degenerative changes in the cells, as they occur in cancer and multiple sclerosis, are chiefly restricted to the people who live in 'civilised societies'. Moreover, it is only in the industrial world that many infectious diseases are rampant, where refined food has weakened the people. Interestingly, more primitive people living near industrialised communities are not affected by many of their neighbours' diseases, even though the causative agents could attack them just as well. I am referring especially to multiple sclerosis, although here is as yet no conclusive evidence that it is caused by micro-organisms. But similar diseases cannot gain a foothold among such people either, simply because they live more naturally and therefore have sufficient resistance to germs and other causes of disease.

Nothing but wholefood offers real sustenance and protection and this is shown by the example we have in whole rice. Everything offered by nature consists of an integral whole and if only a fraction of it is removed, whatever it maybe, we are deprived of something that would otherwise provide us with complete nutrition. The Creator meant cereal to be a complete formula and to benefit fully from it we should prepare our food from the whole grain.

Whole Rice (Brown Rice)
Let us look at a rice grain. The inner kernel, the endosperm, consists mainly of starch, as is the case with all other grains, for example wheat and barley. From this we get white flour. Starch is a carbohydrate, and supplies energy, without which we cannot live. That is why it would be unwise to throw away the starch and use only the bran, for example, because the proportion in which starch is associated with the others substances contained in the grain is intimately related to the needs of our bodies. The proportion matches the correct formula. To meddle with it would be equivalent to altering the proportions of the ingredients of a perfect recipe, the one our wise Creator provided for our benefit and that of other animals.

Besides the starch, the grain contains bran. This, in turn, is made up of layers of gluten, various minerals and trace elements. Research has shown that only the most minute amounts of these trace elements are required, yet if they are missing altogether, the various functions of the system begin to suffer. These known and unknown trace elements are found in the outer layers of the grain, the bran.

Another vital part of the grain is the germ. Fats, proteins, phosphates and valuable vitamins are found in it. Of particular importance is the vitamin E in the germ, because it regulates the functions of the sex glands.

There is yet something else in the grain, cellulose, and some may argue that we can do without this outer preservative layer that envelops each grain as if with a fine cellophane film. True, it is indigestible and cannot be assimilated, but its action is nevertheless a necessary one for the intestinal tract. It cleanses its lining, which is studded with villi, tiny microscopic processes that assist assimilation. These hair-like processes are apt to become clogged up if the food ingested consists of too much material lacking in roughage. It is here that the cellulose-containing bran or fibre, comes in. Its particles scrape along the intestinal walls, cleaning away the filmy adhesions and at the same time stimulating peristalsis, the wave-like contractions of the intestines that press their contents onward and so prevent constipation. In fact, if everyone ate natural wholefoods, containing starch, minerals, nutrients and roughage in the right proportions, no one would suffer from poor digestion or constipation.

The importance of the bran and germ of the rice grain was drastically demonstrated when people in the Orient began to copy those in the West by refining their staple food, their rice. A disease known as beriberi became rife among them and after all the known medicines had been thrown into the combat against the disease without success, a colonial doctor, Dr Eijkman, as well as other researchers, discovered that rice bran alone was able to cure the scourge. This definitely established the fact that beriberi was a deficiency disease, an avitaminosis, not an infectious disease as had been thought previously.

Fortunately, our Western diet is much more varied than that of the Oriental nations and such pronounced deficiencies rarely occur. If our diet lacks one substance or another, the deficiency can usually be compensated for, at least partly, by the substances contained in other foods we eat. However, it is only a partial compensation and we still often suffer from an imbalance in our food intake, as will be discussed in a later section. Many people in the Orient suffered the sad consequences of beriberi, but as soon as they began to take food supplements or returned to their former way of preparing whole rice, their health was restored.

This experience provides a strong argument in favour of changing over to whole cereals, including whole wheat and whole rye. It is incomprehensible how students who have seen films or experiments showing what happens to pigeons when they are fed on refined rice can continue to eat the very food that is responsible for such devastating results. They seem blind and thoughtless in the face of the evidence. Why spend time and effort in tireless research if the findings continue to be ignored by the consumer? Is it not strange that the consumer often prefers to take the consequences and become sick, rather than make a change in his diet?

Remember that natural rice, also known as unpolished, whole or brown rice, contains nine and a half times more minerals than the polished, refined kind. It is these minerals that are of vital importance to us. Observations have shown that whole rice contains substances that keep the blood vessels elastic for much longer and it is for this reason that Asians seldom suffer from hardening of the arteries and high blood pressure.

Whole or brown rice should be prepared in the same way as refined rice, only do not pour away the rice water. The rice should be soaked in as much water as it is able to absorb and cooked in as little water as it requires to soften without the grains sticking together. Then the nutritional elements will not be wasted or lost. Brown rice can be served in a number of ways, and many Chinese and Middle Eastern recipes are excellent for this purpose.

What about the Wheat Grain?
What I said about the rice grain also applies to the wheat kernel. Its valuable constituents are to be found, not in the inner part, but in the outer one, the bran. Like rice, the wheat grain should be used in its entirety, ground coarsely as wholewheat flour or flakes. Groats, coarse meal, are especially suitable for soups, rissole mixes, bread and biscuits. If you have no rough-grinding mill to make you own wholewheat flour, soak the wheat overnight and then put the soft, swollen kernels through the mincer.

This flaky wheat can be added to your muesli. Of course, you can use *Vogel's Wheat Bran and Germ* instead. According to taste, sweeten the muesli with raisins or sultanas, putting these through the mincer together with the soaked wheat. The raisins will give you natural sugar. You see how easy it is to prepare a delicious muesli! Add some honey, perhaps some finely ground almonds or almond purée and a variety of fruit according to what is in season. Berries are an ideal addition. If you tend to suffer from constipation, mix some soaked linseed into the muesli to encourage the bowel function.

A high-energy food can be obtained by keeping the wheat moist and warm so it can germinate. According to the temperature, the wheat takes about two or three days before it begins to sprout; then use the sprouted wheat in the same way you would the ungerminated kernels. Germinated wheat is good for the blood and is a tonic for the whole body. Let the sprouts grow 2–5 mm (up to about ¼ inch) long, but remember to put the grains in a warm place so that they are encouraged to germinate. Do not add more water than the grains can soak up. On the other hand, instead of soaking the wheat in water, you could spread it on a wet cloth; the sprouts will then be greenish in colour. These green sprouts are necessary for people suffering from anaemia, who need chlorophyll.

Bread and cakes can also be made with germinated wheat, or rye, barley, or any other cereal. Bread and muesli prepared in this way are far more nourishing than anything made from flour that has been stored, and that you may have to store even longer before use. The oxygen in the air is harmless as long as the grain remains whole, but as soon as it is milled into flour it begins to destroy many important nutrients, especially the highly active ferments. If used fresh, and if possible germinated, the goodness of the whole grain is available to us. A more detailed account of the uses and benefits of germinated wheat is given on pages 520–21.

So, if you eat wheat raw, either in muesli or using any other method of preparation, you will have at your disposal an energy food that contains all the important vitamins and minerals of the grain in their complete and unchanged form.

It is amazing to see the effect of such a wholefood on sick people. They derive infinitely greater benefits from it than from the most expensive remedies. Natural food is without doubt the best medicine for every nature-oriented person.

Vegetables and Herbs

If you want healthy vegetables they must be grown organically. They depend upon the soil in which they are grown and for the soil to be healthy it must be worked and looked after properly. If you live in the country, take advantage of the various edible plants growing wild in the woods and fields. You will find wild spinach and many other wild vegetables, all tasty and nutritious. Do not neglect to gather and eat them. *Bear's garlic (ramsons)*, for example, is a prized vegetable, one of the best blood-purifying plants there is, and it should be gathered and eaten in the spring. It regenerates the blood vessels, and lowers and normalises blood pressure. The blood pressure problems that often accompany old age, brought on by the loss of elasticity of the arteries, can be effectively counteracted with brown rice, bear's garlic and mistletoe tea, if taken on a regular basis. Young *nettles*, finely chopped and mixed in with salads or steamed like spinach, are also very good for the blood.

Dandelion salad, which is rich in vitamins, cleanses, stimulates and assists the liver to do its job. Every spring this delicious salad should be on the table. If you have a garden you can grow your own dandelions. Dig up some roots and plant them in a trench, fill in with compost, forest soil or peat and then dress the top with a layer of pine needles, if available. The roots will soon begin to sprout and the shoots will show their tender green tips. Then remove the pine-needle dressing or peat, cut the shoots as far as the roots, put the cover back on again and leave to sprout anew. This method will give you fresh dandelion leaves for an extended period, in fact, until well into the summer – and if you are blessed with 'green fingers' you will be able to obtain a continuous supply throughout the growing season.

Watercress is often found growing wild too. As it is rich in iodine, it will benefit your thyroid and all the other endocrine glands, the hormone glands. The iodine in watercress is present in the right amount and combination with other substances. If you have thyroid problems, such as palpitations, oversensitivity to every little influence, or enlargement of the gland itself, you should definitely eat watercress on a regular basis. You will find it a marvellous remedy if you lack vitality and are always listless and tired, symptoms that are usually caused by the poor function of the endocrine glands.

It is also good to add a little *yarrow*, finely chopped, to your salads, but do not overdo it. You can mix it in with your salad dressing, giving it a delicate, slightly bitter flavour. This is most effective for treating the venous system. It would not be a bad idea to mix in a few leaves or flowers of *St John's wort* as well. As we have said before, natural food is remedial at the same time.

In cases of circulatory disturbances, if the veins are responsible, yarrow and St John's wort can be used with good results. Piles benefit too. All these medicinal plants are easily collected from meadows free from chemical fertilisers, unpolluted waysides and even near the garden fence. Even if you are not troubled by any ailments, these plants should be used as a means of preventing disease, thus avoiding the subsequent need to cure one.

Anyone who suffers constantly from respiratory problems, catarrh and sore throats, should take a little *ribwort*, chop it up

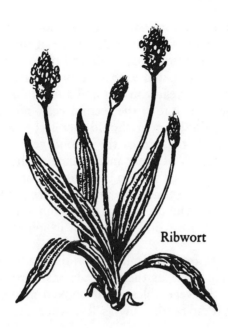

Ribwort

finely and mix it in a salad dressing. When finely chopped, the herb is absorbed in the dressing but still enhances the medicinal value of the salad.

All these herbs are rich in minerals and vitamins. They are beneficial to our health even though used in small quantities.

If you have a garden, the cultivation of culinary herbs such as savory, tarragon, thyme, marjoram, lovage and many others will be found most rewarding. Their effect on the system is second to none.

Further information on these and other herbs can be found in the sections on 'Medicinal Herbs' (pages 338–81) and 'Seasonings' (404–16).

Fertilising and Conditioning the Soil
If you work your own garden, any manure you use should be organic. Compost, bone meal, hoof and horn meal and forest soil can all be used for soil improvement. According to your soil's particular need, if it is loamy or peaty, it may require stone meal. All these natural materials are appropriate for organic fertilising. Strong chemical or artificial fertilisers should be avoided at all costs. The keeping quality and the flavour of produce grown in organic soil are vastly superior to that of produce grown in soil treated with inorganic fertilisers.

If you have liquid manure and dung at your disposal, do not spread it directly on the soil but incorporate it into compost to improve its quality. The compost heap will mature more quickly if layers of dung are alternated with yarrow or pine needles in its construction. In the first year you can add animal dung and liquid manure to the compost. But in the second year, no new material should be added to the heap; it should merely be turned over to let the air get to it. At the end of the second year you will have valuable compost that is of great importance to the plants. Vegetables that require nitrogen will do better if the compost has bone meal added to it, while legumes like peas and string beans, as well as roots and vegetables that are rich in potassium, grow better with wood ash compost, since wood ash is rich in minerals, including potassium.

If we are to benefit from the minerals in the plants we grow we should avoid boiling them, as the minerals pass into the water. It is better to steam the vegetables or, if cooked in water, use the bare minimum so that hardly any is left when the cooking has been completed.

GREEN MANURE

For years now I have no longer simply dug or turned over the garden or a field and spread the manure over the soil, in other words, applied a top-dressing. Rather, I cover the manured soil with grass, carrot tops or other vegetable waste, so that the organic manure, such as compost, cannot be dried out by the sun. I plant seedlings with a dipper, then spread freshly cut grass around them, about 1 cm (about ½ inch) thick. This top-dressing, or cover, is renewed after about three months when the soil is still moist, the bacteria have multiplied and the plants have grown much faster than when treated the usual way. This method has also given good results with berry bushes and shrubs. However, you must take care that the grass or weeds used are still young; do not use them when they contain ripe seeds.

This green manure will make hoeing unnecessary. And since any germinating seeds under the green cover will suffocate and die, weeds will not be able to grow.

CALCIFIED SEAWEED

If you would like to enrich your soil with valuable trace elements from the sea, spread it with calcified seaweed (seaweed lime) from time to time. The soil will then receive potassium bound to iodine.

It has been observed that plants given calcified seaweed are much healthier and less susceptible to mould and similar diseases.

Raw Vegetables and Vegetable Juices
Raw vegetables possess greater therapeutic value than cooked ones. Deficient digestion and assimilation require raw juices. Cabbage juice (green or white cabbage), for example, will improve and often cure such conditions as arthritis, stomach ulcers and metabolic disturbances. Raw potato juice is another superb remedy for stomach ulcers and is most effective when taken in combination with cabbage juice. If you cannot take raw vegetable juices neat or diluted with warm water, you might like to try adding them to soup (vegetable, oatmeal or barley) immediately before serving. Most people find this idea more appealing, apart from the fact that juices usually enhance the flavour. While not everyone is keen on soup, in this case it is a useful means of taking the vegetable juices. You can also add a little raw juice to cooked vegetables or a gruel. Boiled cabbage frequently causes indigestion or flatulence, while raw cabbage, taken finely grated or as juice, will create no such consequences. White cabbage can be made into sauerkraut, another perfect medicinal food, which should be eaten raw, if possible, in order to retain its full value. The cabbage family is rich in calcium and anyone suffering from calcium deficiency should eat plenty of cabbage, including sauerkraut, as a simple and inexpensive source of this mineral.

Although juices are good for us, they should not be enjoyed to the exclusion of anything else; our digestive tract also requires cellulose, roughage, if it is to remain in proper working order. Juices are potent and should not be taken in excessive quantities over long periods of time. After a course of juices, go back to eating the whole vegetables. Raw vegetables demand good teeth and should be thoroughly masticated and properly insalivated to promote the digestive process. The fibres must be broken down if they are to release their nutrients. If your teeth are bad, grate the vegetables or put them through a mincer or blender. The reason why many people do not tolerate raw vegetables is not that they are indigestible, but that they have not been properly masticated and insalivated. Fruit juices and vegetable juices should be well mixed with saliva and not just swallowed. Acid fruit juices need to be neutralised by the alkaline saliva before they reach the stomach. Vegetable juices are more easily tolerated than fruit juices, and even liver patients or people who have a sensitive liver or suffer

471

from kidney trouble have little difficulty in digesting them. Particularly recommended are juices that have gone through a process of lactic fermentation; they also keep better. For further advice on raw fruit and vegetable juices, please read the sections on pages 495–9.

A Good Natural Diet

A good natural diet consists partly of cooked and partly of raw foods. For very serious diseases such as cancer a raw food diet works wonders and is often the only measure that will get to the root of these pathological problems.

The patient who has lost the ability to digest and assimilate his food should begin the diet with juices, then start taking small amounts of finely grated raw vegetables and fruit. Gradually, the quantity is increased until he is able to eat the foods in their natural raw state.

If there is no need to change over to a diet made up entirely of raw food, it would still be beneficial to incorporate small quantities in your daily menus.

Vegetables and fruits should not be served at the same meal, but taken separately, as breaking this rule will mean you are likely to be bothered with flatulence. This important rule is explained in greater detail on pages 493–5.

On the other hand, in spite of contrary opinions, cereals, organically grown and stone ground if possible, are good companions to both fruit and vegetable dishes.

Milk

When milk is uncontaminated and pure, it is a valuable food, providing protein and fat. However, since there are many sick cows and the main causes of sickness are tuberculosis and brucellosis, milk – especially unboiled, raw milk – cannot be recommended without reservation. In cases of cancer, arthritis and many other serious illnesses, it is better to avoid milk altogether. Then there is the question of whether one should drink it fresh or sour. Some say one thing, some another. There is obviously more nourishment in fresh, untreated milk direct from the cow. Sour milk has lost the lactose which, through fermentation, has been transformed into lactic acid, but it is nevertheless easier to digest and more beneficial to the intestinal flora, which it regenerates. From this it will be seen that both kinds of milk have their advantages, whether fresh or sour, or as yogurt, even though the substances contained in them may vary.

More advice on how we can gain the many benefits of milk is given in a later section (see pages 536–40).

Eggs

Eggs should come from healthy, naturally fed, free-running (free range) poultry, if at all possible. When eaten raw, they are more wholesome than any other way. However, since it is quite possible that eggs contain hazardous bacteria, great care should be taken in choosing one's supplier. Sick chickens usually carry these bacteria and can transmit them through their eggs. Duck eggs are known as carriers of the paratyphoid bacillus, although the birds themselves may appear to be quite healthy. For this reason, be especially careful with duck eggs.

Nevertheless, eggs are rich in lecithin, which is a valuable nerve food. Raw egg stimulates the flow of bile. Healthy eggs can be beaten raw into soup before serving, or mixed with honey or some other natural sugar and eaten in this way. Eggs are also rich in protein, especially the yolk, although most people make the mistake of assuming that the protein is found chiefly in the egg white.

Eggs do, however, have the disadvantage of causing the formation of uric acid. This gives rise to the release of sulphuric acid, which can be noticed on the breath after one has eaten boiled eggs. For this reason, people with arthritis, rheumatism or cancer should abstain from eggs in all forms. Yet again this example goes to show that it is always necessary to consider whether any food can be eaten without detriment, or whether it should be avoided altogether. Fruit and vegetables, however, are always recommended, provided one's digestive system tolerates them and the bowels do not react adversely, producing flatulence.

Avoiding Fruit Sprayed with Pesticides

When you buy fruit, make sure that it has not been sprayed with pesticides. Traces of lead, arsenic and other chemicals pose health hazards and will make the fruit inedible. Eating sprayed fruit need not necessarily bring on an acute case of poisoning, but chemical pesticides may have a cumulative effect and continuous doses, however small, can, sooner or later, lead to the development of pathological conditions (see also pages 557–60).

In any case, fruit purchased at the market should always be properly cleaned and it is a good idea to peel it if spray spots can

473

be seen. Many orchards are sprayed with chemicals to which has been added a substance with a special adhesive property so that the rain cannot wash the spray off the fruit. It is true, however, that by peeling the fruit you will lose valuable elements that are found in and under the skin, so it would be much better still to be discriminating when buying your fruit and to look for organically grown produce. If you have fruit trees of your own, make sure that no hazardous sprays are used.

Spices and Seasonings

It is best to avoid nutmeg, pepper and other hot spices and use safe and wholesome seasonings and herbs instead. Yeast extract, especially pure culture yeast extract, can be recommended since it is natural. Pure culture yeast extract contains the vitamin B complex and is about the best seasoning you can use. It is good as a sandwich spread or dissolved in warm water and added to soups and stews as a liquid seasoning. But it should never be boiled, in order to preserve its ingredients.

By now it should be self-evident to every reader that, as our daily bread nothing but crispbread, coarse-grained wholewheat (wholemeal) bread, in other words, bread made from *flour of the whole grain*, should be on our table.

The body will react favourably to natural foods prepared with skill and left in their natural state. Various ailments will disappear without the need for medication of any sort if we feed our bodies in the proper manner. Only natural food, wholefood, contains the elements we need to keep our bodies healthy and in a balanced condition, as it provides all the necessary known and unknown nutritive factors. One does not have to be a dietician to realise that the 'divine formula' embodied in every fruit of the earth cannot possibly be improved upon by man if it is to remain health-promoting. We benefit fully from the food provided only if we eat it in its natural form. If we reflect on the unhealthy state of mankind in the civilised world, we must conclude that man apparently throught himself wiser than the Creator by changing, refining and otherwise adulterating the food that was offered to him in the most perfect condition possible. So then, back to natural wholefood!

Helpful Diets for the Sick

A Low-Protein Diet

A low-protein diet is of paramount importance in treating all metabolic and digestive disturbances, high blood pressure, arthritis, rheumatism and gout, and should be adopted for some time. Protein is found chiefly in meat, eggs, cheese, milk and milk products, peas, beans and lentils, so vegetarians should reduce the intake of milk products and pulses (legumes). People who have previously enjoyed a mixed diet ought to refrain from eating pork, sausages and cold meats and restrict the diet to veal, beef, lamb and mutton.

Eggs and cheese and dishes prepared from them should also be avoided. But if you must eat eggs, have a limited amount and eat them raw. They can be beaten and added to cooked soup. Since eggs produce a great amount of uric acid, sufferers from arthritis are better off without them. Women troubled by insufficiency of the ovaries may eat raw eggs in moderate quantities.

Those who like cheese should restrict their intake and then only eat the mild types, along with vegetables, for their midday meal. Soft white cheese (curds, cottage cheese or quark) is much better than hard cheese, because it has none of the drawbacks of other high-protein foods and assists the function of the liver – a fact of which all liver patients should take note.

Avoid eating high-protein foods in the evening because they are usually the cause of restless sleep. Heavy food is more appropriate for the midday meal, as it generally requires longer periods for digestion than breakfast or tea would allow. If a heavy meal is eaten at night, the digestive system will not be able to cope so easily with the demand placed on it.

Avoid Fried and All Denatured, Refined Food

Fried foods have no place at all in a liver diet, or where a person has a sensitive liver. Of all fats, only fresh butter or a good vegetable margarine is permissible, or a little unrefined oil. Although vegetable oil may be better tolerated when used for frying, it is to be avoided in more serious cases of illness.

To complement a proper diet and support any treatment you may be taking for the good of your health, you would do well to cut out all white flour and refined sugar products, also all canned food and any other refined and denatured food items.

Suggestions for a Health Diet
In planning a healthy diet, the following suggestions should provide some useful guidance.

BREAKFAST

For breakfast to be nourishing and wholesome, the ideal foundation is muesli with apples or other seasonal fruit. Add nuts and wholegrain flakes to enrich it further. A highly nutritive addition is whole wheat, first soaked and then put through the mincer. Raisins or sultanas can be mixed with the wheat before it is minced; these are excellent for the blood. A level tablespoon of ground linseed may also be added if constipation is a problem. Use honey or grape sugar to sweeten.

Crispbread, wholewheat or whole grain bread (for example *Vogel's Whole Grain Flake Bread*) with a little butter, honey or rose hip conserve can follow the muesli. If you like, sprinkle some wheat germ on the bread or over the muesli.

For a drink, make a cup of rose hip tea sweetened with honey or grape sugar. If desired, top the tea with a little cream or even less milk. Cream is better than milk because it contains fat but little protein, although liver patients will find milk or almond milk more tolerable. For a change, you might try some cereal coffee.

These suggestions give you an idea of how to plan your breakfast according to the season and the availability of fruit, as well as your own preferences.

An occasional fruit juice breakfast is beneficial, and grape, orange or grapefruit juice can be recommended. Grapefruit juice is especially good because it stimulates the kidneys, the liver and the entire glandular system.

In cases of impaired liver function take 100–200 ml (about 4–8 fl. oz) of pure, raw carrot juice and a slice of buttered crispbread sprinkled with wheat germ, rather than sweet fruit dishes such as fruit salad with citrus fruits. Muesli with apples is permissible too. If this does not satisfy you, sandwiches as described under 'Supper' can supplement your breakfast.

MIDDAY MEAL

Depending upon the time of year, a great variety of salads may be served. The dressing may be prepared with lemon or *Molkosan* (whey concentrate), which is a great aid to digestion, but never use vinegar. Another tasty dressing can be made with sour cream or yoghurt, and herbs such as savory, marjoram and thyme may be added to give a zesty flavour. Every kind of cabbage is good, but it is best eaten raw as a salad, because cooked cabbage can easily cause flatulence. Cabbage salad (coleslaw) is not only well tolerated, but is also very tasty, healthy and nutritive.

Then you might have vegetables which, when steamed, should not cause fermentation and flatulence.

A third category, food containing starch, or carbohydrates, should also be on the menu. From a dietetic point of view, whole rice is the best choice. It has a good effect on the blood pressure, helping to normalise it and to regenerate the veins. For variation, substitute potatoes, either boiled in their skins or baked. Of course, they can also be served in other ways, but they can harm the liver when fried so this method should be avoided.

Whole wheat also provides an ideal dish and should be prepared in the same way as rice. Instead of a risotto you would then get a 'wheatotto', so to speak. Other good carbohydrate foods containing nutritive salts are millet and buckwheat.

If you like soup, choose a vegetable soup, but only mildly seasoned. Meat soups are not particularly healthy for they promote the formation of uric acid in the system. Vegetable soups, on the other hand, are very beneficial for those who suffer from arthritis. Before you sit down to eat the soup, add some fresh herbs and raw vegetable juices. And if you do not like raw vegetables prepared as a salad, they too can be added to soup, finely chopped or grated. Finely chopped nettles, bear's garlic (ramsons) and other herbs will improve both the nutritive value and the taste of the soup.

For those who like meat, beef or veal may be added to whatever dish they have chosen, but this should be considered as just a small addition to the main meal, for it is best to restrict oneself to a minimum of the protein-containing foods.

A sweet course or dessert has no place in a health diet because it encourages fermentation, that is, flatulence. If you cannot overcome your desire for fruit or some other naturally sweet food after a meal, postpone indulging in your fancy until at least 4 p.m. It is better, however, not to make a habit of such snacks between meals because it is always better to eat a little rather than a lot. A small amount of nutritious food goes a long way towards good health. Eating slowly and thorough insalivation will enable you to obtain the maximum value from whatever you eat; it prevents the pancreas from being overburdened and the formation of intestinal gases.

For your midday meal, instead of soup, you may substitute vegetable juices or natural unsweetened yoghurt. Sugar does not go well with the lactic acid in yoghurt, as it causes fermentation. If you wish to increase your weight, by all means take soup, but if you tend to be overweight and wish to reduce your weight, you would do better to go without it.

EVENING MEAL (SUPPER)

I prefer to call the evening meal 'supper' rather than 'dinner' because it should be a light meal rather than a heavy main one. Nor should it be eaten too late at night. A light meal will be well digested before it is time to go to bed. Supper may be the same as breakfast, but it does not have to consist of sweet food and fruit, although a fruit salad makes a pleasant change, especially if served with any of the whole cereal flakes or corn flakes. A good and inexpensive mixture is one made with ordinary oat flakes, currants or raisins and chopped nuts.

Be careful to use nuts sparingly at the end of the day. True, they are nourishing, but are intended for moderate consumption. Pine kernels make a pleasant change from walnuts and are tasty and nutritive. Crispbread and wholegrain (wholewheat) bread with a little butter or a good vegetable margarine go well with fruit salad, but if you have a problem with your liver, consider using honey or raw rose hip purée instead of fat.

As a change from fruit, a meal of sandwiches and salad can be very enjoyable. If you wish to drink something with it, have some cereal and fruit coffee (*Bambu Coffee Substitute*) with a little cream or milk. Liver patients should have a glass of carrot juice instead. For variety's sake you might have a good vegetable soup.

Sandwiches: You can use your imagination to create quite a variety of sandwiches. Serve wholegrain (wholewheat) bread or crispbread, lightly spread with butter, then perhaps just a touch of vegetable extract such as *Herbaforce* or a yeast extract. A variety of fillings can be used, such as curds or cottage cheese mixed with chives or some other culinary herb. If you like garlic, chop some finely or mince it and spread it on the buttered bread. Garlic, chives and watercress go very well together in a tomato sandwich and so does finely chopped onion in place of the garlic. Grated carrot and a little horseradish is also a tasty combination. There is almost no end to the variety of sandwiches that can be prepared according to your taste and preferences. Herbs mixed with soft cheese and a little cream can be spread on bread or eaten with potatoes boiled in their skins. In the spring, radishes are a welcome addition to the sandwich menu, but they should be used sparingly because they are quite strong and too many can overstimulate or even irritate the liver. The resulting upset would be contrary to the objective of a health diet. Small cucumbers, thinly sliced, are delicious in a sandwich, and even white cabbage, also finely sliced, tastes surprisingly good.

So there are many variations possible; all you need is a little imagination and natural good taste. If you like, fresh tomatoes can be put on the table as well. A juicy tomato is always refreshing and will enrich the meal with its vitamins. Arthritis patients, however, should take great care to eat only the fully ripe ones.

General Advice

A health diet should be planned in such a way that it does not cause unnecessary disturbances in the system. Special attention should be given to the requirements of the individual organs that are weak. The liver and the pancreas cannot tolerate unhealthy fats or excessively sweet things; the kidneys react to too much salt and spices. As regards salt, the latest research has shown that sea salt is vastly superior to mined stone salt because in its unrefined state it contains many of the substances and trace elements that are found in healthy blood. Moreover, if the sea salt is enriched with herbs you have an excellent seasoning. We have such a tasty and wholesome preparation in *Herbamare*. For those who are prone to catarrh and similar infections or inflammations, there is also *Trocomare*. This herbal seasoning salt is also indicated as a prophylactic for infectious diseases. It is a dietary salt made up of natural sea salt and enriched with eight different fresh plants whose antibacterial effects are similar to those of penicillin, but without the danger of the body becoming resistant to them or the intestinal flora being damaged. As with herbal seasonings, *Trocomare* should never be boiled, but should be added after the food has been cooked so as not to destroy any of the active ingredients. Remember, *Trocomare* provides valuable remedial properties as well as flavouring.

Of course, sea salt should not be used indiscriminately either, only in small quantities. Those who suffer from diseases that require an absolutely salt-free diet, for example, nephritis and cardiac oedema, should not even use sea salt. Seasoning has to be done sensibly and always restricted to a minimum. This does not mean that food should be bland. Far from it. If vegetables are steamed instead of boiled, they will retain all their own rich flavour and by making use of the many kitchen herbs that are at our disposal the palate will have no reason to find fault with any dish.

That salads should not be salted almost goes without saying. And as a dressing, use lemon juice or *Molkosan* whey concentrate, not vinegar.

By adhering to a correct diet we can do much to help achieve success with whatever natural remedy or treatment we may be taking. There is little point in swallowing medicines or taking water treatments if, at the same time, we pay no attention to the food we are eating. Actually, our diet should be the first thing to come under scrutiny since it is useless to take remedies to cure, for example, the accumulation of uric acid, if at the same time we encourage its formation by eating eggs and other concentrated protein foods. It is senseless to take kidney and blood-purifying teas and steam baths to eliminate metabolic wastes from the system if we continue on the diet that is responsible for our problem in the first place.

Manure is for the plant what food is for the human body. The gardener or farmer will only be wasting precious time if he uses the wrong kind of manure when caring for his plants. It is the same with our nutrition. If we eat the wrong kind of food we will not achieve our goal of keeping fit and healthy. What we have become used to eating for no better reason than its pleasant taste or convenience, must in the future be considered from the stand-point of what it will do for us. Only then can we expect to benefit to the fullest degree from the food we eat. Moreover, it is only with persistence that health can be restored, for did it not require equal persistence in eating the wrong things that made us fall victim to disease? We should all remember that good health does not depend upon our physician alone; a lot depends upon our-selves. It often takes years to become sick, so it would be foolish to think that good health could be regained in a matter of days. Yet with perseverance many patients have overcome their ailments and recovered their health.

Fasting
One of the best remedies to maintain general well-being is fasting. If we do not feel well because we have eaten too much, or if our stomach is upset because we have eaten unsuitable food, perhaps making us vomit and causing diarrhoea, then fasting is a most natural remedy. Under similar circumstances our domestic animals have more sense than we do; they simply refuse all food. When

unwell, dogs and cats usually eat grass or some cellulose, so as to bring it up again with the mucus. They follow this up by being off their food for at least a day. Animals instinctively know they must not eat until they feel well again. This natural treatment of upsets is even more closely followed by animals living in the wild. They, too, know of no better remedy than fasting if they are ill. They just lie down in the shade, rest and fast until they feel well again. It would also be good for us if we gave the body a chance to purify itself.

When a person fasts the body has an opportunity to rid itself of accumulated harmful metabolic wastes. From time to time it is a good idea to plan ahead to have a fruit juice day and follow this up with one or two days of taking only clean pure water. However, before you begin the fast, make sure the bowels are empty. Mucilage-producing substances such as linseed or psyllium seed, or a herbal laxative, perhaps manna, will help move the bowels. If your liver is in good order you can then begin the fruit juice diet with orange, grapefruit or grape juice, according to what is in season. During the berry season, add berry juice to the list. Any wastes in the body will be eliminated and your organs will begin to function more efficiently.

Should you feel sick during the fast, you will be well advised to speed up the elimination by encouraging the skin function. Friction baths, vigorous washing and towelling or brushing down will stimulate the circulation, while deep-breathing exercises will likewise help to get rid of the feeling of sickness. Short walks in the woods and along country lanes, breathing in the aromatic air, will soon restore a feeling of health and well-being.

If you feel very hungry, chew a few raisins slowly and thoroughly. The Bedouins wandering in the desert often live on nothing but a few dates a day, because they obtain the full benefit from this frugal meal by chewing it thoroughly and so predigesting it properly. In the same way we can help ourselves during our special period of fasting. Spit out the skins of the raisins and just enjoy the grape sugar.

You must observe an important rule when fasting; never begin a fast while feeling disturbed, annoyed or worried about something. A happy frame of mind is a natural medicine that stimulates the endocrine glands and keeps them at the peak of their efficiency. This is one reason why our modern way of life with its constant hustle and bustle, and its problems, worries and upsets, can damage our health so much.

How long should a dietary fast last? The answer to this will be determined by the needs of the individual. Two or three days may be sufficient; however, having kept it up for three days, it is perhaps a pity to stop. The first three days are like climbing a high mountain with all its initial difficulties. Having scaled the hardest part, the worst is over and, to one's surprise, the going becomes easy and enjoyable. So it is after the first three days of fasting. The body will have adapted to the change and can easily stand another five days. An eight-day fast, taking only fruit juice, will give your body a complete 'spring clean'. If you suffer from arthritis, a condition that cannot easily be shifted, you will find it beneficial to continue the fast even longer. Remarkable men like John the Baptist, and a still more distinguished person, Jesus Christ himself, fasted. Of course they did it not for the purpose of cleansing their bodies, but to achieve the utmost mental concentration. As documented in the Scriptures, Christ fasted for forty days. It is an established fact that when great demands are made on the mind, fasting will help to make one's thoughts crystal clear, one's understanding precise and accurate.

If fasting has improved your well-being, do not encourage a friend or neighbour who suffers from Graves' disease (exophthalmic goitre) or tuberculosis to undertake the same treatment. Such a course would definitely be harmful because you cannot cure these two diseases by fasting. Be very careful, therefore, about recommending a fast to others. A long and complete fast might also prove dangerous to people with certain types of heart trouble, even though the fruit juice diet would make it less strenuous since the body is being nourished to the necessary extent while the work of cleansing is going on. If a liver disorder is suspected, take vegetable juices or Vogel's vegetable juice mixture, rather than fruit juices, because the fruit acids do not usually agree with the patient. Carrot juice is particularly good in such cases. You see, then, that each case should be considered individually with respect to what one can or cannot do.

When you are fasting and taking natural medication at the same time, take only a third or even a quarter of the normal dose of your remedies. While on a fast, your system works more efficiently and will respond to medicines much more promptly than usual.

During the fast it is necessary to maintain the normal rhythm of movement and take adequate rest. All extremes are harmful, so avoid them. For instance, do not spend your days on the couch or in bed in the mistaken belief that you must conserve your energy while not eating. On the other hand, do not engage in arduous sports or walks; it would do you no good. The balance of movement and rest during your fast will revive you, restoring vitality and giving you a new foundation for health and well-being. However, I want to stress that it is important to lead up to your fast days slowly and also to return to your normal diet in the same way.

Fattening-Up Diets
Although it should be sufficiently well known that fattening-up diets are anything but sensible, and contrary to the findings of modern nutritional research, they are still occasionally recommended. Lymphatic children with swollen glands and shadows on their lungs are overfed during their stay in Swiss mountain resorts to such an extent that they return home quite plump. It is not surprising that when they are back home in the lowlands and complain of excessive tiredness, show signs of some liver trouble, or even succumb to jaundice. The weight increase achieved by stuffing butter, milk and rich foods into them is no longer the accepted procedure of the nature-oriented, progressive doctor, since it has been found that there are other factors of even greater importance.

The fattening-up diet produces something like an optical illusion. Fat, heavy-bodied children somehow create the impression of being in the best of health, but that this is not always true is borne out by past experience and common knowledge. Excessive feeding usually affects the liver because the diet contains too much fat. This, in turn, leads to other metabolic disturbances which eventually have to be corrected. So forget fattening-up diets. They are not sensible. The resistance to infection is nearly always lowered after such an extreme feeding programme and, all in all, nothing good is ever gained by it.

How Much Food Do We Need?
I have often been asked how much an adult should eat. Should we adopt the system of calories as a measure of our need or is there another way of knowing how much food will prevent us from becoming undernourished?

Like most systems, reckoning in terms of calories is not the perfect system, and should therefore be considered as a purely theoretical guide. An exact method of calculation is not possible because an individual's need for food depends upon so many different and constantly varying circumstances, so that the adoption of a strict and definitive system can do more harm than good. True, a person's body weight or build plays an important part in determining how much food one should eat. Theoretically speaking, a stout and tall person should require more food than a slim one. It is possible, however, that the slim person has a more vigorous nature and burns up more energy than the fat, placid, calm person and in this case our theory already ceases to be valid. A happy, jolly type needs less food than a discontented, unhappy person, because cheerfulness promotes better glandular function and consequently better digestion and improved assimilation. The happy person gets more out of his food. There is much truth in the old saying that one does not live on what one eats but on what one digests.

A person who works in the garden with a spade and a fork has a different food requirement to someone who sits in an office all day. Climate must be considered too, according to whether one lives, for example, in Sweden, Switzerland, Africa or California. It has a bearing on one's need of food as far as quantity and kind is concerned.

I myself never rely on systems that will probably change anyway, like so many other things in life. The only reliable guide is that furnished by the body itself, its automatic mechanisms the Creator endowed it with. Its demands will automatically vary or change with the prevailing circumstances. I fared well by listening to my body's voice when I lived in a cold northern region, in the temperate region of my native Switzerland, and in the tropical regions with their steppes and deserts.

The basic rule to remember is that if you take care to eat only natural foods, wherever you are, you cannot go far wrong. Avoid refined products and imbalances in your diet. If you let nature guide you it will help you to follow your inner urges and interpret them correctly. In this way you will be able to feel more than just hungry; you will develop those finer instincts that nowadays only the more primitive peoples have retained.

Vitamins

Natural Food for the Nerves – Vitamin C
Every year, come autumn and winter in my garden in the Engadine, the little clusters of scarlet barberries between the leafless thorny branches of the berberis shrubs just beg to be harvested. A little earlier it would have been the ripe redcurrants, shining in the autumn sun. So when I am there, I pick some of these berries most days and enjoy their acidic flavour which is due to ascorbic acid, or vitamin C. These berries are, in fact, a natural food for the

nerves. Before long, even the slopes facing south become covered in thick snow, and the birds will be daily guests on the shrubs, feasting on the beautiful red, oblong berries in order to obtain their requirements of sugar, minerals and vitamins. The red fruits of the *Rosa canina* (wild rose), the rose hips, will still be peeping through the snow. When these hips are ripe they are deliciously sweet. Because of their vitamin C content they, too, are a wonderful food for the nerves. No wonder that rose hip purée and barberry purée are a perfect source of vitamins during the bleak winter months. They should be on every table because they fill an important gap in our nutrition, since practically all other foods lose some of their vitamin content during their months of storage. Wild fruits, in the form of fruit purée or conserve, prevent vitamin C deficiency while being tasty and pleasant food. But not only barberries and rose hips are rich in vitamin C, even richer are the berries of sea buckthorn, which grows abundantly in the lower Inn valley, the Tessin and the Maggia valley in my native Switzerland. Their orangy-red colour, bright amongst the olive-green leaves, can be spotted on slopes and along brooks and rivers – a delight to the eyes of every nature lover.

THE MERITS OF FOOD RICH IN VITAMIN C

In order to show someone how important it is to prevent vitamin C deficiency, we would do well to refer to Captain Cook's famous experience. Realising the disastrous effect of a lack of vitamin C in the diet, and to guarantee the success of his expeditions, he carried on board whole barrels of sauerkraut. His farsightedness spared him and his crew from falling victim to scurvy. Every 100 g (about 3½ oz) of sauerkraut contains approximately 20 mg of vitamin C, about the same proportion as in raw potatoes, but the latter, of course, are less palatable when uncooked.

The symptoms and consequences of vitamin C deficiency are muscular weakness, bleeding under the skin, bleeding of the gums and loosening of the teeth, which can even fall out. Resistance to infectious diseases is greatly reduced and susceptibility to catarrh, sore throats and tonsillitis, pneumonia and pleurisy is considerably increased. The capillaries are weakened and damaged, severely affecting the circulation.

DAILY REQUIREMENT OF VITAMIN C

Although there is no unanimous opinion as regards the daily requirement of vitamin C, for adults it seems to be between 75–100 mg, or about one-tenth of a gram (0.0035 oz), and for children about half this amount. The following list will give you some idea of how to cover your daily requirement. The quantity of each food item for this purpose is given in grams (1 g = 0.035 oz; 1 oz = 28 g); for example, you would have to eat 12 g of sea buckthorn berries to obtain the amount of vitamin C needed for one day.

- 12 g sea buckthorn berries or raw sea buckthorn purée
- 20 g ripe rose hips or raw rose hip purée
- 70 g blackcurrants
- 120 g green cabbage salad
- 170 g strawberries
- 180 g spinach salad
- 200 g white cabbage salad or natural sauerkraut without additives
- 300 g dandelion salad
- 500 g potatoes boiled in their skins

The amount of vitamin C contained in each item is only approximate. The actual figure varies according to where the plants grow and the season, but the fresh fruit or vegetable has the highest content when just picked, as a certain amount is lost in storage. It goes without saying that you will only need part of the amount given for each food item containing vitamin C because you will eat more than one category of such foods in the course of the day. If sugar is added to the raw, freshly prepared fruit purée, a larger amount of fruit will be needed to cover your requirement.

To set your mind at rest I would like to point out that the natural vitamin C in our food does not harm the system, even though we might take in more than the indicated daily quantity. However, this cannot be said about the synthetic vitamins. These artificial products should only be taken in accordance with the prescription and are never equal to the vitamins contained in plants or fruit. *Bio-C-Lozenges*, on the other hand, are made from fruit extracts with a high natural vitamin C content and help to prevent vitamin C deficiency. So if you believe the principle that food should be a remedy at the same time, you will not take synthetic vitamins but see to it that your daily requirement comes from carefully chosen and prepared food.

Vitamin A
At one time there was not much one could do about conjunctivitis and dehydration of the cornea caused by vitamin A deficiency.

While it was more common in infants and small children, adults were sometimes affected too. Vitamin A deficiency also predisposes one to pulmonary ailments, pneumonia, inflammation of the middle ear, suppurations and abscesses. So where do we find this important vitamin? In butter, cod-liver oil, dandelion leaves, stinging nettles, parsley, savoy cabbage and carrots. Fruits which contain the most vitamin A are apricots, dates and rose hips.

Vitamin A deficiency in children and adults can quickly be rectified by taking *Vitaforce*, rose hip conserve and date sugar. Children and patients whose assimilation is poor should take the condensed juice of organically grown raw spring carrots (*Biocarottin*), which has the additional advantage of being a liver remedy.

Natural food serves our purpose much better than anything else. To illustrate, 1 g of mother's milk contains 2–5 international units (IU) of vitamin A; the same amount of blackcurrant juice, 3–5 IU, and rose hip conserve, 60–100 IU.

CARROTS, CAROTENE AND BIOCAROTTIN
Carrots are so rich in important minerals and vitamins that they can rightly be called a remedial food. You should eat them every day in one form or another, especially during the low-vitamin winter months and early spring. They should preferably be eaten raw, because when uncooked they retain all their goodness.

Children like to nibble carrots as if they were sticks of rock or candy. So when mother puts them on the table cut up into four pieces, maybe grandmother would not be so pleased with her meal, but this is perfect for the children since their teeth are given a little extra work to do. I remember the time when carrot salad used to mean a dish of cooked carrots, sliced and dressed. However, since the importance of their vitamins has become common knowledge, boiled or cooked carrots are hardly ever served as a salad, instead, grated raw carrots have taken their place. With a little grated horseradish added they taste exceptionally refreshing.

WHY CARROTS ARE SO GOOD
One kilogram (2.2 lb) of carrots contains approximately 2.5 g potassium, about 300 mg calcium, 6 mg iron and 0.6 mg copper. If you consider the importance to our blood of iron and copper in organic form, that is, from plants, you will have every reason to give your children plenty of carrots or *Biocarottin*. Moreover, it is good to know that there are about 300 mg of phosphorus in every kilogram of carrots, and we all appreciate the significance of

phosphorus for the brain, particularly our memory. Carrots are also good for the glands because of their content of iodine. Furthermore, they are a source of magnesium and cobalt, as well as carotene (provitamin A) at the rate of 70 mg per kilogram of carrots.

Carotene is extremely important in our effort to keep the cellular system healthy and the digestive organs functioning efficiently. It promotes healthy growth and the development of strong, resistant teeth. In fact, vitamin A, that is, carotene, together with calcium and vitamin D, contributes considerably to good teeth.

Did you know, too, that carotene, if taken plentifully, is able to prevent the formation of kidney stones? This has been proved by careful observations. And another thing, a lack of carotene is one of the factors that contribute to a greater susceptibility to infections, especially coughs and sneezes.

Taking plenty of carotene helps to achieve a faster and more complete recovery in cases of pneumonia, various heart troubles, eczema and psoriasis. Women should also take greater amounts of it during pregnancy. It is generally known that it is good for the eyes, helping to improve the eyesight and, if taken in sufficient quantities, it can be the means of overcoming night-blindness – a tremendous benefit to pilots and night-drivers. Carotene has another welcome benefit in that it reduces the tendency to form cataracts. In addition, experiments and observations are said to have shown that carotene improves the function of the sex glands because it exerts a certain influence on the production of sex hormones; thus it can be of assistance in overcoming sexual weakness and impotence. This effect may be attributable to the high vitamin E content in carrots, for there are about 25 mg of it in every kilogram (2.2 lbs). Finally, just let me mention some other vitamins in carrots: one kilogram contains 0.5 mg vitamins B_1, B_2 and B_6, as well as the important vitamin K, and about 50 mg vitamin C, the valuable nerve food.

CARROTS IN WINTER

In the winter our diet should include carrots every day, either in the form of a good fresh salad or a glass of freshly prepared raw juice.

An abundant crop of carrots provides the basis for a beneficial use of the surplus. Let me add that we grow our carrots organically. When harvested, we produce juice and condense it under vacuum at a low temperature. The result is our concentrated juice product known as *Biocarottin*. Among its other valuable applications, if Biocarottin is taken together with *Papayasan* it is possible to keep one's intestines free from worms. Biocarottin has also proved its worth as a supplement in a liver diet, since the goodness of carrots is even more readily available in the concentrated juice. So why take chemical medicines, which are unnatural and foreign to our system, when nature has given us so many good raw materials that are of real benefit to our health?

Vitamin B Complex
Vitamin B_1, or thiamine, is considered to be the anti-beriberi vitamin. *Beri* is a Hindustani word referring to a sheep's fetlock; in Sinhalese, *beri* means weakness. The weakness or loss of energy experienced by those whose main diet is white rice leads to a partial paralysis of the limbs, making the patients drag their feet similar to the way sheep do. For this reason the disease, which is caused by a dietary deficiency of vitamin B_1, came to be known as beriberi, a reduplication of the word *beri*.

The anti-beriberi vitamin is contained in the aleurone layer of cereals; a good quantity is also present in yeast. The substance consists of various chemical compounds which, although not related to one another, have the same quality of being water-soluble.

The vitamin B complex is essential to enable the cells of the nervous system to take up oxygen. The primary and best remedy available in biological medicine for the treatment of painful inflammation of the nerves, as well as for strengthening the entire nervous system, is a steady supply of vitamin B. It is also a reliable help for those who suffer from poor stomach and bowel action and the lack of appetite connected with these disorders. If taken in greater amounts, vitamin B will often relieve disturbances during pregnancy. In cases of circulatory disorders and heart trouble and prescribed natural remedies will act faster and better if vitamin B is taken at the same time. In the past, explorers on arctic and Himalayan expeditions took along supplies of yeast extract for the sake of its concentrated nutrients and, not least, its sufficient amounts of vitamin B.

Today we have a fine supplement in *Herbaforce* because of its content of cultured yeast extract and fresh plant extracts. It is very tasty and most suitable as a sandwich spread, for snacks and food for journeys. It enhances salad dressings and is a splendid flavouring for soups, stews and other dishes.

489

VITAMIN B$_{12}$ AND THE BLOOD

A doctor friend of mine told me once that he was of the opinion that a certain patient's anaemic condition had its basic cause in his vegetarian diet. This patient, who was otherwise quite healthy, was unable to overcome his condition, and the doctor was adamant that the man should add meat to his diet because it is rich in the haematinic vitamin B$_{12}$. But when the doctor found out that I have been a vegetarian since I was seventeen, and have a constant haemoglobin count of 100–105 and otherwise excellent blood, he was extremely astonished and had to change his opinion. Mind you, a healthy vegetarian diet must include plenty of green vegetables and all the green culinary herbs, such as all kinds of cress and parsley, because these contain sufficient levels of vitamin B$_{12}$. All these green herbs, in particular parsley, stimulate the kidneys and urination and should therefore be used regularly, and not just as an occasional garnish on prepared dishes. In fact, your health will benefit greatly if you chop up some kitchen herbs daily, mixing them in your salads and cottage cheese and sprinkling them over vegetable and potato dishes. You can ensure a regular intake of these green herbs by always using the herbal seasoning salt *Herbamare*, which is made from fresh green herbs. If you use natural products regularly in your kitchen you will reduce the risk of succumbing to vitamin deficiency.

Vitamin E – the Fertility Vitamin

The Roman gladiators had no idea about hormones and vitamin E, but they knew from experience that they became more energetic and efficient when they ate bulls' testicles the day before their contests. No doubt it needed clear thinking and some degree of biological understanding to come to this conclusion. Not infrequently it was mere chance, an acute observation or clear and logical thinking that led to discoveries that serve us today in our quest to rectify errors in nutrition that plague us in the form of deficiency diseases and avitaminoses.

DEFINITE MERITS OF VITAMIN E

It was many decades ago (in 1922) when the American scientist Herbert McLean Evans discovered vitamin E. Since then it has been proved that there is no better natural remedy for sterility and infertility. Many a woman could have saved herself great heartache if she had known about vitamin E. Not only does this vitamin prevent miscarriage, but it also promotes the healthy, normal development of the foetus, ensuring a normal pregnancy without complications.

However, vitamin E is not only important for women; men too depend upon an adequate supply of it for the normal functioning of the sex glands. In turn, vitality, pleasure in work and stamina are dependent upon the efficiency of these glands.

Vitamin E influences the development and function of the smooth and striped muscles, being able to prevent muscle degeneration. This is of great importance for the cardiac muscles. In fact, vitamin E, together with natural heart remedies such as *Crataegisan* and *Auroforce*, has proved most effective as a tonic for weak heart muscles. It can be added that a vitamin E deficiency is very bad for the nerves too.

In cases of vitamin E deficiency swelling of the intercellular substance in the connective tissue and impaired firmness of the vascular walls have been discovered. Stagnation in the capillaries and bad circulation are connected with this condition, and all of these things lead to metabolic disturbances and increased oxygen consumption.

If these disturbances are diagnosed in the years of development and growth, an increased intake of vitamin E can help. Menopausal problems also respond well to average doses of vitamin E, as do rheumatic ailments. All in all, vitamin E is important in keeping the body functions healthy.

Cows can succumb to brucellosis (undulant fever, Bang's disease), an epidemic infectious disease causing miscarriage, if they lack vitamin E. It can be cured by giving the animals feed that is rich in vitamin E, such as bran that contains wheat germ. Brucellosis can be transmitted to humans, for example by drinking contaminated and unpasteurised milk and by eating infected butter or cottage cheese.

The correct daily dosage of vitamin E has not yet been established. It is assumed that the daily requirement is 15–25 mg. One litre (1.76 pints) of wheat germ oil contains 1 g of vitamin E, so that we would have to take 15 cc (about ½ fl. oz) every day to meet our requirement.

SOURCES OF VITAMIN E
Vitamin E is rarely found in meat, except in those parts that are unsuitable for human consumption, for example bulls' testicles, the spleen, placenta, pancreas and pituitary gland. It is, however,

found in fish and egg yolk, and in small amounts in milk as well as butter.

It is more abundant in vegetable products, primarily in cereal germ, oil fruits and cotton seed, also in corn (maize), peanuts and all varieties of cress – watercress, garden cress, nasturtium and American cress. For this reason the formulae of *Herbamare* and *Trocomare* include these cresses. Vitamin E is also present in spinach, lettuce and alfalfa (lucerne), as well as in most leafy salad greens. That explains why vegetarians probably meet their daily vitamin E requirement more effectively than meat-eaters. If you suffer from a deficiency, make use of the above-mentioned sources. For quick results take wheat germ oil, and if you do not like its taste, use wheat germ oil capsules, which are quite easy to swallow. The gelatine capsule dissolves in the intestine and there is no danger of the taste repeating on you.

Overcoming Protein Deficiency
Lactovegetarians will not find it easy to prevent protein deficiency if they travel in countries where there is little dairy farming. In fact, a vegetarian may have difficulty even in our temperate regions in obtaining his eighteen amino acids every day in the food available to him, yet they are essential building blocks for the protein in his body.

Millet was the staple diet of our forefathers; together with milk and meat it provided the necessary protein. Later, potatoes were added as a valuable source of protein, and in more recent times, soya beans. Soya has proved to be an excellent vegetable protein, and was responsible for saving millions of Chinese from starvation when overpopulation made the production of sufficient animal protein impossible.

Because they are so good for us, we should give much more attention to soya products. The beans contain first-class protein, as well as minerals and other vital substances. Millet proved its worth in the past when it served to satisfy our forefathers, giving them strength and energy. For this reason alone it, too, deserves to be on our table now. Over forty years ago, millet began to go out of vogue and was only used for chicken feed. More recently, however, as a result of the serious efforts being made to enrich our diet with valuable plant products, millet has begun to be revived as a food and it would be to our advantage if we used it regularly in alternation with potatoes and soya.

On travels through tropical regions in the developing countries of Africa and Asia, a frequent sight are many adults and even more children with pot-bellies and skinny limbs. This condition is generally a symptom of protein deficiency. Although it is true that pure calories, that is, carbohydrates, are often plentiful in the form of tropical fruits, and the body is able to produce its own fat, in hot countries it is very difficult to obtain sufficient protein. Because of the great heat, cattle yield less milk. It is therefore not surprising that in those areas all kinds of seeds are considered important for food. In folk museums we can also find that seeds, kernels and nuts stand out as a special feature in the nutrition of ancient peoples.

Seafood – Saltwater Fish and Shellfish

As suggested in the previous section, non-meat-eaters may find it difficult to get the necessary protein in tropical countries. Milk and milk products are usually scarce or unobtainable because the climate is too hot for productive dairy farming. Soya is not grown everywhere and nuts are often unknown. So what can be used to provide protein? Small island populations could not survive if it were not for seafood. Shellfish are a welcome and valuable source of protein in these areas.

Of what benefit is seafood for those of us who already obtain enough protein from other sources? The addition of seafood is then not really essential. Still, we are accustomed to eating many things that are not absolutely necessary; for example, we could live without citrus and tropical fruits, yet we are glad and grateful for the added variety. Seafood contains good quality protein, is easily digestible and many prefer it to animal protein. Important, too, is the fact that seafood contains traces of iodine.

The great progress in civil aviation has made foreign travel easy and has brought us into close contact with people from other parts of the world, who visit us and are pleased when they can get their own food and fruit in our shops. Conversely, many of us venture out and travel to faraway places, where we become familiar with other customs and habits. The result is that we now have many food items in our shops that were rare or even unknown until relatively recently.

Eating Vegetables and Fruit at the Same Meal

I keep receiving letters and reports that confirm the fact that digestive problems often arise when fruit and vegetables are eaten at the same meal. Let me quote the following account as an example.

493

'There has been much talk lately about modern diets, with many lectures being given on the subject. My daughter and I went to an interesting one given by Dr Bircher. The speaker made the point that, before every meal, fruit and raw vegetables or a salad should be eaten. So my whole family started a regime of eating an apple before our meals. The result? My goitre scar from an operation eleven years ago was dreadfully painful for three or four days and a small swelling developed. Then the pain diminished, although it did not disappear entirely. I should also tell you that on the evening of the lecture, I hurried a little and for the first time in my life I was conscious of my heart beating rather rapidly and ever since I have felt sick almost every day. We have now stopped eating an apple before our meals, for it seemed to give us flatulence as well.'

All things considered, what does this account emphasise? It is good to serve a dish of raw food before the main meal, but be careful to stick to one variety of food. Before a vegetable meal eat raw vegetables, never fruit, and before a meal composed of sweet dishes, you may eat fruit. Dr Bircher-Benner's theory may apply to healthy people whose organs function properly, but if there is a tendency to dysfunction of one or more organs, especially the liver and pancreas, the consumption of fruit and vegetables as part of the same meal can encourage further disturbances.

A urinalysis disclosed that the writer of the above letter had trouble with her liver and pancreas, and it was no doubt for this reason that she suffered from flatulence when she ate fruit and vegetables at the same meal. Where the liver and pancreas are working efficiently, the digestive juices are able to break down fruit and Dr Bircher-Benner's theory would be correct. It would then do no harm to eat fruit before a vegetable meal. However, if the organic mechanism is impaired, the enzymes will clearly be unable to digest the fruit acids, resulting in a reaction between the fruit acids and the alkaline vegetable components. The unpleasant consequences are excessive fermentation and flatulence.

We are naturally grateful to Dr Bircher-Benner for his great achievement in the field of modern nutrition, but we regret that he did not see the importance of keeping the two classes of food, fruit and vegetables, separate. For one thing, even taste-wise they do not necessarily go together. Take strawberries and cabbage or radish salad, for instance; the very thought of having to eat these salads after strawberries is far from tempting. Our sense of taste alone tells us not to mix these foods.

In a personal interview, Dr Bircher-Benner told me once that he could find no scientific reason for separating fruit and vegetables. Nevertheless, many of his patients complained about disturbances, especially fermentation or flatulence, in connection with his diet. Of course, if someone follows the Bircher method and experiences no disturbance at all, there is no reason why he should not continue. On the other hand, if upsets do occur, it would be unwise to stick to a regime that causes trouble. Rather, it is better to follow the lead of nature which, after all, is more important than all our theories. The rule about not eating vegetables and fruit at the same meal applies to the combination of food items in general; in particular, it is important to avoid fried food and sweet things when the liver and pancreas are affected, because they cannot cope well with these.

Fruit and Vegetable Juices – their Effects on You

Perhaps you do not know which juice will agree with you. Or the choice may be difficult if you want to recommend juices to relatives and friends. The following hints will provide you with the information you need.

Carrot Juice

The essential oils contained in carrots have an effect on the mucous membranes and stimulate the blood circulation in the stomach and intestinal tissues. Because of its balancing action carrot juice is good for constipation and diarrhoea. With small children it usually stops the dreaded attacks of diarrhoea and vomiting in no time at all, and also eliminates intestinal worms. Other complaints, such as headaches, eczema and skin blemishes (for example acne), may be connected with bad digestion and can be rectified with the help of this juice. Many women prize carrot juice as an ideal natural remedy that acts from within the body, keeping them slim and ensuring a good complexion. Carrot juice is refreshing and soothing if taken during convalescence after an operation or a serious illness, coughs and colds, and infectious diseases accompanied by fever. We owe it to the rich content of carotene (provitamin A) that this juice improves the eyesight and stimulates the production of rhodopsin (visual purple), the lack of which causes night-blindness.

Beetroot Juice

This juice contains betaine, which stimulates the function of the liver cells and protects the liver and bile ducts in cases of disturbance. Every 100 g of beetroot juice contains 5 mg of iron, in addition to a number of trace elements, which, it is believed, encourage the absorption of the iron in the blood. A healthy body needs plenty of iron, especially in the first two years of life, during puberty, in pregnancy, when breast-feeding and during the menopause. Beetroot juice is highly recommended for these crucial periods of life. If your child is pale, do not forget to give him or her a small glass of beetroot juice before meals every day, morning and evening. In the case of infants (six months to two years) one teaspoonful will suffice.

Celery Juice
Celery juice is distinctly alkaline and eliminative. It is therefore recommended for all disturbances caused by the accumulation of wastes and toxins, for example rheumatic and arthritic ailments. Celery juice regulates the water balance and puts new life into elderly people.

Tomato Juice
Tomato juice is recommended as a protection against premature aging, as well as the symptoms of overtiredness and unpleasant body odour. It is refreshing and cleanses the body.

Potato Juice
Unlike the other juices, which are good for health but also delicious taken before meals to stimulate the appetite, potato juice is strictly remedial, and is particularly indicated for the treatment of stomach ulcers.

Vegetable juices enhanced by lacto-fermentation have a stimulating and balancing effect on our vital intestinal flora.

Raw Juices, Medicinal Juices

SCIENTIFIC RESEARCH
While living on 57th Street in New York for a short time during 1950, I used to go for a drink of freshly squeezed orange juice at a certain 'health bar'. Whenever I went there I was amazed to see people drinking cabbage juice from enormous glasses. I had, of course, known the benefits of raw cabbage juice for certain disorders for along time, but I also knew that it was a rather unpalatable drink.

Later I came across an article in the Toronto Magazine Digest, which extolled the virtues of cabbage juice in the treatment of gastric ulcers. Here, then, was confirmation of a treatment we in Switzerland had known for quite a while, based on our own experience with cabbage juice. Dr Garnett, the author of the report, referred to experiments with 'vitamin U' (U standing for Ulcer) which, according to him, is responsible for the curative effect of this juice. What he may not have known, however, is that raw potato juice is even more effective, and it is quite likely that he would have found 'vitamin U' in it as well. Another researcher, however, may advance Ragnar Berg's explanation proposed many years ago. According to him, the alkaline properties of raw juice neutralise the free acids in the system and so rehabilitate the mineral metabolism, making possible the successful treatment of gastric ulcers.

THE EVIDENCE OF EXPERIENCE
It is not essential to know exactly how a cure takes place. The mere knowledge that juices can cure is infinitely more valuable than any scientific explanation advanced in this connection. Science, after all, only confirms the discoveries made decades ago. Many years ago, as a young man, I lectured on this subject and drew attention to the value of raw juices. Today it is easier to convince people because science has, in the meantime, confirmed our assertions of the past that raw juices and raw vegetables are wonderful remedies. It is, and will remain, a fact that the raw juices of potato and cabbage will heal gastric and duodenal ulcers.

Even more interesting is the observation I made in connection with raw potato, cabbage (green and white) and carrot juice in the treatment of gout, rheumatism and allied conditions. If these juices are taken in conjunction with a strictly natural diet, these diseases will eventually respond to the treatment.

A SPECIAL DIET
Before *breakfast*, on an empty stomach, take half a glass of raw potato juice diluted with a little warm water. The breakfast itself should consist of whole wheat that has been soaked in water for a day or two. It can be made more palatable with the addition of a good vegetable stock or fresh butter. If the bowels need special attention, add psyllium seed or freshly ground linseed to the wheat. Crispbread with butter and wheat germ will complete your breakfast. If the liver is not functioning properly, drink a glass of raw carrot juice. Chew all the food well and insalivate it thoroughly.

Midday Meal: Eat a good, hearty vegetable soup with a cup of raw cabbage juice, which is added after the soup has been taken off the heat. Then have a dish of natural brown rice, steamed vegetables and a salad. Never use vinegar to make your salad dressing; use lemon juice, or sour milk or whey concentrate (*Molkosan*) if you cannot tolerate lemon. For variety, in place of the brown rice you can use whole wheat, buckwheat or millet. If you feel nervous and tired out, beat a raw egg and mix it in with your food every other day. On no account should the eggs be cooked because this would destroy most of their vitamins and, in addition, produce too much uric acid. Only when eggs are eaten raw do they have a place in a therapeutic diet, if it is at all advisable to include them. Thus, raw eggs can be used, as indicated, in a diet for stomach ulcers, but those who suffer from rheumatism should avoid eggs altogether.

Evening meal: This can be along similar lines to the breakfast. The wholewheat dish can be varied by taking oat flake porridge or, even better, raw, soaked oat grains, put through the mincer.

Keep off fruit on this special diet, only use vegetable juices.

CHANCES OF A CURE

With this diet it is possible to cure a stomach ulcer within a month. Gout and rheumatic complaints will improve within two or three months and then slowly disappear. Afterwards, continue with the diet but have only fruit every second day. Avoid sausages, cold meats, pork, canned foods, white sugar and white flour and everything made from these. In fact, you would do well to forget these items altogether. You may start eating meat again after six months, but only veal or beef.

If you follow the suggested diet consistently, you will find that even the most stubborn case of gout will eventually disappear. Of course, you can back up the healing process by means of natural remedies. *Wallwosan* or *Symphosan*, applied externally, will give relief; take *Petasites* internally, also *Nephrosolid* to stimulate the kidneys. For gastric ulcers *Gastronol* is recommended, to be taken after meals. But never lose sight of the fact that the cure depends fundamentally on the raw juices.

Since these juices, with the exception of carrot juice, are somewhat unpalatable on their own, try mixing them in thick minestrone soup. The vegetable flavours will neutralise the strong taste of the raw juice. As pointed out already, add the juice only after the soup has been taken off the heat, so as not to lose the medicinal value. If this should make the soup lukewarm, gently warm the juice in a double boiler before adding it to the soup. You will have to eat this soup with the raw juices twice a day and between meals take an additional 200 ml of juice (about 8 fl. oz). In grave cases, 400–500 ml (just under a pint) of raw juice daily is absolutely essential.

Proponents of nature cures and nutritional therapy were advocating the use of raw juices long before scientific research began to confirm their value. Patients should remember the proven effects and be willing to persevere with the treatment until the hoped-for results are obtained.

It is amazing that it was in the United States where these drastic methods of treatment were developed and practised, for it is there, more than anywhere else, that poor nutrition has led to such modern diseases of civilisation.

Patients elsewhere should show the same perseverance in adhering to a raw juice diet that may be relatively unpalatable but will eventually lead to rehabilitation. Mere taste is a small price to pay for health restored!

Which Juices Are Compatible?
Some people assume that it is permissible to combine fruit and vegetable juices, such as orange with carrot juice. This, of course, is no better than eating fruit and vegetables at the same time, which, as already discussed, is apt to cause fermentation and flatulence, especially in sensitive people. Generally speaking, one juice can be mixed with another of the same kind, so that the best way is to take, for example, carrot and beetroot juices at one time, and orange and another fruit juice some other time. This way your digestion will not suffer. As a rule, it is better to drink only one juice, not a mixture. What is more, sipping is much better than gulping it down, because little sips, properly insalivated, will avoid flatulence or any other digestive disturbance. The curative effect will be greater too. Insalivating well helps to warm ice-cold juice in the mouth and so avoid chilling the stomach. A bite of crispbread or rusk with each sip of fruit juice will help to neutralise the acidity somewhat and protect the stomach lining.

If, in spite of all their goodness, you simply cannot tolerate fruit juices, mix them with muesli, while vegetable juices are best incorporated in soups and stews, after these have been cooked.

Difficulties in Adjusting to a Raw Food Diet

High blood pressure, thick blood, venous ailments and similar conditions, demand a change in the viscosity of the blood and this can be accomplished by following a protein-reduced diet. Meat, cheese, eggs and other protein foods have to be cut down to a minimum in such cases. However, it is not always easy to change over to a fruit diet. Elderly people in particular are likely to be troubled because gastric acid does not always mix well with the acids found in fruit. When changing over to a fruit diet it is of prime importance to eat very slowly, insalivate the fruit and fruit juices thoroughly and eat some crispbread, wholewheat rusks, oatmeal biscuits, toast or any other flakes or wholegrain crackers or biscuits, as the starch contained in them will help to neutralise the acids, rendering them more acceptable to the stomach.

Those who change to a raw food diet must take into account that the digestive organs will not immediately adapt themselves to the change from a mixed or one-sided protein diet. A little time and patience are needed before a really successful changeover is achieved, and the body must be given all the help it needs. Let me use a motor car as an illustration. A driver knows that he cannot change from a high octane to a low octane petrol without first making adjustments to the carburettor. Similarly, the digestive organs must be adjusted to the new diet. Many people fail in making this dietary change simply because this point has not been given the necessary attention.

When Raw Food Causes Problems

It is known that crude oil can produce more power than a refined product, but it requires that an appropriate carburettor be fitted. There is a similarity with a diet of raw food. Some people have health problems, weak digestive organs, and are not able to tolerate raw food in its solid form. Their condition may only allow them to take it in the form of juices.

Since raw fruits and raw vegetables contain the highest amount of vital substances, every meal should include at least some raw food, so that we can obtain sufficient quantities of vitamins and enzymes. A weekly raw food day will benefit us if we are able to take and digest them well. Bearing this prerequisite in mind, it will be beneficial to go on a raw food diet for a while, especially when the weather is amenable during the change from winter to spring. The diet will give the body a chance to be properly cleansed.

However, if you find that nuts and salads are eliminated without being digested, a raw food diet is not for you. In particular, children with digestive problems or who suffer from coeliac disease should not be given any food they cannot digest. It would be closing one's eyes to the facts if a diet were continued although the patient was slowly dying of a complete loss of energy – a kind of foolishness I remember seeing once in the case of a girl who would not listen to reason.

It is true that some primitive peoples live almost entirely on raw foods and remain fit and strong. We in the industrialised world, however, should not draw the wrong conclusions from this. Figuratively speaking, civilisation has inflicted many wounds on us, and many of us have acquired extremely weak digestive organs, making it almost impossible, or at least very difficult, to digest raw foods. If this applies to you, you will have to make the food more digestible by cooking it. Only a modest addition of raw food in the form of purée or juice will be permissible. Facing the facts is the answer to keeping your body from being put under unnecessary stress. When the system has recovered sufficiently and the digestive juices are once again able to break down the raw vegetable cells and assimilate the nutrients, you can begin to enjoy some raw foods, but with great care. Even then, you should never forget that proper chewing and thorough insalivation are called for. Never eat in a hurry. So if you want to benefit fully from raw foods, you will have to take more time eating them than you do with cooked food.

THE DANGER OF INTESTINAL WORMS

The danger of ingesting intestinal parasites together with raw salads is not unknown. But if you are able to grow vegetables organically in your own garden, that risk should be eliminated. With bought vegetables, however, you are never quite sure whether they were fertilised with liquid manure and thus infected with worm eggs. Hence the warning to wash salad greens thoroughly in salt water, rinsing them afterwards, to make sure that you have at least some protection. The effects of intestinal worms are most unpleasant and you would be wise to take care to avoid infection. Mind you, some people have had intestinal parasites for years, possibly decades, without realising it. They have no idea why they are always on edge, often unwell and anaemic. Nor do they know the cause of the black rings around the eyes. People who recognise these symptoms should consider the possibility that they may have intestinal worms. As mentioned above, one precautionary measure is to be careful when preparing raw food; another good suggestion is to take a course of *Papayasan*, the plant remedy that effectively eliminates worms.

TYPHOID FEVER, DYSENTERY AND OTHER INFECTIOUS DISEASES
Imported vegetables can pose dangers if they are not 100 per cent clean and so are perhaps infected with typhoid bacilli or carriers of dysentery or some other infectious disease. If you live in a hot country or in the tropics, never eat any raw food or fruit that you cannot peel or disinfect. The same advice goes for anyone who travels to such countries. It as advisable to be scrupulous in this respect, for the damage is quickly done. When peeling fruit, do not forget to disinfect the skin first, since anything adhering to it can stick to your fingers and, in turn, infect the peeled fruit before you eat it. Constant caution is indispensable, even though it may make life a little more complicated.

Conclusions
If, after all the above considerations, you conclude that the value of raw food does not really compensate for the many disadvantages and dangers, you are wrong. I have only made you aware of the disadvantages to show what could minimise the value so that you can exercise the necessary care and draw the full benefit from it. These reflections should stimulate anyone able to do so to take up organic gardening in order to obtain produce that poses no danger. So, if you have a garden or plot of land, there is nothing to prevent you from doing this. It is also gratifying to know that organic cultivation methods are winning more and more advocates.

Berries
If it were generally known how rich in vitamins berries are, they would figure far more in our everyday diet. Most of them contain a considerable amount of vitamin C. The importance of this vitamin is fully realised by those who have had bleeding gums, loose teeth, a tendency to chills and colds and a predisposition to haemorrhaging. All these forms of bleeding become immediately apparent when vitamin C is lacking.

Blackcurrants are rich in vitamin C, although not everyone likes their distinctive taste. But if you ate 50 g (2 oz) of these daily, you would provide your body with its full requirements of vitamin C for a whole day. Rose hip, sea buckthorn berries, raspberries, redcurrants, cranberries and nearly all other berries are excellent sources of vitamin C.

Vitamin A is supplied by various other berries. For example 100 g (about 4 oz) of fresh bilberries (blueberries) contain as much as 1.6 mg of pure vitamin A, and 100 g of blackberries, 0.8 mg. It is clear, then, that during the berry season you need not be solely dependent upon carrot juice and watercress as sources of this vitamin. Various berries will help to meet your daily requirement. This fact should be remembered by all those who suffer from the consequences of vitamin A deficiency, usually showing up in skin diseases, pathological changes in the hair, teeth and nails, softening of the cornea, obesity from glandular dysfunction, night-blindness (nyctalopia) and other conditions (see pages 486–8).

Although much has been done, said and written about vitamins, the last word on the subject has yet to be spoken. We are today catching a glimpse of the intricate interplay between vitamins, enzymes and hormones. Vitamin B_{12} is an indispensable component of the yellow respiratory enzyme; vitamin A, the opponent of the thyroid hormones and so on. Hyperthyroidism can thus be checked by eating plenty of food containing vitamin A, such as the berries mentioned above.

It is generally known that berries are also valuable because of their high mineral content. All berries, with the exception of cranberries, are predominantly alkaline. But in spite of their acidity, cranberries are still valuable, mainly for those who eat a large amount of raw food.

Experience has shown that berries are good for the liver and pancreas. In cases of disturbances in these organs, bilberries (blueberries) will do much to restore their proper functions. Although stone fruit, pears and other fruit can upset people with these disorders, berry juices will have a beneficial effect.

The one fruit that has to be watched is the strawberry. Many people are allergic to strawberries and they can also affect the kidneys, although much depends upon the fertilisers used in their cultivation. If the right organic manure or compost is used, that is, a natural compost, bone meal and natural lime, then reactions such as nettle rash (urticaria) may be avoided. If you are allergic to cultivated strawberries, try wild ones, because there is a difference. On the other hand, you may forget strawberries altogether and stick to the other kinds of berries that do not cause allergic reactions and are just as good.

People of a lymphatic constitution, who frequently have reason

503

to complain of swollen glands, should make the fullest use possible of all available berries. They are excellent for the glands, and may also help to reduce susceptibility to infectious diseases of the respiratory organs.

Mothers-to-be will similarly benefit from berries. When there are sufficient vitamins and minerals in the blood, most of the ailments associated with pregnancy can be avoided. Since vitamin C prevents morning sickness, it is recommended to eat food rich in this vitamin during pregnancy.

Allergic problems and the weariness often felt in the spring, the so-called 'spring fever', will be alleviated or even overcome by eating plenty of berries. Of course, we are referring to berries in their fresh, raw state. Eat as many as possible before preserving or bottling the surplus. You must remember, however, not to use white sugar for preserving, since it is a calcium robber and can cause problems. Rely on the fruit's own sugar instead, which, after all, is the most valuable sugar of all and berries are very rich in it. Since extra sugar is needed to make jam, use unrefined brown cane sugar with at least 10–20 per cent grape concentrate added, to give it still greater nutritional value.

The Curative Value of Berries

The outstanding curative properties of berries come into their own when they are eaten raw. When we let them ripen fully in our garden, their own fruit sugar suffices so that we do not need to add cane sugar or honey. Their vitamin content, their vital substances and natural colouring are an inestimable source of nourishment that is also remedial. When the liver or pancreas is sluggish, bilberries (blueberries) are not only acceptable but can actually bring about a cure.

Wild berries are also good for people who suffer from arthritis, rheumatism, cancer and multiple sclerosis. Those who are allergic to cultivated strawberries can usually take wild ones without experiencing any trouble. Since the endocrine glands, besides the liver, benefit greatly from the curative and vital substances of berries, they are, in a manner of speaking, a food for rejuvenation. This should not really surprise us, because by eating them regularly we can reduce excess weight, along with exerting a favourable influence on the ovaries, the thyroid gland and the hypophysis – in short, on all the endocrine glands. Wild fruits have the advantage of having been grown organically, so that we can be fully confident of their undiminished medicinal value.

The Properties of Sour Berries
Anyone who avoids eating sour berries for fear of ingesting too much acid is mistaken, because not everything that tastes sour is also chemically sour. Even in very sour-tasting berries the alkaline substances predominate. The only berry with an excess of acid is the cranberry. All the others can help to neutralise excess acidity, even in the overacid bodies of people suffering from rheumatism and arthritis.

Berry Juices
We have established that most berries are rich in vitamin C, so when they are in season they can supply us with what our bodies need, and that their alkaline minerals are also most beneficial. So as long as berries are there to be picked we should preferably eat them whole rather than only drinking the juice. We can do the latter once the season is over, enabling us to benefit from the curative properties of berries until the next crop. For those suffering from liver disorders bilberry juice is known to be excellent. Drinking blackberry and blackcurrant juice can be to our advantage. We know that the berries' colouring substances share in their curative effect. For instance, they cleanse and regenerate the intestinal flora. So it is for our good if we do not let the berry season pass us by and during the rest of the year make good use of natural pure fruit juices for the sake of our health.

Be Careful with Stone Fruit
People who have problems with the liver and pancreas must take care not to eat stone fruit, such as plums and peaches, in any great quantity, for if they do, they will probably pay for it with increased discomfort and pain. It is also important to remember that stone fruit should never be eaten on an empty stomach. What is more, be absolutely sure to eat slowly and insalivate the fruit thoroughly before swallowing. If you eat some crispbread, rusks or whole-wheat bread along with the fruit, the gastric reaction to the acids, especially hydrocyanic acid, will be diminished. Healthy constitutions used to raw foods can probably digest stone fruit very well and eat it at any time, but sick or delicate people should not take the risk. It is better to abstain from eating stone fruit than to eat it and suffer the consequences, only because other people might be able to enjoy it. If you should happen to eat some and upset the gastric and intestinal mucous membranes, you can obtain relief by taking a tablespoon of clay in water, morning and evening for a

few days. Should excessive gastric acidity develop, take a teaspoon of wood ash before each meal and the disturbance will quickly disappear.

Rules for Eating Stone Fruit

Stone fruit is known to be more digestible when dried than if eaten fresh. But whether fresh or dried, it is essential that we observe a few basic rules in order to enjoy these tasty fruits without having any problems.

Stone fruit cannot be stored in the cellar, nor would it ripen there. It should always be picked when fully ripe, and should also be ripe when bought. Partially ripe stone fruit causes problems, and also tastes unpleasant. Thus, anyone who buys unripe stone fruit will subsequently be disappointed and feel cheated. You will never see unripe apricots, for example, miraculously ripen. You can wait as long as you like, but they will not become juicy and sweet; rather, to your great dismay, they will shrivel up pitifully. Cherries should be ripe and what is more important, unsprayed, otherwise they will be harmful. When we eat fully ripe and unsprayed cherries together with some wholewheat (wholemeal) bread, chewing everything well, they will not cause fermentation and will exert a good influence on the liver. Another thing, we should never drink water while eating cherries, or immediately afterwards. This rule applies to all stone fruit. Remember, too, that this kind of fruit is not to be simply swallowed before being properly chewed, as is usually done. Stone fruit, if well insalivated will not give any trouble, as long as it is ripe and unsprayed. In the case of dried fruit (see below), it is also important to ensure that it is unsulphurised.

It is true that nowadays it may not be easy to follow through this advice if you cannot obtain your fruit from the right sources. Our own gardens, which we tend ourselves, will provide us with all we need, as will also the produce of farmers who look after their trees in an absolutely natural way, who pick and sell nothing but fully ripe fruit.

Jam-Making and Dried Fruit

An abundant crop of stone fruit is an inducement to use the surplus for making tasty jams. But you must be careful that the fruit's value and taste are not unduly spoiled by boiling it for too long. Well-made apricot jam is delicious. Cherry jam is also always popular, not only that made from the sweet but also from the sour cherry, which is customarily used more for jams than for eating fresh. Those who have no time to make their own will find the natural and carefully prepared *Vogel jams* worthwhile trying.

It is peculiar that stone fruit when dried does not cause any problems; rather, this process brings out its real goodness. However, when buying dried fruit we must make sure that it is natural, unsprayed and unsulphurised, for only then will we enjoy its full benefits. Dried apricots are a wonderful, thirst-quenching food to take with us when out walking, but again they must be absolutely natural and pure.

Health Benefits
Since natural food is indispensable for good health we can count on its benefits. Even if the vitamin content of cherries is relatively low, it is still important, because it is easily absorbed by the body. Cherries contain 0.05 mg per 100 g (2 oz) of vitamin B_1. This anti-beriberi substance, also known as thiamine, is good for vascular problems, circulation disorders and heart trouble, as well as for low blood pressure. This makes even small quantities of these vitamins welcome. Another of the B complex vitamins, known as nicotinamide, which is used in the treatment of pellagra, is also present in cherries at 0.01 mg per 100 g. If a person's gums often bleed or are inflamed, or the teeth are loose, natural food rich in vitamin C is needed. In this case we should eat unsprayed, fully ripe cherries. Sour cherries contain more vitamin C than the sweet kind, but they have 1 per cent less sugar. In spite of their sour taste, these cherries are alkaline-forming. They contain less sodium than sweet cherries, but in comparison they have more potassium and sulphur, and are very rich in malic and citric acids.

Formerly, a specially prepared syrup made from cherries together with the stones, which contain hydrocyanic acid, served as a diuretic for dropsy and as a refreshing drink. The fruits and their stones were crushed together, the pulp was squeezed out, and sixty-five parts of sugar were added to thirty-five parts of juice. Cherry stones were also once used for people who suffered from kidney stones, six to be taken daily. Even cherry stalks, especially those of red and sour cherries, were used for medicinal purposes; a tea was made from them to treat infections of the respiratory tract and to increase the flow of urine.

In former times, dried cherries were a remedy for chlorosis and anaemia. And even today, prunes, soaked and eaten before going to bed and before breakfast, are still used for sluggish bowels.

Continuing this simple treatment over a period of time will help even in stubborn cases of constipation.

Fully ripe and uncontaminated apricots and peaches are a wholesome addition to our food. They are relatively rich in vitamin C, contain some vitamins B_3 and B_2, a substantial amount of carotene and also pantothenic acid, which helps to prevent the hair turning grey.

SLOES – A STONE FRUIT

Not everyone knows that the blackthorn or sloe is a shrub that also bears stone fruit, sloes, although they are not edible. Nevertheless, to complete our list of the various stone fruits that have healing properties, we must not omit to mention it. As far back as antiquity this shrub was widely used. The flowers were picked and the essence made from them was used to cleanse the blood, as a laxative, as a remedy for the stomach, for coughs and for the lungs. A syrup made from its fruits, especially in combination with tormentil, was good for chronic diarrhoea. It is also beneficial for the mucous membranes of the stomach and intestines. Even anaemic persons will find sloe syrup to be a good and natural remedy. So the fruits of blackthorn serve exclusively for curative purposes, while we enjoy the other stone fruits as wholesome and healing food.

Fruit Sprayed with Pesticides

As more instances of poisoning from eating fruit sprayed with pesticides come to our attention, we would do well to consider the different aspects of this dangerous practice.

Some people do not react immediately to poisons such as lead, arsenic and copper sulphate used in sprays, being less sensitive. Others are more sensitive and immediately show signs of poisoning upon eating sprayed fruit. Be it as it may, when buying fruit one should make sure it has not been sprayed. It is common to find blemishes or an occasional brown spot on fruit that has not been treated with insecticides, but the fruit is still edible and its goodness is not impaired, since these blemishes are harmless plant fungi.

If you are uncertain as to whether a fruit has been sprayed, caution commands that you peel it, which unfortunately also removes the phosphates and other valuable materials which lie immediately under the skin. It is better to do without these minerals, however valuable, than to risk poisoning. If the fruit trees are sprayed in winter, when they are bare, the fruit cannot suffer since there is none; the only damage that can then be done is to the ground and the micro-organisms in it. The poison adhering to the bark will not find its way into the fruit later on.

It is hoped that the practice of spraying poisons, chemical pesticides, will eventually stop as there is the possibility of using harmless biological pesticides that will help increase the yield of crops without the risk of harming the consumer. However, such harmless products can only be discovered if an effort is made to find them, as is the case with natural remedies as opposed to chemical ones.

Experiments carried out with herbal sprays, containing extracts of horsetail (shave grass), yarrow and nasturtium have given very satisfactory results and trials are continuing. We also recommend spraying with tobacco extract because it is organic and much less hazardous than chemical sprays.

Rhubarb

I am often asked whether rhubarb is harmful as a food. There are some good things to be said about it, for instance that it is rich in vitamins, acids and various essential minerals. On the negative side, however, it must be said that rhubarb can be hard on the kidneys, especially when there is a tendency to kidney stones. One should always be very careful with rhubarb, as well as asparagus and Brussels sprouts, as all three of these are excessively acid-forming. Although they are beneficial if taken in small quantities, they can have an injurious effect on the kidneys if eaten in large amounts. Particular care should thus be exercised by anyone suffering from kidney stones or gravel, rheumatism and arthritis. For them it would be better to limit their intake of these foods or avoid them altogether.

Furthermore, it is important to choose the right kind of manure for rhubarb. If artificial fertiliser or unfermented liquid manure is used, the rhubarb can actually become poisonous. It is indeed lamentable that what is good for the farmer often turns out to be bad for the consumer. Still, we have to draw attention to these things. And then: 'let the buyer beware!'

Sugar

It is necessary to clarify certain questions connected with the various kinds of sugar, since many people are not sure of the difference between unrefined cane sugar and refined white sugar. In fact, it has been said that brown sugar (unrefined cane sugar) is treated with sulphur and is therefore no less detrimental to health than refined white sugar, which has been bleached and dyed for the purpose of preservation.

However, white sugar is dyed solely to enhance its whiteness, not to make it keep longer. This is done following the same principle as is applied in the manufacture of washing powder, to which is added 'blueing agents' to make the linen appear whiter than it actually is. Without this addition it would soon begin to look greyish. Sugar keeps indefinitely on its own and needs no preservative. If stored correctly, it will last a hundred years and still be sweet. It is 'blued' for eye-appeal and for no other reason.

Refined sugar, like refined flour, is a product of our civilisation, an unnatural 'food' and a contributory factor to ill health. We should keep away from anything that is detrimental to our health and reduces the nutritional value of our food. It is therefore obvious that denatured, refined foods are to be rejected. Unrefined cane sugar, on the other hand, contains various minerals, which are alkaline-forming and, at least, make some contribution to our health. Moreover, the allegation that it is treated with sulphur is untrue.

The best sugar is, and always will be, that found in nature, that is, in fruits, either fresh or dried. Raisins, sultanas, dates and figs are ideal sources of natural sugar. Since it does not need to be digested, it is the best and quickest source of energy. In fact, it is completely wrong to believe that protein foods are the only energy source. And why? Just think of a bull and its tremendous power, yet it does not eat any kind of protein food at all. Or think of a cow and the enormous quantity of fat it produces – all from the grass it eats!

If you wish to sweeten your morning dish of muesli, you do not need either sugar or honey. Currants or raisins will amply sweeten your breakfast dish; just put them through the mincer and add them to the rest. Honey and grape sugar are excellent, nutritious sweeteners. Condensed sugar cane juice, pear or peach syrup and similar forms of sugar, which have not been refined, can also be used with confidence.

The commercially prepared so-called grape sugar, glucose or dextrose, made from corn (maize) starch, does not belong in the category of natural sugars. The chemical formula of synthetic grape sugar happens to be the same as that of natural sugar made from grapes. The two have nothing else in common. In fact, the 'grape sugar' or dextrose that is sold over-the-counter in powder or tablet form is a misnomer. To be sure, it supplies calories, it gives energy, but it lacks the nutritive and curative properties of the genuine grape juice. After all, we are not so interested in the chemical formula of sugar, but in its effect on our health.

So what do we mean by 'grape sugar', as referred to in this book? We refer to the genuine sugar made from grapes, the condensed pure grape juice made from vine-ripened grapes. The manufactured grape sugar is artificial, but the genuine article can be described as nutritive grape sugar or grape concentrate. This syrup can also be made from raisins, sultanas and currants. It is by far the best sweetener available, in many ways equal to honey and in other respects even superior to it because some people cannot take honey, whereas practically everyone can tolerate real grape sugar.

Infants and children, patients with a feverish condition, and seriously ill adults suffering from metabolic disorders should use only grape sugar, rather than white sugar, to sweeten their drinks. It oxidises in the system without any waste and does not impose any additional burden on the body. Unlike white sugar, grape sugar is not a calcium robber. It should be part of the diet of every convalescent and those with weak hearts or frayed nerves because of its soothing quality. Sleeping drops, lemon balm herb tea or heart tonic sweetened with grape sugar in a little water and taken at night encourage restful sleep. Grape sugar has only one drawback: it is relatively expensive. But this is not at all astonishing in view of the cost of grapes nowadays.

Since reports continue to circulate that seek to discredit natural foods and justify the use of denatured, refined products, it is high time that we clarify the question of sugar once and for all, so that the consumer can be sure of what is genuine and wholesome, and what is misleading and false.

The goodness of fruit sugar is not in any doubt, but when you buy dried fruit take care to select only the produce that is not sulphurised, bleached or denatured in any other way. Nothing but natural, pure fruit guarantees the benefits we intend to derive from it in the first place.

The Value of Natural Unrefined Sugar

I shall never forget the Indian children we met in Central America. They would approach us slowly, smiling timidly, while chewing on a piece of sugar cane. This seemed to satisfy their sweet tooth and helped them to overcome their shyness. Practically all children like sugar, the peculiar carbohydrate that gives our taste buds the pleasant sensation of sweetness. The young Indians enjoy raw sugar cane and also the raw fresh juice that is then condensed over a fire, making what they call *pilosillo*. Most astonishing to me was the fact that although they ate a great deal of the sweet brown syrup their teeth were strong and beautiful. In fact, if they had no knife handy, I often saw them using their teeth like one.

JUSTIFIED WARNINGS

More than ever before, we read and hear about the dangers of eating too much sugar. Are these warnings justified? Why are we nowadays told that sugar and sweets are harmful, especially to our teeth and bones? Is the appalling condition of our children's teeth really the result of their eating too much sugar and sweet things? Again, is the assertion true that even unrefined cane sugar is not the healthy natural product it is made out to be?

Being good observers and knowing how to use practical experience, we can draw the following conclusions. We must look for the problem's solution in what our sweets consist of, what goes into their making. The Indian children probably indulge as much in sugar and sweet products as do our young ones, yet 90 per cent of our children have bad teeth in spite of good oral hygiene, using a toothbrush and toothpaste, while the Indians lack these modern implements and have good teeth. However, the sweet things the young Indians enjoy are not refined products, but still contain all their natural substances, a combination of minerals such as calcium, fluoride, magnesium, manganese, iron, silica and phosphorus. And that is the crux of the matter, because what our children eat is refined sugar without the minerals, which is bound to disturb the whole mineral metabolism and result in a mineral and vitamin deficiency. This serious state of affairs is made even worse by our eating other denatured products, for example white flour and white rice. The resulting deficiencies then lead to bad teeth and other damage to our health.

Alternatives to Refined Sugar

People who move to our regions from far away lands and exchange their natural foods for a diet of our refined foods will soon begin to experience dental problems. It is a fact that sweets and refined sugar can cause much more damage to our health than is commonly assumed. Yet there are other good sweeteners around, for example honey, grape sugar syrup made from grapes and dried fruits such as raisins, sultanas, currants, figs and dates. All these fruits contain easily assimilated natural sugar, but with an abundance of minerals.

So, when you prepare a dish of breakfast muesli, a gruel or porridge, think of including raisins; put them through the mincer and then add them to your dish as a sweetener. You may ask, 'Can I use crude sugar?' Sugar made from sugar beet is unsuitable for the table; it would not be a good sweetener for fruit muesli because it often makes it taste like soap. There is another drawback to unrefined beet sugar; it is treated with lime, a process that reduces its mineral content. Unrefined cane sugar, as we know it, is not equal to the *pilosillo* mentioned earlier. *Pilosillo* is simply condensed and crystallised sugar cane juice, whereas the kind we buy in Europe has already been through one refining process, again generally using lime, and is therefore no longer 100 per cent pure. However, it does contain some of the molasses and a total of about 2 per cent minerals, so that it is still more valuable than the white, completely refined, sugar.

Another very good natural sweetener or sugar is maple sugar, which the Indians of North America make from condensed maple syrup. This is very tasty and well worth trying. A further alternative is date sugar, which is discussed below.

If you want to remain healthy, watch what kind of sugar you eat. Parents should heed the advice given regarding sugar and sweets, because it is intended for the sake of their children's well-being. If you observe these guidelines your health will benefit because of eating natural food, and you will save a great deal of money on dentist's bills!

THE GOODNESS OF DATES

The visitor to Mesopotamia and the Persian Gulf is greeted by millions of date palms. Growing in unspoilt, mineral-rich soil, they bring forth thousands of tons of a wonderful fruit sugar year by year, the great benefits of which, however, rarely extend beyond these geographical borders. It is a joy to admire the Arab children's beautiful teeth, but the sight also fills the visitor with sadness. Why? On the one hand we are glad for the Arab children, but on the other hand we are sad because the teeth of our own children and youths, according to the reports of school dentists, are in a very poor state indeed.

When I visited the ruins and vicinity of ancient Babylon, an Arab boy climbed up a date palm, happily and with enviable ease, picked some ripe dates and threw them down to me. It gave him great satisfaction to see that his generosity was gratefully acknowledged, his beaming smile showing a row of healthy white teeth. His firm and strong muscles and his lithe body, which gives those sons of the desert the agility of a wild cat, impressed me greatly. Although these children of nature can be presumptuous and brash, they do leave an unforgettable impression.

While our children spoil their teeth with all sorts of sweets made from refined sugar, the children of those desert tribes have nothing but dates to satisfy their sweet tooth. It is not without good reason that dates are called the 'meat' of the desert Arabs. Their children eat a large amount of date sugar but still have healthy teeth, just like those of the Indian children who satisfy their desire for sweet things by eating green sugar cane or *pilosillo*, the condensed sugar cane juice.

What a pity that we are not similarly inclined and satisfied with simple natural things! If we could avoid the use of refined sugar, which contributes to tooth decay and many other degenerative conditions, our children's teeth would be much better. What is more, refined sugar is now about three times dearer than it was just a few years ago. So there are many reasons why we should try to eliminate it from our diet as much as possible, substituting fruit sugar instead.

Date sugar and grape sugar, made from raisins and currants, are so valuable that everyone who is interested in his or her family's health should make the effort to sweeten all fruit dishes with it. This would provide the entire family with valuable carbohydrates and the vital minerals and vitamins needed to prevent sickness.

In view of my observations I am sure I was right to give consideration to the problem of sugar while sitting in the shade of some Mesopotamian date palms. There and then I made up my mind to experiment with the valuable natural sugar of dates and come up with a product that pleases the taste buds and is also a healthy food. Indeed, every food item, and especially sweets, should be such that they cannot spoil our children's teeth in the future. We want their teeth to be just as healthy as those of the Arab children who obtain their sugar from Mesopotamia's date palms.

The Value of Canned and Bottled Fruit

Some time ago I received a letter with the following query: 'The other day I read in a book on diet reform that preserved fruits and those bottled hot have no nutritional value. I have been wondering about this, because during the past year I have bottled a quantity of fruit, thinking it would have greater food value than fruit commercially canned.'

I would like to answer this enquiry in print because it will be of interest to everyone. It is quite true that in preserving fruits and vegetables by the heat process many of the vitamins are destroyed. However, the statement about preserved fruits having no nutritional value is absolutely untrue. The actual nutrients, such as carbohydrates, sugar, starch and minerals, remain unchanged and for this reason preserved fruits and vegetables do have considerable food value, assuming that a natural process is used to preserve them.

It is quite a different story with commercially canned fruits and vegetables. The bleaching, blanching and chemical additives definitely affect the nutritional value. If I speak out against canned foods, it is because it so often happens that, just for the sake of convenience, factory-preserved foods are used when the meal could, with a little extra effort, consist of at least some fresh fruit or vegetables. Canned foods are served all too often in hospitals and sanatoriums. If sick people are to get well, they must have health-giving nourishment, which can be obtained at its maximum value only from fresh vegetables and fresh fruit. For this reason one should eat fresh foods as much as possible – fresh berries, fruit and vegetables – when they are in season. Eat your vegetables raw in salads and fruit in muesli or fruit salad. Any surplus that cannot be used this way should be preserved and bottled immediately, so that provision is made for the winter.

You can guarantee healthy nutrition if you always supplement a dish of preserved vegetables or fruit with some fresh produce. Not everything you eat need have a high vitamin content; it suffices when part of the meal meets this criterion. The important thing is to make sure that you do not leave out anything essential when planning your menu. Let us suppose that, for lunch in winter, you have yogurt, which contains vitamins, and some fresh carrot or beet salad. In addition you may have some of your preserved vegetables, as well as potatoes or natural brown rice. The body will then obtain its vitamins from the fresh vegetables, and other nutrients from the preserved or bottled food. All in all, you will be adequately and correctly fed.

Preserve and bottle all surplus from your garden produce, but do not make the mistake of depriving the children of fresh fruits and berries just because you want to keep them. I remember as a child having to watch the blackcurrants and raspberries I longed to eat being made into jam. Parents, in their eagerness to preserve them, forget about the value of fresh fruit.

Our Daily Bread

Bread has always played an important part in our nutrition. It is still on our table today and every day as a staple food. The age-old request 'Give us this day our daily bread' illustrates to what extent we depend upon it. We may have an abundance of other foods, but bread remains the foundation of our diet. How much we disliked having it rationed during the war years. Things have changed since then, although the need for good and wholesome bread is as great as ever.

Nutritious Bread

It has always pleased me when, here and there on my travels, I have been served with bread as it was once made in my own country – from the whole grain. I found that the North American Indian women prepared their bread from grain that they had ground themselves with a stone mill. Arabs, Bedouins and other African people still keep up the custom of making their bread from wholegrain cereals. Some use wheat, some rye, others barley and each of these breads tastes good and provides the body with all the goodness of the whole grain, because whole cereals contain most of the elements needed to build up the organism and maintain it in a healthy condition. They abound in minerals, enzymes, vitamins and other essential factors.

The Greek mountain peasants also use good wholewheat bread as the foundation of their diet. Wherever you find good bread, the health and resistance of the people consuming it is better than among those living on white bread. Where white bread and rolls are the common fare, I have always found more bad health. True, white bread may not be the only reason for this, but it does share the blame for lack of good health.

One cannot imagine Ruth, a woman of biblical fame, having gleaned the valuable ears of grain from Boaz' field, only to turn it into refined flour. The Book of Books reports that in ancient times the whole grain, barley or wheat, was ground in a stone mill, then honey was added to it and it was made into cakes.

The Correct Baking Process

We know from the history of ancient Rome that their legionaries were issued a certain quantity of wheat every day. Wheat grain can be stored almost indefinitely without losing any of its value, but this is not the case with flour. As soon as the external sheath has been broken and the grain has been milled, the oxygen in the air begins to take effect, and the longer the flour is kept, the more it will lose of its value. The enzymes are probably the first to suffer from such exposure. These are active elements in the grain, for example diastase, which comes to life during the process of germination and changes the starch of the grain into maltose, then dextrose.

An interesting observation will illustrate this. Make some dough from freshly ground flour and knead it well with your hands. You will notice that the hands become quite red as hyperaemia is produced. It is the active enzymes that are responsible for this phenomenon and these are found especially in the bran and the germ. If you make dough from the same flour after it has been stored for 5–6 weeks, this reaction will no longer occur to the same extent, if at all, because the enzymes will have decreased in effectiveness or died off during the long period of storage. That is why it is better to use a stone mill for grinding – as our forefathers did and certain primitive peoples still do – then prepare and bake the bread immediately. Thus the full value of the enzymes is preserved and the bread will be more nourishing, for it contains the healthy substances of the wholegrain cereal.

Wholewheat or any other wholemeal bread should be prepared in the way just described, and we should make it a point to make or buy bread which is prepared and baked according to this natural method. When we consider the great demands placed on our system today, it is only sensible that we should prefer bread that retains its full nutritional value and reject the less valuable.

The Milling Process
The manner in which bread cereals are ground is quite important. Some time ago I visited an old miller, who showed me an old-fashioned stone mill, now unused, beside the beautiful new machinery that replaced it. Without any prompting on my part, the miller began to tell me that his old mill had produced excellent flour, while the other two modern machines seemed to take all the goodness out of it. At first I thought this was rather exaggerated, but in the light of subsequent observations I was forced to agree with him.

The ancient Romans, who knew something about metallurgy, were certainly in a position to make metal rollers or discs, if they had not been convinced that the use of stone was more appropriate for milling grain. Every metal mill, if it creates too much friction heat, does something detrimental to the flour which, ultimately, is reflected in its taste and quality.

Today it is known that copper destroys most of the vitamin C content of food that is brought into contact with this metal. Similar effects take place with other metals too. Thus it is possible that an iron or steel mill could affect the taste or composition, or both, of the flour, even though this has not yet been proved conclusively.

The Question of Bread – a Solution

All these deliberations urged me to find a solution to the bread question that would comply with all the requirements I have mentioned. Many years ago I carried out a series of experiments with the help of a master baker. I decided to use not only wheat, but also rye, because of its high fluoride content. As a rule, the bread we eat is mainly made from wheat, but rye is particularly important for the teeth and bones. In areas where much rye bread is eaten, good teeth and excellent bone structure stand out as a characteristic among the people. There is no doubt that rye bread and rye cripsbread lay a healthy foundation for this.

On the other hand, wherever white bread is now consumed, deficiencies have developed to such an extent that dental caries and other problems affecting the teeth and bone structure are very much in evidence, sometimes as early as in the first generation after the changeover.

On account of this definite link between white bread consumption and poor dental health, I decided to bring out a natural bread, called 'Risopan'. It is, in content, comparable to the bread eaten by primitive peoples, being made of whole rye, wheat, barley, rice bran and rice germ for the sake of their richness in vital minerals. Unfortunately, for the most part, we are used to eating refined white rice instead of the whole brown rice and it is advantageous to compensate for the deficiency somewhat by means of bread that contains all its nutritive substances. 'Risopan' is prepared in accordance with the principles I have just outlined. The grain is ground in a stone mill and the flour is immediately made into a dough and baked. It keeps very well and is most suitable for taking on long journeys. The new Vogel wholegrain flake bread is also made in a similar way to 'Risopan'.

It would be a good thing if other wholegrain or wholewheat bread were always made according to the same natural method. If you eat such bread year in and year out, it is reasonable to assume that your body will benefit greatly from it. Remember that nature is not guided by our palates, moods and appetites, but works according to its eternal laws. If we ignore or reject nature's dictates, we will have to suffer the eventual consequences, or at least our children will. So make sure to serve nothing but good and wholesome bread. It alone is the foundation of natural and healthy nutrition.

Whole Wheat and Other Cereals

However intensively one may campaign against the use of white flour and other refined foods, there is still far too little attention given to the fact that cereal deprived of its germ and bran is no longer a health food. Vitamins, minerals, highly valuable oils and other substances are no longer present in refined flour. As a result, it is not the least bit surprising that the general standard of nutrition is decreasing despite the abundance of other varieties of food. Even though many may not want to see that the health and physical strength of the people are drastically reduced when white flour, white sugar and other refined products are the common fare, the facts cannot be denied. Modern nutritionists and researchers tell us clearly that minerals and vitamins are essential to good health, yet what do we do? Most of us simply ignore such clearcut statements based on scientific research.

Our grandparents could certainly tell us a thing or two about the more natural way of life. Their diet, simple though it was, did not produce the deficiencies of today, because it consisted of wholefoods, lacking none of the vital elements. In the country bread was baked in the home and this good, old-fashioned cereal bread formed the basis of their daily diet. We really should abandon the lamentable custom of refining and canning food, a custom of our civilisation that has been nothing but detrimental to our health, and return to the simple, natural ways of our forebears.

You, the individual, can do something about this for yourself. Eat whole wheat, which is no doubt one of the best foods available, containing just the right amount and combination of elements, and should be used in its entirety. You will find it very tasty and wholesome. Soak the grains, then steam them with a little butter or oil and onions, and season with one of the many culinary herbs. If you prefer not to use onions, they may be omitted. The dish can also be prepared 'au gratin' in the oven, or you can add soaked wheat kernels to soups, stews, casseroles, etc. Wheat prepared in

519

the same way as a risotto makes a delicious 'wheatotto'. Why not use whole wheat in every form possible? If you like, you can even sweeten it with almonds, raisins or currants.

Whole rye and barley can be used in the same way, although they are not quite as palatable as wheat. Seasoned with fine culinary herbs, the soaked grains can be put through the mincer and made into rissoles. There are many possible methods of preparation and the resourceful cook will never be at a loss to find and make many cereal dishes that are tasty and healthy. A dish made with whole wheat is an energy food for growing children and ravenous youths, as well as for those who do heavy work. Add vegetables and fresh salad and you have a combination of foods that provides the basis for first-class nutrition. Since it is amazing what strange combinations of food are sometimes dreamed up, I would like to stress that you should never eat a salad or vegetables together with a sweet wholegrain dish; it is better to combine sweet things with stewed fruit or grated raw apple muesli and cream. For a good effect, grate some fresh fruit and mix it in with the *compote*. A cup of rose hip tea also goes well with a sweet wholegrain dish.

Germinated Cereals – an Inexpensive Tonic

It is quite common to spend good money on expensive tonics, so you will be pleased to learn that there is something much cheaper within your reach. I am referring to germinated cereals, whether it be wheat, rye or barley. These cereals offer us what many an over-the-counter potion promises but does not provide.

So how can we obtain germinated wheat? Well, all that is necessary to make grains sprout is moisture and warmth. Place a wet cloth on a plate, sprinkle it with grains and put it in a cupboard or similar warm place. Be sure to keep the cloth damp or germination will be retarded or even stopped altogether. When the sprouts have grown to a length of about 2–5 mm (up to about ¼ inch), put the grains through a mincer and use as a foundation for muesli. Or eat the mince just as it is, but remember to chew it thoroughly and insalivate well.

As soon as germination takes place, the enzyme diastase becomes active and transforms the polysaccharide starch into disaccharide sugar, or malt, which is easier to digest than starch. This process, by the way, is used to turn barley into malt. If you chew the germinated grain you will notice its sweet taste. This fresh 'malt' is rich in enzymes, especially diastase, and this is what makes it such a wonderful tonic food. It can be eaten together with linseed as is done in Sweden, where the dish is called *kruska*. It aids the digestion of other starchy foods and is recommended for those who have poor assimilation and have trouble gaining weight. It is a simple, inexpensive and excellent tonic food and is also good for the blood. If, at the same time, you eat plenty of raw carrots or drink fresh carrot juice, perhaps going on a grape diet as well, you will be able to build up your strength without having to pay a fortune. Together with plenty of grapes or fresh grape juice, this diet is recommended for people with heart trouble. Anyone suffering from constipation should avoid the skin and pips of the grapes. The advice also holds true for those who tend to suffer from fermentation and flatulence, since not eating the skin and pips prevents these intestinal problems.

Good results with germinated wheat encouraged Dr Bircher-Benner to recommend it to his patients too.

Wheat Germ

Wheat germ – those tiny yellow flakes – is far too little valued and used. If people only realised how wonderfully nourishing and curative these flakes are they would serve them every day in one way or the other, including in their breakfast muesli. Girls and young women in particular would eat more wheat germ if they appreciated what marvellous properties it has to offer.

Wheat germ contains a first-class protein and much oil. More important, however, are the phosphates in it, and we should all know the vital role phosphates, and their combinations play in keeping our nervous system healthy. Still more important than phosphates is the high content of vitamin E in wheat germ. Let me briefly remind you of what vitamin E means to us.

It is not for nothing that vitamin E is also called the fertility vitamin, since it plays a considerable part in the development and function of the reproductive organs. But the ovaries and testicles are more than just reproductive organs, they actually discharge their secretions into the bloodstream and therefore belong to the category of organs known as the endocrine glands. Vitamin E is of great importance for the correct functioning of these glands and thus for the entire metabolism.

Provided there is no physical disability, vitamin E often acts as an aid to conception when a woman eats foods rich in this vitamin. Due to its high content of vitamin E, wheat germ is the single most indicated item for this therapy. Every 100 g (4 oz) of wheat germ contain as much as 30 mg of pure vitamin E.

Wheat germ is one of the best remedies that can be recommended to help overcome a tendency to premature birth. In fact, if pregnant women were to eat sufficient wheat germ or take wheat germ oil capsules, the painful experience of miscarriage could often be prevented.

Brucellosis (undulant fever, Bang's disease) has been successfully treated with vitamin E preparations and there is no better specific remedy than wheat germ and wheat germ oil for this purpose. For years, farmers have observed that feeding their cattle with good bran, which contains wheat germ, reduces the incidence of brucellosis and abortion. The results of experiments in which cattle suffering from brucellosis were fed with wheat germ have confirmed that sufficient quantities of vitamin E in time enable the body to build up resistance to the germs which cause this disease.

Girls and women who become obese because of ovarian insufficiency should take *herbal sitz baths* and eat plenty of wheat germ, as this will stimulate the ovaries, increase the metabolic rate of the body and so dispose of undesirable fat. In addition, they should take the seaweed preparation *Kelpasan* for even faster results.

Lack of vigour and stamina, tiredness because of overwork and neurasthenic conditions call for foods rich in vitamin E, which have a better effect than all expensive medicines if taken over a period of time. Anyone suffering from impotence should not give up hope, but take a long-term course of wheat germ or wheat germ oil capsules and, at the same time, *Kuhne treatments* (see pages 436–8), which will certainly help, if not cure the problem completely. In addition to wheat germ, other sources of vitamin E are *lettuce, watercress* and *soybeans*. So make sure to eat enough of these natural products if you suffer from any of the above-mentioned conditions. Moreover, it is interesting to note that experiments on vitamin E have shown that no side effects have resulted if too much of the vitamin is taken.

Thus there are many reasons why we should ensure that our families eat wheat germ regularly. Among other things, it will ensure that our children's most important glands will develop properly. Wheat germ has a delicious taste, not only when sprinkled over muesli and in soups, but also on bread and honey – a much healthier snack than sugary buns from the baker's.

Wheat germ as a concentrated food is an absolute necessity in our modern world, where so much low-value, denatured food is eaten, causing an increasing prevalence of deficiency diseases. People living in areas relatively untouched by modern development and those of us who live on natural wholefoods, generally speaking may not need to take concentrated food such as wheat germ on a regular basis. If you make it a habit to eat whole grains and other wholefoods, you will obtain the essential substances in the right proportion. In wheat germ they are in a concentrated form.

Wheat Germ and Bran
If we slice a wheat grain lengthways we will find that the white inside is mainly made up of starch. White flour comes from this part. The yellowish germ is located at one end of the kernel. Years ago the wheat germ was not fully used because no one knew about its great value as a source of vitamin E. The outer protective cover over the starchy part is the bran, consisting of a tough sheath which, being pure cellulose, is indigestible. This roughage should not be eaten if one suffers from gastritis and stomach ulcers, for it is so tough and sharp-edged that it would actually irritate and inflame an already damaged stomach lining. In the case of ulcers it may even trigger pain and light bleeding.

A number of valuable minerals are found in the layers between the starch and the outer cellulose sheath. These layers contain vitamins of the B complex, gluten and amino acids essential for the building up of body protein. It is exactly these valuable and important parts of the wheat kernel that are usually fed to cattle, the bran together with its roughage or cellulose and germ. It is quite an achievement that modern milling machines are able to separate the valuable layers without including the indigestible cellulose, so that we can actually obtain the important elements of the grain and include them in our diet. This product is sold as 'wheat germ and bran.'

Buckwheat (*Fagopyrum esculentum*)
If you travelled down to Pusciavo during the war you could have seen in the districts adjoining the Italian border many fields sown with buckwheat, a crop which is almost unknown to this day in other areas. Our fellow citizens in the south were smarter than we in the north when it came to looking after themselves. There was a government requisition order on wheat flour, but buckwheat, a wild cereal, was exempt. So the farmers started to grow buckwheat, which was known to be highly nutritious and wholesome.

Buckwheat is satisfied even with poor and sandy soil and has a short growing period. In fact, the crop matures within three months and for this reason it is cultivated in northern climates where the seasons are short, as in Siberia. The plant attains a height of half a metre (1½–2 feet) and has reddish white flowers which provide a good supply of nectar for the bees. American buckwheat honey is known far and wide.

The French name for buckwheat, *blé sarrasin,* seems to indicate that buckwheat must have been brought to France from the south by the Saracens, whereas the Russian name, *gretsikha, grikki* suggests that the Greeks probably introduced this valuable food into their neighbouring lands. In many parts of Russia it is a national dish and the people prepare a most delicious oven-baked buckwheat.

Whole buckwheat can be cooked in the same manner as rice, and buckwheat groats are excellent in soup and for rissoles. The flour makes what is called a 'short' pastry and is good for mixing with wheat flour. The resulting pastry is better than that made with wheat flour and a high proportion of butter.

German biologists have discovered that buckwheat reduces high blood pressure, a finding that has since been confirmed by American scientists. An extract of buckwheat is thus claimed to combat high blood pressure and arteriosclerosis (hardening of the arteries). Unpolished brown rice has the same attributes as buckwheat in this respect. It would be to the advantage of older people if they were to change their menus slightly, to include more natural brown rice and buckwheat, but fewer eggs, cheese and pulses (legumes), for these two cereals have a rejuvenating effect on the blood vessels, especially the arteries. The intake of protein and salt should also be reduced to a minimum as one advances in age or if one suffers from high blood pressure.

Buckwheat Dishes
Whole buckwheat: Precook some buckwheat in a little water or vegetable stock. Make a sauce from two teaspoons of wholegrain (wholemeal) flour, finely chopped herbs and unseasoned tomato purée and mix with the buckwheat. Add some stewed onion and a little oil, and cook until the grains are soft but still whole.

Cold buckwheat: Prepare some buckwheat as above, pour it into a mould and leave to cool. When cold, remove from the mould and garnish with parsley and tomatoes. Serve with a green salad.

Fried buckwheat: Prepare a buckwheat gruel, then add some finely chopped onions, garlic and a little marjoram. Form into small shapes and fry in oil on both sides until golden brown.

What You Should Know about Potatoes

What else is there to know about potatoes other than that they are tasty? That is about the extent of most people's knowledge about the peculiar solanaceous plant we call potato and botanists call *Solanum tuberosum*. Because potatoes belong to the same family as the deadly nightshade, our forefathers had some rather unfortunate experiences with them when they were first brought to Europe. No one knew this strange plant native to Peru's highlands.

If ever you get the chance to visit the mountainous areas of that country you will be surprised to see how many varieties of potato actually grow there, many not even known to us. In the Altiplano, from Cuzco as far as Puno on Lake Titicaca especially, the Indians cultivate some beautiful vegetables.

It was as late as the sixteenth century when Spanish sailors and Sir Francis Drake first brought potatoes to Europe, with the intention of cultivating them as a food on the European continent. They gave them to their friends but did not explain anything about the new plant. Why not? Well, it often happens, does it not, that someone knows something but does not tell it to another person simply because he thinks that he will be aware of it already. That is exactly what happened with the potato. No one who planted the tubers seemed to realise that the unknown plant was a member of the deadly nightshade family and had poisonous properties. Neither could anyone imagine that it was the tubers themselves that served for food and not the round green berries growing on the plant. In fact, no one took any notice of the actual potatoes. Of course, the result of eating the berries brought only trouble, because anyone who tried the new vegetable from overseas soon suffered from diarrhoea and vomiting.

The story goes that, very upset and disappointed, some of those participating in one of the potato meals went and uprooted the plants, tops and all, and flung them onto a bonfire. Involuntarily, they had also pulled out the potatoes attached to the roots. Meanwhile, these roasted nicely in the fire and one or two rolled out of the embers. In anger, someone stamped on them, but they smelled so appetising that the person picked one up. A little hesitant, he tried it and to his surprise it tasted as delicious as it smelled. So that was it! What they were to eat were not the green berries on the plant but the tubers that grew under the ground! The mystery was solved and Europe had gained a new food, one that is not only a source of protein, starch and vitamin C, but also a remedy.

Potatoes as a Remedy

Raw potato juice has proved its worth in the treatment of arthritis and it is also a fine remedy for stomach ulcers. Patients are advised to drink the juice of a medium-sized potato (about one-third of a glass) before breakfast on an empty stomach. The ulcers usually disappear within 3–6 weeks. If a little fresh *carrot juice* is added to the potato juice the taste will be improved, making it easier to take. If the patient is unable to prepare his own juice because of lack of time, he can take the lacto-fermented juice sold in health food stores.

Raw potato juice, together with *centaury*, is a splendid help in neutralising excess acid in the stomach, which is generally the cause of heartburn. The simplest way to do this is to add fresh centaury drops to the potato juice. It has not yet been discovered whether the remedial effect is attributable to the solanin content (about 0.002 per cent) or to the alkaline mineral salts.

An interesting letter informed us recently that *Solanosan*, together with *Petasites*, helped a stomach and liver patient to find relief from pain, providing restful sleep, an improved appetite and weight gain. Solanosan complex is made from the potato plant, which can have a poisonous effect, but the remedy is in homoeopathic potency and therefore efficacious in treating the indicated illnesses. Large amounts of Solanin, however, can cause poisoning and even endanger one's life.

BEWARE!

The green potato leaves contain approximately 0.06 per cent solanin, the flowers 0.6 per cent and the fruits, which look like green berries, about 1 per cent. The white eyes or sprouts on the potatoes themselves are very dangerous, the green ones even worse. As soon as they begin to appear, in winter or spring, cut them out carefully. They are especially bad for the eyes. When the tubers grow a little above the soil and turn green, make sure to cut the green part off since it is poisonous. These rules are simple and can be followed without any difficulty. However, this need for care does not mean that a plant which is considered dangerous cannot also be most useful, even contain food and remedial properties – as the potato clearly proves.

Oils and Fats

Their Role in Degenerative Diseases
In the search for contributory causes of gout, arthritis, cancer, multiple sclerosis, liver trouble and other serious diseases, investigators always discover something new after years of research. Almost all experts agree that hereditary factors play an important part in the predisposition to certain diseases. Mental and physical strain, overwork, constant hurry, irritations, fears and worries cannot be ignored as contributory causes, or they may even trigger the diseases. Poisons finding their way into the system through drugs and unnatural foodstuffs, preservatives and additives, must be recognised as detrimental to health. Modern refined and nutrient-deficient foodstuffs also share considerably in the blame and invariably undermine our health. We are thinking especially of canned foods that are prepared in such a way that they retain none of their original nutritional value. Then there is a particular substance that has so far received little attention, but the absence of which may lead to degenerative diseases. I am referring to the polyunsaturated fatty acids that are contained in natural oils and fats but are destroyed by heating, refining, hardening and other factory processes. A lack of these acids gives rise to disturbances in the metabolism of the cells, and it is obvious that this must have a bearing upon other pathological processes as well. A few years ago, little was known about the unsaturated fatty acids and few, if any, references were made to the importance of natural oils and fats in a balanced diet. Only recently has it become possible to see what part these substances play in degenerative diseases or their prevention.

The Nature and Properties of Oils and Fats
Oils and fats do not have a highly complicated chemical formula: on the contrary, they consist of the common elements carbon, hydrogen and oxygen. All fats and oils used for food contain one or more of the three types of fatty acids, the saturated, the unsaturated and the polyunsaturated. If we consume an excess of saturated fatty acids, as found in refined fats and oils, too much energy is required to digest them and for this reason we feel tired and sleepy after a meal.

The saturated fatty acids are chemical compounds that are exceedingly poor in oxygen and their consumption would require us to exercise and breathe deeply – something we feel no inclination to do after eating such foods. These heavy fats, are mainly of animal origin and have a high melting point, while the unsaturated oils occur chiefly in seeds and have a low melting point. Vegetable oils are richer in unsaturated, even highly unsaturated fatty acids. For this reason natural, unrefined oils are better for you than others. Oils with a low melting point are hardened or hydrogenised because transporting and stocking them in bottles is more difficult and costly. So the oil industries prefer the method of hardening because firm slabs of fat can be more easily packed and transported than liquids.

However, the hardening process has a detrimental influence on the quality of the product since metallic compounds can remain in the fats, even if only in homoeopathic dilution. Furthermore, the unsaturated fatty acids are transformed in the process into high-melting stearic acids, which do not have the same health value. If you want to remain healthy, avoid the hardened fats, even though they may be easy to use and store.

Why, then, do the unsaturated fatty acids have the above-mentioned advantages, whereas the hardened fats have lost them? The answer is quite a simple one. They are not saturated and therefore able to become saturated. That is, the unsaturated fatty acids are still able to combine with other elements. Figuratively speaking, they are still single, unmarried, and therefore ready and willing to enter a relationship. They will combine with the minerals, proteins and oxygen in the body and in this way encourage normal cell metabolism and oxidation. If these functions are interfered with over a period of years, even decades, the cells degenerate and disease will inevitably manifest itself. Cell growth may become abnormal and malignant, cancerous. The phospholipoids may degenerate and this can lead to thrombosis. Where there is a lack of polyunsaturated fatty acids and in their place an excess of saturated ones, the cholesterol in the blood will combine with the fats and deposit itself on the walls of the blood vessels, giving rise to hardening of the arteries (arteriosclerosis), high blood pressure and the danger of apoplexy or a stroke.

Considering all these factors, it will be seen how vital it is to change over to unrefined fats and oils, such as those made from sunflower and safflower seed, olives, poppy seed and linseed. Also, fresh tree seed products, or nuts, are suitable for meeting our vital requirement of unsaturated and polyunsaturated fatty acids. A first-class source of highly unsaturated fatty acids are sesame seeds, which contain up to 43 per cent of these oils, in addition to interesting combinations of minerals and proteins, making these seeds a valuable food item indeed. Sesame seeds and products made from them serve millions of people in the Near East as a daily health food. So it would be quite appropriate to include them in our diet. It would help to rectify a deficiency in our unnatural diet that has been permitted for much too long.

Evaluating Fats and Oils Today

When an Arab friend and I walked through the olive groves in Upper Galilee, taking pictures of gnarled trees that might have been several hundred years old, I began to realise why olive oil was considered so important even as long ago as in biblical times. The South Sea islander looks at his coconut palms with the same reverence, seeing that they provide him with clothing and food. To the Russian peasant in the Caucasus his sunflowers are equally valuable, providing him with necessary oil. When he eats the seeds, spitting out the husks, he knows that this food will give him strength and tenacity. The Egyptian peasant feels the same way when he harvests sesame in fields irrigated by water from the Nile.

A TOPICAL QUESTION

Which of all the oils and fats provided by nature is the best for our consumption? This question is a difficult one to answer. To start with, the criteria for judging or evaluating an oil or fat must be clear in our mind.

Today, oils and fats are primarily rated according to their content of unsaturated fatty acids. It has been found that these are necessary to guarantee the normal growth of many body cells and also to keep them healthy. Furthermore, we know that premature aging of the vascular walls, above all, the arteries, can be caused by a lack of unsaturated fatty acids. Even a cancerous degeneration of the cells has been attributed to this deficiency. Unsaturated fatty acids are therefore a vital factor, and we cannot remain healthy without them.

But it has not yet been proved that an oil or fat should be judged only by the amount of unsaturated fatty acids in it. It almost goes without saying that when a vital substance is discovered, it is at first highly overrated, such as once was the case with vitamins and the great fuss that was made over them. While this fanfare was going on, it was all but forgotten that minerals, the nutritive salts, are just as vital as vitamins. For example, olive oil has only a modest content of unsaturated fatty acids and therefore tends to

be unjustly downgraded. In contrast are the interesting findings of
one scientist, who observed that the composition of the fat molecules of olive oil compare the closest to those found in mother's
milk. Hence it could be assumed that olive oil is probably the most
acceptable kind for human consumption, because the body will
find it the easiest to process for assimilation. Whether this
researcher's view is right or wrong, his findings make us sit up,
listen and think. It should also prevent us in the future from being
too quick and one-sided in judging a natural product. The benefits
of a single constituent, in this case the value of unsaturated fatty
acids, should never lead us to ignore the others – which may prove
equally important in the end.

REASONABLE EVALUATION CRITERIA
The Creator made all natural products with a rich and varied
content. All are extremely valuable in their original composition.
But man has often overlooked this wisdom and learned little or
nothing from it. In this connection I remember one of Professor
Kollath's expressions: 'Let nature be natural.'

However, it has been quite a while since nature's produce was
left simple and natural; instead it has been violated by refining,
denaturing, devaluing, colouring and flavouring, often with chemical additives. While enumerating these violations, we cannot help
thinking of Kurt Lenzer who speaks in his writings about 'poison
in the food'.

REFINING AND SOLIDIFYING
Oils and fats have not escaped being tampered with either. By
being refined and solidified, and by having emulsifiers added, they
have received a bad name, and rightly so. Not only polyunsaturated
fatty acids, but the whole structure of natural products with all
their known and still undiscovered qualities, has been thrown off
balance. Every oil or fat, left as nature made it, would provide us
with what we need to meet our nutritional requirements. It is only
when we interfere by introducing chemical and technical methods
in the manufacturing process that damage is done and loss of
value ensues. More often than not these interferences cause health
problems. Of course, oils have been refined, and their taste
improved, for many years, but simpler methods were used in the
past. Oil was refined by means of wood ashes, because their alkaline substances removed some of the excess acid in the oil, thereby
improving its taste. A further advantage of the old methods was

that large quantities of oil were not stored, but a fresh supply was pressed from time to time. Oil-bearing fruits keep longer than the oil once extracted.

It is especially harmful when fats are hardened by electrolysis, as metal salts are used in the process. Although this method destroys much of the goodness in the natural product, this is not the only bad result. The traces of metal salts remaining in the oil can cause further damage to health by acting like poisons in homoeopathic potencies. Scientific research, as well as information disseminated by groups promoting a more natural way of life, have accomplished a great deal of good by encouraging greater awareness of these problems in recent years.

FIRST THE SMALL, NOW THE LARGE MANUFACTURERS BECOME
MORE NATURE-ORIENTED

Forty years go there were not even a dozen health food stores in Switzerland selling natural, unadulterated foods and only very few manufacturers produced such items. It was around that time that Mr Klaesi founded the company 'Nuxo-Werk'; besides this company I knew of only Messrs Phag in Gland who made an effort to market unhardened natural fats.

Subsequent research and an ongoing campaign of enlightenment have resulted in even larger manufacturers producing unhardened, naturally pure oils and fats, and it is most gratifying to see that substantial progress has been made in the field of fats. In all these necessary innovations, health food stores must continue with their pioneering work, so that in the future they will become even more popular as specialists. However, providing healthy natural and pure food cannot be left just to the health food stores; everyone has a right to be able to obtain such food from his local shops. It is the duty of large companies and manufacturers to rectify the neglect so far shown in this respect, because commercial interests have taken precedence over those of health for too long. However, since oil and fat manufacturers are clearly beginning to see the light, it can be assumed that other food industries will soon wake up too. As far as the chemical industry is concerned, it should stay where it belongs and not get mixed up with the food business! The growing tendency of people to suffer from liver disorders and cancer should suffice as a warning signal to encourage us to remove at least some of the causes that are closely connected with nutrition.

A sensible solution to the fat problem is at the same time an important solution in the fight against the diseases I have mentioned. This is a clearly proven fact. With the exception of fresh butter, the sale of animal fats has rightly fallen to a minimum; this can no doubt be attributed to the consumer wisely beginning to take his health into consideration. As far back as 3,500 years ago, Moses demanded that all animal fat be burned sacrificially. Without doubt this law would have benefited the health of the entire nation. I find it gratifying that the tendency these days is to make vegetable oils and fats in their natural form available to many more people, permitting them to meet their dietary requirements with wholesome products. Nevertheless, our total fat consumption is still too high, and too much fat is bad for us. Although the increase in serious diseases is certainly regrettable, we do want to discover the various causes and possibly combat anything that contributes to their development. It is a fact that fats contribute to this problem. Thus there is need for a change in this respect, a change that can only be to our benefit.

The Importance of Oil Seeds and Fruits

It surprised me to find that among many primitive peoples, seeds or fruits from which oil is produced appear to play an important part in their diet. Not only do they use the oil, but also the whole fruit, which is crushed or cut up and added to another dish. People who live close to nature, untouched by civilisation and its corrupting habits and customs, usually have good health, which most definitely has something to do with their natural diet. Science is slowly being forced to admit that natural wholefoods, among which we can certainly count the oil-bearing seeds or fruits, are of great value and importance to our health.

The Whole Seed

Throughout my many decades of practical experience I have always noticed that it is far more beneficial to utilise food in its entirety, as a wholefood, if at all possible. We should use not just the oil extracted from the seeds, but we should also consume the residual matter, the oil cake, adding it to our food. If the liver is sensitive and cannot tolerate certain oils, especially those that have been refined, it will usually accept the unrefined ones. It is even more beneficial for the liver if the whole oil seed or fruit is eaten. This observation has been confirmed in many cases and will no doubt become a universally accepted fact in the near future following its endorsement by scientific research. It is obvious that, as far as modern nutrition is concerned, new ways should be found and followed in the interests of everybody's health.

Meanwhile, we can at least take advantage of our present knowledge and make a dish of oil seeds and honey. In doing so we will prevent oxidation and the deterioration of the nutritional value of the oil seeds. Creamed into a spread, poppy seeds, freshly ground sunflower seeds or any other oil seed and honey, is about the healthiest and most strengthening food that exists. Furthermore, it is a splendid food and remedy for those who suffer from liver problems.

Linseed

First, let us consider linseed, the seed of the flax. People who are used to eating linseed regularly have no problems with their livers. Indeed, recent experiments have confirmed that linseed is important for good liver function.

Before eating linseed, grind it with a small mill or mincer. If you buy it already ground, make sure that it is fresh because after four or five days ground linseed begins to go rancid. The reason for this change is the effect of oxygen on the ground seeds and, after just a few days, although their goodness is barely reduced, the unpleasant taste is most off-putting. Thus, it is better to buy the seeds to grind yourself and use them right away. Take care to select good linseed, rich in active substances and highly unsaturated fatty acids. A small mill or a blender can be used to grind; set on the lowest speed for the best results. There are various ways of using linseed, for example, mixed with honey or curd cheese and herbs, all nourishing and delicious. These seeds can be called a strengthening food, a tonic, and once you have become used to their taste you will not want to do without them.

Sunflower Seeds

It is regrettable that these oil-bearing seeds receive so little attention as food for human consumption. They are delicious when mixed with raisins, for example. In fact, sunflower seeds are much more valuable than sunflower oil because the seeds contain a first-rate protein, besides highly unsaturated fatty acids. Unfortunately, the sunflower oil we buy is usually refined and although it is still relatively valuable, it cannot be said that it has the value of unrefined oil with its full content of highly unsaturated fatty acids. So if you use whole sunflower seeds you will have a food that is beneficial because of its oil and other elements.

Poppy Seeds
What has been said about sunflower seeds applies equally to poppy seeds. As part of the diet these seeds are worthy of far more consideration than they have hitherto received. One should not be content with making a poppy seed cake once in a while, or on certain holidays during the year as they do in Hungary. Instead of putting them in cakes, poppy seeds should be eaten regularly. They do not contain opiates as some people think, as the opium is obtained from the seed capsule and not from the seeds themselves. It sometimes happens that fruits or nuts do have a slight trace of a harmful substance, for example the hydrocyanic acid contained in plums. However, this is no cause for worry. The substance is an integral part of the fruit and, as such, does not act in the same way as the pure, extracted acid would. It is only found in infinitesimal quantities, in what one could say was a homoeopathic potency, and far from being harmful, it can actually do some good.

Sesame Seeds
These small oil-containing seeds of the subtropical sesame plant are comparatively little known worldwide, although in parts of Europe and North America they are commonly used. They contain an abundance of minerals and high quality protein. As these are partly combined with highly unsaturated fatty acids, they are directly transported to the cells and assimilated. The same fatty acids also supply the body with oxygen necessary for the combustion of calorific foods and so contribute to more efficient metabolism and to proper elimination. Sesame seeds will be found useful in preventing constipation and in combatting suppurations, cradle cap and eczema, and even tumours. They strengthen the nerves, stimulate the heart muscle and, because of their vitamin E content, can be taken with confidence during pregnancy. Patients afflicted with liver and gallbladder problems will welcome not only the seeds, but the raw oil as well, because both can be easily tolerated.

Because sesame is beneficial to health in so many ways, it is good to make use of the seeds themselves and also the different sesame products on the market, which children especially like to eat as snacks, only at the same time they actually provide the extra nourishment needed during their growing years – unlike sweets. Sesame seeds can be considered a perfect wholefood.

Almonds

Few people know about the high quality of almonds as a food, and they are hardly ever used by anyone who lives in the country. Almonds were quite expensive during the Second World War and so they went out of vogue. It is quite understandable that their excellent nutritional value has also been forgotten. However, almonds are cheaper today and it is well worthwhile reconsidering their food value. No doubt they will then receive more credit than they do at present.

About a quarter of the total weight of an almond consists of a high-quality protein and approximately 60 per cent is a fine oil, the almond oil. This oil can be recommended to liver patients who may not be able to tolerate any other fat. Almonds are also rich in minerals, especially potassium and calcium. They also contain valuable magnesium and, last but not least, nerve-nourishing phosphates.

It is necessary to masticate almonds thoroughly if the body is to digest them and obtain the full benefit. A particularly practical way to eat almonds is in the form of a purée. This is easily digested and assimilated and can be recommended to anyone who has problems with the liver and pancreas. Pour the almond purée into a blender to make almond milk, a nourishing drink that is rich in vitamins and easily digested.

Almond purée is a suitable food for babies, and almond milk should be substituted for ordinary cow's milk in cases of cradle cap. Only very rarely does almond protein not agree with a baby and more than 90 per cent of them tolerate it much better than the protein found in cow's milk. Many grateful mothers are aware of the fact that it was this milk that helped their babies to overcome cradle cap, as well as gastric and intestinal disturbances. Almond milk, if given regularly, will eventually rectify even the most stubborn disturbances. It is especially beneficial in the spring, when cow's milk does not always agree with some babies because the animals feed on fresh grass. Couple almond purée with a good *biological calcium preparation* and *Violaforce* in homoeopathic form, and cradle cap will soon disappear in most cases.

Because of their outstanding value and properties, almonds should find an esteemed place in every modern kitchen.

Walnuts

The walnut harvest is an unforgettable experience for all those who have had the privilege of growing up in the country. It was always a red-letter day for me when, armed with a stick, I was allowed to climb the high walnut trees and beat down the nuts, which, though ripe, were not quite ready to fall out of their green outer shells. Even the bravest climber had fearful moments sometimes, when some outer branch would not release its precious load, and it was neither safe nor easy to persevere until the last nut dropped to the ground.

Searching for walnuts in the leaves under the trees, piling them together, then prising the nuts out of their shells, although not the cleanest thing for the hands, was great fun. Such work was not for the ladies with their delicate fingers and polished nails, because for more than two weeks afterwards the yellowish-brown stains would still be impregnated in the hands.

Many of us will be familiar with the good fresh taste of newly harvested walnuts. Eaten with wholewheat bread and sweet apple cider or freshly pressed grape juice, they are both delicious and nutritious. But did you know that walnuts are especially good for those suffering from metabolic disturbances and constipation? When drugstore laxatives do not produce the desired results, walnuts may solve the problem. Walnuts are recommended for people with liver disorders and although most liver patients cannot tolerate fat they will find that moderate quantities of walnuts will agree with them quite well.

So, do not wait for the festive season to eat walnuts. They should be eaten all the year round. Make a point of including them with fruit dishes and snacks.

Milk and Dairy Farming

While milk is a valuable food for growing children, is must be free from impurities and pathogenic matter, which it may contain if the animals are housed under poor hygienic conditions. The quality and biological value of milk also depend upon the animals' feed. Some farmers use excessive quantities of concentrated feed or artificial fertilisers for their fields. Milk produced by their cows is not 100 per cent safe and the consumer would be advised to boil it. Since in some countries there is still the danger of brucellosis, in this case, too, it would also be advisable to boil milk. However, if you are fortunate enough to live, or spend your holidays, in the mountains where the cows roam freely, no such safety measures will be needed and you can drink the milk without any hesitation or risk. Good pure milk and wholewheat bread, and of course vegetables and fruit and other natural, wholesome foods, are essential to good growth and health.

Milk – a Recommended Protein Food

If we meet our requirement of protein with meat, including processed and cold meats, the body will respond by producing more metabolic wastes, but this will not happen if we concentrate on milk as a source of protein. Most people can take and assimilate milk protein quite easily, which is why milk products are excellent protein foods; for example, the soft white cheese known as 'quark' in German-speaking lands, or curds and cottage cheese in other areas, are excellent foods. Quark is ideal for making cheesecake, a tasty and wholesome sweet addition to our menu. Many Swiss families enjoy sweet quark, that is, quark mixed with almonds, berries or other fruits. Other healthy dishes are potatoes boiled in their skins, or jacket potatoes, and quark with horseradish. If you cannot obtain this type of soft cheese, cottage cheese or curds are equally good. They can be enriched with vegetable juices and are very popular for stuffing fresh tomatoes.

Another milk product is hard cheese, which satisfies the hunger of the labourer very well. From the point of view of health, however, soft white cheese is better. It is recommended that hard cheese be eaten together with salad and raw vegetables, so that it can be chewed and digested better, causing less disturbance to the stomach. They say that cheese is like gold if you eat it in the morning, like silver at noon, and like lead in the evening. In other words, you should watch what time of day you bite into a piece of hard cheese.

Milk – a Nourishing Drink

Although milk is a popular food in Switzerland, it should be used much more for drinking. Many other countries have a much better arrangement, for everywhere you go in the United Kingdom or the United States, for example, milk is available in small cartons, so that workers, schoolchildren, travellers, in short, anyone who wants a cool, nourishing and strengthening drink of milk can obtain one without difficulty. I have even seen some railway stations where milk automats have been installed. It is definitely better and cheaper to enjoy a cool, fresh drink of milk in the heat of summer rather than alcoholic beverages or sweet soft drinks with artificial additives.

Milk is a natural product with many benefits. It is only regrettable that not every dairy farmer is well enough equipped to produce and supply uncontaminated milk, but efforts are being made to improve the quality.

Unfortunately, deliberate interference in nature can reduce the value of the best quality milk, especially when the cows are inoculated. It is necessary, therefore, to raise this subject and draw the dairy farmers' attention to the problem.

The Consequences of Inoculation
When cows have been inoculated against tuberculosis, on no account should their milk be drunk raw for at least four or five days. It would be best to discard such milk altogether, at least for human consumption. Unpleasant consequences from drinking this milk may be experienced, such as liver and digestive disorders, headaches and feverishness; those who live on a natural diet are especially affected. The strange thing is that the feverishness does not cause a loss of appetite and the affected person continues to eat normally. The problems can be counteracted with *Echinaforce, Usnea* and *Urticalcin*. It is advisable to stimulate elimination through the kidneys and liver, thus enabling the toxins to be disposed of. Be careful then, if you do not want to harm your health. The best thing you can do is not to drink this contaminated milk.

Dairy farmers who deliver milk from sick animals should think twice and consider the health of their fellowmen as more important than the small financial return they might gain. But it is unfortunately true that monetary advantages often take precedence over a farmer's sense of responsibility.

Other Factors that Impair the Quality of Milk
Poorly kept cowsheds can result in tubercular cows. Only good housing conditions for the animals will avoid their contracting disease.

The incidence of tuberculosis is reduced considerably if the animals receive sufficient exercise in the fresh air, because even the best fodder is not enough to keep them healthy if they are cooped up inside all day. They should be allowed to enjoy the benefits of light and exercise in the fresh air, for this is an absolute necessity for their health and well-being.

The danger of tuberculosis is often minimised, and although it is true that it is only when the udder is affected that the disease is directly transmitted to the milk, who would dare to assert that tuberculosis of the lungs, or of any other organ for that matter, would not reduce the quality of the milk. Only healthy animals can produce milk that is safe and wholesome. The milk of a diseased cow must be affected in some way, even though the animal might not be tubercular. This is not difficult to understand because it is the same with humans. If a mother is sick, suffering from mineral and vitamin deficiencies, she will be unable to pass on these vital elements to her baby because she lacks them herself. Only a healthy mother can transmit healthy nutrients.

What do we learn from these considerations? That certain basic principles must be put into practice. We have to go full circle if we want to eradicate any mistakes. We have to provide healthy conditions before we can successfully combat today's nutritional problems. First, we must see to it that the soil is healthy and provides healthy food for the animals. Then we must make sure that their housing is adequate if we want them to produce safe milk. By observing these requirements we can be more certain of better health for the consumer.

American Dairy Farming
It would be a salutary thing to compare Swiss dairy farming and its various deficiencies with American dairy farming. The Swiss farmer, and, no doubt, those from many other countries, can learn much from the organisation, installations and hygienic conditions and rules found in the average American dairy farm. There are many American ideas that could be applied elsewhere for the benefit of producer and consumer alike. Admittedly, the American dairy farmer has larger herds and more extensive facilities, but with a little good will, some improvements could be made. If milk is to be wholesome, it must be equal to the requirements demanded of healthy food.

Dairy Farming and the National Economy
There are vegetarians who assert that they can get by quite well without dairy products. True, this is perhaps possible in the lowlands where practically all the land can be used for farming and vegetable growing. A typical example of turning pasture land into arable land is provided by China, where the huge increase in population required the conversion of much of their pasture land to allow the cultivation of more grains and vegetables, which yield more protein, minerals and vitamins. The Chinese example, however, would be impossible to apply to mountainous regions where fruits and vegetables will not grow. With very few excep-

539

tions, dairy farming is usually the only activity that can be successfully undertaken for the production of food. In my own country, Switzerland, the best milk comes from the mountainous regions and is instrumental in stabilising the national economy through the production of various kinds of cheese and other dairy products.

WHEN FINANCIAL CONSIDERATIONS ARE OVEREMPHASISED
The subject of dairy farming leads me to comment on a strange policy among some dairy farmers. There are some farmers who muzzle calves to prevent them from eating hay or aftermath. By feeding them only on milk their flesh will remain white, the idea being, of course, that white meat fetches a better price. This view of things, aided and abetted by the consumer, is extremely shortsighted, because red meat is of better nutritional value. However since the white meat is more tender, it is also more expensive.

The same principle applies to white bread, white rolls and other white flour products, showing once more the power of advertising and how demands are created to spoil the palate so that artificially prepared foods with all their additives seem to taste better. The knowledge that they are greatly inferior to products made from whole cereals is simply ignored. If one continues to eat white bread, lack of fibre will soon weaken the peristalsis of the intestines and lead to constipation, which, in turn, encourages a host of other troubles that will ultimately be dealt with by injections and all sorts of harmful drugs and medicines. One mistake after another is made and, sooner or later, the price for choosing one's food according to the dictates of the palate will have to be paid for by chronic ill health and physical suffering.

How much wiser it would be to adapt oneself to the more healthy foods, which give a true sensation of taste, instead of the cultivated taste for the artificial. It is not only the individual who would be the ultimate beneficiary from eating natural health foods, but the economy of the land would be boosted as well.

Yogurt
Yogurt reminds me of the old Bulgarians, whose longevity and health have commonly been attributed to their eating plenty of this healthy dairy product.

What is yogurt? One usually receives the answer that it is a kind of curdled milk. In a certain sense this is correct, the difference being that ordinary sour milk contains approximately 6 g of lactic acid per litre while yogurt contains only about 2 g.

Lactic fermentation does play an important part in the preparation of yogurt, but its particular properties and flavour are due
to the Maya bacillus, which works in symbiotic association with
the ordinary oriental lactic acid bacillus.

Is yogurt better for you than ordinary sweet milk? Sweet milk
coagulates in the stomach into curd. The same process is used in
making cheese, when rennet from the stomach of calves is added
to warm milk, which then turns into curd. The process of turning
milk into curds imposes quite a bit of work on the stomach,
which it accomplishes only insufficiently, or not at all, if there is a
disturbance in the secretion of the gastric fluids or if the stomach
lacks tone. Some people find it difficult to digest sweet milk if the
stomach is not performing well. On the other hand, most people
can tolerate yogurt or sour milk, the reason being that yogurt
enters the stomach in a predigested form, that is, a fine curd. Proof
of this can be seen when a child vomits after having drunk some
milk and the milk returns in big white lumps, whereas yogurt or
sour milk is brought up as a flaky fluid.

Yogurt benefits the intestines most of all. It will cleanse the
intestinal mucous membranes and encourage the development of
healthy intestinal flora. The yogurt bacillus will eliminate the
pathological kind. All this promotes better digestion and assimilation of food.

Yogurt should be eaten as the first course of a salad meal, that
is, first the yogurt, then salad and finally, vegetables. It is often
eaten with fruit but this is less beneficial because it can lead to
undesirable fermentation. Anyone inclined to flatulence should particularly avoid taking sugar or fruit with yogurt.

Intestinal putrefaction, which manifests itself by offensive smell-
ing stools, can be gradually overcome by eating yogurt. I would
emphasise the qualification 'gradually', for there are some people
who think that an occasional bowl of yogurt will rid them of all
their digestive disorders. This, of course, is not so; it will take time.
It is a good idea to keep a stock of yogurt at home; in fact, you
may find that it pays to make it yourself. Yogurt has an even
greater health value if *Lactobacillus acidophilus* is also used in its
preparation.

Lactobacillus acidophilus
Milk is an ideal culture medium for all kinds of bacteria. If you
leave unpasteurised fresh milk in a normally warm room in summer
it will turn sour. The curdling is caused by lactic acid bacteria

whose spores were either present in the milk or invaded it while it was in the kitchen. We do not recommend using milk that cannot turn sour because of chemical additives that make it stringy and go off if left outside the refrigerator.

There are various species of lactic bacteria, each one playing an important part in the preparation of special cheeses. Yogurt is made by inoculating the milk with lactic acid bacteria. Some of these bacteria should not be ingested constantly because they affect the intestinal flora. Thus yogurt is good for you if you eat it occasionally; if, however, you take it regularly all year round, its influence on the intestinal flora is one-sided and therefore detrimental. Some researchers claim that yogurt, if eaten every day over a long period of time, will cause the essential coliform bacteria in the intestines to degenerate. For this reason it is not recommended to eat yogurt continuously.

Acidophil bacteria help to build up new intestinal flora in cases of dysbacteria and the connected destruction of useful bacteria. American researchers also claim that acidophil bacteria are important in the formation of vitamin B_{12} in the intestines due to intestinal biosynthesis.

We know that vitamin B_{12} is important in the formation of red blood corpuscles, so we can conclude that the *acidophilus* is a tremendous help in cases of anaemia, as well as in the fight against pernicious anemia, in a supportive role. The intestinal flora is impaired when there is too much or too little gastric acid. Flatulence and poor digestion may occur. Acidophil bacteria have done much to relieve this condition as well as easing other problems too. For example, they are helpful in treating enteritis and similar inflammations of the intestines, and some causes of constipation. In view of these beneficial effects, it is recommended to take *acidophilus* two or three times a year for about a month on a regular basis. Any problems with the intestinal flora will then be rectified.

Coffee

The Effect of Coffee

Coffee, as a product of the coffee tree, has such a general acceptance all over the world that millions of tons of beans are consumed annually. Because of its composition, it is not surprising that many people concerned with their health are talking about it in conferences and in the press and other media.

Coffee can damage our health, for it has been shown to have an injurious effect on the nerves of those people who are already 'living on their nerves'; it peps them up. Although I disapprove of the regular use of this nerve poison, I drink coffee to stay awake and alert on occasions when I am forced to drive long distances at night. Still, I know it does not do my nerves any good. True, I cannot justify drinking coffee except that on such occasions it is better than falling asleep over the steering wheel and causing an accident. If one is not a regular coffee drinker and only takes it occasionally as a stimulant, that is, a medicine, its immediate effect is amazing. If, however, you have been drinking coffee regularly, perhaps three or more cups of a strong brew every day, you will be used to it and the effect will be weaker or not apparent at all. Caffeine dilates the blood vessels and coffee, used as medicine, is therefore indicated as a chemical vasodilator.

Coffee the Arabian Way

Generally speaking, coffee has the dilatory and stimulating effect described above; however, I learned an interesting fact with regard to coffee as the Arabs drink it. It surprised me that it can be prepared in a way that is much less harmful than the coffee made in the European or American home. In fact, I was quite astonished to see that the usual stimulating and insomniac effect was barely noticeable when I had coffee in Arab lands.

The Arabs serve it as the Turks do, in little cups together with the grounds. As a rule, they do not keep it roasted and ground but prepare it when the guests arrive. They roast the beans and grind them shortly before use, bring the ground coffee rapidly to the boil, let it bubble briefly, and pour a little cold water over the froth to settle. Then it is served very strong and thick with plenty of sugar.

In comparison with regular coffee, which I normally take with milk or cream and without sugar, the Arabic coffee did not cause me any trouble and seemed less stimulating. The unfavourable side effects of the coffee somehow appear to be eliminated by the Arabian method of preparation. After many observations and experiments I found that the grounds contain certain materials that, to a certain extent, neutralise the soluble substances in coffee, including caffeine, weakening its stimulating properties.

If you like the pleasant taste and aroma of coffee, why not try the Arabian method and take only a small cup, together with the grounds. However, you should only indulge if your nervous system is in good working order; sensitive or nervous people should leave coffee alone.

Bambu Cereal and Fruit Coffee Substitute

Since most coffee drinkers should give up drinking coffee completely for the sake of their health, the question arises as to how they can achieve this. Efforts to find a satisfactory substitute for coffee have been continuing for a long time, with the result that there are several good cereal and fruit mixtures on the market today, including our own *Bambu Coffee Substitute*.

These substitute coffees are healthy and have none of the undesirable effects of the coffee bean. Even the milk in fruit coffee suffers none of the drawbacks it encounters in ordinary coffee. Milk taken in 'bean' coffee coagulates or curdles in the stomach, with each mouthful becoming a little ball of curd in the acid medium of the stomach. However, if ingested in cereal and fruit coffee, milk curdles in fine flakes, making it much more digestible.

Bambu coffee also mixes well with raw milk for a cold drink in summer. Its bitter constituents, which come from acorns, and other minerals, are all of importance to the body in general and the liver in particular, which may well apply to bitter elements in other foods too. However, the principal benefit of this coffee is its coagulating effect on milk, as described above. Of course, if you are fit and healthy, none of these considerations will mean much to you, but if your health is not so good, or you are nervous, sensitive and highly-strung because of a life-style that is contrary to nature, it is a different question. In that case, you should definitely choose only mild food and drink.

THE BENEFITS OF CEREAL AND FRUIT COFFEE

It is not unreasonable to suggest that a modern health diet should be accompanied by a good coffee substitute, one that is pleasant to the taste and has none of the side effects of regular coffee – important factors when choosing any food product. A confirmed coffee drinker might think that it would be impossible to get used to a substitute, no matter how badly regular coffee affected his health. Fortunately, it is possible to train our palate and even use a trick to help us change its likes and dislikes. Those who feel that making such a changeover might be difficult should at first try drinking their coffee with only a slight addition of the cereal and fruit mixture, then gradually increase the quantity of the substitute and decrease that of the regular coffee until eventually they are

THE NATURE DOCTOR

drinking only the cereal and fruit coffee. A coffee addict who suffers from insomnia because of drinking too much will gradually effect a change in taste and then really enjoy his cereal and fruit drink. The health benefits will be obvious, especially for those who are accustomed to drinking their coffee with milk. By drinking a good cereal and fruit coffee substitute rather than regular bean coffee, the heart and nerves will benefit tremendously.

These substitute coffees are usually available at health food stores and delicatessens and, interestingly, the modern substitute is often similar in taste to regular coffee. Moreover, the availability of instant cereal and fruit coffee, such as *Bambu Coffee Substitute*, makes its preparation an easy matter: simply put a teaspoon of Bambu in a cup, pour hot water or milk over it, and serve a fine and aromatic beverage to your family and friends.

Sauerkraut (Fermented White Cabbage)
We gratefully accept all the information science can supply us regarding effective substances found in natural foods and medicines. However, more important than long-winded dissertations on the subject is the practical application of such knowledge – at least to the patient. Anyone who has seen people suffering from scurvy, in camps and institutions and on ships, will appreciate why foods containing anti-scorbutic elements are so necessary for them. Their diet may be adequate in all other respects, but if certain vitamins are missing, their food alone cannot overcome the deficiency.

Apart from lemon, sauerkraut is the best anti-scorbutic remedy and it was sauerkraut that enabled the daring explorer James Cook to sail the farthest seas for years without any of his sailors falling victim to scurvy. Of course, in those days, such things as anti-scorbutic vitamins were unknown, but through trial and error men like Cook, who observed and understood the ways of nature, eventually discovered the remedy for the insidious disease. Captain Cook always made sure that there were sufficient barrels of fermented cabbage on his ships. The supplement of sauerkraut with the sailors' meals provided them with food and medicine at the same time, so that the devastating effects of scurvy were avoided and Cook could carry on with his explorations and discoveries.

If your gums bleed easily or become soft and spongy around the teeth, if you constantly have small ulcers or sores on your gums and oral mucosa, if your skin bleeds easily, if you notice swellings near the joints, or if you suffer from a general feeling of weakness

545

and weariness, then you must add raw sauerkraut to your daily diet and make your salad dressing with lemon juice. The old Central European saying that 'sauerkraut every day keeps the doctor away' is undoubtedly true, for raw sauerkraut is a wonderful remedy and should have a place of honour in every home. If you have no opportunity to make it yourself, go and buy some at a health food or delicatessen. In addition to vitamin C, its content of natural lactic acid and other effective enzymes makes sauerkraut a remedial food.

Sauerkraut water or juice is an excellent remedy for many gastric and intestinal disorders and ailments, but beware of the highly salty, factory-made sauerkraut, which cannot be considered good for health. Remember, too, that only when it is raw does sauerkraut have the above-mentioned anti-scorbutic elements, supplementary substances and healing properties.

Making Sauerkraut at Home
If you want to make your own sauerkraut, you might like to try the following recipe for *sauerkraut with onion*.

Shred a head of white cabbage, not too fine, not too coarse. Spread a layer about 2 cm thick (a little less than 1 inch) on the bottom of a container, preferably one made of wood or glazed earthenware. Scatter some juniper berries and mustard and coriander seeds over the cabbage and add a small pinch of salt. You can leave out the salt, but then add more mustard seeds to compensate. On top of this, place a layer of sliced onions about 1 cm (about ½ inch) thick. Add another layer of cabbage and seasoning, then onions; continue until the container is full. Press the cabbage and onions down firmly and cover the vegetables, using a lid or plate that will fit inside the neck of the container. Place a heavy stone on the lid to weigh it down, and allow the cabbage to ferment. If you want to speed up the fermentation process, dilute some yogurt ferment or whey concentrate with water and pour over the cabbage.

Of course, sauerkraut can be made without the onions. It is important, however, that the preparation is done in a warm room and that the cabbage it left to stand for two or three weeks in a room not under 20 °C (68 °F). After that, place the container somewhere cool so that there is no butyric acid fermentation, which could ruin the contents. If you prepare sauerkraut without salt, you must make sure that you exclude all air from the container and that everything is scrupulously clean so that it will keep well.

Formerly 1–2 per cent salt was used, in other words, 100–200 g for every 10 kg of cabbage (4–8 oz for every 20 lb). Nowadays, 0.5 per cent salt or less is considered enough, since it has been found that too much salt reduces the lactic acid fermentation, resulting in an inferior product.

The Art of Cooking Depends upon Proper Seasoning
If you have been able to travel extensively, your judgement in many things will be better than that of the person who has been used to looking at everything from the limited experience of his immediate environment and local events. Through travelling, we become acquainted with the art of many cooks and come to appreciate those who know how to prepare healthy and nourishing food and not only tasty dishes that merely appeal to the palate. In this respect, three entirely different types of cooking have impressed me no end: the French, Arabic and Chinese cuisines. Each of the three follows the principle that the art of cooking is based on the correct use of spices, seasonings and flavourings. Food that is naturally bland needs careful preparation and seasoning if it is to be made palatable so that we will want to eat it again. Simply adding plenty of salt will not achieve the desired result and cannot produce the flavour that the food lacks in the first place. Cooking is an art that some people develop naturally, but others have to learn it. What helps to make our food healthy and tasty are the herbal or vegetable seasonings that are added to it, certainly not just the use of salt.

The Characteristics of Chinese, Arabic and French Cuisines
Chinese cooks prefer not to boil vegetables until they are soft; instead, they leave them about 20 per cent raw. In this condition they may taste somewhat bitter and so must be properly seasoned to make them more palatable. But the Chinese cooks know their job and prepare their food in such a way that you will enjoy it, even though you may have to chew more than with food prepared the European way. They also use a wider variety of spices and condiments, for example, curry and soy sauces, various kinds of peppers and all sorts of spicy pods that resemble red and black chillies. Moreover, they almost always include a little seaweed, which, although not much of a taste in itself, adds something to Chinese dishes that is unique.

Centuries of tradition lie behind Chinese cuisine and its habitual use of seaweed, and this ingredient is appreciated for the sake of its minerals and trace elements that are so necessary to our health. This goodness is present in very small quantities, or not at all, in other plants, and the ancient Chinese must have used seaweed instinctively as they would not have known about these substances. However, they must have been good observers and noticed that nature offers us many things that may not be visible to the eye, nor tangible, but are nevertheless of vital importance to us. This precious gift of observation has no doubt contributed to the way in which Chinese cuisine has developed. Even though much else has been forgotten that once was an intrinsic part of their culture, the Chinese people still benefit from this tradition, as they have for thousands of years.

The distinctive nature of Arabic cuisine also depends upon its use of various seasonings and condiments. Arab cooks, however, indulge in one habit of which many Europeans are not so fond: they mix spicy things with sweet ones, and bitter with mild aromas or flavours, creating peculiar contrasts of taste that may indeed tickle the palate of some but, as a rule, put us off. It often takes a while for outsiders to get used to these contrasts, but the Arab is not bothered in the least by eating peppers together with oranges or other fruit, whereas it would take me a long time to enjoy the combination of these contrasting tastes. On the other hand, it must also be said that the Arabs do not just salt their food but season it. And this is to their credit.

French cuisine is famous, not least because its secrets are found in the kitchen garden where a great variety of herbs abound and beg to be used. Escoffier, the modest Frenchman of small stature, came to be known as the King of Cooks because he mastered the use of culinary herbs in our European gardens and markets in a way that no one else has been able to match. No wonder his skill and art enabled him to produce the tastiest and most stimulating sauces, gravies and dressings that inspired the enthusiasm of even kings and princes!

Practical Experience Put to Good Use
When travelling abroad, any useful experiences and observations in connection with food should be recorded and utilised, if necessary adapting them to suit our own circumstances. I have tried to put this suggestion into practice by experimenting at home with new blends of herbs and spices according to specific rules and principles. The combination of fresh herbs, fresh vegetables and sea salt, as

in *Trocomare*, and partly also in *Herbamare*, is an example of my efforts.

Years ago, herbs were dried and powdered before use, but today we know and appreciate that fresh herbs are much more active and effective for seasoning. A fresh herbal seasoning is therefore more savoury and full-tasting. Herbamare and Trocomare seasoning salts are available in convenient shakers and offer you the goodness contained in the fresh vegetables and herbs from which they are made. The plants are organically grown, gathered from the garden and used immediately in the manufacturing process, while still fresh. A wonderfully green mush is made first, to which pure sun-dried sea salt is added. The salt dissolves and absorbs the juices, while the mush is dehydrated without heating. When ready, the seasoning is packed into the shakers. Modern nature-oriented families appreciate having these seasonings on their tables every day.

Another product for daily use is the seasoning sauce *Swiss Alpamare*, also called *Kelpamare*. This product is made from the juices of fresh vegetables and herbs and is also manufactured by means of a special fermentation process. For this purpose suitable herbs are fermented in accordance with old Chinese and Japanese methods, using edible fungi (mushrooms), which develop in an absolutely natural organic way. When fermentation comes to an end we have a seasoning sauce similar to the soy sauce found in Japan and China.

Instead of having to extract the salt using hydrochloric acid, which destroys a number of vital elements, the natural method makes for quite a different product that is far superior in taste and content to the products made according to our old-fashioned methods. Furthermore, Swiss Alpamare (Kelpamare) also contains seaweed, which is added during the manufacturing process and therefore integrally mixed and blended with the herb extracts.

The sandwich spread *Herbaforce* has the same herbal base and, in addition, is enriched with yeast extracts containing vitamin B. *Plantaforce* vegetable concentrate makes a delicious vegetable bouillon or drink. A teaspoonful of this added to a cup of hot water is enough to provide our guests with a nourishing and strengthening drink. We will also be glad to enjoy a cup of hot vegetable broth when we come home hungry and thirsty but it is not yet time to sit down to a wholesome meal. This drink is prepared in a jiffy and is invigorating as well. Plantaforce thus saves time, and time saves energy.

This brief discussion of how we can put our experience and observations to good use will no doubt help everyone to prepare tasty meals that benefit our health at the same time. Neither special knowledge nor ability is necessary, and this is most welcome for all those who have little time and a busy schedule. On the other hand, even if you have enough time to prepare your meals with care, the seasonings and flavourings we have just considered can bring you nothing but natural goodness and will enhance the goodness of your food.

Cooking Salt

How Much Salt Do We Need?
It is appropriate to consider this question, since many people hold mistaken views about salt. We were taught in school that a person requires 7 kg (about 14 lb) of salt a year in order to stay alive. It is true that man and beast cannot do without it, although it is also acknowledged that certain diseases demand a low-salt or even a salt-free diet. This apparent contradiction resolves itself when we realise that our salt requirement need not necessarily be obtained from the crystalline kind of salt known as common or table salt, but can equally well come from our food. Cases in point are the inhabitants of the Asiatic steppes and the Indians living at the headwaters of the Amazon River. They have never heard of salt, nor do they have a word for it, but as they could not survive without it, it is obvious that they must cover their requirement by means of their food.

Adequate Salt Intake
How can we solve the problem of obtaining enough salt without overloading the body with too much common or table salt? We can take advantage of the vegetables that contain plenty of it, for example leeks and onions. All plants contain salt, for when we talk about salt we mean sodium chloride, which is found in plants. Nevertheless, the fact that fresh, raw vegetables are a source of salt is frequently overlooked and many believe they must use ordinary salt to avoid deficiencies. But doing this puts a strain on the kidneys. Many well-known physicians, such as Gerson, Riedlin, Hermannsdorfer and the noted surgeon Professor Sauerbruch, have discovered that in cases of tuberculosis of the bones, too much salt has a markedly bad effect, whereas a low-salt diet or abstinence

from salt improves the general condition and stimulates the healing ability of the body.

Those who suffer from kidney ailments know that little or no salt is one of the important rules of their treatment if they are to recover rapidly. So, even for those in excellent health, it would be sensible to reduce our salt consumption as much as possible so as to avoid overburdening the kidneys. We should definitely give more consideration to these facts, since many other diseases and ailments also require a low-salt or salt-free diet in order to protect the kidneys or effect a cure.

Yeast and Yeast Extract

Earlier this century, the British began to experiment with yeast and yeast extract as a concentrated food for various expeditions. From the point of view of weight and size, they turned out to be most suitable for this purpose. An individual can keep going longer on a pound of yeast extract than on a pound of any other concentrated food. In the beginning, the value of yeast was known only by the results that were obtained from its practical use, as little was known of its vitamin content. If today yeast and yeast extract are looked upon as the most valuable concentrated foods at our disposal, scientific research and experiments have amply justified this opinion.

Yeast contains various vitamins of the B complex, especially vitamin B_1 (thiamine), and is very important to the cells, helping to take up oxygen supplied by breathing (vitamin B_2). The vitamin B_1 content of yeast is also most beneficial to the nervous system and the process of burning up carbohydrates.

Professor Abderhalden has discussed yeast and yeast extract in his publications, even calling them a kind of vegetable insulin. Yeast and yeast extract have a stimulating effect on the pancreas if it is not functioning properly and the internal secretion is upset, that is, if the islets of Langerhans are weak and do not secrete sufficient amounts of insulin. Diabetics should therefore use yeast extract for seasoning and as a sandwich spread, with a topping of sliced onions, in order to benefit from the sulphur they contain.

Yeast extract and yeast itself should only be taken in small but frequent quantities.

I would like to stress that 'live' yeast has certain disadvantages for those whose intestinal flora is disturbed. When the yeast cells, a kind of fungi, reach the intestines they usually cause fermentation and flatulence, although this is not a problem when the intestinal flora is normal. If you are sensitive, take yeast extract, which is also much more convenient to use as a spread and in stews, soups and the like. Simply dilute the extract in warm water.

It is well known that yeast taken regularly in small quantities has a medicinal effect upon furunculosis (boils) and wounds that refuse to heal. It is worthwhile mentioning that small quantities may cure the condition, while large amounts can actually provoke the problem, thus confirming the homoeopathic principle that any substance that leads to pathological conditions when taken in excess, will act as a curative agent if administered in attenuated or potentised form.

Yeast and yeast extract relieve disturbances of one's general state of health. Yeast extract is also good for neuralgic pains, trigeminal neuralgia and similar aches caused by inflammation of the nerves. Owing to its high vitamin B content, it has also been found to be of special benefit during pregnancy.

Those who suffer from stomach and intestinal problems and those with circulatory disturbances have a splendid food supplement in yeast extract. In fact, yeast fulfils the requirements the ancient medical researchers looked for in food: that food should be remedy and a remedy should be food.

At one time barm or beer yeast was used to produce yeast extract, but its bitter taste, which cannot be completely eliminated without altering its health value, led to this method being replaced by a precultured and special control method, usually using molasses as a base. So, if possible, obtain the cultured extract.

Herbaforce and *Plantaforce* are yeast extracts enriched with juices from organically grown herbs and vegetables. Their taste and flavour are superb. Herbaforce is especially suitable for use as a sandwich spread.

Miscellaneous Topics

Impoverished Earth, Rich Sea

How many rivers annually rush into the seas, their mighty waters carrying tons of minerals, lost to the earth forever. True were the words of ancient Solomon, who clearly recognised the water cycle: 'Every river flows into the sea, but the sea is not yet full. The water returns to where the rivers began, and starts all over again.' Untiring is the journey and untiring also, therefore, is the disappearance of minerals. In spite of the water cycle, they are not returned to the earth. The water that evaporates and returns in the form of rain or snow is like distilled water, lacking minerals. When we consider not only the rivers that have their sources in the Alps, but also the far mightier ones, the Amazon, Rio Grande, Mississippi, Ganges, and Nile – all the powerful rivers of our planet – we can begin to appreciate how much the earth must have lost in the form of minerals over the millenniums. Rain and snow continue to dissolve potassium, calcium, magnesium, manganese, iodine, boron and many other mineral substances found in the earth. They are washed into the rivers and thus carried into the seas and oceans. As a result, our earth becomes poorer in minerals and the seas correspondingly richer.

Efforts to Retrieve the Loss

Such reflections have caused some far-sighted people in various countries of the earth to reclaim at least something from the sea. We only have to think of the different kinds of seaweed that grow in it, their rich mineral content being most beneficial. In the first place, seaweed should be used to fertilise the soil, in order to return to the soil some of the substances that it lacks. In California seaweed has been used for quite some time as a fertiliser, for cattle feed and as a food supplement, sometimes even for medicines. Since the 1930s sea-foam and seaweed have been used for fertilising

553

in Holland. And for centuries farmers in France have been spreading a calcium-rich seaweed onto their fields.

The success of these farmers caught the attention of scientific circles and Professor Boucher reported amazing things about the effectiveness of a reddish-coloured seaweed powder, known as 'Calmagol', that has been used as a fertiliser on the isles of Glénan, south of Brittany. It was found that the plants not only grew better, but were healthier because of the addition of seaweed meal. Subsequent experiments with vegetables, fruit and berries provided good results. Mildew, fungi, scab and even pests such as greenfly were said to have disappeared when the plants were dusted with seaweed meal. It was therefore not only good for the improvement of the soil, but had the additional benefit of serving as a plant remedy, so to speak. While kelp is rich in iodine, the iodine content of the seaweed preparation 'Lithothamne Calmagol' is low, although the latter is rich in easily dissolved calcium.

Professor Boucher claims that one region in France escaped an outbreak of foot-and-mouth disease because the farmers treated their land with seaweed meal. Since these reports come from a reliable source, one can rightly expect them to be true. It can therefore be assumed that seaweed is good not only for fertilising and improving the soil, but also for regenerating exhausted, sick soil. It would be worthwhile if more farmers and gardeners made their contribution to improving the soil by adopting the use of seaweed.

No Life Without Iodine

I once read a fairy story about a prince who was never happy, and nothing seemed able to relieve his melancholy. Finally, the king prepared a feast to which he invited princes from all over the world. The guests enjoyed themselves, dancing and applauding the amusing performances of the entertainers and jesters, as it was the custom at court in those days. Although most of the people present gave way to laughter and merriment, our prince remained indifferent and sad. When the king promised a large reward to anyone who could make his son happy, a goatherd from high up in the Alps came forward. He had noticed how frisky and playful the chamois became whenever they licked at a certain area of the rock where salt deposits were located. So he had scraped some off and brought it along, thinking that it might bring good luck to the prince and himself. He gave some to the prince, who made a face as he put it in his mouth, but then slowly began to liven up and join in the fun. His disposition was improved and he felt happy once again. Were this story true, five millionths of a gram of iodine could have performed the same miracle.

Correct Dosage
Scientists have calculated the daily iodine requirement of the entire Swiss nation to be only 25 g (less than 1 oz). Perhaps this small estimate is correct. At any rate, only minute amounts of this mineral are necessary to meet our needs. On the other hand, if it were lacking, an abundance of the best nutrients and vitamins could not prevent the stupefaction and death of the Swiss people. It is a fact that a deficiency of iodine especially affects the thyroid gland and triggers strange symptoms. For example, a goitre can form, or myxoedema can result, leading to mental stupefaction. Conversely, an iodine disorder can cause exophthalmic goitre. This problem is recognised by the symptoms of hypersensitivity accompanied by frequent heart palpitations and nervous internal fluttering, which uses up nervous energy through overstimulation of the sympathetic nerves. The intestinal glands, the liver and pancreas, indeed most organs, will thereby be overstimulated. Even the perspiratory glands will be affected, and excessive perspiration can break out and weaken the body. Depression, characterised by mental imbalance and emotional ups and downs, is often the unpleasant consequence. This condition only deteriorates and becomes insupportable if massive doses of iodine are given.

We can see, therefore, that the intake of the miracle substance iodine has to be measured carefully, for both deficiency and excess mean trouble. Thus, to avoid harm, it is imperative to give iodine only in high potencies of homoeopathic dilution.

Some years ago, since the Swiss and the inhabitants of other land-locked countries often displayed signs of iodine deficiency, Dr Eggenberger from Herisau, a noted goitre specialist, supported the idea of adding iodine to common salt. This was meant to help those people in Switzerland who tended toward goitre, but it caused those with a tendency to Graves' disease having to put up with an increased heart beat and other unpleasant side effects.

Sea salt and sea water both contain iodine, and for many people these can have the effect of a specific medicine. But those who have a predisposition towards Graves' disease will find it better to take the small amounts of iodine found in plants, which will give them no trouble.

555

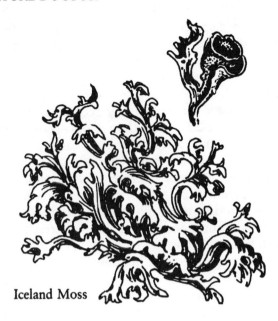

Iceland Moss

Plants Containing Iodine

In Switzerland very few plants contain iodine. Iceland moss, lung moss, reindeer moss, larch moss (*Usnea*) and carrageen (also called Irish moss) are some of the plants that do contain vitamin A and a reasonable amount of iodine, as has been proved by the pharmacologist Professor Gessner. In Switzerland there are thirty-eight different varieties of these mosses, which are described in botanic terms as lichens. Professor Gessner reports that these additionally contain antibiotic substances with a strong tuberculostatic effect. Some of these lichens are used in *Usneasan drops* and *Usneasan Cough Lozenges*. Genuine eelgrass (*Zostera marina*) and thrift (*Armeria maritima*), which can be found on the shores of the North and Baltic Seas, contain iodine, fluoride and bromide, three essential trace elements. Small amounts of iodine are also found in watercress.

All seaweeds contain iodine, the amount varying according to the kind and where it grows. The species known as bladder wrack (*Fucus vesiculosus*) grows to a size of 5 cm (2 inches) wide and 1 metre (3 feet) long. Its iodine content varies between 0.03 and 0.1 per cent, and it is used to treat obesity, struma and scrofula. However, it is unsafe for some people to take large amounts of this seaweed, especially those with a sensitive thyroid.

Kelp is the longest seaweed, reaching up to 700 metres (over

2,100 feet) in length. It is probably the longest known plant in existence. Kelp has the advantage over other seaweeds of having a fairly predictable iodine content, so that it is relatively easy to gauge the correct dosage.

By regularly taking very small quantities of seaweed or food items made with it, it is possible to eliminate an iodine deficiency without running the risk of taking too much. For this reason it is beneficial to include small amounts of seaweed in our food, above all in soups and vegetables. Doing this, especially in land-locked countries, would gradually overcome any deficiency of iodine and other trace elements.

These logical considerations caused me to add seaweed, kelp to be more specific, to a number of my food products, for example *Herbamare* and *Trocomare*, the two popular herbal salts, as well as *Herbaforce*, the practical and tasty sandwich spread. The seasoning sauce *Swiss Alpamare (Kelpamare)*, and the vegetable soup concentrate *Plantaforce* are also enriched with it. In this way it is possible to make use of varied and different food items in order to counterbalance an existing deficiency. The more the population increases and the prevalence of diseases of civilisation grows, the greater becomes the necessity to recognise and make use of the sea, with its rich mineral content, as a source of food.

Poisons that Are Difficult to Eliminate

The virulence of poisons should be judged not merely on the basis of their specific effects, but on their long-term influence. Poisons that trigger typical symptoms such as vomiting and diarrhoea but are easily expelled from the body or neutralised may be unpleasant and considered dangerous by the person so affected; however, poisons that produce none of these symptoms but remain in the body, causing degenerative or insidious conditions, are really much worse. In fact, they may have a considerable role to play in the development of cancer, and it is unfortunate that physicians and the health authorities in general find it difficult to recognise them.

We have not forgotten the disastrous results when a large number of women took the thalidomide drug, in good faith, during the 1960s. It seems that only after hundreds, or even thousands, of people have suffered from taking such drugs, the real danger is discovered. Experience has shown that no one knows the long-term effects of any strong chemical medicine. No chemist, experienced physician or pharmacologist can predict the effects with any degree of certainty. Granted, laboratory and animal experiments do give a limited idea of the general effects in each case and this may help in the specific or symptomatic treatment of a certain disease. However, how is the drug to be judged and what is to be done when suddenly deformity, sterility, and neural and genetic damage is observed, as was the case with thalidomide? If legal proceedings are taken, will it not be difficult even for a very alert and observant doctor to prove his point? What is more, he will have to think very carefully about whether he dare take on a mighty chemical or pharmaceutical company and sue them successfully.

To illustrate this point further, I know of one representative of the chemical industry, involved in the manufacture of pesticides and insecticides, who challenged the opponents of the industry to produce evidence of fatalities resulting from the application of such chemicals. No one would deny that arsenic is a dangerous poison, nor that opium is a hazardous drug. But it would not be easy to provide conclusive evidence that, say, the death of a woman who had eaten arsenic to improve her complexion and looks had been caused by her doing so. Even if it were possible to discover such a case, another expert would almost certainly stand up and prove a different cause of death. The same holds true of opium addicts.

The More the Better?

Preservatives, pesticides and herbicides can be highly dangerous, but if the proper care is taken there will be no acute symptoms of poisoning. Normally, if the directions for use are observed, there will be no evidence of chemical damage. However, what happens when farmers follow the opinion of those who say 'the more the better'? What are the consequences when they use too much poison and spray too late, or when the poison cloud also covers the plants growing under the trees or the neighbour's cultivated garden or field?

I have seen the results of tests conducted in Switzerland and elsewhere that even the experts considered disturbing. I once visited an American institute that operates with government support where the professor in charge acquainted me with the results of experiments conducted with animals, and the things I saw and learned were more frightening than impressive. No one should simply close his eyes to the lasting effects of chlorinated hydro-carbons such as DDT, Duldrin and Aldrin, and it is irresponsible if the damage caused by them is hushed up. I do admit that these chemicals have saved the lives of a number of people, especially in tropical regions. On the other hand, one must face the fact that one cannot shoot sparrows with cannon balls. Honestly, I would not like to eat vegetables and fruit every day knowing that they contained measurable traces of these poisons, which actually remain in the body. For this reason they steadily accumulate in the system until a certain degree of concentration is reached that puts the person's health and life in jeopardy.

Eichholz, a well-known and outspoken professor from Heidelberg, Germany, has stated that in large cities hardly an autopsy takes place where the fatty tissue does not show traces of DDT. People who lose weight during a severe illness are in danger when poisons begin to settle in the fatty tissue, because the body will draw on its own tissues and the toxic matter will enter the bloodstream and trigger reactions that not even the physician is able to explain.

Vegetable Feed for Babies

It is certainly a sign of progress that babies are today given vegetable juices to supplement their usual gruels and milk food. I am sure that this is one reason why vitamin deficiencies are much rarer now than years ago. Infant mortality has also decreased considerably, and it is quite possible that better nutrition has contributed to the improvement.

But what happens when the loving mother has prepared the juice with such care but the carrots, for example, contain poison? How puzzled she must be when her baby does not put on any weight or, worse, loses weight, despite her constant attention. The baby's stool becomes thinner and thinner, but the doctor is unable to diagnose the cause, having eliminated the possibility of its being coeliac disease. Not long ago, on a visit abroad, I was shown the results obtained from tests on carrots grown in Germany, Switzerland and Italy; they all contained considerable amounts of poisonous chlorinated hydrocarbons. The implications of this are quite frightening. The offspring of animals that had been given these carrots to eat did not live beyond the age of babyhood.

Now the thing is, if a mother presented her dead baby in court to prove that the poisoned carrots were responsible for her baby's death, she would be hard pressed to find even one scientist willing to back up and prove her case. The short-sighted farmer is unable to realise the consequences of the excessive use of pesticides, or their application at the wrong time, so the question of poisonous sprays and the people's general health is more acute and urgent than ever. It is the responsibility of our governments to do something about this danger, to subject the poison-spraying to government inspection and to see to it that the problem is judged without prejudice; after all, our governments have the power to introduce appropriate legislation and give the necessary direction whenever damaging practices come to the fore.

The Call for Safe Pesticides

The call for pesticides that do not harm our own health or that of our children is more urgent than ever before. If it is really impossible to fight pests without some kind of poison, then we should at least employ plant poisons that are easily eliminated, neutralised and made ineffective. When I was in South America I came to know of certain roots that were used as an insecticide. They had hardly been discovered when the industry replaced them by synthetic chemicals. Systematic research, I am sure, would no doubt find ways of using tobacco extract, products made from derris (of the *Artemisia* family), and various tropical plants. Such products could be used without disturbing the biological balance in nature or harming our health. It is possible that plant pesticides may be considerably more expensive than chemical products, but it is only right that people's health should come before financial considerations.

ORGANIC FARMING

The call for organic farming will have to be given more and more attention, and it is good to see the results so far. No longer is organic farming palmed off as eccentric or a dream. Organically grown vegetables, for example carrots, are absolutely essential for children. If you have your own garden, however small, you can be truly happy because you will be able to cultivate it organically and ensure the growth of pure vegetables. Our condensed carrot juice is made from organically grown carrots. However, if you are unable to grow your own vegetables, they are now available at most health food stores, an increasing number of supermarkets and from farmers who have changed over to organic methods.

Poisonous chemical sprays are detrimental and a health hazard not only when used on the land, but also on fruit trees. This practice still demands careful investigation and we should always remember that the consequences can be disastrous when financial profits are put before health and safety in the production of food.

DOES ANYONE REMEMBER THE BEES?

Having become used to disregarding the health of human consumers, who worries about the welfare of the bees? Hardly anyone gives a thought to the fact that millions of bees and other useful insects are killed every year by poisonous sprays. Perhaps we will realise one day the extent of the damage that has been done. We should never forget that insects have other functions besides pollinating our fruit trees. To give one example, the ichneumon wasp is able to keep millions of the larch roller (tortricid moth) larvae, or caterpillars, in check before they can destroy all the beautiful greenery of the larch trees. On occasions, when insufficient DDT is available, the trees are cleaned up and saved from these pests by these small wasps, which finish them off.

DEVASTATION IN THE JUNGLE

I became aware of the ruthless manner in which some enterprises are conducted through some friends in Guatemala. For years, our contact in that country, a Canadian married to an Indian woman, has produced honey for us. One day, quite unexpectedly, a powerful cotton company established itself in his neighbourhood and began to clear vast forest areas and plant cotton. Without any real necessity, only because of habit, the owners had their cotton plantation dusted, not manually of course, but on the generous lines the Americans are accustomed to, by plane. The finely distributed poison was intended to prevent supposed pests from settling on the cotton plants. It did not worry the commercial giant that various other insects, including bees, were killed as a consequence of their dusting. In fact, our contact lost 300 colonies of bees! Moreover, he was forced by these circumstances to pick up what was left and move to another area. The beekeeper, a simple, uninfluential man, has decided not to sue for compensation; he could not risk losing the case and facing bankruptcy as a result.

Today, totally untouched places in nature are few and far between, and their number continues to decrease, so that we wonder where it will all end. I remember talking to a zoologist I met in Guayaquil, Equador, as he was preparing to travel to the Galápagos Islands to study the iguanas, large lizards, living there. He poured out a tale of woe about the devastation being inflicted and how, soon, he would hardly know where to go anymore to study certain animals in their natural habitat. Wanton destruction and killing and the advance of civilisation were changing the environment so drastically that these animals were being robbed of their habitat and chance of survival. Something or someone has to pay when short-sighted, one-sided measures are taken and the biological balance of nature is disturbed.

Look Out – Metallic Salts Are Hazardous

More than twenty years ago, Dr E. Eckmann gave a lecture in which he pointed out that metallic salts, especially of heavy metals, become deposited in the lymphatic system. Other scientists have proved that these salts can form a barrier in the kidneys and that they also become lodged in the spine, causing problems even decades after originally settling there, as is the case with arsenic.

Plant poisons can also do us harm, but it is usually much easier to expel them, whereas metallic poisons remain in the body and do extensive damage, as a rule, years later. It is not quite clear yet how far metallic poisons contribute to the onset of paralysis, muscular dystrophy, lymphogranuloma and all kinds of conditions connected with the spinal column and cord.

How Do Metallic Salts Get into the Body?

You may wonder about the answer to this question. Well, there are various medicines that contain metals, for example Salvarsan. If this is taken, the patient will be ingesting mercury and arsenic, since both of these are ingredients of Salvarsan. There are also certain medicines for the blood that contain iron and copper.

Secondly, metallic salts are used in some old-fashioned preserving processes and, of course, in pesticides; these contain copper, lead, arsenic and so forth. In the case of pesticides the danger arises even as they are being sprayed or dusted, because they can thus be inhaled. They then settle on vegetables and fruits, posing an added danger, since it is difficult to remove the traces even by washing the produce.

It is still not fully known which of the new and frightening diseases are connected with the insidious effect of toxic metallic salts. Some of these diseases cause partial or total paralysis, confronting the doctor with an unsolvable problem and subjecting the patient to painful infirmity. Most likely this is due to poisoning through metallic salts, in addition to the influence of radiation. It is for this reason that we cannot be too careful in our efforts to ensure that we do not take into the body dangerous poisons in the form of metallic salts that undermine our health and future.

Chemical Sprays Are a Health Hazard

Only recently I heard from a mother whose child came down with an extremely dangerous form of poisoning after eating sprayed grapes.

Another report came from a woman in her sixties who loves the grapes from the Ticino canton in Switzerland. Although she should have known better, she would eat the grapes that obviously still had traces of pesticide on them and then, without fail, would suffer from digestive upsets accompanied by strong fermentation in the bowels. At first she thought that the problem was caused by eating too much raw sauerkraut, but as soon as the grape season came to an end so did her intestinal trouble, even though she continued to enjoy eating sauerkraut regularly. Moreover, she only consumed sauerkraut obtained from a reliable source, which was prepared in a natural way and not detrimental to health. These facts pointed directly to the sprayed grapes from Ticino as the cause of her upset.

I received another account from a woman who had observed similar reactions in the case of an old friend in her eighties. This old lady had been bedridden for twelve years following a stroke, paralysed from the spine to her chest. For eight weeks her organs failed to function, but then her digestion returned to normal. Still, the patient could not eat berries or stone fruit brought by her visitors, because half an hour after eating such fruit she began to feel a tightness and dragging pain in the bowels and experience flatulence, followed by diarrhoea. This condition lasted for about one or two days and the patient, understandably, felt miserable all the while. So she avoided all fruit which she felt might have been sprayed or fertilised with chemicals. The point was that she experienced no problems whatsoever if she ate cherries, strawberries, plums, grapes, currants, raspberries or blackberries that had been organically grown and not treated with chemicals. But whenever she did experience some disturbance, the cause was always the same – chemical sprays and fertilisers.

The lady who reported these findings had read an article in our magazine *Gesundheits-Nachrichten* (*Health News*) dealing with 'sprayed grapes' and was now sure of her observation and conclusion. She was glad to have discerned correctly the cause of her friend's problems, even though she had been laughed at by some, who were of the opinion that the patient had simply been imagining these things.

Although the above causes of poisoning can be avoided if proper care is exercised, there are still other, undiscovered, sources that can be even more disastrous because their potential danger is not discernible.

AN EXAMPLE OF POISONING THROUGH CHEMICAL SPRAYS

I recently visited the family of a farmer whom I knew through friends. It was a chance visit, and the farmer's wife, who had heard of me and had also read some of my publications, took advantage of the opportunity to talk to me about her little daughter's condition. She described the girl's symptoms, and how she usually lay in her bed quite listless and apathetic, and it occurred to me immediately that this was probably some form of poisoning. The little girl had been treated with penicillin in hospital, yet her condition had deteriorated. It so happened that I knew the senior consultant of the hospital personally and would say that he is an excellent physician, but unfortunately he was looking for the pathological cause in the wrong places.

I asked the unhappy mother about the circumstances she could still remember from before her little daughter fell ill and whether she could think of any influences that might have been responsible. Sure enough, what she remembered confirmed my suspicions because she told me that her husband had been spraying the trees round about that time; in fact, the girl had walked straight into the poison cloud. From that moment onward, her mother said, the trouble started. I was in no doubt at all that the circumstances and symptoms proved what the cause really was.

Now all I wanted to know was whether the doctors had been told of the incident, and she said that they had. Yet only one doctor at the hospital considered pesticide poisoning to be the cause of the girl's condition, whereas his colleagues flatly rejected this opinion. It was perfectly clear to me, however, why penicillin could not even relieve the symptoms, because it would have given at least temporary improvement if bacteria, instead of chemical poisons, had been the cause of the illness. Having made the correct diagnosis, I had no problem in choosing the appropriate treatment and remedies, and I suspect, no, I am convinced, that the natural treatment and necessary natural remedies helped the little girl to recover.

EARLY WARNING

I have always been against the spraying or dusting of crops with poison. But if anyone is of the opinion that he cannot do without it, he should at least ensure that it is done in the winter. Moreover, it is important that farmers take their responsibilities seriously and protect their workers and, especially, children from any possible harm. The consequences are not always immediately recognisable, because the chemicals may contain slow-acting poisons, such as copper, lead, arsenic and tar. The modern products, chlorinated hydrocarbon compounds and phosphoric acid esters in their various forms, are even more dangerous, since these poisons do not merely stick to the outside skin of fruit but actually penetrate the leaves and circulate in the sap. It is too late to sound a warning when a farmer or farmworker comes down with lung cancer ten or fifteen years after exposure to poison. Telling him that he should have worn a face mask when spraying his trees will be of no help or comfort to him then.

Never think that the body becomes used to the poisons so that in time they will do no harm. This, unfortunately, is untrue. A quarry worker does not become used to stone dust either and it will be of no use to inform him of the danger he is exposed to when he has already fallen victim to the incurable condition of silicosis. It is certain that this disease will end his life prematurely. It does no good to become careless or complacent as regards obvious dangers, or to lose one's fear of occupational hazards and neglect to take the necessary precautions.

ANOTHER CASE OF PESTICIDE POISONING

Pesticides can cause other disturbances when, for example, sprayed fruit is eaten. The headmistress of a girls' boarding school telephoned me during one cherry season because all but one of the girls were suffering with diarrhoea; some were even feeling so unwell that they had to stay in bed.

My first question concerned the menu, as I wanted to know what the girls had eaten the day before. The answer pointed straight to the cause of the problem, the girls having eaten cherries fresh from the trees at 4 o'clock in the afternoon. The one girl who had not been affected was also the only one who had not eaten any cherries because she did not fancy any. It will be quite obvious how this circumstance led us directly to the cause of the trouble.

I asked the headmistress to let me have some cherries for testing and recommended her to check with the farmer about spraying. And indeed, the investigation brought to light that the farmer had sprayed his trees shortly before the cherries were ripe for harvesting; in fact, they still had spots of dried pesticide on them.

How much simpler it would be if people of responsibility were to continue the search for harmless, nonpoisonous pesticides. If sought with patience and perseverance, no doubt such substances could be discovered among the great number of plants available to us. What a boon and blessing this would be, circumventing all kinds of damage and upsets.

Copper Cookware

Disadvantages and Possible Danger

Copper vessels were used much more in days gone by than they are today. Copper pots and pans were the pride of every prosperous home. But since the knowledge of vitamins has become widespread, the use of copper cookware has gone out of fashion. It was found that copper is a catalyst and, as such, destroys vitamin C. If rose hips, barberry purée or other vitamin-rich foods are cooked in copper pans, only a small amount of this vitamin remains intact. The same foods, if cooked in an enamel or stainless steel pot, will retain a much higher content of valuable vitamins. As far as health is concerned, copper pots and pans have no place in the kitchen. What is more, copper oxidises easily and forms harmful verdigris.

I have observed many cases of problems with the mucous membranes of the stomach and intestines resulting from eating food that has been prepared using copper utensils. The liver may also be affected since everything that passes the portal vein from the digestive organs comes into contact with the liver, the poisons having to be broken down. It is nothing unusual that jaundice results when large amounts of such metal oxides and metallic salts are regularly taken into the system. Changes in the blood are also possible and certain forms of anaemia may be connected with them. Kidney damage is another possible result of poisoning with metal oxides. And it has been noticed that copper, just like aluminium, can trigger a mild disturbance of the central nervous system.

The Question of Health

All these factors are important enough to make us look at our pots and pans and check whether some should be discarded in the interest of good health. Certainly all copper pans should be removed from your kitchen and no longer used for cooking. Homoeopathy prescribes *Cuprum* (copper) in potencies of up to 20x. So, if such high dilutions produce a medicinal effect, surely it is most appropriate to consider the potential danger of your cookware.

Copper has an interesting effect on microscopic organisms. Put some copper shavings in a cloth bag, place this in some water and watch what happens to the microscopic protozoans, algae, fungi and bacteria living in it. They all die. Without losing much of its weight, copper can produce such a powerful catalytic effect that it kills these microscopic organisms.

Silver-plated or nickel-plated copper can cause upsets when they are used for toys, because once the plating has been abraded, the oxidised metal can harm the child playing with such a toy.

All these considerations should make us want to keep away from copper. If you wish to cook and live in a way that is conducive to good health, you must take care to choose safe cookware. Why add to the already existing detrimental influences in our modern life? As it is, our food loses much of its natural value because of chemical additives, preservatives and the refining processes, apart from other influences such as chemical sprays and fertilisers used in its production. You are merely following a course of wisdom if, in your kitchen, you take care not to add to all this pollution but keep the standard as high as possible so that your health will benefit.

Are Synthetic Fibres Detrimental to Health?
Professor Jaeger devoted much time to the question of fibres, or materials, some fifty years ago. The main point of the arguments current at that time was whether silk, wool or cotton were to be preferred. Dr Lahmann of Dresden, at the 'White Hart', joined in the controversial debates on underwear and fibres. Those who had the money wore silk, which was considered the healthiest fibre of all. Depending on its quality, wool may cause itching and not everyone can wear it next to the skin. In particular, women in the change of life and after are usually very sensitive and cannot stand wool; it may be that even cotton causes itching and they have to resort to buying expensive pure silk lingerie, which produces no reaction and feels pleasant to the skin.

The Arabs and Bedouins living in the desert prefer to wear wide, flowing woollen clothes and coats as a protection against the heat of the day and the cold of the night. Cotton had many opponents at first, but in time it came to be accepted and established itself as a good, inexpensive material, especially as a substitute for linen, which was much more expensive. Eventually, cotton began to replace linen more and more.

All these fibres are produced by nature, yet each one has its own characteristics and qualities. Wool and silk are better insulators than cotton and linen, making them more suitable for winter weather and cold days. Interestingly, however, silk is also pleasant to wear in the heat of summer because it has a cool feel.

Synthetic Materials

For several decades now there have been new materials and products on the market, based on fibres that are made synthetically by machines. The principle of manufacture is similar to the one used by the silk worm in making its fibre or thread. Indeed, every time man intends to produce a substitute for a natural material he has to learn from the marvels of nature. A liquid pressed through fine nozzles hardens into a tough thread when exposed to the air. The thread is then spun and woven like silk. The resulting artificial fibre, called nylon, perlon or other names, is of great importance to industry. However, is wearing such synthetic materials healthy and can it be recommended? The answer to this question is of great interest to the many patients whose letters have so often made this enquiry.

We can only base our answer on experience and observed facts; for example, these artificial fibres had hardly been on the market any time at all when many women began to complain of aches and pains after wearing stockings made from them. Synthetic lingerie produced the same unpleasant reactions, such as pain similar to that experienced with rheumatism. Yet it is strange that not all people are affected in the same way when wearing synthetic materials.

It seems that artificial fibres are able to influence or partially destroy the body's electric field. Adults and children who notice such disturbances should wear only natural fibres. It is careless when symptoms of pain are ignored only because it is easier and more convenient to look after synthetic fibres than it is to treat natural ones. Wearing artificial fibres can even trigger spasms. Those who suffer from rheumatism and nervous problems should not wear artificial fibres, nor should people who have circulatory problems, since these may be aggravated. It is, however, impossible to give a general rule and each person must find out for himself which fibre suits him the best, because personal experience is of greater value than a whole series of well-meaning suggestions and advice.

Every material develops or possesses energy of the electromagnetic kind, which can be easily observed in the evening when undressing. Some pieces of clothing and underwear may crackle and spark, depending on the kind of fibre worn. Science does not understand everything involved in this area, and research is still in its infancy. For this reason we ourselves, in the interests of our own well-being, must watch our physical reactions to certain fibres, draw the right conclusions and then act accordingly.

Animals and Insects as Carriers of Disease
Some years ago, on my arrival in La Paz having travelled from Cuzco, the Swiss consul warned me to be careful of the Indians on the Altiplano, saying they were riddled with parasites. However well meant the advice was it actually came too late, since I had been living among the carefree native Indians for quite a while and had seen for myself that many individuals had lice.

From the reports of German doctors who had accompanied the troops on the German campaign in Russia I knew that lice can transmit typhus. Of course, not all lice are infected with this disease but they are an awful nuisance anyway. I have often had to give medical advice to patients who returned from foreign countries complaining about intense itching, especially in the hairy parts of the body. Mind you, I could not be so blunt as to tell them outright that the itching was caused by lice.

Parasites, Tropical Leeches and Mosquitoes
In tropical countries there are many tiny parasites, such as mites, that penetrate the skin and cause cold or hot fevers. I myself once caught such an infection in the tropical jungle and only DDT was able to save my life. These tiny parasites are not visible to the naked eye. They stick to plants and when touched with bare arms or other parts of the body they attach themselves to the skin and enter through the pores. The resulting infection is referred to as 'cold death' because the body temperature progressively decreases until life ceases if no help is forthcoming in good time.

When you are roaming through the jungle, leeches may fall from the trees, drop onto you and attach themselves to your skin. These tropical bloodsuckers, however, are not harmless like their cousins in temperate zones, because they can cause blood poisoning. The mosquitoes in those areas are also dangerous and able to transmit malaria. This disease is rampant near the headwaters of the Amazon and no traveller there should dare to sleep without a mosquito net. Even so, these carriers of disease are equipped with a peculiar instinct that enables them to find every chink in a hut and tear in a net and so torment their victims. When I was visiting that area I often discovered some mosquitoes under my net in the morning and, on squashing them, would find them to be full of blood. It could have frightened me, but perhaps I am immune to malaria or the modest quantities of quinine I took to be on the safe side were enough to protect me. In Sri Lanka I came across another type of mosquito dreaded by everyone because it transmits the fateful disease called filariasis, or elephantiasis.

Rats, Mice, Domestic Animals and Flies

Some time ago I visited San Francisco, where I met a scientist with whom I discussed a number of problems. Among other things he told me that in the dock area rats are often caught that are infected with cholera. In such a way it is possible for international ports to be endangered by foreign ships even though no sick person is on board, the reason being that rats and mice are disease-carriers. If more efforts were made to eradicate not only mice and rats but also flies and mosquitoes, I am sure that foot-and-mouth disease would spread much less. It is a documented fact that in the tropics, the jungle and the prairies more people die from diseases transmitted by insects than are killed by tigers, leopards, snakes or any other wild animal.

On the other hand, our own domestic animals are not necessarily safe either and can also transmit disease. For instance, it is possible to contract brucellosis by drinking infected raw milk. This animal disease, which is characterised by a recurrent or undulating fever is by no means pleasant and is difficult to cure, unless powerful doses of vitamin E are given. Most people know that cats and dogs can easily transmit worms to humans if no care is taken and close contact with the animals maintained. For one thing, never let these pets lick your hands when they try to show their joy and enthusiasm. Then there are some forms of eczema that can be transmitted to humans by cows, mainly the calves. Beware of these conditions too, since it is often very hard to cure them. Dab the eruption at once with diluted *Molkosan* (whey concentrate). It usually helps to kill the causative agents.

Even if pets and animals are dear to you and you love them, remember the reasons why it is necessary to keep them at a proper distance. Moreover, do not think of flies and mosquitoes as being harmless and entitled to fly around your home. Make a determined effort to rid the home of these and other insects and you will be much less likely to suffer from infectious diseases.

Climatic Influences

Today, many unnatural influences undermine our health and we often lack enough strength and energy to put up with the vicissitudes of the climate. To be exact, many of us are much more sensitive than were earlier generations. This should not surprise us if we look at our modern circumstances, yet it is more difficult to understand why the influence of climate can be so strange and inexplicable in its effect. Perhaps the laws governing climate and weather may still elude us despite scientific and meteorological progress.

On a visit to Sri Lanka I had the opportunity to make an extraordinary discovery in connection with the climate and its miraculous effect on us. The case in question concerned a nurse who had suffered from severe asthma attacks in her native Australia. The hot and humid climate of Colombo should, on all counts, have aggravated her condition but, instead, it had such a favourable influence that her asthma disappeared altogether. This change in her condition was in complete contrast to the usual experience with the disease, since dry, warm climates, particularly mountain and desert climates, generally have the best curative effect, or at least help to alleviate it. However, when this nurse visits her brother in the dry and cooler air in the higher altitude of the island, her health problem returns immediately. Once back on the hot and humid coastland, the trouble is as if blown away. For this reason the nurse has been living in the low-lying area for some years without as much as a twinge of her asthmatic problem.

No Rule without Exception

The above case shows that rules formulated on the basis of experience and observation do have exceptions and that some people respond well to something to which they should not. Most people suffer and experience intense disturbances when the seasonal winds blow, for instance the föhn, khamsin and monsoon, but there are some who feel well in this kind of weather. The sea air may not agree with some individuals, while they may feel good in the mountains, perhaps when engaging in winter sports.

Whatever good advice the doctor can give you, it would be

appropriate to get to know yourself a little better, to find out what your body needs in order to feel fit and well. You cannot always go by what others think or tell you. It is useful to watch yourself and see what benefits your well-being so that you can be guided by the favourable effects and so be able to choose the best place for your holidays or work. I can tell you from experience that some people suffer from liver trouble in Europe but the moment they change their habitat and move to the United States they are completely rid of their disturbances. Then I know patients who simply did not feel well while living in Basle, but after moving to the Appenzellerland where the föhn is often blowing, they had no complaints whatsoever. The opposite is also true, for many people feel unwell in areas with much föhn, but when they go to the Jura where it is unknown, or stay by Lake Geneva, even with a northeasterly wind, they remain fit and well.

Unfortunately, there are not many books that deal with bioclimatic influences on general well-being and the various illnesses. The only such manual so far published that I am aware of is one by the American physician Dr Manfred Curry.

The Sun Means Life and Death

If we put a hot-house or indoor plant outside in the blazing summer sun, it will probably die. Remembering that the sun throws out powerful radiation can save us from experiencing such a disappointment. The sun's rays consist of different wavelengths, a bundle of rays that can be likened to a cable made up of many wires, each one with its own frequency. We should not forget that the ray complex of the sun puts a great strain on plants, animals and humans. The effect can be illustrated by considering the sun's energy in terms of electric voltage. For example, if a power point has been set for 380 volts and we plug in an appliance that is adjusted for 220 volts, the difference in voltage will create heat and can burn out the appliance. Similarly, a destructive effect can result in unhealthy plants because, figuratively speaking, the higher voltage will damage the weak plant. Instead of charging or invigorating the plant, the sun's energy will destroy it. Plants that are damaged, maggoty or infected with insect pests will live longer if they are not exposed to intense sunlight, better still if they are kept out of the sun altogether.

The Sun's Effects on Humans

Animals seem to know about the sun's effects instinctively, because you will never see a sick animal lying in the sun. They carefully avoid sunlight and rest in the shade. We, too, should know and understand that we cannot expose ourselves to the sun if we are not well; in fact, doing so could lead to death. When a friend or acquaintance dies suddenly we invariably wonder about the actual cause of death. Recently a lady with whom I was acquainted had a stroke and died. Now I know that she had suffered from high blood pressure, yet just prior to her stroke she had been working outside in the blazing sun without a head covering; this, of course, would have raised her temperature considerably. The same kind of thing is repeated in hundreds of cases every year.

Patients who suffer from, or once had, tuberculosis should also avoid sunbathing. It should always be remembered that sunlight may even have a stronger effect in the winter when it is reflected from the snow. Intense sunlight may cause a focal reaction; increased circulation or hyperaemia can trigger bleeding and have serious consequences, even causing death. Inflamed parts of the body, infections and latent infections in the lymphatic system should never be exposed to strong sunlight because they could be caused to erupt or become acute, leading to serious reactions that place the patient's life in danger.

APPROPRIATE PRECAUTIONS

Even if you are healthy you should not expose yourself to the sun's rays indiscriminately if you want to avoid trouble. You will have to be patient and adjust your body gradually, staying in direct sunlight for only short periods at a time. And another thing: it is much better for you to move around in the sun rather than lie in it passively. Sunbathing in half-shade is far healthier and can even be recommended for the sick.

In low-lying areas the sun has little power in the winter months and more and more people prefer to spend their holidays in the mountains. High up in the mountains amidst the snow and ice it is quite common to see girls and young women in their bathing suits. They hope to get an even better tan in winter through the reflection of the snow than they would in summer. Watching this effort could really be a great comfort to the dark-skinned populations of the earth, especially those among them who strive to look as light-coloured as possible and escape the contempt they think white people might have for them because they are dark!

Both healthy and sick people should take the same precautions in winter and in summer. If you have never had the opportunity to see for yourself the amount of care taken by desert dwellers in order to find protection from direct sunlight, you would be surprised to find them walking around in voluminous woollen gowns and thick head coverings in spite of the heat. As a rule, it is quite cold during the night in desert areas and a warm head covering is no luxury, but the fact that the natives do not go without it in the daytime either shows that it is pleasant, comfortable and a protection. There are still some natives who wear little or no clothes at all, but remember that this is less dangerous for dark-coloured skin than it is for white, since dark skin absorbs part of the rays.

Anyone who knows how to appreciate nature's gifts recognises the sun's value as a source of energy. At the same time, however, no one should forget to exercise caution and show respect for its power. Every year we hear of cases with tragic consequences and these remind us of the absolute necessity to familiarise ourselves with both the good and bad effects of sunbathing. As with any other therapy, we should be guided by our personal condition and decide on the most beneficial length of exposure. Take the example of water treatments where we have to take into consideration the individual's predisposition in order to know whether hot or cold would be better. Similarly, it would be foolish to decide on taking some physical treatment if we know that medication would give better results, or vice versa. Five minutes in the sun may do us real good, whereas an hour's exposure may be disastrous, even more so for those who are sick already.

People in today's industrialised society should never forget that they cannot expose themselves to the sun's energy indiscriminately. We have not been used to walking around in nature since infancy without much clothing, exposed to all kinds of weather without fear or trouble. Instead, for generations we have been trained to protect our bodies from inclement weather by sitting and working in heated rooms and wearing thick clothing. We are not toughened-up, but reared more like hot-house plants, and this is a great disadvantage when we want to let the full impact of solar rays work on our bodies without any protective measures. So, do not do it, or you will have to reckon with the consequential damage to your health.

Intense Heat and its Dangers

I am always reminded of visiting a hospitable desert Bedouin in his tent whenever someone complains about a hot summer's day in my native Switzerland, where cold and rainfall are well known but not real drought. In the shade of his black goat's-hair tent the temperature must have been around 40 °C (104 °F) and the air outside was shimmering in the heat. In spite of this the bearded man, whose deeply lined face betrayed his advanced age, served me hot tea. I was astonished and wanted to know the reason. His answer was quick. It was completely wrong, he said, to drink cold water in the intense heat; it would only increase the thirst instead of quenching it. And so would sweet drinks, he added. It would be asking for trouble and not healthy either. At the time of our conversation I was still doubtful about his conclusion, but eventually it was confirmed by my own personal experience. It is really true that a hot drink or juicy fruit are better than anything else to quench one's thirst in the heat. What is more, they may prevent you from catching a cold, but there is no guarantee for that if you gulp down ice-cold beverages.

It is also important to breathe through the nose when it is very hot, not only when you are in the cold. The nose is equipped with a built-in air-conditioning system, or temperature control, which warms up the incoming air in the winter and cools it down in the summer.

Additional Advice

People who live in the desert keep themselves fit in spite of the continuous heat and we would do well to learn from them and imitate their habits and customs. Since not only hot beverages are important but also the way they dress, we might try comparing their ideas to ours; in so doing we will be surprised to find that the desert people do not at all agree with our custom of wearing light clothing when it is very hot. On the contrary, in the desert they wrap themselves in loose woollen robes that are more like cloaks and keep their heads covered. Watching these people you can see that they feel comfortable and seem to suffer much less in the intense sunlight than we do when wearing tight clothes or swimwear. The loose robes protect the Bedouins wonderfully and we obtain the impression that they do not perspire. We give much too little thought to the fact that the sun's intense rays are extremely damaging to anyone who has not sufficiently adapted to them. There is the danger of sunstroke, and sunburn can set off permanent or prolonged damage to the peripheral nerve and vascular systems.

The Bedouins do not feel the need to lie around motionless in the hot sun for hours on end; they do their work and moving around early in the morning or in the evening. We can also take a look at animals and their habits to see wheth r such exposure is beneficial. In fact, no animal, domestic or wild stays in the direct sunlight when it is hot, preferring instead to seek a shady spot or half-shade.

What do all these observations teach us? They suggest that we, too, should use common sense. The sun's rays have a stronger effect in the mountains than in the lowlands or by the sea, and if you are used to living at a high elevation you will be able to stand the sunlight there better than in low-lying areas. The converse is true of people who are used to living in lower areas. They would do well to avoid the sun's rays in the mountains but become less tired when exposed to the sun in their habitual lowland climate.

Let me tell you an experience from Sri Lanka that confirms my point. Together with our friends who lived by the sea we went to visit some other friends in the beautiful hills. How amused the hill dwellers were when they saw the lowland folk quickly make for the shady places because the mountain sun was too much for them. Not so with us Swiss; we felt much better than we would by the sea, where our lowland friends were at home and on their best form. The conclusion we must draw is that we should never go beyond what does us good. Brief spells of indirect sunlight are more beneficial and healing than the more common sunbathing. Moving around in the half-shade is a healthy exercise. People who suffer from high blood pressure and heart trouble should never expose themselves to intense heat or strong sunlight. Doing so could lead to sudden death.

When it is extremely hot you must be careful to avoid cooling down suddenly. Bathing in very cold water, for example in a mountain lake or a river with glacier water, can pose a great risk. Although I have mentioned the matter of drinking before, I would like to reiterate in this context that it is bad for us to drink water that is too cold. So, if you are on a mountain tour and nothing but cold water from a spring is at hand, add a little thirst-quenching *Molkosan* but no sugar and sip the water slowly while insalivating well. In this way you will avoid the chilling effect your body would otherwise experience and your thirst will be quenched much better than if you had taken a sweet soft drink. It is thus worthwhile putting a small bottle of Molkosan in your rucksack when going on a hike in the summer.

Breathing Means Life

The peculiar connections between our psychological and physical life are reflected in the sentence 'Breathing means life'. Again and again we find this concept discussed in journals and lecture halls and it may be of benefit from a scientific as well as a practical point of view if we examine and analyse what lies behind it.

It is a fact that mental stress can have a potent effect on our general health. I have experienced that myself. If one's profession requires one to be in the public eye, hostile people will engender malice and slander and make life difficult. Not everyone has a 'thick skin' and is able to shake off any and every kind of attack without feeling hurt, letting storm and the sound of ruin blow over him without upsetting his inner balance. You may think that you know your own strength and believe that your mental health is greater than it really is, but some problems can upset you so much that, in spite of having a healthy body, your organs begin to weaken, and may even give in and stop functioning. Anger, worry, disgust, disappointment and frustration are bad companions for health as they gnaw at our nerves and, eventually, the liver and pancreas become affected. This is what happened to me. My stomach began to play up in spite of my maintaining the best possible diet. Flatulence followed. Breathing became difficult and heart problems appeared. And, to top it all, appendicitis set in. A colleague examined me, confirming the diagnosis and expressing concern and fear. He advised me to have an operation.

Instead, I fasted, drank only carrot juice, and took hot water treatments. I felt slight relief, but the condition did not really improve.

What was I able to do to regain my resistance and get rid of the disturbances?

Breathing Exercises

Thinking things over, I hit on the idea of exercising the abdominal organs by rhythmic breathing. At first I practised this by drawing in the abdomen when I inhaled, and pressing it out when I exhaled. On further consideration, however, I decided to reverse the order of things and draw in the abdomen when I exhaled and press it out when I inhaled. This resulted in considerable relief after a little while. The gases escaped and I felt better.

It is true to say that the exercises made me a little tired to begin with and gave me light pains that reminded me of aching muscles, but soon I noticed a peculiar warmth surge through the body. The pain in the heart region disappeared. I increased the breathing exercises daily, doing them once, twice, three times, four times a day, very briefly at first, then for five, ten, fifteen minutes. I exhaled slowly and steadily while pulling in the abdomen at the same time, then inhaled and slowly pressed out the abdomen. If this is done vigorously, the chest really fills up well and, in time, can hold twice as much air as before.

First thing in the morning I would do my breathing exercises, repeating them at noon during my lunch hour and again at night before going to bed. I began to sleep better, as the intensive breathing exercises gave me a feeling of pleasant tiredness and relaxation. Sleep became more restful and worries, sorrows and anxieties were no longer able to wake me up in the middle of the night. What a marvellous thing it is that breathing exercises have such a profound effect, even being able to influence our mind!

From a physical point of view, my abdominal muscles seemed to be the first to benefit. They became stronger, my diaphragm developed and my digestion improved. I no longer felt any trace of pain and the inflammation which had plagued me for weeks disappeared.

No doubt the natural remedies I took also helped, but without the breathing exercises it would have been difficult to achieve such success.

Some time after this experiment I saw a chiropractor, who was a friend of mine. The X-rays he took showed a normal spine, no arthritis, in fact, no signs of degeneration. Happily he assured me that my diaphragm muscles were exceptionally well developed, better than average, which I attributed to the breathing exercises. Slowly, I began to realise that the exercises had contributed to relieving the mental pressures that had bothered me. It only took five, ten or fifteen minutes each time, but eventually I began to feel more cheerful. It was now easier for me to bear the problems that had weighed so heavily on my mind. Light and sunshine entered my life once more. Indeed, in my case, 'breathing meant life'!

Breathing through the Nose

Many years ago I had an experience when, quite by chance, I applied the same breathing method. My lungs were damaged in a car accident and the resulting problem could have posed great difficulties for me.

I decided to go to the mountains for the sake of pure air, adopted a natural diet and was making satisfactory progress. The 'finishing touches', however, were provided by regular deep-breathing exercises. I concentrated on thorough exhalation, followed by equally thorough inhalation. I began these exercises in front of an open window in fairly cold weather. In time, my condition became so good that I was able to do the breathing exercises in a temperature of −10 °C (14 °F), in front of the open balcony door, with the curtains drawn and without clothes, for fifteen minutes. In spite of the cold, the strenuous exercise made me perspire.

At the same time I combined the breathing exercises with a relaxation exercise. While standing on a carpet, I tightened and loosened my muscles again and again, tightening when I inhaled and loosening when I exhaled. I then took a short rest before starting the exercise again. The air seemed to flow through my body like a warm, pleasant stream. If I had been breathing through my mouth, I would have undoubtedly caught a chill, with the possibility of pneumonia developing. Thus I became aware of the importance of breathing through the nose and could appreciate why this is recommended in all health books.

We possess a heating element in our nose which warms the air as we breathe it in; thus air below freezing point will be warmed up to natural body temperature as it passes through the nostrils. Our lungs would suffer if we breathed in cold air all the time and it could not be warmed before entering. That is why it is important in cold climates to breathe through the nose and when it is really cold to wrap a woollen scarf over the mouth and nose to protect the membranes. In extremely cold weather no one likes to breathe through the mouth anyway, but if you did, you could become so ill that you would have to stay in bed and not be able to enjoy yourself in the mountain snow. If you persist in this lack of care, you might eventually suffer to such an extent that you stop breathing altogether and then, of course, will never again benefit from your vacations in the mountains!

It is different in the tropics, where the nose acts as a thermostat in the hot and humid air, cooling down the hot air that passes through it to approximately blood heat.

This air-conditioning system in our nose is a marvellous thing. It maintains the air temperature at a level that is appropriate for our needs.

Correct breathing exercises, always breathing through the nose, will help to relieve certain types of headaches. If, in spite of having had a good night's rest, you are still tired in the morning, or if you wake up with cartarrh in the throat, then you must pay particular attention to breathing through the nose. You can tie a handkerchief around your mouth, or put a piece of adhesive tape over it at night, until such a time as breathing through the nose comes easily and naturally. Once you establish the habit of breathing with your mouth closed you will no longer catch cold even in an unheated bedroom and will wake up refreshed for the day ahead. Also, if you snore, you will soon overcome this tendency through nasal breathing.

There is no doubt that correct breathing has a salutary effect on the brain, since the air passes beneath the bony roof of the post-nasal cavity over which the important brain cells lie. Every anatomical detail of the human body serves a specific purpose. For example, why is the nasal space divided into three corridors through which air must pass before it can enter the nasopharyngal canal and the bronchial tubes? In flowing past the blood-vessel-lined interior of the nose the air is warmed and prepared for the lungs. In addition, the anterior nostrils are considerably smaller than the posterior nares and this causes a partial vacuum in the nasal interior, which sucks the warm air from accessory nasal cavities and mixes it with cold air coming in with each breath. With what extraordinary ingenuity the construction of the nose has been designed! Even the smallest detail has a purpose.

This finely tuned detail of anatomical construction becomes more obvious to us when we consider the ear. If the smallest detail in its structure is changed, the acoustic requirements, the reception of sound waves and the transmission to the auditory nerves, will be disturbed and our hearing impaired. Any deformation produces damage and problems. Of course, the same thing applies to our nose.

The Influence of Correct Breathing on Illness
Correct breathing is not only good for the head, abdomen and the whole body, but it influences and stimulates the activity of the sympathetic and parasympathetic nervous systems. These interesting anatomical mechanisms, which could be described as being able to function without a brain, are responsible for the involuntary or subconscious functions of the body. All depend upon correct breathing. In fact, if deep-breathing is practised, you will notice

that the sympathetic nervous system works more efficiently, also influencing the activity of the heart.

Even conditions such as angina pectoris may be improved and perhaps even rectified with the help of deep-breathing, if other curative measures are employed at the same time.

If the bronchial tubes have not degenerated beyond repair, deep-breathing can sometimes even cure asthma. If not a cure, then at least a significant improvement is possible.

While constipation requires the regular intake of natural food for improvement, it is put right with correct breathing. If you breathe in and out correctly and sufficiently you will notice that the bowels begin to function better. Five, ten or fifteen minutes, each morning, afternoon and evening should be devoted to deep-breathing exercises. It may take a week, two weeks or even four weeks before the bowels will begin to function more efficiently, but regular movement will not fail to come.

A slim figure can be obtained or retained by correct breathing. A 'spare tyre' will disappear more quickly if, at the same time, attention is given to the diet. Even if one is careless with the diet, correct breathing alone will ensure a 50 per cent success rate in achieving a good figure.

Anyone suffering from enlarged adenoids may do so because of faulty breathing, since it can lead to the formation of these growths of lymphoid tissue. On the other hand, correct breathing, day and night, will prevent them and even make existing ones recede.

Some people lose their sense of smell. For them we recommend a diet of natural foods, for a time perhaps even raw food, and correct breathing exercises. This combination can slowly bring back the sense of smell. Indeed, no illness or disease exists that will not benefit from correct breathing techniques.

If women would but breathe properly, most of their abdominal complaints, tumours and growths could be prevented. Confinements would be much easier because nervous congestions would disappear. Tight clothing, belts and tight-fitting elastic girdles should be avoided if abdominal breathing is to be unrestricted. It is preferable to exercise the abdominal muscles to maintain their elasticity, rather than to control their shape by girdles that restrict and only serve to weaken the muscles. As soon as such an artificial contrivance is removed, the muscles which have been kept in place by pressure alone will again bulge out and the whole purpose of maintaining a pleasing appearance will be defeated.

If children were to be taught correct breathing at school, their lungs, chests and diaphragms would develop properly and respiratory problems of the chest and lungs, as well as obesity, would remain practically unknown. At the same time, they need to be given calcium-rich foods. All these things make for healthy growth of the internal organs and prevent the lungs from weakening.

Singing teachers take great care in helping their students to achieve success by training them in proper breathing techniques. This is why professional singers never lose sight of the importance of correct breathing.

How much time should we spend on breathing exercises? To begin with, one minute may be sufficient. Gradually the time should be increased, to two minutes, then five minutes and so forth, until the correct way of breathing becomes habitual and automatic under any circumstances. As already stated, the exercises should gradually be extended to fifteen minutes. Regularity in practising the exercises is of the utmost importance because it helps the body to become accustomed to a new rhythm; in this way we will find that deep-breathing is better than any other form of exercise. This is a 'medicine' that is within the reach of everyone and costs nothing but a little effort, concentration and perseverance.

We recognise with gratitude the help obtained from natural remedies and food, from rest and proper exercise. But are we aware that it is only through correct breathing that we will crown the other therapeutic successes, adding the finishing touches to them? Once this is so we will then prove the principle that 'breathing means life' to be true.

Fresh Air

The benefits of fresh air are far too little known and appreciated. One so often enters a bedroom, living room, study or work room and finds the air so heavy that it is almost impossible to breathe. These rooms should be aired frequently. A sickroom, in particular, requires a regular change of air because the exhaled gases and germs are harmful to both the sick person and those who care for him. Fresh air must be let in regularly. However, the question might arise as to whether it is wise to air rooms at a time when fuel is scarce or expensive? Heating engineers will answer that our concern is not at all warranted. The fire in a stove will not burn efficiently if it is deprived of oxygen. That is why we will benefit the fire if the room is ventilated frequently, though quickly, letting oxygen-rich air in. The room will heat up more quickly because fresh air becomes warm faster than stale air lacking oxygen.

In the case of a sick person, never deprive him of fresh air, even though he may have a fever. If he is properly covered he will not become chilled, and do not be surprised if I tell you that a fever patient cannot catch cold easily under normal circumstances. He is in fact overheated and a quick cold breath of air will do him no harm, so that you will have nothing to fear on this account. See that the sick person is well tucked up in bed, then open all the windows for a few moments. Nothing untoward can happen when this is done; on the contrary, the fresh air will help the patient on his way to recovery.

Oxygen as a Healing Factor

Cancer specialists will tell you that cancer cells are cells that lack oxygen. Doctors specialising in rheumatism, arthritis, diabetes and similar diseases have also pointed to oxygen deficiency in their patients. We must therefore conclude that modern man may have money and all sorts of conveniences but he lacks oxygen. In fact, many diabetics would not enter a coma if they were made to increase their oxygen intake early enough.

Let me illustrate this by an experience I have already mentioned elsewhere in my publications. A doctor once spent his vacations in the mountains together with a diabetic friend. When he realised that his friend's condition was threatening to send him into a coma he resorted to a ruse to save his life. Having no insulin on hand, the doctor could see the patient getting weaker and more listless and knew that the only way he could help was to oblige the man to walk faster, or better still, run, in order to get rid of the acetone in the lungs and make him inhale more oxygen. To force his friend to do this, the doctor had to try and make him angry and did this by whispering something in his ear! As expected, the sick man turned on his doctor friend furiously and then ran off as fast as his legs could carry him. The excitement and movement provided the man with the oxygen he needed to prevent him going into a coma. Later, when he found out that his friend had made him angry only in order to save his life, he was most grateful and both men rejoiced over the successful outcome.

A Simple Remedy

Monotonous work can be so tiring that our limbs feel heavy, while an interesting activity can involve our whole being to such an extent that we forget to breathe properly. The deficiency, however, can be rectified in a simple way if we take an evening walk in the fresh air in order to unwind. For the best results go uphill because this will necessitate deeper breathing. Our feeling of tiredness will soon vanish, faster in fact than if we decided to lie down and rest in a room with little oxygen.

The healing processes will proceed much faster in the case of illnesses that enable the patient to move around, if he increases his intake of oxygen by walking briskly in the fresh air, possibly through an aromatic forest or woodland, on a regular basis. Anyone putting this 'prescription' conscientiously into practice will enjoy positive results. As a rule, even depression can be overcome by taking a brisk walk in the fresh air for as little as an hour. Mind you, a slow walk will not have the same effect or benefit as would a strenuous march requiring vigorous breathing, which results in oxygen rushing to the brain cells and normalising their function.

Patients who are unable to go for walks should have their sick-room aired regularly in order to allow oxygen-laden fresh air to replace the stale air and so accelerate their recuperation. Lack of oxygen will retard their progress.

Those who practise winter sports will benefit more healthwise if they climb uphill with their skis for an hour rather than using the ski-lift. The lazy or convenient way does not benefit them as much as they would like it to. Modern means of transport have a similar effect, hindering us from using our legs. We appreciate our legs when we use them vigorously, letting them benefit our health. Walking briskly makes us breathe more thoroughly and this, in turn, supplies the body with plenty of oxygen. Our daily activities and work deprive the body of oxygen, yet it needs this vital element to keep it fit and healthy and to recuperate from illnesses. How good it would be if we resolved not to fill up with more petrol but, instead, with more oxygen! Better health would surely follow.

The Effects of Smoking

When a young person first starts smoking, how unpleasant he or she usually finds it. To be honest, it is far from enjoyable. On the contrary, the young person must fight all the way through nausea, disgust, nervous shock, dizziness and a general feeling of natural aversion in order to overcome the ill effects the learner smoker is subject to.

As with all harmful practices, the person trying to enjoy smoking insists that the pleasure outweighs the risks involved and that it can't be all that bad anyway. He may even point to his grandfather who, although an inveterate smoker, lived to be eighty years or more. It is true that a person with a strong constitution may be able to stand poisons without any apparent damage to his health. However, if there are people who can take drugs and grow old in spite of doing so, that does not mean that everyone has the same strong powers of resistance. On the contrary, millions of people have died prematurely because of tobacco or nicotine, narcotics, alcohol and other drugs.

Focusing on smoking, however, what are the dangers inherent in nicotine? It is the arterial system in general and the coronary arteries in particular that are affected by nicotine. If the addict has constitutionally weak blood vessels to start with, the danger of smoking will be all the greater for him. The vessels lose their elasticity, become progressively narrower and thus restrict the flow of blood to the heart, the walls of which are poorly nourished and begin to deteriorate.

If we could see through the chest and look at the heart we would be shocked to notice the change in its appearance under the influence of chronic nicotine poisoning. The delicate, toned muscles become relaxed and their beautiful red colour gradually changes to a dirty brown. If a person's heart muscles constantly suffer from lack of adequate nourishment, they will begin to look like those of a very old person. Pathological anatomy speaks of 'brown atrophy' in describing such cases, because the worn-out brownish pigments are deposited in individual cells of the heart muscles. In addition, a number of small white streaks are noticeable. These indicate that minute particles of the muscle itself have been destroyed and are now replaced by connective, or scar, tissue. Once the tissues of the heart muscles have been ruined, they cannot be replaced, not even by the best possible natural remedies. All one can do is to strengthen whatever undamaged tissue is left so that it can now do the work that had previously been done by the scarred tissue.

So, if one values life, the heart muscle ought to be well cared for. This brings to mind some words of ancient wisdom: 'More than all else that is to be guarded, safeguard your heart, for out of it come the sources of life.' Even though these words have a deep symbolic meaning, they indicate nevertheless that our heart is an organ that demands our whole attention, for if the heart fails what else remains but death? When the liver or the kidneys fail the patient is able to stay alive for a little while, but when the heart suddenly stops beating the person will drop as if struck by lightening and death follows instantly. Anyone who has witnessed a case of heart failure is extraordinarily affected by the tragedy – the sudden transformation from life to death. The pathologist will probably say that the heart muscles had been starved of blood for many years and were therefore terribly changed. The information that nicotine had been responsible for the fatal damage is then, unfortunately, no longer of any use. It is too late. Fortunately, it need not come to this, because the mere fact that the effects of nicotine poisoning become apparent long before the possible fatal consequences should make the addict decide to give up the habit before it is too late. Or would it not be better to give up smoking long before disturbances arise?

The blood pressure and the pulse rate also react adversely to nicotine, as has been proved in extensive tests undertaken by the Americans Mathers, Patterson and Levy, who investigated the link between circulatory disturbances and smoking. It was found that the average rise in blood pressure after inhaling one cigarette was 15 mm, while the pulse rate increased by fifteen beats per minute, and in cases of special sensitivity to nicotine, by twenty-five beats. The results of the tests varied according to the nicotine content of the respective cigarette brands and the individual smoker's sensitivity.

Tobacco smoke can also damage plants, as a simple experiment will prove. Put some cress seeds in two small dishes and when they begin to sprout, place a clear glass cover or jar over them. When the plants are about 2½ cm (1 inch) high, under one of the glass covers blow cigarette or cigar smoke; repeat two days later. Within a week the smoked plants will be dead, completely shrivelled up, while the ones in the unpolluted dish will be perfectly healthy.

Any gardener will tell you that tobacco extract kills insect life and that he uses it to destroy aphids. This particular use of tobacco can be recommended, but you must watch that the plants are sprayed when the fruits have not yet developed or are very small, so that the rain can wash away the extract.

How Dangerous is Tobacco Tar?
There is a general idea that tobacco is only dangerous because of its nicotine content. This view is incorrect. There is yet another evil inherent in tobacco and that is the phenols and tarry substances that are released in the process of smoking. The latter are, to a

great extent, responsible for the development of cancer. Smoker's cancer of the tongue or throat results directly from tar contamination rather than nicotine. Experiments with rabbits have shown that tobacco tar can cause malignant ulcers. The ears of some rabbits were brushed with tobacco tar every two or three days, and within a few weeks or months most of the animals developed cancerous ulcers. If these experiments are repeated using ordinary tar, the same form of cancer develops, thus proving that it is not the nicotine but the tar in tobacco which is responsible for cancer. Thus, it is wrong to draw the conclusion that low-nicotine or nicotine-free tobacco is safe to smoke.

Smoking – a Vice of Modern Times

If someone maintains that our ancestors were tobacco smokers too, he is actually quite mistaken. The widespread habit of smoking is not very old. True, we know that the North American Indians used to smoke and so did the people who lived where tobacco was grown, on the various Pacific islands, but tobacco was brought to other countries only through maritime traffic. Our ancestors in the West did not know the tobacco plant, and it is amazing how fast it spread over the globe and got a hold on people, making them think that they could not live without smoking. Somehow the idea developed that you are not 'with it' or lack credibility if you do not indulge in smoking. It is not surprising that Dr A. H. Roffo, a university professor, wrote: 'I consider tobacco a narcotic such as cocaine, morphine, opium and other drugs. In my opinion, tobacco is much more dangerous, for the number of people who are addicted to cocaine, morphine, etc., is ridiculously small in comparison to the ever-growing number of tobacco users. Besides, cocaine and morphine addicts, more often than not, are sick people, while tobacco, for the most part, attracts healthy young people.' Although narcotics are much more dangerous than tobacco, the latter is a far greater menace to our health because it has become so widespread. Since the 1970s the proportion of women smoking has grown steadily, but the female body is even more sensitive to such poisons, posing great risks and producing disastrous consequences during pregnancy and lactation.

Stress – a Disease of Modern Times

Leisure, a cosy home atmosphere, tranquillity and contemplation, as well as a period of relaxation at the end of a working day, are things that will soon only be known from reading descriptions of the past. Even at mealtimes modern man is in the grip of restlessness connected with his busy schedule. Mind you, the body cannot stand this pace of life for ever and the natural outcome is seen in the constant increase of gastric disturbances. We should not be in a hurry when we sit down to eat; in fact, we should rest for a few minutes beforehand and then enjoy our meal with a calm mind and a healthy appetite. Most gastric problems will disappear if we make an effort to be relaxed at mealtimes, eat slowly and chew the food thoroughly. It will then be better assimilated and cause fewer disturbances in the intestines. Also, when chewing thoroughly you will be less tempted to eat too much, giving you a chance to combat excess weight more effectively. It is an undeniable fact that in the Western world more people become sick and die as a result of overeating than because of going hungry. We would do well, therefore, to reduce our intake of food and so benefit our health.

A Miscalculation

If you have been so infected by a hurried pace of life that it becomes a habit and you cannot even slow down when you should rest and relax, the end result of rushing about will not be what you expect. It will not save time and enable you to relax for longer. If the spare time is not devoted to relaxation but sacrificed to other business activity or intense efforts, do not be surprised to find your interest in work declining.

Our ancestors used to start the day at 4 a.m. in the summer and, as the poet Johann Peter Hebel wrote: 'The work you do at four in early morning light, will not affect your health and rest at nine at night.' A working day was not an eight-hour period in which certain work had to be done; but rather, the day was long enough to make work a pleasure and the evening hours a time for 'recharging one's batteries'. Because people today want to get more out of life and enjoy it in a different way, all these former pleasures have gone. However, the calculation has misfired. The outcome has not provided a beneficial basis for relaxation. On the contrary, a shorter working week has demanded greater effort from us, often taxing the energy reserves beyond capacity.

An overtired person derives less benefit from a longer period of inactivity than those who work steadily, without hurrying and feeling under pressure, because they prefer to spread their workload over a longer period of time.

The shorter working week has given us more free time and if

this time were used to relax and unwind, there would hardly be anything wrong with it. However, since the hurried pace has also invaded the most popular forms of entertainment and pleasures, sooner or later there will have to come a collapse somewhere. So far, the willingness to work has been greatly impaired, and the long weekend has led to people turning their backs on work, showing open dislike for it. The German poet Goethe observed that rest from work can be detrimental to the work ethic, saying, 'Everything in life we can endure, except too many free days, to be sure.' Many people find it much easier to stop work than to start it again. This is understandable, because work that does not give pleasure is like a punishment. On the other hand, if you use your free time in a leisurely manner, slowing down the pace, you will be able to return to your place of work with renewed vigour; the week will pass enjoyably because fresh strength will make your tasks and duties easier and so lead to happiness. A steady, persistent and joyful pace of work, and shorter rest periods, are better for our life, for our physical and mental health, than the unnatural change of pace that modern life has forced upon us.

Housing Problems and Sickness

Years ago, rich people who were able to build large houses and mansions had a peculiar custom that helps us to understand why it is necessary to let the humidity and chemical processes going on in the new building settle down for some time before taking up residence there. For the sake of their own health, they allowed poor people to live in the new building rent-free during the first year. Even if the house was built of natural and quarried stone, this precaution was considered necessary in the interests of health. Of course, it was the health of the rich that benefited; the poor derived only financial benefit.

Concrete Structures and their Dangers

What about modern concrete structures? Do they not represent a far greater hazard to health than buildings made of stone? If so, there are still some strong people around who, apparently, are not affected by living in concrete buildings. At least they are not aware of any disadvantages healthwise. Not everyone is so favourably endowed, however, and some people notice twinges of rheumatism and neuralgia after only a few weeks – a more accentuated stiffness of the limbs, or a stiff neck. The gouty nodes one may already have become more painful, perhaps even depression may set in, even if not experienced previously. If you notice these or other disturbances shortly after moving into a concrete building, you should experiment by spending a holiday with friends who live in a brick, wooden or stone building. If the symptoms disappear while you are there, it would be reasonable, in the interests of health and if you are able, to move from the concrete structure, despite its modern conveniences, to a healthier dwelling place.

A humid home with little sun can damage your health just as much as a concrete building. We often calculate incorrectly, economising on the wrong things, for what good does it do us to pay less rent if we have to pay more than what we save on doctor's fees and medicines! Pain and psychological suffering can also be avoided if, when deciding where to live, we consider not only the cost but also the possible effect on our health. Living in a healthy home is of greater value than having modern conveniences and should take priority. Unfortunately, neither the authorities nor the individual are sufficiently interested in solving the question of housing from the standpoint of health. How people's health would benefit from this knowledge if those in positions of responsibility could be moved to transfer a few million from the military budget to that of health. Such a humane action would definitely be worthwhile, especially if some of the money were to be used to improve the housing conditions in the poorer sections of our towns and cities, where there is little sun and where insect pests, even rats and mice, can still contribute to the transmission of infectious diseases. It would be most appropriate if every country had an effective programme for healthy housing as one of its main targets.

Taking Health into Consideration when Building a House
Thousands of years ago the Chinese princes would order their builders to test the ground of a new building site before work commenced to see that it corresponded to the requirements for healthy living. We do not know exactly how they went about it, but we can see from old records that the order was carried out each time. In order to provide the healthiest possible conditions, it is important to consider whether a house is to be built on rock or gravel, on clay or marshy ground, whether the foundation is laid in wet earth with a high groundwater level or whether the ground is dry. One might have no other choice but to accept the plot of land that does not have the best conditions, in which case it is up to the builders to minimise the existing deficiencies and

590

disadvantages by means of technical devices, perhaps by drainage and insulation or lagging.

You may have never given any thought to the importance of checking a building site from the standpoint of whether it provides a basis for healthy living. Watching animals in their habitat can help you appreciate this point. You will notice how careful they are in choosing a spot where they want to spend the night, and where they intend to build their burrows, nests or whatever. You will never see wild deer choose wet and marshy ground to sleep on. No fox or marmot will built its den in wet marshland. Even dogs and cats are often quite choosy when it comes to selecting a place to sleep if given the opportunity. A dog will not stretch out on a concrete floor, even though it may provide a cool spot on a hot day.

Exhaustive scientific research and subsequent discoveries have brought to light many aspects of bioclimatics, electromagnetic waves, electric fields and other things that sensitive persons have always experienced reactions to but had no plausible explanation for. Our ancestors based their approach on experience and observation, taking into account many of these things even though they probably knew nothing of their exact nature. We still do not have all the explanations, but modern technology and science have come up with many a revelation that years ago had been perceived instinctively or intuitively, or simply on the basis of supposition.

Where to Build or Buy Your House

If you want to move house, you should check the location you have chosen from the standpoint of bioclimatology; of course you will also wish to see whether the area is suitable, that is, whether you actually like it and it suits you. For this reason it would be useful if you could live in the selected area for a while before finally deciding to build or buy a property there. In accordance with our constitution and sensitivity, various circumstances can be significant, for example atmospheric humidity, elevation, and whether the area is known for the föhn or any other influential winds. You should also take into account whether you feel the cold or the heat, your preference as regards food and exercise or movement, or whatever type you are. In view of the different idiosyncracies and natures we have inherited and from which we cannot escape, it is by no means of little importance where and under what conditions we live. The various members of a family often differ in their needs and preferences, in which case it would be advisable to be guided by the more sensitive ones, choosing your site to suit them.

Of primary importance is a dry building site. The foundation must be sound, and it is essential to provide adequate insulation. The choice of building materials has a bearing on health, wood being the healthiest of all, especially in a dry climate. In second place is brick, fired clay; next follows natural stone as a third choice. Concrete, especially the reinforced kind, must be considered as the unhealthiest building material there is, so one should keep one's distance if at all possible.

The Electric Field

Every person and every material has a certain connection with electricity. When undressing at bedtime you may have noticed that some items of clothing crackle, or you may even see them momentarily light up in the dark. The electric charge causing this varies with different people; some have more than others. Not only every human but also every animal, and even dead matter, is electrically charged. The electric charge can be restored or increased. Since we use up energy through life's processes and functions, it is necessary to replace it constantly. We do this by eating food, taking tonics and food supplements, as well as by breathing deeply. The electric field and charge are also influenced by where we live and in what conditions. It is even possible for those factors to upset the natural balance.

Once the balance of the electric field is upset, all kinds of disturbances may manifest themselves; for example, we can be overcome by an unnatural heavy fatigue, or persistent headaches, sometimes leading to troublesome migraine and depression. A lack of vigour and initiative often comes in its wake. Worry and nervousness may set in, bothering the sufferer so much that he does not know what to do with his fidgety limbs. He may fall victim to an unpleasant nervous condition, coupled with inner discontentment.

Since modern technology enables us to measure this electromagnetic field, we know that concrete, and reinforced concrete in particular, is able to rob much energy from those people who have to live in concrete buildings, the amount depending upon their individual sensitivity. For this reason, if you have the choice, select instead natural stone, brick or, better still, wood as the main building materials if you plan to build your own house.

The place we live in is very important to our health in these modern times. For many, though not all of us, where we live depends largely upon our own personal decision, whereas we may not be in a position to influence other important health factors. For instance, we are more or less left to accept the levels of air and water pollution and the frightening increase of radioactivity in the atmosphere without being able to do anything about it. Since we have to eat contaminated food and inhale polluted air, the accruing influences progressively weaken our bodies, to our detriment. Taking care that the house or apartment we live in is as healthy as possible is therefore a sensible and well-founded decision.

Questions of Health and the Protection of Nature
In the not too distant past, the Swiss were generally trained to keep their land clean and tidy. They were brought up with this attitude from earliest childhood at home, and when they started school, strict order and tidiness continued to be taught; in fact, teachers took great care that on outings and excursions the children never left litter lying around.

However, this order was soon disrupted when other habits and influences found their way in. I remember a beautiful wooded area in the Rhine valley, a delightful place where one could always relax. But one day, I found that the scene had changed and the picturesque landscape was littered with paper and wastes. Many a person resented this untidiness, but during the following year their anger could turn to gladness because a litter bin was installed – a quiet hint to put the rubbish where it belonged. This preventative education allayed our fears for the future and impressed upon observers that the Swiss were not inclined to let the beauties of nature be spoiled by thoughtless people who threw their rubbish just anywhere.

Nevertheless, in spite of local efforts, the new habit spread faster than the protective defence could educate. There is an awful attitude and saying that poisons the minds of children, youths and adults alike: "That's the way it's done today. Someone else can clean up after us!' Just take the following experience. While waiting for their train, two fresh-looking girls from the Engadine littered the whole platform with peanut shells. An observer's remark of 'Well, now!' caused nothing but the weakest indication of embarrassment on their part and the thoughtless excuse: 'Everybody does this nowadays; the cleaner will sweep it all up anyway.'

If this is the attitude of modern youths, it is no wonder that we encounter a lack of concern and love for untouched nature even in the most beautiful areas. Today, it is quite common to see rubbish in gorges and streams. A campsite, picnic area or wayside frequently tells us that visitors have enjoyed themselves without giving as much as a single thought to the fact that other people want to enjoy the beauty unspoiled. How can they do so if they have to sit down in the midst of empty cans, bottles, paper and all kinds of rubbish? Neither meadows nor forests, not even rhododendrons and the white snow escape this antisocial behaviour! It is amazing how quickly good habits become forgotten when bad influences take over. How superficial the sense of beauty really is when it can close its eyes to ugly disorder!

Whenever I travelled abroad to faraway places and had to watch how thoughtless and ignorant some people were in treating their surroundings, I felt pride in knowing that tidiness prevailed in my native land. Such actions upset and often repulsed me, and I would never have thought it possible for things to change so much in my own country. I vividly remember an incident in Central America where I saw a stream full of rubbish and dead animals. The same contaminated water flowed downstream and was used to irrigate gardens, for people to bathe and wash their clothes in; it was even used in their kitchens. Maybe the natives were tougher there, but they nevertheless suffered from infections on an epidemic scale, as I saw for myself. The blatant lack of hygiene among people living in such conditions, has led to rampant infestation with worms, so that in certain areas all the inhabitants can be infected with intestinal worms and amoebas. The authorities care little or not at all about taking the necessary precautions, even though such unhygienic conditions are responsible for damage to health, and can even contribute to a slow death.

Water Pollution in Europe
Are the waterways and lakes in Europe any better than elsewhere in the world? I have it first-hand from the experts that people in Europe are exposed to ever greater dangers. I once saw a good film on the preparation of the Upper Rhine for commercial navigation that provided eloquent examples of the appalling condition of our rivers and lakes. It was clear that the exploitation of this river for economic advantages was not worth all the accompanying disadvantages. But it is not enough to inform the people; governments should also be quick to take remedial action in order to

stop the pollution and killing of our lakes and rivers. The entire fish population is put in jeopardy and may die if the water continues to be poisoned. Soon it will be impossible for the aquatic animals and birds that live on these fish to survive. Most of us know that in many areas bathing is no longer permitted because of contaminated water.

Those who are aware of the existing problems can help by joining in the protests, which are gaining strength all the time. All of us can contribute personally by doing everything in our power to care seriously about tidiness and order with a view to preserving the beauty of the land, things that used to be automatic and taken for granted years ago.

Air Defence in Another Sense

There is also another thing which needs to be protected in the interest of health. It is our right to breathe good, unpolluted air, is it not? Clean air is necessary for life, and the sanitary measures taken everywhere should definitely embrace this important requirement. Appropriate laws should be made and enforced. For is it not still possible for anyone to pollute the air without anything being done about it? We all know that air is just as important as water. So if industry is not allowed to poison the water, it goes without saying that the many factory chimneys should not be permitted to belch out their fumes into the atmosphere without any consideration for the well-being of the human race.

Think of those people who have built their homes and picked the spot carefully so as to enjoy it, only to find that in time the increasing traffic brings an endless stream of cars and lorries passing right outside their front doors, forcing them to inhale stinking exhaust fumes instead of clean and healthy air. Since the motorways have already been built, it is imperative that remedial measures be sought and taken in order to protect the health of people who now live near them but did not choose to do so. If every motor car had to be fitted with an exhaust emission control device, the costs of installation would certainly not ruin us economically, but would improve our environment.

Each and every one of us should remember that the air is free and belongs to all, being a valuable gift we cannot do without. Yet how many people blow foul-smelling cigarette or cigar smoke into the air, completely oblivious to the fact that the atmosphere also belongs to their fellow human beings, who all have a right to inhale pure air. To all those people we could put the same question an American friend of mine once asked a smoker, saying with a tone of surprise: 'I didn't know that you couldn't stand clean air.' The poisons in our body change our natural sensitivity, yet great apathy has taken over regarding the things that merit special protection and care. Instead of being given greater protection, the air is expected to absorb all kinds of poisonous gases!

Nansen once said with regret that everybody is on the move and everything is possible when it comes to making war and destroying life, but when life and health demand protection, no one and nothing is forthcoming to help!

Television and Health

Living with Technology

During the last eighty years or so, the inventions made have been truly amazing. According to biblical chronology, thousands of years have passed since the days of Adam and Eve, yet during all those millenniums, until the turn of the last century, the achievements of technology amounted to nothing like the progress that has been made in my lifetime.

The modern developments have opened up a vast field of knowledge and the great number of inventions are certainly useful to us if we apply them in the right way and learn to strike a happy medium. However, many of us find this very hard to do. Already we feel lost without a motor car, because our business has to be done quickly. We have become so used to rushing around and the convenience of driving that, in time, we almost forget how to walk. That is a great pity. It is all very well to move quickly when there is a need, but it should not extend to our whole life. We should retain the pleasure of walking in our leisure time. Similarly, the modern business world is unthinkable without the telephone – it being a major disaster when the telephone is out of order, even for a short time. However, if the telephone worries us at all hours of the day and night, the otherwise useful invention turns into a nuisance which we could describe equally well as a 'worriphone'. No wonder we look forward to our holidays without the constant ringing to disturb the peace. The blare of the radio can be another undesirable disturbance when it intrudes relentlessly from a neighbour's apartment without any consideration for our peace. In such circumstances even this useful invention becomes annoying.

The Pros and Cons of Television

Let us now consider the television, an invention that most of us could not imagine being without. This is no exaggeration, for no sooner has it cast its spell than people rush out to buy a set, whether it is necessary or not and whether they have the means or not. Those who can ill afford a television set are often the ones most interested in acquiring this costly form of entertainment come what may.

Let us now examine this desire to be entertained by what we watch on the screen from the point of view of our health. No doubt it is a marvellous invention that can transmit much valuable knowledge and broadcast many important world events. Could one ever forget observing the animals in Kruger National Park? We are amazed at the giant lizards on the Galápagos islands, those surviving animals that give us an idea why legends tell of dragons. Although we may be sitting comfortably in our armchair, television transfers us to those distant shores, making us believe we are actually there, so engrossed do we become in the life of some strange creature. And what about the presentation of a heart operation in a well-equipped modern operating theatre – a gripping experience for anyone who is interested in the human body. Such educational programmes can fill many a gap in our knowledge and give us pleasure and enjoyment. At the same time, moderation is called for if we do not want to run the risk of losing time and control and suffering as a consequence.

DANGERS TO HEALTH

I learned about the danger of television to our health some years ago when staying with friends in the United States, where I noticed that their children sat in front of the screen for hours at a time. The parents usually had great difficulty in persuading them to come to the table to eat or to go to bed. The consequences of this unnatural enthrallment were not in the least welcome; in fact, they were disturbing and difficult to combat and overcome. The children were in an overwrought state, with a poor appetite; their scholastic achievements had dropped; they were absent-minded, lacked concentration and were much more subject to infectious diseases. Indeed, even at such a young age their health had already been undermined.

Scientists have pointed out that watching television puts a great strain on the eyes and that the oscillations harm the nervous system, especially in the case of children. I do not want to go into details here about the additional mental and emotional harm inflicted by programmes that are inappropriate for children, since that has been done elsewhere. Every person is impressionable to a greater or lesser degree, but children in particular are easily influenced because they have not yet acquired a firm position and are therefore receptive, and vulnerable, to everything that rushes into their minds. As it is, our modern times with their frequent changes and innovations in every field, their dangerous radical changes with respect to moral codes and values, do more harm than one can bear. Whether we want to or not, we transmit unrest and bad impressions to our children, who are entitled to protection from these things. So why should we let television programmes put additional stress on them and divert them from their wholesome course through life? Parents should be constantly aware of these factors and take great care.

IT IS EDUCATION'S TURN TO SPEAK

Years ago people were highly selective in the choice of intellectual nourishment for their children's minds. Today, however, we have become spoiled with the great variety of things on offer, unfortunately not all for our good. The demand, even need, for constant saturation with ready-made entertainment suggests that we no longer appreciate what it means to relax in tranquillity and peace. Having reached this point ourselves, we cannot expect to retain an educational hold on our children, for they are good observers and covetous copiers of enjoyment, wanting the same things they see their parents indulge in. A child begins to be demanding when he notices that his parents exercise no self-control. The parents may want to be strict in determining what programmes their children can watch and for how long, yet they are frequently powerless in the face of their children's disobedience. All these reflections have to do with education, and if we adults let ourselves be influenced by advertising and other pressures we should not expect that our children will want to be any different.

Yet, today, obedience is more necessary than ever before if a child's desires are to be curbed and not become too demanding. A child who has learned to be obedient and comply with his parents' wishes will only have to train himself in the practice of moderation, whereas badly brought up children who always get their own way succumb hopelessly to the gripping power of television. This is much more dangerous than many parents may think, because a growing child who is allowed to absorb anything he likes, without restrictions, is left to the mercy of bad influences. So, if parents do not set a good example in all they do and say, they can hardly expect self-control from their children. Where self-discipline is lacking it would be much better not to have a television at all.

The Need to Relax
If there is one thing the busy person finds difficult to achieve, it is the ability to relax correctly. Whether we are conscious of it or not, our modern technological age transmits its restless rhythm to everyone. Whatever we do has to be done quickly because we have so many other things waiting. The modern procedure of concentrating on one job enables a person to become skilled and adept in his field, but at the same time it is apt to kill one's interest in the whole thing to be made or done – the overall picture. The individual does not, or will not, see how his part fits in with the rest, so that the immediate consequence of his attitude is an unsatisfactory condition of joyless existence. Where interest in work and verve are missing, the job itself will not prevent boredom from encroaching into our lives, and we feel that our free time must be arranged so that it is more eventful, rather than used to provide wholesome relaxation.

It is different, however, with the person who enjoys his work. The time will fly, instead of drag by and he will derive pleasure from what he is doing. However, because of his good disposition such a person may be asked to fill in here and there and, in time, he will become overloaded. So beware!

Shorter Working Hours – No Solution
Working shorter hours tends to cause more stress because less time is available, and more concentration and haste has to be packed in. The change to a five-day week implemented some years ago has, in the main, failed its original purpose. The working week lost another day so that more effort had to be crammed into five days, resulting in greater fatigue which, together with the increased tension, is difficult to shake off and the additional day of rest cannot be enjoyed fully.

In addition to work there are usually too many other obligations, not to mention the diverse opportunities to engage in new and exciting activities, crowding out the intended relaxation. Years ago, people came home from work and were happy to sit on a bench in front of the house and relax until it grew dark. Nothing exciting happened to disturb the peace and pleasure hours of leis-

ure. No noise and no radio programmes subjected the body to
further tension and no television shows demanded the undivided
attention of the viewer. In the place of these canned programmes
there was often heard rising from the valley a beautiful song that
refreshed the singer and the listeners alike. These aspects of life led
to wholesome relaxation which we search for today but seldom
find in spite of all the money spent. Often, sound sleep escapes
those who did not retire early enough, not wanting to miss out on
some nocturnal pleasure. For them the hours of the night become
more arduous than even their work during the day, but sleep is an
indispensable and natural requirement.

While some people are never able to relax, there are others who
cannot do enough to make money. Some workers, for example in
the catering industry, do not enjoy their days off as a time of rest
and relaxation, but to make more money they accept casual work
as well. Such demands on the body may be possible for a little
while but they will sap the person's energy reserves in the long
run. We must recognise that the rhythm of life consists of periods
of tension and relaxation, the latter being necessary to recharge
life's batteries. Another modern tendency is to seek the necessary
relaxation in sport, but unfortunately this often degenerates into
competition and the body is overtaxed once again.

A Programme to Unwind
As well as having a work schedule, I recommend that you also
have one for relaxation. If you are a housewife, you can plan your
time quite well after your husband has gone to work and the
children to school. When your housework is finished in the morning, take a break for five or ten minutes. You will be surprised to
discover the benefits resulting from such a short rest period. The
same relaxation can be observed at midday, and if it becomes
habitual, you will build up a store of energy, enabling you to deal
with daily problems more easily. Whether you stay at home or go
out to work, you will have more opportunity to relax if you do
not feel obliged to scrutinise every little item in the daily newspaper
whenever you have a break. There is better nourishment available
for the brain – things that edify – and it is this you should turn
to in order to supply the mind and spirit with food that fortifies.
The right kind of upbuilding material will also serve to relax the
body, proving the truth of the saying 'Man does not live by bread
alone.'

There are many people who believe that it is beneficial to have a lie in after a hectic week's work. But unless you are ill, spending the whole morning in bed only makes you feel worse. It is much better to go to bed early the night before, get up in the morning soon after you awake and take a long walk through the woods or forest, or along a bubbling stream. Doing this will do wonders for your nerves. Once in the aromatic air you will automatically breathe more deeply and soon feel wonderfully refreshed. Doing some gardening is also a great way to relax after engaging in strenuous mental or office work. Then there is the possibility of berry-picking and gathering medicinal herbs, a meaningful distraction that helps you to revive.

So you will see that in spite of all the modern hustle and bustle and the air and environmental pollution, there are still a number of opportunities to unwind in a natural way. As a rule, these opportunities are inexpensive. All you have to be is content with them and they will benefit you in every way.

Tiredness – a Natural Symptom

In a medical book I read recently it said that man is not a machine and has to rest after making a strenuous effort. If the author, a medical doctor, had a proper understanding of technology he would have known that even machines cannot go on running forever, but need rest periods just as much as we do. It is not without reason that engineers speak of fatigue and stress in the case of machines. In fact, many railway and aeroplane accidents happen as a result of metal or mechanical fatigue. The molecules lose their strength and resilience when the metals remain in constant use, creating a greater risk of them breaking. So when a lifeless machine or engine is subject to symptoms of fatigue, how much more so is the living human body!

It is possible that a person cannot eat or sleep because he is just too tired. His condition is then one of exhaustion. But what can be called mere tiredness, and where is the border between tiredness and exhaustion? Normal activity is good for the mind and body, but laziness and idleness are harmful. An engine that runs at a reasonable pace has a longer life than if it is hardly ever used; mechanical parts that are left idle become rusty, oxidise and seize up due to hardened lubricants; in other words, they suffer damage. An engine runs best at a certain number of revolutions per minute and an adequate temperature, and it becomes damaged if it is overheated. This is the reason for installing gauges that tell you the best temperatures for running the engine so that its life can be extended. We humans also possess a reliable gauge that indicates whether our 'body engine' is running properly or whether we are overtaxing it. This motor is, as we all know, the heart. When running at high speed, it should not be left to a colleague or the 'motorist' to decide the maximum rate, or speed; let the heart itself tell you. As soon as it beats considerably faster than usual, this should be taken as a warning that you must slow down. It is true that we can let our 'heart motor' run at a higher speed for a short time, but when the exertion continues over an extended period, our energy reserves become drained, fatigue sets in and our health is adversely affected.

The normal strain of work stimulates the circulation and, with it, the entire metabolism, so that the body is kept resilient and healthy. Of course, a normal and healthy metabolism also produces wastes, resulting in a feeling of tiredness when these waste products reach a certain concentration. This symptom of tiredness should always be met with rest and relaxation, even by young people who are usually able to work 8–10 hours a day with ease. A healthy, properly nourished body experiences the sensation of pleasant tiredness in the evening, and 7–9 hours of sleep, the exact amount depending on our individual needs, will be quite enough to restore a feeling of refreshed well-being. We will then be able to carry out our duties quite happily the following day if our body has had sufficient rest during the night.

The Need for Common Sense
It is mainly young people and athletes who find it difficult to be sensible and not go beyond what is physically good for their health. There are times when they do not seem to understand the importance of warming up in order to help the muscles and internal organs to acquire sufficient elasticity. Sports physicians, gynaecologists and other specialists are well aware of this since they have to deal with the consequences of carelessness. We should not overtax ourselves to the point of exhaustion in our work, and how much less should this be done in sports activities! Those who go beyond what is reasonable when they are supposed to relax and restore their energies show a lack of knowledge and understanding. In some cases they are driven by ambition that, strictly speaking, creates an attitude which has nothing to do with sportsmanship.

It is impossible to establish general rules that would constitute an exact standard or yardstick regarding the energy we can safely spend, because each person has to take into account his constitution, his physical and mental reserves and, last but not least, his age. It really depends upon our individual capabilities and need for rest and sleep, which can vary enormously from one person to another. For this reason, what follows are only guidelines, intended to point you in the right direction regarding how much you can do.

How to Judge your Capabilities

Let us take an example. A twenty-year-old has at his disposal 100 per cent energy, of which he may spend 80 per cent on work and sporting activities without damaging his reserves. He will not be so tired at the end of the day that he would speak of exhaustion. When calculating one's potential it is necessary, according to age, to deduct the years of one's life from the 100 per cent starting point. This means that a forty-year-old can risk spending 60 per cent of his energy potential, while a sixty-year-old will have to be satisfied with spending a mere 40 per cent. It would obviously not be good for him if circumstances forced him to spend as much energy as he could if he were only twenty years old. The result would be that instead of feeling normal tiredness in the evening, he would be completely exhausted. He would not find proper rest in sleep and would wake up still tired. This condition of exhaustion reduces vitality and shortens life expectancy, which means that the individual would have more years to look forward to if his use of energy were to be more sensible and moderate.

The Beneficial Rhythm of Life

In modern times the normal rhythm of life that once was a hall-mark of country life has been turned upside down. You can only expect to wake up feeling bright and breezy in the morning if you refuse to follow the spirit of our times and, instead, go to bed early, well before midnight, in order to do justice to the body's need for rest. Those who fall victim to the modern trend of indulging in nocturnal pleasures will not dream of leaving them to retire early. Radio, television, the cinema and so forth keep them prisoner and demand an even greater amount of their energy and strength than would have been lost in the course of their daily occupation and consequent normal tiredness. These additional nightly demands at the expense of sleep upset the balance that is maintained by a normal pace of life. Even young people who extend the day into the night in order to get more out of life will, in time, suffer from a form of fatigue that manifests itself in irritability, feeling uptight and, in the end, insomnia.

How wise it would be to interrupt this deteriorating condition in good time before it takes over one's being, leading to the need for strong sleeping pills that can become addictive! People who feel overtired should decide to spend their holidays in the country, where they can go on easy excursions and for walks in the forest or woods and the hills or mountains, rather than choosing a travel programme that would involve great strain and effort. They need to breathe deeply in the fresh air, enabling them to feel naturally tired in the evening and so enjoy restful sleep once again. Anyone who thinks that he can get rid of overtiredness by sitting in an armchair all day is mistaken, because he needs more than rest: he needs sufficient exercise and deep-breathing. This will eliminate the tiredness and metabolic wastes from the body. Townsfolk would benefit more from their holidays if, instead of lying around, they helped the farmers make hay and went for short walks, besides eating and drinking well.

If you do not want to become overtired, you should observe and become familiar with the rhythm of exercise and rest. Plan to have sufficient time to get ready if you work away from home, so that you will arrive at your place of work without having had to rush. Moreover, it will be of special benefit if you choose, not the shortest way to work, but the most pleasant – perhaps passing through a park or some gardens. Remember, this can be a protection from exhaust fumes at the same time. Following this advice, anyone can derive physical benefits from his daily walk to and from work and this cannot be appreciated enough in view of the limited opportunities to move about in our jobs. If the distance is too great or walking to work presents other problems, why not train yourself to get up a little earlier in order to go for a brisk walk before setting out to work? It would also be to your advantage if you repeated this in the evening. A balanced combination of exercise and rest maintains our efficiency and well-being and helps us to avoid getting overtired. So why should anything prevent you from putting this advice into practice conscientiously and with perseverance?

No one can prevent the process of aging, nor waning vitality, which can take place at different rates for different people. There is little point in being too grieved about it; just remember that you have gained experience, wisdom and skills in those past years, things that can help you to replace the decreasing energy to the extent that the achievements of an experienced man are able to surpass those of a youth still full of vitality. Even in the area of technology it is not so much the existing knowledge and power but their skilful use that raises its potential to the maximum heights.

Beware of exerting yourself to the limit, leading to complete exhaustion, because every violation of biological laws will find its revenge and you may have to pay a bitter price.

What Is Exhaustion?

The human cell is a marvel made by the Intelligence that has shown endless ingenuity in technical design, forever presenting scientific researchers with surprises.

Although each kind of cell is different in structure from the others, they all have basic similarities. The cell's most important part is the nucleus, just like the yolk of an egg. The nucleus is, as a rule, surrounded by a nutrient reserve, similar to the egg white that envelops the yolk. The cover holding everything together in the cell is the cell membrane. The cell itself is a small state within a state and enjoys a certain independence. There are even cells that circulate or wander for the purpose of being on hand wherever their help may be needed. That is why they are called 'wandering cells'. We can say that every cell has it own internal regulations, and absorbs and releases certain substances. This process is called metabolism. The cell uses the absorbed nutrients and changes them into energy, or it converts them into a new substance that serves the body, especially in its growth.

The breakdown and conversion of nutrients produces wastes, in the same way as wastes are formed in the process of combustion or oxidation. We are talking about the so-called 'metabolic waste products'. Exercise, breathing and rest are responsible for the elimination of wastes from the body, and if these processes are restricted, hindering their removal, then congestions and deposits occur that lead to rheumatism, gout and arthritis. Besides the nutrient reserves, the body has other reserves that can be so substantial that they influence the body weight. Active cells retain their elasticity, and work and exercise that requires plenty of movement maintain the health of individual cells, therefore benefiting the whole body.

The Use of Energy

In accordance with effort and demand, cells use up nutrient materials during the day, which are replenished during the night. This is the normal rhythm of life. In the evening, when the cells

605

have exhausted their supplies, we become tired. If we use up more energy than normal, the cells draw on their reserves. If the energy consumption is excessive over a period of time, we have to spend more than can be replaced during the night. The inevitable result of this mismanagement is a deficiency that gets progressively greater. The normal reserves diminish and are finally used up; the cells are now completely exhausted. We suffer from a kind of fatigue that is like a sickness, in time leading to a condition of painful tiredness. People who are constantly on the move, always doing something, can easily reach this state, and if nothing is done about it, or if it is stepped up by increasing the overexertion, this senseless condition can trigger a sudden reaction and suddenly snap, like a short circuit. This explains the cases of sudden death that may puzzle even the doctor.

Activity and work produce a natural tiredness which should not be resisted but given in to. We do this by taking a break or going to bed to obtain the necessary rest.

This natural rhythm refreshes, letting the preceding exercise of the muscles serve to strengthen the body. However, if the strain and effort are not followed by the necessary rest, the consequence will be exhaustion, causing the opposite to happen, because constant overexertion damages the cellular system and thus the whole body. It is important to avoid exhaustion in our daily life as well as in sport and exercise. Those who ignore this advice will often have to reckon with permanent damage that may be far greater then they imagine or would like to be true.

Natural Sleep

How Much Sleep Do We Need?
The question of how much sleep a person really needs has occupied the minds of many clever people who, try as they might, have never arrived at a satisfactory answer. Some say that seven or eight hours sleep are necessary if one wants to be rested and ready for work, while others seem to think that they can manage quite well with four or five hours. Regarding those who sleep fewer hours, it is questionable whether the nerve cells will have sufficient time to become regenerated and whether, in time, some deficiency will become apparent. An unusual failing of strength, shorter attention spans and becoming easily tired are definite indications that one is not getting enough sleep, no matter what kind of theories anyone has on the subject.

When should we sleep and for how many hours? There are many different answers to these two questions and it is better if we ask, not other fellow humans, but nature itself – the most appropriate teacher. Nature sets before us a splendid example in the lively, ever-active world of birds. What can we learn from our feathered friends? When and for how long do those cheerful little singers sleep? Well, we all know the answer, don't we? They begin their songs at the break of dawn when the average person is wasting the sunny hours of an early spring morning lying asleep in bed. They are already about their business and do not return to rest until the last traces of twilight have gone. For the birds this seems to be a natural and proper way of life and, indeed, primitive man adopted it.

Our eyes were given to us by our Creator to enjoy and explore the light and what each day unfolds. They are a miracle and we should look after them well. The daylight opens them in the morning, and when night falls it is natural to close them in rest. For what other reason were we given alternate light and darkness? Modern man, however, came along and invented artificial light for himself, allowing him to prolong the day indefinitely. First he used kindling and candles, then paraffin and gas, until the invention of the electric light bulb made it even more simple to switch on the artificial light and continue working at any time of the night. No longer can we say, as once was said: 'Come, let's make an end to the day and go to bed, for we have endured its cares for long enough.' Now we can think of other ways, besides sleep, for banishing the cares of the day – by doing more work or by dissipating our night hours in pleasures to help us forget our troubles. Thus, although artificial light seems useful and practical to us, we have forgotten that we have changed the natural rhythm of life to suit our own transient mood, personal need, or perhaps just to comply with a certain set of circumstances.

Instead of waking with the first rays of sunshine so as to use every moment of natural light, we sleep through the most beautiful hours of the day and, of course, it it impossible to get our work done before the departing light invites us to sleep once more. In the summer, could we but follow the natural rhythm of life, like the animals in the wild, we would have longer working hours; we would then have a wonderful opportunity for resting and becoming regenerated in the winter. We do not have to hibernate, but by enjoying sweet sleep before midnight, we should be well enough rested to rise with the dawn and work during the daylight hours, giving in to the body's natural demand for sleep at night. Perhaps you have never wondered why daylight appears and then disappears. We should do our business during the hours natural light is available, because this is nature's way and rhythm. Natural sleep lasts from sunset to sunrise.

What would our civilisation say to such a way of living? Obviously a resounding 'No!'. How could habits and customs be changed so drastically? From a social and economic viewpoint it would, at this time, seem impossible to adapt to this once natural pattern, although it would be healthier for us.

Try this way of life as an experiment either during your holidays or when you are convalescing from an illness. Instead of going out in the evenings on some social occasion that may last far into the night, take the opportunity to enjoy some natural sleep several hours before midnight. If, during our holidays, we accustom ourselves to this way of life, perhaps when we return home we may succeed in cancelling our social obligations on two or three weekday nights in order to enjoy the regenerative power of natural sleep. Our business and social life will actually benefit, for our energies and strength will be renewed. If, on the other hand, we behave like most people on holiday and stay up all hours of the night indulging in social life to the full, then we should not be surprised if our body and mind are still tired once it is over.

As I have said before, sleeping far into the day does not compensate for those hours lost before midnight. An old rule of country folk says: 'One hour of sleep before midnight equals two hours after.' This is no delusion but a fact confirmed scientifically, and one that anyone can prove to himself over a two-week period, by going to bed when the sun goes down and getting up when it rises. He will find his nerves have become regenerated and his general health and vitality greatly improved. A clinical experiment carried out for one week produced interesting results. One person went to bed every night at midnight and slept for twelve hours until midday, while another slept from seven or eight o'clock in the evening until four or five o'clock in the morning. Even though the second person slept three or four hours less than the first one, it was found that he was more refreshed, more rested and in better physical shape. This was obvious proof that hours spent in rest before midnight are far more beneficial than the hours after midnight, since they recharge the system with energy more effectively.

Natural sleep is a simple and easy way to help the body stay strong and healthy. All that is needed is a little willingness, a little determination and perseverance.

Sleep and Salutary Conditions

You may never have thought about it, but did you know that it matters where we sleep, whether in a healthy environment and bed or not? It strikes you first when travelling and your customary routine and sleeping place are not possible. The first time I slept in an Indian hut in the jungle I looked around in vain for a mat or some other soft surface to lie on. In the end I had to sleep on the bare bamboo floor like the Indians themselves, but at least I had my jacket, which I rolled up and used as a pillow. The only luxury I found was a mosquito net to keep out the malaria-carrying insects. If it had not been for the screeching sounds of monkeys and parrots or the cries of wild animals that kept rousing me, I would have slept comparatively well, because lying on a hard base is actually healthy. But when one is not accustomed to sleeping on a hard surface the old bones do rather object! Nonetheless, I did sleep better in that hut than the time I used a farmer's bed that was too soft and gave me the feeling of being smothered under a mountain of downy feathers.

A HEALTHY BED

It used to be the custom in country homes to cover the mattress with a quilt for greater warmth and softness. But it is hard to understand how it was possible for the habit of sleeping on a soft foundation to creep in, especially in areas where the people are usually tougher. Soft beds that sag when you lie down are not healthy. And if there is a bolster and thick pillow as well, do not be surprised to find that the spine will adopt a distorted position. If the sleeping person could be X-rayed from the side, this would be seen quite clearly. That is why old beds in country homes, where great-grandmother had had difficulty in sleeping, are far from ideal for healthy sleep today.

A good bed must have a certain degree of firmness, because if it is too soft the blood vessels, in particular the veins, become congested and this impairs the circulation. Many people do not sleep properly on foam rubber, and those who suffer from rheumatism may find metal springs unfavourable to their condition.

Blankets should be light and porous. A duvet filled with down provides beautiful warmth but a heavy old eiderdown is uncomfortable. Woollen blankets are popular in many places, but in really bad weather anyone who feels the cold will probably need an additional duvet. On the other hand, those who become warm easily will find a light duvet is better in the summer, as opposed to a woollen blanket that keeps in the heat and is heavier. Our choice, then, depends upon our individual disposition and the time of year.

In Guatemala, where two woollen blankets did not keep us warm enough during the cold nights, they gave us newspapers to use as insulation material between the blankets. True, it made us feel warmer but the constant rustling of the paper disturbed our sleep. Blankets made of pure wool, especially camel and angora, are excellent; for instance, they provide good insulation and create an electromagnetic field. Less favourable are synthetic fibres since many people, including those who suffer from rheumatism and arthritis, are susceptible to their unpleasant effect.

Bed linen, too, has its place in providing the basis for healthy sleep and should be changed frequently. While in use, we should hang it out to air in the sun from time to time. Well-aired sheets will help to stimulate the skin pores so that they will function more efficiently. In fact, it is no idle imagination to feel a sense of pleasure and well-being between fresh sheets, but a clear sign that the frequent changing of bed linen makes for healthier sleeping.

OTHER REQUIREMENTS

In the past it was considered important to sleep with the windows open. Today central heating is the accepted norm in many homes and it is therefore essential to open all windows before going to bed, letting in fresh, cool, oxygen-rich air. Unfortunately, this may have other drawbacks because in modern industrial towns there are many pollutants present in the air. Should you be fortunate enough to live in a relatively unpolluted area, keep a small window open for ventilation if your bedroom is heated. Draughts can be prevented by closing the curtains. It is important to realise that stale air in the bedroom disturbs the normal exchange of gases and sleep will not provide the rest it should. No wonder so many people still feel tired in the morning!

It is one thing to take care and change the bed linen frequently, but it is equally important to keep the body clean by daily washing. Never go to bed when the body is hot and sweaty; first take a shower or at least wash yourself down and remove all sweat and dirt. Sweating is healthy because it brings out toxins, but it also demands thorough washing. Dried up sweat clogs the pores and the toxins stick to the skin. Therefore, a clean body is part and parcel of salutary sleep.

Poor blood circulation can be helped with a hot water bottle or bed warmer if you cannot warm up naturally. Better still, take a foot bath, or alternate hot and cold baths, to warm your feet. A warm shower or bath is recommended when the body has cooled down considerably and just does not get warm. If you do have poor circulation, never go to bed with cold feet because they can keep you awake for hours. In that case it is better to make the effort and have a warm bath.

Sleeping drugs are the worst thing anyone can take because they do not cure insomnia, unless you use natural remedies. A person who does not subject himself to the laws of nature as regards sleep and rest can become a slave of chemical drugs when constantly resorting to sleeping pills.

Salutary sleep means learning to go to bed early. Soft harmonious music, not loud noise, may send you to sleep, and uplifting reading has a calming effect, in contrast to some exciting television entertainment. Quietly meditating on the deeper meaning of life can free us from the sickening happenings of our times and help us find the necessary rest.

So then, salutary sleep is based on many small necessities and requirements. Give due consideration to them before you consult your doctor about insomnia, because the answer to your problem is generally to be found simply by observing them.

Sleep, the Remedy We Cannot Do Without
The best medicines, money and possessions cannot take the place of sleep. When travelling it may overcome us on a train or plane, to the homeless it may come as a relief in open fields, and at night it gathers the more fortunate ones among us into its soothing arms on soft pillows. It is always necessary when it comes, and we should not drive it away; otherwise it may one day take revenge by avoiding us.

Do we really know what sleep means to our senses? Do we show understanding for its necessity? Have we ever stopped to think how it recharges our batteries by letting us rest and relax? While we are asleep we forget everything. When a day has been full of heavy burdens we can bring it to an end by means of merciful sleep. For the nerves, brain, muscles and blood vessels it is an important break. While we sleep, millions of our body cells can rest and renew themselves. In its wonderful effects sleep remains

611

a mystery, a phenomenon of nature, in spite of all that has been written about it.

Since it is said that every cell is subject to a rhythm of tension and repose, it is astonishing to hear that millions of heart cells, from before our birth to the last moment of our life, never stop working. It is strange that not all cells have been given the same potential. While some require the regular rhythm of rest, others are capable of working throughout life with untiring pliability, without ever resting. What miracle makes this possible is known only to the One who put the building blocks of life together and imparted the life force to them in the first place.

AN EXTRAORDINARY THING – THE NEED FOR SLEEP
One thing we know for sure from experience: we must not let the body go short of sleep since there is simply no substitute for it. Experience and observation also tell us that bedtime has something to do with the coming and going of daylight. We are aware of the fact that sleep before midnight is more refreshing and relaxing than sleep afterwards. If we postpone our bedtime to the hours after midnight we will not derive the strengthening benefits from sleep that we would by going to bed earlier, because the hours before midnight provide double the benefits. Not everyone needs the same amount of sleep. Individual requirements generally lie between six and ten hours.

If we want to derive the most from sleep as a source of energy we must definitely make sure that we allow ourselves the time we individually need. Anyone who cuts sleep short so that he can work more will soon notice that he has calculated wrongly. During the day his energy will decline and his efficiency will diminish. If we need a great deal of sleep in order to feel fresh during the day we should not compare ourselves with those who get by with less. We must by all means obtain the amount we personally need. May we therefore never forget the mysterious renewing power of sleep. It is essential for good health.

What Do Dreams Tell Us about Ourselves?
If you watch a dog asleep on the floor after an exciting chase, you can often see his legs twitching and hear him making strange noises. The dog is dreaming and the chase or something similar is still going on in his subconscious mind.

After telling a child a story about the wolf who wants to devour it, or some other exciting story, do not be surprised if the child wakes up screaming from a nightmare and runs to his mother or father because he is frightened. Modern teachers avoid exciting childrens' minds unnecessarily, but what about some of the television programmes children watch that are really inappropriate for them and can lead to real addiction?

Life Goes On While We Are Asleep

Strong impressions, agitation, fear and panic usually disturb the sleep pattern. The reflexes of the subconscious mind prevent quiet relaxation during sleep. After all, not every part of the body is asleep, many functions such as the circulation and, with it, the activity of the heart and the lungs, never stop to rest. If they stopped working our life would stop too. Digestion and everything linked with our metabolism continues working during the hours of sleep. Part of the brain rests, consciousness in particular being switched off, but other parts continue their function at a reduced rate.

We should not eat much in the evening and should avoid heavy or indigestible food completely; neither should our last meal of the day be taken late if we wish to prevent the subconscious mind, with its reactions and reflexes, giving us excitable and restless dreams that rob us of valuable energy for no good reason at all. It is of equal importance to try and forget the day's happenings, perhaps by listening to some soothing music before going to bed. Another means of unwinding is to read something pleasant or take a leisurely walk where we can take in calming impressions from nature around us. The result will be a relaxed state of mind leading to undisturbed repose. I am in no doubt that exciting radio broadcasts and television programmes that last until the early hours of the morning are the worst enemies of restful sleep.

On the other hand, not all dreams are troublesome; indeed, some dreams are quite pleasant and may let you experience some beautiful things you may never have had the chance to see in real life. As a result, you will wake up happy and contented after your 'trip' to far-distant lands. A feeling of joyful surprise may fill your being as you visit the jungles and other sights of nature, without having to spend the time and money that would have been necessary had it all been reality.

Diagnosing Illness

Dreams can, in a limited way, betray our condition of health and help us discern what illness may lie dormant in us. Dreams of being chased while the facing wind holds one back from escaping can indicate blood congestions that require attention. Oppressive dreams may be the result of lying uncomfortably so that the limbs go to sleep, or indicate that the bedroom is too hot or badly ventilated. These dreams often wake you up and you are then able to solve the problem.

The Interpretation of Dreams

The general interpretation of dreams as practised by private individuals or by psychologists usually goes too far. It is interesting, however, that you may find an answer to some problem you have been looking for in vain while awake, the reason being that the rested brain is able to draw more logical conclusions. Some researchers and inventors have even found the solutions they were seeking while asleep and dreaming. The solutions were proved to be correct on subsequent examination of all the details involved.

According to God's inspired writings in the Bible, the Creator revealed his purposes on several occasions in the form of prophetic dreams way back in antiquity. On the other hand, dreams can also be inspired by magic, metaphysical powers that are neither in harmony nor accord with the Almighty. Dreams have always had an important place in ancient cultures, as can be clearly seen from Daniel's reports about King Nebuchadnezzar of ancient Babylon, as recorded in the Bible. However, the memorable dream in question, telling of a mighty tree, came in fact from God Almighty, and the King's magicians and interpreters of dreams were unable to understand its meaning. No one but Daniel himself, with God's help, succeeded in presenting the correct information to the frightened ruler. A similar thing happened to the Egyptian pharaoh in the time of Joseph. In that case, too, no one but Joseph knew the divine dream's interpretation.

PRECAUTIONARY MEASURES

Based on this difference between divine and magical dreams, we must bear in mind that God has not used dreams to transmit the progressive steps of his purpose since the conclusion of his inspired Word. The fulfilment of his written prophecies is sufficient to reveal his purposes. Knowing this will protect us from falling victim to metaphysical influences. Once you understand their real origin you will reject them in the interests of your own well-being, guarding yourself against their evil intent. The disastrous influence of metaphysical powers to which some people open their minds can be clearly seen in India and other Far Eastern lands, where dreams and visions have been known to plague and mislead the population.

As regards modern interpretations of dreams, it would be better to treat the subject with healthy scepticism and sobriety. In spite of scientific research, dreams are still a borderline area of unexplained processes and it is most advisable to observe a healthy, natural way of life that will keep your sleep as free as possible from vivid dreams.

The Symptoms of Old Age

Medical textbooks dealing with the signs of old age mention all kinds of conditions that have as their cause the progressive deterioration of the body. Ossification of the cartilages increases, elasticity of the ligaments decreases, and the whole body becomes stiff, the entire bone structure bent. The joints are less flexible and moving them becomes more difficult, often painful. Walking becomes less safe and the person feels as if the joints lack lubrication, easily said after hearing them creak and crack! The memory deteriorates and the increased hardening of the blood vessels leads to high blood pressure. Strenuous physical effort and exposure to strong sunlight can no longer be tolerated but cause giddiness and the danger of a stroke.

This description is enough to make you lose a little of the joy of life if you are past sixty. But does it have to be like this? Is this fate immutable? Have a look at those who are much older and you will meet many eighty-year-olds who are full of vitality and energy, sometimes more so than other people who are only fifty. This reminds me of my grandmother's sister who, at the age of ninety-six, was still able to read the newspaper without glasses. Her memory and mental alertness were so sharp that I had great admiration for her when I was a young man.

A Sensible Way of Life

On examining the life-style of such people we can gene: ʻ₁, find the following basic characteristics. Their life is simple and they are moderate in their ways. They work, but do not go without time spent in rest and relaxation. They do not go short on sleep and know how to retire, in the proper sense of the word, when night falls; indeed, they are able to shut out the impressions of the day and forget whatever worries there might be. In fact, such people have the ability to overcome the ups and downs of life with a calm

615

and cheerful spirit and without worrying themselves sick. Any problems are tackled with determination and are soon solved.

Admittedly, this way of life cannot prevent old age but it does keep one young and flexible inside. Such people are content with the experience and maturity age has given them, knowing that these qualities compensate for their former youthful agility and energy. This attitude helps them to use their energy reserves moderately even at a highly advanced age, rather than squandering them in senseless pursuits. It is no doubt an art not to let the many worries and annoyances irritate and upset us too much and, instead, think more about the good and beautiful things, showing grateful appreciation for them. But this art can be learned and it is worthwhile doing so, since it helps to make the twilight of one's life more pleasant and happy.

Some old people take a constitutional walk every day, inhaling a good supply of oxygen in the fresh air, even though it is almost impossible nowadays to find a quiet country road free of all traffic. Everywhere you go there are cars, leaving only narrow meadow paths and remote trails in the forests where they have not yet been able to advance. So, if older people escape from the motor exhausts and flee to nature's solitude, the exercise, healthy air and available oxygen will be a boon to them. In addition, older people should eat natural food and in moderate quantities, with only a little fat. Their protein intake should also be limited, which avoids the formation of too much cholesterol.

Experience teaches us that the normal signs of old age can be put off by years, even decades, if the right and natural measures are taken in time. But this is only possible if we do not let the speed of our times infect us; rather, we should remember Goethe's advice and take things slower and calmer as we get older. The transition from a fast pace of life to a quieter one may not be easy; on the contrary, many people complain as different physical problems crop up and they find it increasingly difficult to cope. They confirm Solomon's observation that the years of old age are far from welcome. For this reason the wise man of biblical fame admonished the young: 'Remember, now, your Grand Creator in the days of your young manhood, before the calamitous days proceed to come, or the years have arrived when you will say: "I have no delight in them".' All those who maintain the right attitude towards the Creator throughout life will not moan about the difficulties of old age, because their heart will remain young.

Gratitude – a Remedy

I was made aware of the importance of gratitude in our life some years ago when a good friend who was an instructor at a missionary school in the State of New York asked me whether I had expressed thanks for the air I had inhaled that day. In a way, this unexpected question startled me, because I had never before thought of expressing gratitude for this indispensable gift, but had for years taken for granted its being there to receive daily. Of course, I am sure that I am not alone in having been thoughtless in this respect. At the same time, I realised that I had reason to be grateful for many other precious gifts. Moreover, I became conscious of the fact that everyday life with its hectic demands and its various joys, but also its many obstacles, often crowded out the invaluable precious things we receive from the Giver of all good and perfect gifts at no cost to us whatsoever. Once we have begun to realise that, in spite of many difficulties, we have reason to be grateful for all the indispensable things that we cannot produce ourselves, then the awakening gratitude will permeate our being with a warm feeling, and this inner warmth is a gift of which we can always avail ourselves without cost.

Many years later I was living among the carefree inhabitants of a small South Sea island. I was curious about the cause of their happiness and found that they subscribed to gratitude without thinking. They never forgot to express gratitude for all the many little and greater joys the Creator gave them day by day. Without tiring they felt grateful for the sunshine, the warmth, the blue sea with its abundance of food, the coconut trees, various other fruit trees and many other things. Gratitude not only transmits warmth, it also produces contentment, which in turn awakens happiness. It stimulates the endocrine glands, promotes good circulation, and thus influences the metabolism for better health, with all the important body functions being activated. The German poet Schiller once described joy as an animating spark, believing that joy in fact makes the world tick. With two world wars behind us, and all the subsequent wars, we realise that the spring in the world clock can be equally well wound by destructive powers. However, since these powers are never able to rob us entirely of the divine gifts of light, sunshine, air and others, we have reason enough to express our joy about them daily.

THE NATURE DOCTOR

Maintaining a Positive Attitude
One of the worst enemies that could be unleashed on the primitive peoples of the world was greed. It made them lose contentment and their inner balance, and it is therefore not without reason that many dangerous conflicts resulted. The same consequences may be triggered in children. Take an unspoilt child who is happy and content when playing with fir cones, pebbles and bits of wood. If the child is suddenly given purpose-made toys they arouse a feeling of desire and craving in him that cannot easily be allayed but demands satisfaction. In time, the desire inevitably increases. In the end, even an abundance of such toys will no longer be enough, because contentment will have been rejected and his greed will have become insatiable. Of course, this process is not confined to one child, it can take hold of whole nations, permeating them with discontent. It is this evil process which the 'civilised' world introduced to the developing countries, resulting, inevitably, in conflict and unrest.

Fortunately, there are still some people left who resist being infected by discontent but know how to remain cheerful in spite of difficulties. I remember a very sick farmer's wife who suffered from multiple sclerosis and had been paralysed for fourteen years. When she achieved a slight improvement with great effort and was able again to use her arms and eat without help from other people, she was so happy and grateful for the fact that she could cope so well with her still deplorable condition. Whenever I had to face some unpleasant jolt such as cannot be avoided on our bumpy earth my mind always returned to this lady and her quiet contentment.

Especially when we are tired we tend to look at the present, future and past with a negative spirit, but this does not contribute to a contented attitude by any means, nor will it provide the basis for restful relaxation and refreshing sleep. Therefore, we would do better to think of all the positive things that have happened to us and are still going on every day; in other words, we should count our blessings. This attitude will allow a pleasant sense of gratitude to enter our heart and will help to restore the mind and body to a state of well-being. We must admit that every person has sufficient grounds to feel upset, to worry and feel unhappy. However, if you place these negative factors on one side of the scales, then the same quantity of active, positive factors should be placed on the other side in order to balance them. So when you feel depressed and beset by problems, think about all the valuable things you have,

618

the good you have been able to do in your life, your successes, the many gifts nature offers you day by day. All these encouraging memories and experiences are able to fill your heart with gratitude so that life's burdens, all your complaints, appear small indeed.

Even sick people and those who are seriously ill can relieve their frame of mind and, in so doing, ease their suffering by adopting a positive attitude. Why should your disturbed condition of health dominate the whole spectrum of your life and emotions?

Should a sick person not be happy because at least some of his organs still function well? Could he not think up ways of how he may contribute to a quicker recovery by taking the proper measures? An illness that is properly treated and cured can, in fact, help to eliminate wastes from the body and thus improve one's general well-being. However, if a morose attitude is taken and the pain is dulled by means of chemical drugs instead of proper treatment leading to cleansing and a cure, you should not be surprised to see your hopes of success vanish. Gratitude and contentment during an illness are the best basis for recovery. Often, when you think you have good reason to give free rein to sadness and despair, why not remind yourself of the dangerous times of war or the millions of refugees who lost, and continue to lose, their homes and possessions. These thoughts would awaken gratitude in you for what blessings you have and make all your little sorrows disappear. For is it not wonderful to have a roof over your head that protects you from the rain and cold, and to live in a reasonably orderly environment and land? Gratitude and appreciation for all the many things we take for granted, that embellish our daily life, can cheer us up and dispel any feelings of depression. Try it out and you will see that it works.

The Therapeutic Power of Music

If harsh, clashing sounds such as those made by machines get on our nerves and can damage our health, it is easy to believe that harmonious music would do just the opposite for us. Science has studied the effects on humans of various kinds of sound, and the consensus is that the right sort of music definitely has a beneficial effect on our state of health.

The lullaby a mother or grandmother sings at a child's bedside is a good example of how a soft melody can have a calming effect. On the other hand, is it not true that the loud blare of pop music coming from a neighbour's open window, when one is trying to relax and rest, has just the opposite effect? How often have

Mozart's delightful melodies boosted our morale? How many troubled and wrinkled brows have been smoothed by listening to the works of the great composers? The power of a Beethoven symphony has quietened many an agitated heart. Even the twittering of birds is often able to disperse worry and anxiety to such an extent that those who see no solution to their troubles return home from a walk in the woods comforted and strengthened, hardly realising from what source the power came. A child might fall and immediately begin to scream to attract attention and assuage his pain. If, just then, a robin or blackbird in the garden hedge starts to sing, the child invariably stops wailing. At first he is interested to know where the voice is coming from, then is comforted by the cheerful little minstrel; soon the pain is forgotten and the little face is all smiles again.

It is not surprising that intelligent doctors assert that music has a soothing influence on their patients when under stress and in pain. It relaxes cramped muscles, improves the function of the glands and influences good digestion, which is directly dependent on glandular secretions.

The Choice of Music

It goes without saying that not every sort of music has the same effect. Some lovers of light music might think it strange that classical music has the best effect on some sick people. It may also seem odd that musicians often do not react to music in the same way as those who do not make music a part of their daily lives. Perhaps this can be attributed to a sort of professional diffidence.

Music for the invalid must be chosen just as carefully as medicine, even with regard to 'dosage', so that its therapy can work properly. We should bear in mind the homoeopathic principle that strong stimulants are destructive but weak ones vitalise.

It is interesting to note that there is a resemblance between all biological laws and principles. Just as a stimulating and invigorating medicine is given in the morning and a sedative at night, in the same way, lively music will be found suitable for the mornings and soothing, soft music for the evenings, helping to relax the patient and induce sleep. It is understandable that the choice of music and the volume must be right if the patient is to benefit.

Great care should be taken that someone suffering from Graves' disease (exophthalmic goitre) and others with an increased heart beat are only exposed to soft harmonious music, which will be of greater benefit to them than fast, exciting sounds. On the other hand, a slow heart that can do with perking up will benefit from a little more movement and rhythm, so as to catch a little of the enlivening spirit.

As with all biological methods of treatment, it is necessary to apply intuition, understanding and feeling. Those who lack such sensitivity and do not have the ability to develop it, should at least be considerate and spare the patient at home or in the neighbourhood from the worst of the blaring noises that go under the name of 'music' today. It is sad to see the abuse that has been inflicted on us since radio has been invented.

In summary, try the influence of some healing music with your family, friends and acquaintances, at the same time not forgetting to show consideration for your neighbours and especially those who are ill.

The Therapeutic Power of Peace and Quiet

Have you ever stopped to think about the great healing power that dwells in tranquillity, in undisturbed peacefulness? Have you ever got to know it and sought refuge in it from all the noise around us? Did you know that there are, in fact, some people who are afraid of quiet and solitude? They are not used to seeking rest and relaxation in peacefulness. They need noise, the unsettling rushing and chasing around, the feverish restlessness that does not give them even time to think. They flee from tranquillity, the healing power that could do so much for them if they only would trust in it. But they do not know it and it passes them by. So they drown in the noisy hustle and bustle of our times, letting the wondrous relaxing power of peace escape them, though with mixed feelings and suspicion. How strange that it is often the very people who are in urgent need of peace and quiet as a remedy that often shirk it!

Where to Find Peace

It is increasingly difficult to find peace in certain areas and lands, or only in such remote and inaccessible places that might frighten even those who love it. But in those areas where it still displays its beauty and serenity it should be taken advantage of as the wonderful recuperative remedy or tonic it really is. If you have not yet come to know peace, do not ignorantly shut it out or reject it. A good opportunity to become familiar with it is in the wintertime.

Imagine, for a moment, that you are walking home alone one wonderfully clear starry night. The delicate hoarfrost on the shrubs

621

and hedges glistens in the cool moonlight. The snow under your feet sparkles and in the stillness around you the crunching of your shoes sounds almost deafening. Without thinking, you stop to take in the peacefulness and the glistening beauty. You feel as if you are in another world. No sound disturbs the enchanting silence and stillness. Have you ever before realised the beauty of the birch trees in their white winter coats? It is as if you are seeing everything for the first time.

How many gifts of nature have you passed by without even looking? But look at your garden, how everything shines and sparkles. As you contemplate it, the beauty and splendour grows on you, the silence and peace take a hold of you. Involuntarily, you cast your eyes up to the sky, the Milky Way with its millions and millions of solar systems – what a tremendous, silent, quiet wonder! In fact, have you ever wondered how long the twinkling stars have already been in their places? For millions, or billions, of years they have been shining in silent peacefulness. What are you in comparison? Your life has gone on under their light for twenty, thirty, forty or fifty years, yet you have never before seen them so beautifully still, so remote but so majestic. Slowly you begin to meditate on the meaning of life, wondering whether you actually fulfil its purpose, or even whether you know and understand what that purpose is. Perhaps hitherto you have merely let the noisy current of the modern world propel you along.

Somehow you may feel weak, possibly even ill, and you ask yourself whether the noise, the hustle and bustle, the restlessness of our world have contributed to your condition. Does sickness make sense at all? Is it part of the purpose of life? There is something in you that just cannot accept the idea of sickness being inevitable. Was there not a man in antiquity who also could not accept it, doubting that sickness served a sensible purpose?

Slowly you walk to your study, still turning these thoughts over in your mind and, without prompting, you reach for a book on the shelf, the book that tells you about Job and his painful disease. Your room is quiet too. Nothing disturbs your meditation, and your reading tells you that the man Job was able to prove his devotion and integrity to God despite his suffering.

You put the book back on the shelf and now turn your eye to the pictures of your parents and grandparents that look at you from their places on the wall. They have been hanging there for years but never before have you noticed their calm, benign expressions. Of course, you know that their times were quieter times, even though the people in their day had to work hard to be successful. But there you have it, an easier life is not always a successful one. You cannot help pondering over all this. You may have come to know just the tail end of their days, before humanity was plunged into wars and many disastrous cravings, putting an end to peace and quiet.

You eye the radio in the corner as if it were an enemy. Why, is it not a source of noise? Does it not force foreign thoughts on to you, robbing you of your peace? And what about television? From the moment you let it in through the front door, it is in the home like an intruder, like some evil thing intent on stealing your time and tranquillity, while parading before your eyes all the disastrous happenings in the world. How fortunate are those of us who never let it in and have never become used to it! However, it is up to you to keep your room quiet and peaceful if you want to!

THE AWAKENING OF GRATITUDE
You are tired and decide to go to your bedroom. There is your bed in front of you. It is cold outside but you have a roof over your head and own many other things that millions do not have at all. You remember the pictures you have seen, pictures of refugees with nothing but the clothes on their backs. You still have it quite good. So why be sad? How many people go on living without a bed, or even a room, of their own. Poor people, herded together somewhere in the world, feeling cold and afraid, hungry people with no way out of their predicament – these thoughts cause you to reflect on what you have and can be grateful for. It is wrong to take everything for granted. Indeed, even the air you breathe suddenly appears to be worthy of gratitude and so does the peace and quiet around you. You feel it surging through you with a warming kind of joy and you go to bed feeling content.

You are still alone, your family has not come in yet, and they cannot know what has gone on in your heart and mind. You pull up your blanket, still deep in thought, comfortable in the calmness surrounding you. You fall into a sleep that has not been so good and restful for a long time – and all because of those moments of peace and quiet, solitude and gratitude you had enjoyed before closing your eyes. The healing powers at our disposal would make our stressful times much more endurable if only we could recognise and use them.

Happiness Means Health

Promoting health through happiness is an interesting pursuit. The poet Conrad Ferdinand Meyer thought deeply about this subject and concluded that a heavy heart is not cured by unrestrained hilarity but responds very quickly to even a little happiness. Was he really right? Can life's problems be sorted out by just a little happiness, even though our everyday demands, worries and sufferings continuously erode our energies?

Imagine a beautiful peach tree espaliered against the wall of your house. Each spring it blossoms anew and a few months later it brings forth delicious fruit. Why should we think it could be otherwise? Yet suddenly the unexpected happens. The peach tree flowers as usual, but just as the flowers open they fall to the ground. The bark of the tree dries up and the tree dies. What has happened? The tree was the pride of the household; its healthy growth, its beautiful blossoms and delicious fruit were the talk of the neighbourhood. How could this tree die so quickly and unexpectedly? What malicious enemy could have attacked it? You ask yourself all these questions but you can only find the answers by digging up the tree. It is then that you discover the cause: field mice have eaten the roots and so killed the beautiful tree.

What a joy it would have been to see the tree recover and again send forth its blossoms. Sometimes it is only by losing things, either material or spiritual, that we become aware of their value. Young people would not be so casual about their health if they could but know that they might soon lose it. How bewildered we are by the loss of health and until we know the cause there is not much we can do about it. Good health should be treasured and never abused, for good health leads to happiness.

Negligence, ignorance, inexperience, ineptitude, often force of circumstances, as well as a lack of knowledge on how to sustain health and prolong life, are all, metaphorically speaking, rodents that are gnawing away at our life and bringing us eventually to ruin. So does the little word 'happiness' imply that having it will bring back health and save our lives from an untimely end?

If you inherited good health and vigour you should always cherish and appreciate these valuable gifts. Inherent advantages should be enjoyed and used to make others happy too. An old proverb puts it this way: 'The happiness we give to others will return to make our own hearts rejoice.'

Life is like good garden soil. It brings forth nothing if we do not sow, till, water and care for it. Without good seed even the best soil will not produce a thing. If we do not put anything into life, we cannot hope to get anything out of it. Again, the poet's words come to mind: 'Know that the noble mind puts goodness into life, but does not seek it there'! All the things that raise our spirit and give us strength are like valuable and beautiful plants in our lives. The useless things that hang about us, imperfect beings that we are, are as weeds, which should be pulled out and destroyed.

Undoubtedly one of the best and most useful plants or attributes we possess is happiness. This not only brings peace to our spirit but also healing to our body.

Happiness as a Remedy
Happiness can indeed be spoken of as a remedy. Mysterious functions take place in our bodies, which are responsible for equally mysterious and inexplicable effects. No less puzzling is the interaction between the mind and the nervous system. In what a wonderful and simple way the central nervous system executes the orders of the mind! Millions of muscle fibres work like obedient little horses, harnessed and driven by millions of reins and guided by our will, the driver. To this wonder-system of divine design we owe the movement and rhythm of life.

How differently the sympathetic nervous system works! Unguided by the cerebrum and uninfluenced by the will, it performs those functions that could not possibly be maintained and attended to by our conscious minds. The circulation and digestion, as well as all the organs involved in these processes, are regulated by the autonomous nerves on which our physical and mental well-being depends. Although the will has no power over them they can nevertheless be influenced by our imaginative faculties, by our feelings and emotions. Joy will get hold of the hidden switches of the sympathetic nerves, and release cramps and flood away congestions in the liver, the kidneys and the pancreas. Even the heart cannot escape the positive influence of joy and happiness.

By helping those around us to see and appreciate the beautiful things in life, to achieve happiness, we are administering to them the best biological medicine possible. Showing them the meaning of life and the opportunities to do good to their fellow human being will bring joy and happiness into their life.

If you know a diabetic patient, you can be of great service if you teach him to enjoy the good and beautiful things in life. Point out the beauty of the spring buds and blossoms; encourage him to rejoice in the golden splendour of the ripe wheat fields of the summer, to take pleasure in the autumnal symphony of colours and to admire the ornate beauty of wintry ice and snow crystals. To experience this happiness will touch his heart, improve his breathing and instil him with a vitality that will carry him through the woods and over the hills with opened eyes and a thankful heart. The pancreas will begin to function better; the secretion of digestive enzymes and consequently the digestion, will improve. A lower intake of food will be of advantage to him in his condition, since better digestion means better utilisation of the food eaten. The inner secretions will be stimulated, the islets of Langerhans will increase their production of insulin and the sugar in the blood will be oxidised. Aided by physical measures such as hot abdominal packs and good natural wholefoods, especially by plenty of raw vegetables in the diet, all eaten slowly and well insalivated, his health will visibly improve. If joy and happiness are added to the diet, before long he may be fortunate enough to have regained his health.

You can help people who suffer from liver disorders, too, by telling them of this happiness cure. They will have reason to be grateful to you. If your own liver, the most important gland in your body, is not working as it should, let happiness set about casting out trouble and anxiety. It can wage a successful war against these saboteurs and will effectively counteract the damage done by them. Take and use this help which, though sometimes buried deep within you, is always ready to come to your assistance. Be filled with the rhythm of the pulsating life of happiness; be glad, even if the gladness at first is somewhat artificial and forced. Breathe deeply and at the same time concentrate upon something of beauty and value. Eventually you will find that happiness will pervade your whole being and so master your body and all its functions.

Happiness is like warmth. Even the coldest heart must melt if this warmth is allowed to penetrate for long enough. If whatever you do can somehow help your neighbour, the resulting happiness you receive will permeate your entire being. Whether you are a farmer, salesperson, housewife, office worker, doctor, lawyer, butcher, candlestick maker, or whatever, your fellow human being needs your skill and by rendering a service to him it should bring happiness to you. Do not go about your work sullenly, thereby spoiling the blessing of it. If you are a teacher or a doctor and perhaps you feel that what you do does not receive proper recognition, at least take comfort and happiness from the fact that you are in a position to help those who need and want to be helped. Those who work only for the sake of making money, or are forced to because of circumstances, gain very little, if any, satisfaction from their work. If there is no pleasure to be found in what you are doing or in your achievements, then you are cheating yourself, to be sure. If your eight- or nine-hour working day is pervaded by ill-will and discontent, and you sleep for another eight hours, it is fairly certain that you will not have many happy, cheerful and thankful feelings during whatever time remains. Such a life is one of slavery and drudgery. Your work would be so much easier and enjoyable and it would make fewer demands on you if only it could be permeated with happiness. In the evening you would be much less tired, your dinner would taste better and your morale would be higher. The hours of leisure spent with your family and friends would be filled with pleasure and peace of mind. Even though others contaminate the atmosphere with hate and discontent, your happiness would be strong enough to triumph over such discord.

Envy and jealousy are powerful enemies that corrupt the mind. They can destroy and gnaw away at the plant of happiness in the garden of your heart and lay hold of your innermost being.

There once was an Indian prince who marvelled at one of his fellow believers, a poor man, who could rejoice without envy at the beauty and gracefulness of the prince's wife. The prince, puzzled, questioned him and the poor man explained happily: 'Why should I not rejoice in beauty, especially if it does not occasion me any worry or responsibility? You have the burden of overseeing all your wealth and of providing for all your wife's needs while I, on the other hand, can rejoice in just looking at her, without any worry or dismay.'

Those who can enjoy looking at the good fortune of others without feeling envious have passed their first big test, which will ensure them happiness and peace throughout their lives. Possessions always mean responsibility but there are many things we can relish without such cares. Our walks can be taken not only for the healthy exercise they give but also for the joy of seeing the beauty of the flowers, the distant mountains, the fine woods and rich fields. We need not consider the fact that the cool, blue lake and the rushing stream do not belong to us. We can rejoice in the graceful gambols of someone else's young animals without fearing that, by some mischance, we might lose them. We can enjoy all these things so much better than their owner, because ownership is a heavy burden that demands work and care. Many who strive for it with envy or jealousy in their hearts perhaps could not enjoy such a burden successfully. So, if you wish to enjoy beauty to the full, do not let envy and jealousy encroach upon your joy in appreciating the possessions of others.

If, one day, you find yourself robbed of happiness, just exert yourself by doing something to please others and you will find that it will return. A kind, friendly word, an understanding smile and a comforting look or remark are the things that can do much good in giving pleasure to others. If you have the capacity to comfort someone in his sorrows, you will undoubtedly find comfort for yourself, for it is well known that one derives more pleasure from giving than from receiving.

Is not every day a gift from heaven? Why spoil it with grumbling and discontent? How much more sensible it would be to fill the day with useful thoughts and deeds, for each day comes but once and by nightfall it is gone forever. Even though troubles may arise, happiness and thankfulness can offset them and thus the day never needs to be lost and wasted.

If you are alone, you can rejoice in the quiet and collect your thoughts. If you are among friends, then rejoice in their company and make good use of the occasion to profit by such companionship. Build one another up by conversation that gives moral improvement and mutual benefit, like the echo of a beautiful symphony. Empty chatter produces spiritual emptiness that craves for distraction. Boisterous laughter does not generate joy but is like darnel, a weed whose ears are empty.

When you go to bed – when the sun sets if at all possible – the last thing you should do before going to sleep is to thank your Maker for the day he has given you. Rejoice in the good you have been able to do and if you have received a kindness, then remember it with quiet happiness and breathe deeply, for joy comes from the depths of the spirit and is carried on the breath of life. When borne aloft to higher spheres by this feeling of joy, you will realise how small and insignificant your everyday troubles really are. You will gently slip into the land of unconsciousness, like an aeroplane crossing from day into night. The higher the flight path the safer the flight because there is less danger of coming into contact with the obstacles on earth, the air currents and gusts. It is the same with us; the higher we reach in the spiritual realm of joy and peace, the more peaceful our inner lives will be, and thus our sleep. Our dreams, if they appear at all, will be quiet and no longer based on our former restlessness.

To change our way of life so that we can find this deep, satisfying joy in the midst of our everyday life, must of course take a little time and practice. Our nature is not used to controlling our mind and spirit as it is to ordering our muscles and sinews.

When the new day dawns, do not hurry agitatedly into the unknown, wondering what new worries it will bring. Try to remember that it has been given to you completely new, to do with it what you will. After all, should we really take it for granted that light and sunshine return day after day for our benefit? So thank your Maker for these important gifts of everyday life, as thankfulness always fills the heart with joy and this happy frame of mind will never nourish the hard-hearted attitude that there is no divine Power interested in our welfare. On the contrary, it will prompt you to express thanks to your Maker for the wonderful gift of light and warmth. Full of joy, your first step in the new day will be a happy one. Whatever problems that arise to worry you can be dealt with more easily; in fact, you will look at them in a different light, giving you a better chance of success, whereas sadness and discontent will rob your time and drain your strength, or they may even lead you into further trouble. Those who begin their day in a happy frame of mind are more likely to end it in the same way.

If you are not in a happy mood when you wake up, think of something joyful. Open your windows, breathe deeply for about five minutes and the lingering tiredness will soon leave you. This exercise will put a different, happier face on things, even though you got out of bed on the wrong side. Moreover, if you do something for the body at the same time, you are well on the way to acquiring a positive mood. According to your nature, this may be washing yourself down with hot or warm water or taking a shower. Additionally, it would be useful to do some exercises, resulting in a pleasant feeling of warmth and a good start to the day. You will enjoy breakfast more than usual if you clean your teeth properly beforehand and gargle to cleanse and refresh your throat thoroughly.

Take pleasure in your food and make sure that it is both tasty and natural. Do not be a slave to time with one eye always on the clock. Eat peacefully and slowly, chewing your food well. In this way you will extract all the nourishment possible and your internal organs will benefit from the work your teeth and salivary glands have done for them. Those who enjoy and value what nature's garden so generously gives us should remember to be grateful and not take the well-laden table for granted. There are so many things in which we can rejoice that there is really no time left for discontent.

If, however, some sorrow strikes you down, face things bravely with determination to overcome it. Eventually you will reach the place where the warm sun of peace and happiness will once again soothe or even heal your pain completely. Always look ahead with optimism.

Should the enemy of all living things rob you of one of your loved ones, try not to be overwhelmed by inconsolable grief. Prophetic words have been written, which promise us a time when there will be no more sorrow, when pain and death will no longer exist. These are not empty illusions. The God of Life will put a stop to evil and destruction and the resurrection of the dead will become a reality. This faith in a happier future brings a warm glow of comfort and hope to our hearts. Nothing can strengthen our morale as much as the thought of the restoration of all things to a state of perfection. What a comfort it is to know that our pain- and fear-ridden world will one day be freed of all destructive forces! No one who wilfully wielded evil power will be allowed to return from death to spread sorrow and anguish once more. Those who mourn their dead, a result of inherited imperfection, should not stubbornly reject joyful hope and faith in the resurrection. True, the superficiality of our lives and the cares of day-to-day living are apt to obscure our understanding of such matters. We think that things have always been and always will be the same. We cannot envisage a time when blood will no longer be spilled, when swords will be turned into ploughshares, spears into pruning knives and man will no longer learn the art of war. This must now seem a quite unbelievable blessing for our war-weary and war-mongering world. However, the God of Life, the God of Peace, will make good his promises. Each one will have his own vineyard and sit beneath his own fig tree, at peace with the world and without fear for the future. These are sacred words of hope and comfort spoken under inspiration by the prophets of old and can be considered as good as fulfilled. The kingdom for which we learned to pray as children is no Utopia, no matter how much the worldly wise may scoff at the idea. Those who believe these words must eventually be filled with hope and positive happiness, even though they may have many trials and tribulations to overcome.

'Yes,' some sigh, 'if only we could understand and believe.' Because many love the dissipations that have become common and seemingly necessary to their superficial lives, they cannot achieve real happiness in life and the joy of worthwhile things. For them the future is gloomy and will remain so, to the extent that they seek a way out with drugs. While they think it is pleasurable, there is no health and joy in this escape.

Our pleasures should be salutary so that they can impart health. Some people become slaves to a passion and regard it as their real and only pleasure in life, yet it is quite possible that indulging in it is doing them great harm. This applies very much to the passion for sports. From a healthy pleasure in movement and rhythm, sports have now become so exaggerated and competitive that they can damage and sometimes even destroy your health. Anything that can harm you is not a true pleasure, which should always make for good health.

If you take pleasure in the beauties of nature you will find that other passions cannot make too many demands on you, especially those that blind you to all true happiness. Concentrate on and enjoy the bounteous riches of creation, which are limitless and offered to you for your delight. Only the normal biological rhythm of a healthy way of life can ensure for you the happiness that strengthens and regenerates. For example, you will not be able to enjoy the fresh, clean mountain air, nor the scent of the meadows and the larch or fir trees if you have ruined your sense of smell by smoking.

Happiness is a soothing balm for a sick heart and the best remedy for a wounded spirit. Even when you lose all that you thought was worth living for, or when the friends you thought you could depend upon desert you, you will still find that happiness is inexhaustible, once you know where and how to find it. A ray of sunlight coming through the window can make you happy. It can transform the unnoticed spider's web into a silver diadem. Light, air and sun are possessions that we place too little value on, yet they enrich our lives by scattering many joys in our path. All we have to do is open our eyes to these things. Even when the sun's light is withdrawn, the inner light which we should have stored in our hearts should continue to illuminate our lives.

Unfortunately, it does not seem to be a characteristic of our times to seek out and enjoy the little things in life. So much unhappiness has embittered people's hearts, too many hopes have been raised and shattered, and peace – that great giver of happiness

— has too often been destroyed. It is very difficult for an overtired nervous system to be relaxed and at ease so that strength and peace-bringing happiness can enter and do its good work. It is never easy to rid oneself of unhappy memories and impressions, but if you wish to regain your health through happiness, then you must do your utmost to forget. Happiness can then take root and a healthy, joyful spirit will provide the best conditions for making and keeping your body healthy.

Recommendations for Breakfast

If you want to do justice to the physical and mental demands of today's world, you must do all you can to obtain and eat natural wholefoods containing plenty of nutrients and vitamins. Many people think that it is enough to watch their intake of calories, as this is generally recommended. However, that this consideration is not the only important one can be seen in the resulting deficiencies and various other disturbances, as well as tiredness, not to speak of sudden symptoms of illness. It is necessary to change to natural, organic wholefoods in order to stem the tide of environmental pollution, and the stress of our modern unhealthy life-style.

You can begin by making the right start with your breakfast. In Continental Europe coffee or tea, white bread, white rolls, butter, jam or marmalade, perhaps some cheese spread, is usually considered sufficient to keep one going until midday, whether in hotels or at home. The idea is that a more substantial lunch will supply the necessary balance. In the United Kingdom and the United States, however, it is often customary to have a quick 'bite' in the lunch hour in order to interrupt the work schedule as little as possible. For this reason people tend to eat a substantial breakfast including plenty of protein (just think of the English breakfast), because the meal has to last until the evening when, on returning home from work, the main meal of the day is served.

Years ago it was the custom in rural Switzerland to eat either specially prepared sauté potatoes, polental, (a dish made of cornmeal) or porridge. This kind of breakfast was more nutritious, even though it can still be described as one-sided, not balanced. Then, in Switzerland, the idea of the now widely known 'muesli' arose, based on the nutritious rolled oats, *mues* (meaning dish). Muesli is a mixture of uncooked cereal flakes with grated nuts or almonds, dried fruit, and grated raw apples or berries. Dr Bircher-Benner became one of the early advocates of muesli and his recommendations were so convincing that the expression 'Bircher Muesli' established itself, especially in Switzerland.

A Special Wholefood Muesli

The experience I gained on my travels encouraged me to formulate a special muesli that contains all the nutrients we need, as well as many vitamins and all trace elements. No wonder it deserves the name 'Vollwertmuesli' (Full Value Muesli) and is on sale in every health food store in Switzerland. It contains six cereals – whole grain rye, wheat, oats, barley, brown rice and millet – all made into flakes. Another ingredient is sprouted soybeans (the sprouting takes away the bitterness and makes soya more digestible), to provide a valuable source of protein. Chestnut flakes are added for flavouring and nutritional value. It is sweetened with granulated dried grapes (organically grown); the valuable grape sugar, like honey, is directly absorbed into the blood. The granulation is achieved using pure lactose and this is a boon for the digestion and intestines. Dried, organically grown fruits enhance the taste of the muesli besides giving it valuable fruit sugars. Ground almonds are another ingredient. A further addition to this nutritious muesli is rather exceptional: it is the tropical fruit known as durian which only grows in rain forests. The natives eat this fruit for its nutritional value, giving them the strength to achieve exceptional tasks. In my own case, by eating durian I was able to keep up my energy and endurance all day long in spite of high humidity and heat. If it were not rich in vitamins and other nutrients it would hardly be so effective. Most of my friends like *Vogel's Breakfast Muesli* so much that they would not be without it in the morning and some even have it for supper as well.

According to the season, I recommend enriching the muesli with berries, fruit and a little milk or cream; you will then have a nutritious breakfast that will keep you going even if you have to do strenuous work. Additionally, I would recommend as a drink a cup of rose hip tea sweetened with honey, or *Bambu Coffee Substitute* with milk or cream, if you prefer it. A piece of whole-grain bread with butter and honey is also appreciated by some. Those who feel more hungry in the morning may appreciate Vogel Bread, if it is available where you live.

A breakfast based on such a nutritive muesli provides the body with enough energy to cope even with hard work without the need to draw on its reserves. Vogel's Breakfast Muesli is also an ideal food for growing children, as well as for young people who have to study or work hard.

Recommendations for Lunch (Midday Meal)

The consequences of unhealthy nutrition are usually felt more keenly when we are older, although nowadays more and more young people suffer from 'diseases of civilisation'. Listeners at my well-attended lectures in Europe keep asking me to what I owe my remarkable vitality and vigour, in spite of my advanced age and heavy work load. I have already explained what I eat for breakfast and, for the benefit of my questioners, I will here outline my nutritious lunch at midday.

Salad, vegetables and starch for lunch supply minerals, which we should never overlook, in addition to vitamins. The salads are made up of what the garden offers fresh, so that the variety depends upon what is in season. The salad dressing is usually made with soft white cheese (cottage cheese or quark), sunflower oil and *Molkosan* (whey concentrate), and possibly horseradish and seasoning herbs. The vegetables, too, depend upon what is seasonally available in the garden.

I recommend wholefood items such as *A. Vogel's Soya Dinners* in place of meat, especially for those who wish to eat a vegetarian diet or need to reduce or eliminate their intake of animal protein for health reasons. These soya dishes are meat-free, being made from carefully selected vegetable products. As they are available in a variety of different flavours they will definitely enrich your lunch table.

The range of easily prepared ready-to-serve dishes has been increased by the new range of *Soya Mixes*. These too contain no meat, and are therefore valuable food supplements for those who are on a meat-free diet. It is possible in this way to supply the body with purely vegetable protein by means of a delicious and pleasant lunchtime meal.

The Soya Mixes are especially indicated for vegetarian diets. Vegetable fats rich in unsaturated fatty acids help to reduce and stabilise the cholesterol level in the blood. The mixes are enriched with important trace elements and their fibre content has a positive effect on the movement of the bowels.

In these restless times, every person interested in health should never forget that proper nutrition is a key factor in protecting one's health and that it is possible to prepare tasty dishes that please the palate while being absolutely natural.

It is important, however, that a person makes sure to eat food that contains protein, starch and vital substances (vitamins and minerals) at least once a day.

Suitable protein foods other than meat are dishes containing soya, or cottage cheese (quark) or other soft cheeses.

Starchy foods are mainly potatoes, brown rice or wholegrain cereals, including millet and buckwheat.

Foods that contain vital substances (vitamins and minerals) are vegetables and salads.

Recommendations for Supper (Evening Meal)

As a light meal is better for you in the evening, the menu should possibly be the same as in the morning. You will sleep better after it than if you eat a lot of food that is hard to digest.

What is more, high-value wholefoods satisfy even in smaller quantities and keep you going to the next meal without feeling hungry, so that you can actually eat less. Every meal should be a happy family occasion and it will be just that if everyone appreciates the companionship as well as the food on the table. If you partake of it with gratitude you will forget the haste and bustle of the day and automatically chew it more thoroughly. The body will then be able to obtain the full benefit of the goodness in the food, all the nutrients and remedial properties.

The laws governing healthy nutrition are the same for man and beast and similar for plants. A healthy diet is especially important for older people and so is moderation in eating. So, if you want to learn the art of how to stay healthy as you grow older, remember that the right mental attitude and diet are of paramount importance.

Important Basic Rules for the Healthy and the Sick

The rules I outline below will help the healthy in a preventative sense, and the sick will find them beneficial when followed in addition to their therapeutic treatment. In fact, a patient who takes these rules into account will have greater success with his medical treatment.

1. Since overfeeding with protein is one of the principal causes of the 'diseases of civilisation', you should conscientiously observe the optimum intake of protein, that is, not more than 40 g (1.4 oz) daily. This is about half or a third of what people usually eat in the course of the day.

2. Your choice of foods should be restricted to natural foods, so avoid eating refined or devalued, denatured products. At the same time, see that you select organically grown cereals, fruit and vegetables.

3. The evening meal (supper) makes healthy sleep difficult if it consists of heavy protein foods. You will find it quite easy to become used to 'Full Value Muesli', enriched with fresh fruit according to the season. Some *Risopan* crispbread with a little butter and a cup of *Bambu Coffee Substitute* or rose hip tea will be enough to complete the meal.

4. I recommend a weekly fast day when you only drink vegetable juice, made from organically grown vegetables. Drink half a litre (just under a pint) of juice and about 1½ litres (about 2½ pints) of a mild kidney tea in the course of the day.

5. Eating correctly will aid the digestion. Always insalivate your food well. Anyone who does not wish to take the time to chew his food thoroughly will one day be forced to take time to stay at home sick.

6. Natural remedies should be taken regularly. In cases of a strong reaction take a smaller dose than indicated, until the disturbances disappear.

7. There are already enough poisons in our environment to upset your body, so take care to avoid as many of them as you can; nicotine, drugs and alcohol all weaken the body.

8. The order for every day is: 'Fill up with oxygen not petrol.' By this I mean that you should make a point of getting enough exercise in the fresh air every day.

9. Do not forget that the usual mad rush and demanding stress of our times not only overtax our nerves, but can also cause painful tension and circulatory disturbances. Therefore, do not let yourself be affected by more than what cannot be helped. A useful antidote is internal peace and calmness. They protect us, save energy and are an aid to beneficial relaxation.

10. Worries, anxiety and discontent harm the liver. So try to be generous and forbearing as regards human weaknesses. Those who can bear such loads preserve the peace that builds up, whereas strife and conflict destroy the things that are valuable.

11. The peace of the twilight hours provide relaxation and time for quiet meditation. When the day has had its fill of necessary duties and obligations, we should not let television programmes unnecessarily whip up our emotions still further. Uplifting spiritual food is soothing. Listening for a little while to soft music can also

help us to relax. Years ago the day was usually rounded off by singing songs of praise and gratitude, but the problems of our modern times have fundamentally changed all that.

12. Sleep is the best and least expensive remedy for good health and relaxation and should not be cut short for the sake of night-time pleasures. The hours before midnight count double and help one to go to sleep quickly. Before going to bed, a short walk in the fresh air can be relaxing, so that even the most tiresome day can end in wholesome rest.

Fasting – a Means to Combat the Damage Caused by Civilisation
People advanced in years tell us that life before World War I was more natural and hence more healthy than it is today. If the statistics of those days are correct, in the industrialised countries one person in thirty died of cancer or a heart attack, whereas today it is already one in four. The reason for this difference is mainly to be found in a change of nutrition as the simple demands people had in the past have given way to greater demands today. This applies especially to the increased consumption of protein foods and low-value carbohydrates, in particular, products made with refined sugar and refined white flour.

Comparing these nutritional trends with the modest require-ments of more primitive peoples who had not yet become familiar with the diet of our advanced industrial society, I discovered that for this reason those people had as a rule, been spared the dangers and sorrows caused by our 'diseases of civilisation'. They knew neither rheumatism nor arthritis, hardening of the arteries accompanied by high blood pressure, or cancer. The symptoms of these insidious diseases appeared only when the traditional and natural diet gave way more and more to one made up of food produced by our commercialised society. As long as people living in their natural, untouched environment were used to eating only a little protein every day – about half or even a third of the quantity consumed in more advanced societies – they were able to maintain their biological balance and good health.

This observation made a strong impression on me in every case I studied and as long ago as the 1920s I published my findings of those days in a booklet that is now out of print. In 1935 I followed this up with the publication of my first book on nutrition, entitled *Nahrung als Heifaktor (Food as a Healing Factor)*. It was clear to me that refined, denatured foods had to lead to deficiencies and could give rise to serious diseases. So why not overcome the problem by means of natural wholefoods that have not been robbed of their goodness?

Eating food as it is presented to us by nature, without anything removed, helps to avoid physical problems and can also contribute to a cure, if some harm has been done already.

At first the World Health Organization (WHO) held the opinion that a relatively high daily intake of protein was necessary. This advice was generally followed, but since the view was in fact incorrect, what was done has led to ill health. On the basis of experience the WHO later changed its opinion, recommending a daily protein intake of only 0.7 g per kilogram of body weight. In more recent times even this recommendation has been further reduced to only 0.5 g. For a 100 kg (15½ stone) man this would mean a consumption of 50 g (about 2 oz) of protein per day. Taking an average weight of 60–70 kg (9½ stones), the daily intake should be approximately 30–35 g (just over 1 oz).

More and more attention has been given to nutrition and efforts are being made to overcome or rectify existing damage to health. In an effort to renew the body fluids, some hit on the idea of fasting. A little time before that, the Austrian farmer and nature healer J. Schroth recommended a diet of solid foods without liquids. However, when it was observed that this diet had dangerous side effects, the 'cure' was given up and small quantities of liquids were taken during the period of fasting. Eventually the use of purifying teas was started, without adding sugar but sweetening them with a little honey. Pure spring water was then employed, as well as mineral water low in carbonic acid or, better, without it. The body reacted wonderfully to this cleansing cure of drinking 1–2 litres (2–4 pints) of pure spring water.

The idea of these fasting cures was to refrain from eating proteins and starchy foods over a period of time, with the benefit that the bowels could rest and the kidneys and liver had the opportunity to cleanse the body, getting rid especially of metabolic waste toxins. By observing the rule of reduced protein consumption, the diseases resulting from an increased intake would decline considerably too, and success in treating existing ones would undoubtedly be greater than when the various recommended medicines, treatments and therapies were taken.

It is with reservation that I mention the fasting treatment with tea, spring or mineral water, because it is, in a sense, a starvation diet and the person is forced to live on his body's own protein. Interestingly, the pH value of the blood changes, becoming more acidic. Anyone who wishes to undertake such a fast for any length of time should have the necessary reserves and attitude or else it could be detrimental.

Fasting with fruit or vegetable juices, on the other hand, places less of a strain on the system, avoids the starvation effect and can more easily achieve the desired cleansing of the body fluids. In South Africa I observed good results achieved by a diet based on freshly pressed grape juice. However, the grapes must be unsprayed in order to avoid taking in blue vitriol and residues of other chemicals. If the juice is contaminated the poisons will enter the system and thwart the purpose of drinking it. You need absolutely pure, organically grown and treated juice if you intend to bind and eliminate toxins that have accumulated in the body.

Since the juices must be made from biologically pure fruit and vegetables, there is yet another important factor to be considered. The soil where they are grown must on no account by subjected to chemical fertilisers because they harm the otherwise good foundation, resulting in a decrease in useful micro-organisms; the bacterial flora suffers and the entire condition of the soil becomes imbalanced. Soil that has been saturated with chemicals, with nitrates, phosphates and nitrogen compounds is definitely 'sick'. But how can soil that is itself 'sick' produce healthy fruit and vegetables? Obviously its produce is by no means 100 per cent. Moreover, chlorinated hydrocarbons, such as DDT, Aldrin and other dangerous chemicals, are bad for the soil.

The many detrimental influences attributable to environmental pollution must also be considered responsible for the deaths caused by cancer and vascular diseases. Then there are the mental pressures resulting from increased stress and constant hurrying, as well as other circumstances. Even though juice diets can work wonders because they cleanse and renew the body fluids, you must take care that the unfavourable influences of our times do not cause additional harm to your health. Be cautious, therefore: never go beyond what the generally weakened condition is able to cope with. If you suffer from heart trouble, you cannot embark upon such a ruthless diet without being cautious. I knew the doctor in charge of a well-known clinic in South Africa. He was a clever man but also quite fanatical as regards encouraging his patients to fast. Having failed to take into consideration the weak heart of one of them, the eventual death of the patient in question was really the fault of the doctor. A patient has to be strong enough before starting a juice diet. The doctor in attendance should act with great caution since a patient with heart trouble may not always be able to take the strain of such a diet.

Protecting the Body Cells
It is true that our cells are wonderfully made, with each one in the system being autonomous, independent. When healthy the cell possesses a marvellous metabolism as well as the remarkable ability of internal regeneration. What occurs inside the cell could be compared to the work of a computer, one that has come from the Creator's hand. It is also true to say that we understand very little about the workings of the cell. Still, the cell's ability to repair or regenerate damage is always ready in its defence. This readiness on the part of millions, indeed billions, of cells is most important to the whole cellular system. In fact, a cell can fight off unfavourable influences for years and, supported by the lymph and enzymes, it is able to absorb the best nutrients from the blood.

If, however, in the course of time it no longer receives the things it urgently needs, it will gradually give up. The cell is then like a business person who is in the red because of unfortunate circumstances and can no longer escape bankruptcy. However, with a cell the situation is far more tragic, because its condition is then what we know as cancer. The cell is forced to give up its normal functions. Since it can no longer hold off the influence of poisoning, it becomes antisocial and begins to act, we might say, like a person who has lost his reason. It becomes a sick giant cell. Juice diets have often proved effective in such cases, but, again, they should not be undertaken without careful thought.

An important rule demands that any treatment should only be given after first considering the patient's physical condition. I remember an occasion when I ignored this rule and went on a carrot juice diet without actually needing it. After two weeks my body suffered a peculiar reaction: I turned yellow, as if I had jaundice. At the time I happened to visit an eminent haematologist from Innsbruck, who was amazed at the excessive amount of carotene in my skin. An analysis brought to light that the haemoglobin count had been increased by 100 per cent. The effect was like a strange fire in the body, as if I had a high temperature, yet the examination showed no fever at all. I stopped the diet and two weeks later the disturbance had subsided.

This experience led me to be more careful and future experiments did not play such tricks on me. For my own purpose, I found a blend of about 30 per cent carrot juice, 60 per cent beetroot juice and about 10 per cent cabbage juice to be most satisfactory. In cases of dysbacteria sauerkraut juice, which contains lactic acid, is excellent; dilute it with half the quantity of spring water or non-carbonated mineral water. Lactic acid is a fine healing factor for the intestines. Juices that are fermented with lactic acid are more easily tolerated than freshly pressed ones, and it is possible to take at least one-third more of the lactic-fermented juices than of those prepared from fresh produce at home. You have to go by the experience gleaned from experiments and then be guided by what your body finds the most effective.

Scheduling Occasional Juice Days
A beneficial way to get used to a juice diet is to go on a one-day fast each week. If this juice day is successful and does not make you feel ill, then you can extend it to two days a week, later on even three days. As time goes by and your body becomes used to juice days, you may be able to go on such a diet for two weeks. But do not forget that you need to get plenty of oxygen during this time.

Grape juice diets are beneficial even in serious cases of cancer, since the juice is able to renew the body fluids to a great extent. For those who respond well to grapefruit, a juice diet using this fruit will be most beneficial, but not everyone tolerates grapefruit, for which reason it is important not to be fanatical as regards any form of treatment.

Whenever you go on a juice diet, a trustworthy, biologically oriented doctor should supervise its progress and the patient himself should carefully monitor his condition and reaction. The doctor must keep a check on the heart, blood pressure and other physical aspects so that the diet will produce the desired effects. In the fight against the diseases of our industrialised society, especially cancer, I have seen the best results when the patient is given the following mixture of lactic-acid-fermented juices: 60 per cent beet, 30 per cent carrot and 10 per cent sauerkraut.

Emptying the Bowels – Indispensable for Juice Diets
Never go on a fast without first eliminating all faecal matter. This applies with greater force to those who already suffer from constipation. If you ignore this advice you may have to reckon with unpleasant, possibly even disastrous, consequences. The peristalsis of the intestines is stimulated by the ingested food and if this stimulation is lacking, as is the case during a fast, the encrusted

materials will keep sticking to the villi of the intestines. Of course, this is extremely harmful to the body; it can even poison the system and cause serious consequences. This can be avoided, however, if the right measures are taken. The patient is therefore advised to consider these words carefully if he wants to escape the detrimental effects of such negligence. Do not forget to undergo a thorough cleansing of the bowels before going on a diet, even if it is only intended to be a short one, lasting a few days.

There are some good botanic laxatives you could use to stimulate the intestines. Some people like *Linoforce*, a tried and tested linseed preparation; others prefer to take *Rasayana No. 1 or No. 2*, or the mucilaginous *psyllium seed*. All these remedies are purgative but do not exclude the need for an enema before beginning the diet. For this purpose it is usually not enough to use an ordinary enema syringe, but a douche should be able to clean out the colon very well. Clinics and sanatoriums use a special douche for irrigation. For the duration of the diet it is advisable to give an enema every morning. This has been found to be very beneficial, because impurities are still eliminated often four or five days after beginning the diet. This faecal matter will have been encrusted in the villi but is softened, dissolved and finally eliminated by means of the treatment.

It depends on the health reserves and the condition of the heart whether a longer period of fasting is advisable. Some people extend the diet up to three weeks, if not longer. Let me add that with this long fast it is still necessary to give an enema every morning. In order to prevent the mucous membranes from drying out, use a decoction of *mallow*, instead of just water, or you can add to the water a little mother tincture of *Symphytum officinalis*, which is made from comfrey. If you happen to have some comfrey in the garden prepare a decoction from it and use this for the enema.

There is also another good suggestion. Add the mucilage prepared from *quince seed* to the water for the enema; or a mucilaginous infusion made from mosses such as *carragheen* (Irish moss). The addition of *Usnea* is recommended too, especially because of its excellent disinfectant action for the colon at the same time. Disinfecting can also be done with the addition of 10–20 drops of *Echinaforce*; this has a good effect on the intestinal bacteria. A tablespoon of Molkosan is beneficial to the intestinal bacteria since the lactic acid promotes their growth and health. When on a fast it is indispensable to follow the advice just given in order to protect the colon.

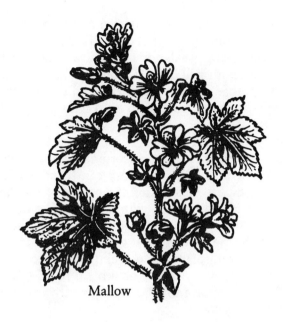

Mallow

At the end of the diet it is important to make a slow transition to your normal eating pattern. Begin with a soup made with oat-flakes or barley. Rice gruel is also to be recommended. However, meat, egg and cheese dishes should be left off the menu during the first week after the diet. Instead, it is preferable to take light vegetable dishes, brown rice, mashed potatoes, corn and millet. Also, have salads and soft white cheese (cottage cheese, quark) mixed with a little garlic and parsley.

It is important to pay proper attention to the transition from your normal food to the fasting diet and from the diet back to normal food again. This is essential to give the body enough time to adapt gradually to the new situation.

Health Benefits from Taking Vegetable Juices with a Specific Purpose

Are vegetable juices really indicated as a curative therapy for various diseases? What is their benefit to our health? These questions are a waste of time to those who do not think that nutrition plays an important part in keeping healthy. At the same time, observation tells us that the diseases resulting from life in our industrial society are on the increase. These illnesses have been termed 'diseases of civilisation' because they are caused by the diet or nutritional habits of people in the more affluent countries. In particular, the daily consumption of protein is generally too high, leading to a condition of overfeeding. Thus, if we are able to achieve a proper dietary balance by a purposeful intake of vegetable juices our health will definitely benefit. In fact, a day a week on a diet of vegetable juices will be beneficial to anyone. If we can see the reason why, it will be easy to keep one day a week reserved for this purpose.

A total of 500–700 ml (18–25 fl. oz) of vegetable juice during one day may be sufficient, but according to the physique of a person, up to 1 litre (1.76 pints) a day can be taken. It would be wise to take the juice in sips during the course of the day, making sure to insalivate it and not just gulp it down. The body will then obtain the full benefit of the vital substances, the minerals as well as the vitamins. At the same time, it will have a rest from the usual intake of carbohydrates, fats and protein. It is especially successful when you reduce the daily intake of protein to 35–40 g (1½ oz). This may be only half or a third of the quantity you are probably used to having every day.

Since 1935 I have been prescribing vegetable juices with notable results. The juices I have used are beetroot, carrot, cabbage and sauerkraut, either pure or mixed. Whatever the disease concerned, these juices have helped to solve the dietetic difficulties. However, since not everyone finds it easy to get the quantities right when mixing the juices, I thought it well worth using my experience and produce a ready mixed combination of juices, known as *A. Vogel's mixed vegetable juice* containing 60 per cent beetroot, 30 per cent carrot and 10 per cent sauerkraut, all three being fermented with dextrorotatory lactic acid. Only organically grown vegetables are used in the normal, biological manufacturing process.

This excellent mixed vegetable juice has an additional benefit in its content of provitamin A, which is important for the eyes. For this reason it is a dietetic help for night-blindness, xerophthalmia and other eye problems. It is suggested that you begin by diluting the pure juice with still mineral water until you are used to the hearty taste of A. Vogel's mixed vegetable juice. This is advisable because excesses should be avoided when on a diet. I have also been successful in helping many people with gastric ulcers by prescribing raw potato juice. It is best to press the juice fresh and drink it right away.

A vegetable juice diet achieves a reduction of protein, fat and sugar consumption without harming one's health. It is therefore an alternative method in the treatment of diseases brought about by modern civilisation. These findings, after years of practice, have prompted me to recommend juice diets for the benefit of all those suffering from these diseases.

In order to step up the elimination of wastes through the urine, it is of paramount importance to drink 1–1½ litres (2–4 pints) of weak *rose hip, goldenrod or kidney tea* daily throughout the duration of a juice diet or fast.

The Excellent Effect of Juice Diets on Various Diseases

The general advice for a prescribed juice diet is especially applicable in cases of rheumatism and arthritis, and following it carefully can only bring good results. For this purpose, go on a vegetable juice diet for two or three days every week and you will ensure that the body obtains plenty of alkaline substances in an easily assimilated form. No strain is put on the body through having to deal with breaking down fats, carbohydrates and proteins while taking only juices. The juices are highly alkaline, able to bind the acid elements and eliminate them through the kidneys and urine. In this way it is possible, figuratively speaking, to balance the acid/alkaline composition, since acid elements, which are partly responsible for causing pain, crystallise and are gradually eliminated. This apparently unimportant process alone is able to effect a considerable improvement in the patient's condition after only a few months. The elimination can be stimulated and the results accelerated if the patient takes *Solidago, Nephrosolid* and other good kidney remedies at the same time.

The use of a good *oil* that stimulates the skin functions is further recommended, as well as the external application of *Symphosan* following a warm shower in the morning or an invigorating herbal bath. If you follow this advice, your skin will benefit and the treatment can have greater success.

If so far you have not bothered much about proper nutrition, you should definitely make an effort to eat only natural wholefoods, avoiding white flour and white flour products. With respect to cereals eat only wholegrain products. The right way of eating your food is important too, because it benefits the digestion. For one thing, forget the usual hurry. Before sitting down to eat, relax and let your insides calm down. Eating slowly and chewing the food thoroughly, with good insalivation, will then be easy. This advice is worth remembering in order to achieve good results.

Then you should give attention to another important requirement, sufficient exercise in the open air. It provides fresh air and the necessary oxygen, essential for those of us who are healthy and even more so for the sick who want to get better. This is another step in the direction of recovery. Painful myogelosis, hardening of tissue, is not uncommon nowadays. Massage by a skilled practitioner can help to remove the problem. If you follow the advice given, the treatment can be taken at home with the same success as in an expensive clinic or sanatorium. So then, remember the various possibilities at your disposal to reach the goal of recovery.

The same treatment applies to those who suffer from various vascular problems and especially when a heart attack is in the offing or has already occurred. If you are in this position you should by no means think that everything is lost and there is no reason left to change your habits. It would be much more intelligent to strengthen your determination to improve and accept whatever help is available. Vascular diseases are often a symptom of a potassium and magnesium deficiency in the body, so it is appropriate to change one's diet to a protein-reduced and vitamin- and mineral-rich one.

A. Vogel's mixed vegetable juice made from carrot, beetroot and sauerkraut juice is a superb means of preventing such deficiencies, since these three vegetables are known to be rich in potassium and magnesium. Its alkalinity is three times as high as its acidity. People prone to heart attacks should have at least two juice days a week, one at the beginning and the other in the middle of the week. The body will soon benefit from doing this because of the reduced intake of fat and protein, and also because of the added provision of minerals and vitamins contained in the juices.

However, heart patients still need plenty of oxygen, which they can obtain by inhaling good air when walking or hiking or by doing some moderate work in the garden. Be careful, though, to avoid direct sunshine; cover the head with a light hat. Any existing congestions should be treated by reflex zone massage and moderate but regular exercise therapy. The heart muscles and nerves can be strengthened if the hawthorn fresh plant preparation *Crataegisan* is taken at the same time. Conscientious efforts to follow the advice given will enable the patient to prevent the disaster of having a heart attack.

An apopleptic must be careful, too, in order to counteract the degeneration of the blood vessels successfully. In this case, there is the danger of a stroke caused by high blood pressure. Such a person should also take the aforementioned advice seriously and follow it as a preventative measure. It is not enough for him to rely on mistletoe preparations or rauwolfia extract alone. The right diet is absolutely essential, because it was poor nutrition that undermined his health over the years and decades. If he does not want to succumb to the consequences of increasing high blood pressure, he must avoid everything that caused the problem in the first place. This means reducing the intake of protein to the normal and reasonable optimum quantity of about 40 g a day, or 0.5 g per kilogram of body weight, in accordance with the quantity established by the WHO (see page 638). The reduced quantity of protein and starch should be replaced by vegetables and salads. Soft white cheese (cottage cheese, quark) or soya protein are best suited to cover the protein requirement. As regards starch, apoplectics should take advantage of the goodness brown rice has to offer. A natural brown rice diet comprises three rice days a week, and this is most appropriate since brown rice has a regenerative effect on the blood vessels, as has been proved in the case of many patients. So do not overlook the great benefit of brown rice.

The question of fats and oils must also be solved in a sensible way. When one's health is endangered it is no doubt advisable to do without fats and oils in cooking in order to avoid the temptation to use heated fats and fry food in fat or oil. The use of fat will then be restricted to cold pressed oils for salads, which is all you need.

Pay careful attention to seasoning. Cooking salt should be avoided; use moderate amounts of the herbal seasoning salts *Trocomare* and *Herbamare*. Healthy and wholesome substitutes for salt and other seasonings are small amounts of garlic, horseradish and parsley. Do not use vinegar to dress your salad but wholesome *Molkosan*, which aids the digestion. While on a diet or treatment it goes without saying that you should really cut out all alcohol and nicotine. If you follow this general advice conscientiously you will notice an improvement in the blood pressure after only a few weeks, and after some time your doctor will be happy to confirm that the pressure has returned to normal. Such a result based on natural treatment is to be highly appreciated, but the method of reducing blood pressure by means of strong medication always presents a risk that has led to disaster for some patients. As with heart attack patients, it will be of great benefit if an apoplectic goes on a juice day at the beginning and in the middle of each week.

Those who suffer from a disturbed lymphatic system tend to be bothered by catarrh. They keep having trouble with their respiratory organs and are prone to anaemia. In view of this they would do well to go on a vegetable juice diet two days a week. At the same time, their general condition should be built up by taking *Urticalcin* every day. This preparation increases the calcium level and is therefore of importance to the patient with lymphatic trouble. Refined sugar and products made with it must be avoided at all costs, even in the case of children, who are usually sweet-toothed. It would be a mistake to give in to their craving during the treatment because it would be detrimental, reducing the up-building and regenerative benefits of the cure.

Besides the wholesome effect of carotene, A. Vogel's mixed vegetable juice contains vitamin B_{12}, which is important for the blood. In order to overcome their susceptibility as quickly as possible, those suffering from lymphatic problems should become used to taking about twenty drops of *Echinaforce* regularly every morning and evening. This remedy helps the body to improve its own powers of regeneration and build up natural resistance against infections, which is most beneficial to the patient.

Diabetics and those who suffer from obesity can also derive benefits from juice days. In addition, diabetics should acquire the habit of taking a glass of A. Vogel's mixed vegetable juice with every midday and evening meal.

As far as obesity is concerned, it can be of the normal kind or hypophysial, although the latter is very rare. A. Vogel's mixed vegetable juice diet is of great benefit in the case of normal obesity. It is recommended to take nothing but juice, together with rice crispbread, such as Risopan, for two or three days every week. At the same time, support the stimulation of the endocrine glands with a seaweed preparation, preferably on an empty stomach in the morning. Good results have been gained with *Kelpasan*, taking 1–2 tablets every morning before breakfast. This, incidentally, helps to combat early-morning tiredness too.

A fast day, eating only apples and grapefruit, besides the vegetable juice days, is also beneficial and helps to reduce weight. At any rate, grapefruit is well suited to reducing excess weight. For this reason always add half a grapefruit or the juice to your muesli in the morning and evening. If you are prone to obesity, make it a point to eat half a grapefruit with your breakfast every morning. Furthermore, reduce your intake of protein to 40 g (1½ oz) and also limit that of carbohydrates considerably; try to meet your daily requirements by eating wholegrain products. On the other hand, you may eat salads to your heart's content without any restriction as to quantity, since they do not share in building up the body weight. However, keep away from white sugar products and sweets; your craving for something sweet can be satisfied with dates and figs in moderate quantity. Brown rice dishes are to be preferred to those made with flour and potatoes.

The Influence of a Vegetable Juice Diet on Cancer and Leukaemia
Why are cancer and leukaemia, as a rule, unknown among more primitive peoples? As long as these people live on food that is rich in vitamins, minerals and high in alkalinity, without any items produced according to our 'civilised' ideas, they are able to maintain their biological balance. Another factor is the ease of obtaining plenty of exercise in the fresh, unpolluted air, and with it, deep-breathing, which provides the lungs with more than enough oxygen. The same factors are important in our own case, if we are to arrange our life in such a way that prevents problems. Should there be cases of cancer and leukaemia in our family we must be especially careful.

Whenever the problem runs in the family, it is definitely indicated to change one's eating habits, that is, to replace the foods of civilisation with full-value natural wholefoods. We can only endeavour to regain and maintain the biological balance in our body if we follow a strict diet that is high in alkalinity and vital substances, vitamins and minerals. If cancer is suspected, or someone suffers from leukaemia, or is recovering from a cancer operation, a low-protein diet is urgently recommended. In preparation for the actual therapy, which requires a very strict diet, not more than 20 g (0.7 oz) of protein daily are permissible. In such a case, an extended vegetable juice diet makes a virtually protein-free diet possible. However, it is most important for the therapist or doctor to check the patient's heart carefully before putting him on the diet, because the heart must be strong and healthy in order to stand the recommended protein-free juice diet.

Whether the diet is based on fruit or vegetable juices, in every case the body will be forced to obtain the necessary amir. acids from somewhere. According to experience, it draws them rrom the cancerous cells rather than the healthy ones. For this reason it is possible that cancerous tissue shrinks and is absorbed after a protein-free diet extending over three or maybe even four weeks. This is possible where the juice, rich in vital substances and highly alkaline, attacks the cancerous tissues with such force that these cells are unable to withstand the violent action. Even in serious, sometimes hopeless, cases surprising changes for the better have been reported. It is additionally beneficial to take plant preparations that tend to prevent cancer, such as *butterbur (Petasites)*, *mistletoe, garlic, horseradish* or another plant containing *germanium*. *Symphytum*, the wild comfrey plant, is also helpful in this connection.

It is not always advisable to extend a juice diet over a period of three or four weeks only because the patient wants to see quick results. It is much better to go on a juice diet for one week and then follow it up with a low-protein natural diet, and then another juice week. If you do decide on an extended juice diet, you should only tackle it under the supervision of a qualified therapist or practitioner. A good choice would be a doctor who specialises in holistic medicine and nature cure methods.

Before embarking on a juice cure, the colon must be thoroughly cleansed. Use *psyllium seed* or a *linseed* preparation such as *Linoforce* for this purpose. It is sometimes advisable to support the cleansing process by taking *wheat bran*. The diet will be more successful if the prescribed quantity of juice is sipped during the day, rather than taken in large amounts each time. Should you feel heartburn at the beginning of the diet, neutralise the acid right away by means of *wood ash*, best of all birch wood ash; take a teaspoon of ash in a glass of water.

Years ago it was the practice in the United States and in South Africa to go on grape juice diets for the treatment of cancer. I remember hearing of excellent results that were achieved to the astonishment of everyone. Unfortunately, it is today no longer advisable to go on such a diet because it has become universal to spray the grapes with pesticides. Naturally, this procedure is responsible for contaminating the grape juice with an excess of copper and chemicals. However, unsprayed grapes still produce a fine juice that can be used for grape juice diets.

The danger of poisoning is minimised in the case of vegetable juices, since the vegetables for juice diets must be organically grown anyway. *A. Vogel's mixed vegetable juice* made from beets, carrots and sauerkraut, all fermented with lactic acid, is especially recommended in the fight against 'diseases of civilisation'. The results have been outstanding even in cases of cancer and leukemia, although it is not at all easy to be successful in treating these two dreadful diseases. Constant vigilance and careful observation of the condition in each individual case are indispensable.

A. Vogel's Rheumatism Cure

Simple treatments are often more effective in curing troublesome diseases than those that require a lot of bother and are costly. So why does not everyone readily acknowledge their worth and take them? The reason is that they require certain sacrifices to be made. The treatment recommended for cases of rheumatism, arthritis and gout is only successful if followed for at least six months or, better still, for a whole year, and involves cutting out completely any food with excess acidity, replacing it with foods that are high in alkalinity. In other words, the patient must go without meat, fish, eggs and cheese.

You can see why this idea does not appeal to everyone and is often considered too difficult to follow. On the other hand, is it really a pleasure to suffer constant pain which may also become twice as bad when the weather changes and the humidity in the air increases? Of course, no one really relishes this idea. True, it may be that the transition period of changing from one set of dietary habits to another requires effort and determination, but the palate is able to become accustomed to such a change, even though it may be reluctant at the start. A little good will goes a long way and it is not, in fact, so difficult to adapt oneself to a special diet; all it means is that the taste buds must be re-educated. Moreover, dietary food, if prepared properly, can be made so tasty that you will want to continue with it after the treatment has ended. What is more, if an improvement in one's condition is noticed within a few weeks the patient will not regret having taken the plunge and changed his diet. Feeling that the aches and pains are actually beginning to recede is a most welcome relief and makes the personal sacrifice well worthwhile.

In the morning, on waking up, the first thing to do is to follow a routine of invigorating personal hygiene. As a rule, a warm shower is recommended; slowly get used to it by gradually increasing the temperature of the water. Then use *Symphosan* to rub down the whole body. The principal ingredient of this herbal preparation is comfrey and it stimulates the skin functions, helping it to become more supple and soft.

After completing this general hygiene and body care have breakfast consisting of 3–5 tablespoons of high-value muesli (*A. Vogel's Breakfast Muesli*). Mix in the juice of half a lemon. According to need, you can also choose half a grapefruit or the juice of 2–3 mandarin oranges or clementines, if available. Next, add half a tablespoon of pure honey, three tablespoons of coffee cream or

651

half a tablespoon of almond purée. Then add two or three grated apples, depending on their size. Instead of apples you could mash and add some berries when in season. These ingredients make a juicy, refreshing muesli. In addition to this dish, have one or two slices of wholegrain (wholewheat) bread with butter or a good vegetable margarine. A cup of rose hip tea is excellent as a mild stimulant for the kidneys. If you need to activate the kidneys a little more take a *kidney tea* and add ten drops of *Nephrosolid* or *Solidago*. For a change, you may prefer to have a cup of *Bambu Coffee Substitute* with a little coffee cream.

Lunch should be prepared without any frying, for the benefit of the liver. For every meal it is enough to have a 100 per cent natural food containing starch, such as brown rice, potatoes, millet, buckwheat or corn. Soya can be considered a source of starch as well as protein. The choice of our starchy food determines what is to accompany the meal. Whichever you choose should first be steamed, then browned without fat in an earthenware pot in the oven. Most vegetables are suitable for this method, for example leeks, fennel, courgettes, aubergines, cabbage stems and kohlrabi (turnip cabbage). Tomatoes grown in your own garden and ripened on the plant should be eaten raw in salads. For a change, however, you can cut them into three and prepare them *au gratin* in the oven. Fresh green beans and peas supplement the protein foods. The beans are very tasty when prepared with the appropriate herbs.

Salads constitute food with healing properties. According to the season, use cress, tender dandelion shoots or lamb's lettuce. White cabbage makes an especially refreshing salad (coleslaw) but should be served without bacon or ham. Equally valuable is raw sauerkraut. Carrot salad is also very popular, and beetroot salad is usually preferred when made with cooked beetroot. Beetroot salad is a good substitute for raw salad. Many people like chicory salad made with the white variety. The Brussels variety can be made into an appetising dish too.

The salad dressing is also important; it should be stimulating and tasty. Soft white cheese (quark or cottage cheese) is a good base, but yogurt (natural, without any fruit), *Molkosan* or lemon juice can be used to give slight acidity, with the addition of a little cream or cold-pressed oil. Season with crushed garlic or grated horseradish and culinary herbs, but everything in moderation so that the dressing is pleasantly seasoned. Such a dressing is valuable because it whets the appetite and so aids the digestion. If you want to put on weight have an additional supplement of cottage cheese or quark every day, seasoned with herbs, garlic or horseradish. Or you may prefer curd cheese.

To drink, choose a good mineral water, a still or slightly carbonated type; add some Molkosan for the sake of the digestion. Instead of wine, try A. Vogel's mixed vegetable juice, 100–200 ml (4–8 fl. oz) with each meal.

The total food intake per meal should be moderate. In fact, when eating wholefoods it is possible to eat 40–50 per cent less and yet be better nourished than before. The evening meal should be similar to breakfast because a lighter meal is easier to digest and guarantees restful sleep.

If you want to speed up the results of the treatment go on a vegetable juice diet for one or two days a week. Take one litre (about 2 pints) of juice during the day, sipping it regularly every hour. You may take a slice of Risopan crispbread with it, since this bread has the highest mineral content.

If the treatment is followed properly it will regulate the functions of the bowels and kidneys. But if you suffer from constipation, especially the chronic kind, do not neglect to take *Psyllium* or *Linoforce* daily at the beginning. After a while you will no longer need to take it because the bowels will respond to the diet and begin to function efficiently, even more so when the food is eaten slowly, chewed well and insalivated.

These rules have been tried and tested. Now and then during the treatment have your urine tested so that you can see what is being eliminated from the body. The urine test is, in a manner of speaking, a test of the treatment's success. Improvement and cure depend upon the alkaline/acid balance being restored.

Are Nitrates Poisonous?

We could also ask whether phosphorus, fluorine and chlorine are poisons, for they are all important to the growth of plants and neither human nor animal life would be possible without them. It was not idle talk when Moleschot said, 'No thought without phosphorus.' Phosphorus is necessary for the brain and the bones. Like fluorine, chlorine and iodine, it is an element, but only when it is combined with other elements, for example potassium, calcium, sodium or magnesium, are nutritive salts formed.

Nitrates are just as necessary as the other substances; in fact, they are actually a harmless source of nitrogen. Plant life would be impossible without any one of these salts or substances, including nitrates. What does matter, however, is the quantity of these sub-

653

stances contained in a plant. If the level is too high, they are detrimental to health and therefore dangerous. For example, it is possible to achieve an excess of acidity in plants that normally are high in alkalinity when artificial fertilisers containing too many phosphates are spread. All minerals existing in nature and necessary to life are detrimental, even poisonous, if they are so highly concentrated and used in order to produce greater yields in an unnatural way (massive fertilising). This cannot possibly happen when the land is worked organically; there will be no overdose of phosphates, fluorides or nitrates. Organically grown vegetables indicate a more balanced content of nutritive salts than those grown with artificial fertilisers. The nutritive salt content varies from plant to plant; for example there are, more nitrates in beets than in carrots or other tubers.

For people who eat too much protein, large quantities of nitrates can be harmful because the nitrates are changed into nitrides in the body, forming dangerous nitrosamines (carcinogenic substances). But even these compounds are rendered harmless when sufficient amounts of vitamin C are taken. Even though beetroot absorbs a relatively high amount of nitrates in a natural way, beetroot juice is one of the best plant remedies for providing cancer cells (which are known to lack oxygen) with plenty of oxygen, thus opening up the way to regeneration and a cure. At the same time, it is essential to adopt a low-protein diet, forcing the body to derive its amino acids (component molecules of protein) from pathological cell tissues such as growths, myomas, even malignant tumours. The vitamin D and betacyan, the nitrogen-containing colouring of beetroot, actively help to regenerate the deteriorated cancer cells. Nitrates are therefore not harmful even in cancer therapy, as long as they are used as outlined above. In this regard we agree with Paracelsus who said that 'Everything is poison; it all depends on how much you take.' It also depends on the circumstances connected with ingesting it.

The 'Nature Doctor' Takes His Leave
Much advice has been given in this book and I hope that it will help many of you. There is so much we can do for ourselves by natural means. With the proper intelligent attitude perhaps we can live with the things that cannot be remedied by leading as healthy a life as possible, by permitting our spirit to rise above our physical suffering.

More could certainly be said about our mental attitude towards life and health but this would take us into another book. The important thing to remember is that we should live our lives according to nature's rules. The more we feel and think in a healthy way, the less will those damaging influences, which are so difficult to disperse, make their way into our bodies.

If we admit the value of the good, which is always at hand for ourselves and those around us, we will achieve something for our health and spiritual balance in these insecure and restless times. How we react to life depends upon our innermost selves. The hurrying stream of time tries to blot out the healthy habits established in the past and thus lead us along strange paths that make it so easy to go astray. But once you have peered into the rich treasure chest of *The Nature Doctor* you will never be deceived again. You will know that there is an answer in nature.

So, open this book when you need advice on matters of health. It will save you many disappointments and you will avoid useless and perhaps harmful treatments. In any event, the advice given here can never do any harm, unless you go your own way contrary to the suggestions. I would encourage you, however, to follow the advice carefully and you will find the balanced middle way, neither being fanatically extremist nor indifferent.

On the other hand, let me say that there is one little 'herb' I do not know either, the one referred to in an old proverb:

There's many a herb to cure,
Not one, however, for death, to be sure.

I am fully aware that my medical advice is but a help for dealing with the times in which we live.

A Special Note
The quantities or doses of natural remedies indicated in this book are based upon the author's experience acquired in many years of practice. The adequate quantities prescribed can vary according to the sensitivity of the patient. More robust persons may take larger amounts to achieve the desired result, whereas children and more sensitive patients may achieve the full effect with half the quantity or even less. Since botanic remedies and homoeopathic medicines are given in order to rectify and cure the cause of an illness, not merely the symptoms, it is more important to take the remedies regularly and for some time than to watch the exact quantity.

655

Index

Index

The Index will help you locate the subjects of interest at a glance. The page numbers in bold print refer to more explicit information on the listed subjects. This makes the answers to your questions about certain diseases and health problems much easier.

Abdomen, organs, 55, 430–1
Abdominal disorders, 5, 62, 79–81
Abrasions, cuts, wounds, 1, 358, 364, 377, 402, 413–414, 444, 450, 455
Abscesses, boils, 13, 32, 395, 396, 401, 455, 487, 552
  focus on tooth, 9, 262, 302, 307
Achillea millefolium, see yarrow
Acidophilus, 89, 219, 226, 541
Acid. phos., 56
Acne, 400, 495
Aconitum napellus, see Monkshood
ACTH (hormone product), 268
Addiction (to tablets), 353
Adenoids, polyps, 72, 581
Aesculaforce (tonic for the veins), 27, 34, 69, 99, 116, 120, 135, 139, 152, 163, 198, 261, 270, 358, 399, 402
Aesculus hippocastanum, see horse chestnut
AIDS, 106, 297–299
Air, fresh, 582, 595
Albumen, 24
Alchemilla vulgaris, see Lady's mantle
Alchohol, 10, 31, 42, 112, 116
Alchohol compresses, 137
Alderbuckthorn, 232
Alfalfa, 111
Allergies (oversensitivity), 182, 183–184, 503
Allium cepa, see Onion

Allium sativum, see Garlic
Allium ursinum, see Bear's garlic (ramsons)
Almonds, Almond cream, milk, oil, purée, 41, 43, 52, 84, 102, 177, 535
Aloes, powdered, 232
Alpine plants, medicinal, 344–347
Amalgam, 307
Amoebas, amoebic dysentery, 233, 235, 240, 446
Anaemia, 19, 111, 368, 447, 542
Angelica (Angelica archangelica), 347–9
Angelica liqueur (Vespétro), 348
Angina pectoris, 151, 153, 384, 581
Anise (Pimpinella anisum), 38, 263, 408
Anthriscus cerefolium, see Chervil
Antibiotics, natural, 88–92, 171
Antimonii sulph, aureum, 49, 98
Antiseptic, 38, 77
Antispasmodic, 98, 353
Aphids, 90
Apomorphinum, 29
Appendicitis, 215–217
Appendix, 108, 215
Appetite
  lack (loss) of, 38, 53, 348, 418, 438
  uncontrolled, 205
Apples, 7, 52, 218, 249, 301
Apricots, 487
Arabiaforce, 50, 423
Armoracia rusticana, see Horseradish

INDEX

Arnica montana, see Arnica

Arnica, 12, 26, 27, 33, 50, 120, 122, 129, 135, 139, 144, 152, 186, 324–5, 349, 358, 384, 395

Arsenicum album, 79, 98, 176

Arsenicum iodatum, 49

Artemisia absinthum, see Wormwood

Artemisia vulgaris, see Mugwort

Arteries (blood vessels), **114–117**, 414
  hardening of (Arteriosclerosis), **115–117**, 120, 124–8, 152, 366, 383, 409, 411, 524, 528

Arteriosclerosis, diet for, 125

Arterioforce capsules, 116, 122, 129

Arthritis, 11, **262–272**, 306, 357, 367, 397, 444, 445, 455, 475, 496, 505, 526, 651

Artichokes (Cynara scolimus), 206, 253

Ascarid, see Roundworm

Asthma, 96–99, 153, 353, 385, 401, 457, 581

Asthmasan, 98, 354

Athlete's foot, 325, 449–450

Athlete's heart, 150

Atropa belladonna, see Deadly nightshade

Atrophy, 585

Atropinum sulph., 167

Auroforce, 131, 147

Autumn crocus, see Meadow saffron

Avena-sativa, 95, 188

Avenaforce, see also Oats, 69, 81, 188

Avitaminosis, disease caused by vitamin deficiency, 47, 273, 274, 308, 310, 319, 453, 489

Autonomic nervous disorder, see Neurodystonia

Backache, bad back, 336

Bacteria, bacterial flora, 24, 80, 81, 107, 108, 218, 219, 412

Bacterial infections, 83, 88, 107, **293**, 301

Bacteria and viruses, **293–299**

Bacterial toxins, 51, 54, 76, 165, 175, 177

Balance
  mental (psychological), 7
  disturbances of, 451, 592

Balm (Melissa off.), see Lemon balm

Bambu Coffee Substitute, 125, 126, 127, 256, 257, 544, 636

Bang's disease, see Brucellosis

Baptisia tinctoria (Wild indigo), 57

Barberry (Berberis vulgaris), 263, 292, **382**, 418, 484

Barberry purée (how to make), **382**

Barefoot, walking, 3, 190, 196, **332**

Barley, 41, 520

Barley malt, 520

Baryum carbonicum, 74

Basal metabolism, 155

Basedow's disease, see Graves' disease

Basil (Ocimum basilicum), 94, 407

Bath herbs, **35–37**

Baths of long duration, 4, 13, 164

Baths of alternating hot and cold, 3, 33, 123, 199, 323, 329, **429**

Baunscheidt treatment (revulsion method), 75, 197, 260, 335, **439**

Bear's garlic (Allium ursinum), 116, 126, 129, 349, 409, 419, 420, 467, 477

Bear's garlic Tonic, 122, 129, 350

Bed-wetting (Enuresis), **171**, 393

Bee pollen, see Pollen

Bee sting, 14, 15, 407

Beet (red, beetroot), 57, 94, 111, 131, 157, 204, 216

Beet juice, 226, **495–496**

Belladonna (deadly nightshade), 47, 49, 75, 98, 213, **391–3**

Berberis, vulgaris, see Barberry

Beriberi (Vitamin deficiency disease), 128, 465, 489

Berries, edible, 94, 502–505

Bilberries (Vaccinium myrtillus)
  leaves, juice, 8, 52, 57, 178, 211, 216, 503, 505

Bile duct, secretion, 400
  vomiting (bilious), 6, 249

Biocarbosan, 8, 226

Biocarottin, 39, 52, 69, 176, 221, 232, 250, 252, 261, 417, 459, 487

Biochemical remedies, **398–402**

Bio-C-Lozenges, 29, 293, **419**, 486

Bio-Sanddorsan-Conserve (Buckthorn), 388, 418

Bircher-Benner, Dr., 494

Birch Hair Lotion, 311

Birch leaves, tea, 24, 252, 263, 441, 442

Birthmarks, moles, **282**

Blackberries (Rubus fruticosus), leaves, juice, 178, 249, 420, 422, 503, 505

INDEX

Bladder, 38, 397
  bleeding, 27
  bladder drops, Cystoforce, 171
  inflammation of (cystitis), 170–1, 385,
    430
Bladder wrack (Fucus vesiculosus), 556
Bleeding gums, 383, 418, 502
Bleeding, staunching of, 5, 461
Blood, 58, 105–107, 132, 490, 521
  circulation, also disorders, 69, 82–3, 357,
    468, 611
  cleansing treatments, 422–424
  corpuscles,
    red, 24, 404
    white, 24, 215
Blood
  a mysterious fluid, 105
  poisoning, 15, 107, 109, 137, 395, 460
  pressure, high (hypertension), 59, 62,
    124–9, 152, 349, 366, 383, 409,
    459, 425, 464
    low (hypotension), 59, 62, 128–9,
      129–132, 406, 459
Blood supply, 11, 33, 69, 82, 360, 429, **452**
  normalising rush of blood to head, 27,
    190, 392
Blood sugar, 449
Blood transfusion, 106
Blood vessels, 418, 543
Blueberries, see Bilberries
Boils, **13**, 455
Boldocynara, 57, 69, 226, 250, 252, 292
Bones, 29, 52, 100, 104, 398, 401
  broken, 355
Bowel function, 24, 54, 95, 100, 119, 175,
    219–222, 399, 405, 465, 466
Bowels, sluggish, 7, 119
Bracken, fern, 14
Brain, 57–60
Bran, 1, 12, 44, 464, 517, 519, 522, 523
Brazil nuts, 84
Bread, 516–519
Breast, cancer, 32
Breathing, abdominal, 577
  deep, 61, 95–96, 123, 577–582
  difficulty in, 367
  exercises, 96, 420, 481, 577–578
  through the nose, 578
Breakfast, 125, 256, **476**, 497, **632**, 651
Breakfast Muesli, Vogel's, see Muesli

Bronchial asthma, 96
  catarrh, 85, 394, 415, 455, 457, 462, 348
Bronchials, 71, 78, 348, 415, 455, 581
Bronchitis, see Bronchial catarrh
Brown rice, natural, see Rice
Brucellosis, 491, 522, 536, 570
Bruises, 13, 444, 448
Brush massage, 83, 123, 163
Bryonia dioica (Red Bryony), 57
Buckthorn bark (Rhamnus frangula), 232
Buckwheat, dishes (Fagopyrum esculentum),
    41, **127–8**, 208, **523–524**
Bugleweed (Lyopus europaeus), **144–5**, 155
Building a house, **590–593**
Burns and scalds, 1, 460
Butter, unsalted
Butterbur (Petasites off. Petasites hybridus),
    91, 95, 98, 111, 186, 261, 263, 270,
    292, 350–5, 526, 650
Buttermilk, 43, 256

Cabbage
  white, 29, 94, 102, 178, 418, 471, 486
  juice, 94, 211, 497
  leaf packs, poultices, **1**, 4, 6, 10, 13, 15,
    56, 62, 78, 158, 175, 252, 271, **442–444**
Cactus grandiflora, see **Cereus**, nightblooming
  (Selenicereus grandiflorus)
Calcarea carbonica (calcium carbonate), 73,
    81, 144, 177
Calcarea fluorica (calcium fluoride), 39,
    141, 299, **398–9**
Calcarea phosphorica (calcium phosphate),
    39, 49, 399
Calcification, **120–128**
Calcium, 15, 29, 94, 100–105, **120–124**,
    157, 177, 191, **192**, 363, 397, 487
  complex, see Urticalcin deficiency, **29–30**,
    38, 43, 45, 52, **83**, 101, 105, 109,
    144, 155, 225, 301, 471
  flouride, see Calc. fluor.
  level, 191, 648
  phosphate, see Calc. phos.
  powder, 1, 2, 13, 72, 102, 105
  preparation, biological, see Urticalcin
  problems in older people, 122
Calendula off., see Marigold (calendula)
Camomile (Matricaria chamomilla), 10, 17
    25, 36, 52, 68, 73, 80, 163, 216,
    251, 311, 430, 456

661

Camphor, tincture, leaves, 73, 335
Cancer, patients, 87, 91, 110, 211, 219, 264, 274–293, 288–292
  prevention of, 351, 354, 367, 402, 434, 450, 528, 649
  remedies for, 292–293
  spectre of, 276–278
Cancerous cells, 108, 113, 273
Cane sugar, 94, 509, 511–512
Canned foods, fruits, 514–516
Cantharis (Spanish fly), 169, 171
Capillaries, capillary system, 111–112
Capsella bursa pastoris, see Shepherd's purse
Caraway (Carum carvi), 38, 408
Carbohydrates, 244, 256, 455, 464
Carbon dioxide, 113, 114
Carbuncles, boils, 13, 395, 396, 401, 455, 552
Carcinogenic influences, substances (cancer-producing), 34, 45, 275, 279–280, 286–291
Cardiac asthma, 96, 98–99
  insufficiency, 151
  valves, 76, 85
Cardiaforce, 56, 214
Carica papaya, see Papaya
Carotene, 487, 495
Carrot(s), 78, 84, 94, 131, 157, 271, 417, 487, 521
  juice, 39, 41, 43, 48, 52, 56, 69, 99, 102, 111, 131, 169, 204, 211, 214, 216, 249, 252, 263, 417, 476, 478, 495, 497, 521, 526, 577, 640
  salad, 91, 92, 169
Cassia fistula, see Purging Cassia
Cassia sticks, 224
Catarrh, colds, 2, 30, 37, 71, 81–83, 90, 375, 348, 381, 394, 416, 418, 448, 455, 468
Cat thyme (Teucrium marum), 72
Celandine (Chelidonium majus), 56, 69, 221, 250, 252, 292
Celery, celeriac (vegetable juice), 8, 16, 84, 204, 404, 496
Cell(s), 113, 143, 272–276, 528, 640
Cell metabolism, 112, 273, 428, 527, 605
Cell nucleus, 143
Cellulose (fibre, roughage), 212, 465, 471, 523
Centaurium erythraea, see Centaury

Centaury, 206, 208, 526
Central nervous system, 60, 102, 258, 566
Cereals, gruels, 212, 516
Cereal and fruit coffee (Bambu), 544
Cereus, night-blooming (Selenicereus grandiflorus), 144, 152
Chanca piedra, 170
Change of life, see Menopause
Charcoal, powder, 5, 10, 208, 209
Cheese, cottage (quark, soft white), 1, 78, 118, 125, 169, 177, 212, 244, 259, 321, 448, 459, 478, 537, 541
Cheese poultice, 11
Chelidonium majus, see Celandine
Chemical medicines, 31, 112, 279, 289
Cherries, 506
Chervil (Anthriscus cerefolium), 408
Chicken (meat), curative powers of fat, 5, 460–461
Chickweed (Stellaria media), 16
Chicory, vegetable, 8
  salad, 253
Chilblains, 3, 133, 138–139
Children's diseases, 46–54
Chives, 408–409, 478
Choking, danger of (insect stings), 15
Cholesterol (formation of), 116, 528, 616, 634
Cider, fermented, 153
Cinnabaris (cinnabar), 73, 75
Circulation, circulatory disorders, 3, 27, 134, 138, 198, 261, 428, 430, 435, 452, 552, 568, 586
Citric acid, 103
Clay/Healing earth (how to use), 6, 8, 13, 15, 50, 69, 213, 219, 249, 252, 400, 439–441, 505
  packs, poultices, 11, 13, 15, 69, 78, 158, 175, 182, 252, 271, 408, 439–441, 445
Cleansing, internal, 419–424
Climate, influence of, 97, 571
Club moss (Lycopodium clavatum), 177, 255
Coccus cacti (cochineal insect), 49, 393
Cod-liver oil, 30, 39, 100, 487
Coeliac disease, 51–53, 501
Coffee, tree, beans, 542–545
  charcoal, 8
Colchicum autumnale, see Meadow saffron

INDEX

Colds, 2, 3, 9, 37, 79, 81–85, 394, 408, 415, 488, 495
  (in the head, runny nose), 2, 72, 82, 412
Cold water applications, 190, 191, 437
Coltsfoot (Tussilago farfara), 420
Collapse, 152
Comfrey (Symphytum off., peregrinum), 216, 263, 270, 293, 319, 323, 336, 343, 355–357, 431, 498, 642
Compost, 469
Compresses, packs, 9, 33, 76, 182, 251, 438
Conducting away from focus (elimination), 46, 75, 85, 152, 189– 190, 385, 438–439
Congestion (head), venous, 3, 5, 25, 27, 35, 139, 411, 430, 436
Conjunctivitis, 69, 392
Constipation, 6, 24, 41, 69, 140, 214, 217, 219–222, 274, 399, 459, 476, 495, 521, 534, 536, 581, 641
Constriction across chest, 395
Contraceptive pills, 34
Convallaria majalis, see Lily of the valley
Convallaria complex/convascillan, 365–366
Convulsions, 16
Copper, copperware, 487, 566–567
Coriander (Coriandrum sativum), 94, 408
Coronary thrombosis, 117
Cortisone, 267
Couch grass, witch grass, 24, 250, 252
Coughs, tickle in throat, 2, 50, 78, 84–85, 393
Cowslip (Primula veris), 422
Cradle cap, 42–44, 177, 449, 535
Cramps, spasms, 6, 16, 25, 53, 185, 392–393, 407
Cranberries, 503
Cranesbill (Pelargonium spp.), infusion, 36, 329
Crataegisan, 99, 152, 187, 384, 435, 646
Crataegus oxyacantha, see Hawthorn
Cress, alpine (Hutchinsia alpina), 412
  See also watercress, garden cress, nasturtium, 84, 478
Crow's foot, 357
Crusta lactea, see Cradle cap
Cuprumacet, 49
Currants, red (Ribes rubrum), 503
  black (Ribes nigrum), 256, 486, 502, 505
  juice, 57, 505

Curry, 125
Cynara scolimus, see Artichokes
Cysts, formation of, 398
Cystitis, 170–171, 385, 430
Cystoforce/bladder drops, 171

Dairy farming, see Milk
Dandelion (Taraxacum off.) salad, tea, 56, 249, 253, 263, 419, 421, 468, 486
Daphne mezereum (Daphne), 184, 395
Dates, 481, 487, 513
Deadly nightshade (Atropa belladonna), deadly poisonous, see Belladonna
Deep-breathing (exercises), 83, 163, 173, 255, 334, 428, 578
Deficiencies, 637
Depression, 555, 592
Dermis (inner skin), 314
Detoxification (cleansing), 419, 420
Diabetes, Diabetics, 12, 87, 167, 194, 241, 254, 256–258, 368, 372, 374, 413, 449, 551, 648
Diaphragm-breathing, 255, 577–578
Diarrhoea, Diarrhoea and Sickness, 7, 38, 42, 95, 156, 213, 217–219, 235, 249, 364, 368, 400, 441, 459, 480, 495, 565
Diastase, 253, 520
Diet, 45, 52, 116, 124–128, 183, 192, 201–202, 208, 212, 218, 256–258, 475–480, 497–8, 651
Digestion, 52, 206, 348, 372, 400, 449, 471, 495, 542, 578, 636
  poor, 36, 38, 254, 289, 348, 457, 475
Digestive organs, 499–500
Digestive problems, 6
Digitalis, see Foxglove
Dill (Anethum graveolens), 38, 408
Diphtheria, 74, 86, 165
Disease, causes, 527
Diseases of civilisation, 86, 258, 262, 359, 637–641, 643
Disinfectant, 77
Dizziness, dizzy spells, 59, 130, 131, 367, 396, 452, 459
Dock, giant (Rumex alpinus), 343
Dormeasan, 188, 200
Dreams, 612–615
Dropsy, 400
Drosera rotundifolia, see Sundew

Drosinula Cough Syrup, 84, 98
Duodenal ulcer, 210
Durian, 633
Dysbacteria, 225–226, 413, 449, 542, 641
Dysentery, 233, 240, 502

Ear, inflammation of the (otitis), 73, 410
Eating technique, 6, 218, 224
Echinacea purpurea, see Purple coneflower
Echinaforce, 33, 44, 56, 68, 72, 84, 137,
     139, 169, 171, 175, 178, 216, 249,
     261, 270, 321, 324, 326, 455, 538,
     642, 648
Echinococcus, see Tapeworm
Eczema, skin eruptions, 12, 42, 46, 48, 55,
     175–182, 395, 397, 400, 401, 435,
     449–450, 495, 570
Education, upbringing, 598
Effusion, bloody (haematoma), 358
Eggs, egg dishes, 2, 16, 177, 245, 473, 498
Eggshells, powder, 103
Elderflower tea, 55, 318, 435
Electric field, 292–293
Electrocardiogram (ECG), 142
Elephantiasis, 234, 236
Eleutherococcus (taiga root, Siberian ginseng),
     69
Embolism, 26, 119–120, 124, 216
Endocarditis, 19, 85
Endocrine glands, see glands
Enema, 20, 47, 50, 168, 214, 251, 252, 642
Enuresis (bed-wetting), 171, 393
Enzymes, ferments, 229, 253, 494, 516, 520
Epidermis, 314
Epilepsy, 191–193
Equisetum arvense, see Horsetail
Erysipelas, 395
Eucalyptus (Eucalyptus globulus), 271, 335,
     441
Euphrasia off., see Eyebright
Evening meal (supper), 126, 475, 478, 498,
     635, 653
Exercise, as therapy, 6, 31, 61, 82, 113,
     123, 135, 163, 221, 420, 431
Exercise, early morning, 83, 334
Exercise, keep-fit, 431
Exhaustion (fatigue), 602, 605
Eyebright (Euphrasia off.), 68
Eye(s), 66–69
   inflammation, 2, 411

problems, 68, 69, 407

Facial neuralgia, 9, 357
Fagopyrum esculentum, see Buckwheat
Fainting spells, 407
Falling sickness, see Epilepsy
False Sea Onion, Healing Onion
     (Ornithogalum caudatum), 15
Fango mud cure (treatment), 271–272
Fasting, 242, 249, 255, 480–483, 577, 636,
     637–640
Fats (oils), 24, 94, 243–244, 479, 483, 519,
     527
Fat metabolism, 61, 449
Fatigue (exhaustion), 53, 459, 592
Fattening-up diets, 483
Fatty acids, unsaturated, essential, 117, 208,
     243, 248, 251, 289, 451, 453,
     527–530
Feet (care of), 3, 133, 326–332
Feet, hot, cold, 3, 72, 82, 95, 133, 326–332,
     367
Felon, see Whitlow
Fennel, (Foeniculum vulgare), 8, 38, 408
Fenugreek seeds (Trigonella foenumgraecum),
     13, 440
Fermentation, putrefaction (in bowels), 30,
     94, 127, 218, 274, 408, 411, 472,
     477, 494, 499, 521, 541, 551
Ferments, see Enzymes
Fern, bracken, 14
Ferrum phosphoricum, 47, 49, 75, 250
Fertilising (fertiliser), 469–470
Fertility vitamin, see Vitamin E
Fever (high temperature), 19–23, 46–50, 55,
     154, 235, 390, 411
Fibres, artificial (for clothing), 567
Fiebrisan, 56
Figs, fig paste, 7, 84, 85, 138, 251
Fish poisoning, 245
Fistulas, 401
Flatulence, 349, 400, 406, 412, 494
Food, quantity requirement, 483–484
Foot
   athlete's, 326, 329, 450
   bath, 95, 329
   care, 329
   sweat, sweaty feet, 318, 330, 401–402,
     410
Formic acid, 11, 79, 97, 176, 183, 352

Formisoton, 184

Foxglove (Digitalis purpurea) deadly poisonous, 365

Fresh plant (herb), extracts, 27, **343**

Fresh plant poultices, 441–442

Friction treatment (according to Kuhne), **436**

Fructus juniperi, see Juniper berries

Fructus sorbi, see Rowan berries

Fruit acid, 208, 494, 500, 505, 507

Fruit, as food, 94, 200, 498
  raw, 55, 127
  sprayed with pesticides, 473, **508**
  juices, 22, 41, 48, 54, 471, 496–497, 499
  sugars, 94, 510, 514, 633

Fucus vesiculosis, see Bladder wrack

Furuncles, furunculosis, see Boils

Galeopsis ochroleuca, see Hemp nettle

Gallbladder, 251, 422, 452, 495
  inflammation of the, 448
  trouble, infections, **249**

Gallstones, 167, **250–252**, 415
  oil cure for, 250–252

Gangrene (due to senility), 134, 139

Garden cress (Lepidium sativum, 90, 91, 92, 412

Gardening, farming, organic, **560**

Garlic (Allium sativum), 7, 116, 127, 408, **409**, 478, 650
  milk, 226, **410**
  perles, 122, 129

Gastric acid, 208–209, 210, 449, 500, 506, 542
  mucosa (mucous membranes; lining), 207, 208, 210, 215, 348, 445, 499, 505
  inflammation of mucosa (catarrh), 207, 208, 372, 445
  ulcers, 187, 207, 210–212, 445, 462, 471, 497, 526

Gastritis, 207, 208, 368, 372, 445

Gastronol, 209, 211, 445, 498

Gelsemium, 54

Germs, 82, 83, 108, 250

Giant dock (Rumex alpinus), 343

Ginkgo biloba (maidenhair tree), 62, 74, 116, 130, 139, 152, 198, 359–362, **452**

Ginsavena, 156, 185, 200, 372

Ginsavita, 150–185

Glands, 29, 30, 40, 49, 50, 363, 398, 401, 415, 427, 504
  endocrine, 123, 142, 155, 192, 201, 203–204, 290, 388, 457, 468, 504, 648

Glauber's salt (sodium sulphate), **400**

Glaucoma, 9

Glycogen, 253

Goitre, **156–161**
  post-operative treatment, **158**

Goldenrod (Solidago virgaurea), 20, **38**, 55, 57, 69, 78, 85, 165, 169, 176, 184, 250, 252, 270, 318, 358, 397, 435, 442

Gout, 87, 105, **262–263**, 266, 356, 385, 391, 404, 455, 497, 651

Granuloma (tooth abscess), 9, 302, 306

Grapefruit juice, 52, 57, 99, 178, 204, 249, 476

Grape juice diet, 9, 56, 99, 204, 249, 521, 641

Grape sugar, concentrate, 56, 94, 152, 510, 514

Grape diet, 521

Graphite, 179

Gratitude (healing power of), **617**

Graves' disease (exophthalmic goitre), 19, 158, 400, 424, 428, 459, 555

Grazes, 1, 364, 358, 448, 455

Greenfly, aphids, 90

Green manure, 470

Growths, tumours, 351

Guaiac (resin from wood of Guaiacum off.), **393–394**

Gums, bleeding, 383, 418, 502

Haemophilia, 5, 400

Haemorrhages, 5, 502

Haemorrhoids, 27, **140–141**, 399, 418, 468

Hair, care of, colour, 309–313, 401
  diseases of the roots, 401
  loss, 156, 312, 412
  restorers, 313, 401
  tonic, 313

Hamamelis virg., see Witch hazel

Hamamelis Soap, 319

Hands, sweaty, 401

Happiness (remedy), **624–632**

Hawthorn (Crataegus oxyacantha), 99, 129, 144, 147, 152, 349, 383–384, 420

Hay fever, 78, 97

Hay flower, hayseed, infusion, 4, 25, 51, 153, 185, 336, 430

Headaches, 9, 15, 24, 53, 62, 186, 219, 302, 307, 367, 392, 399, 407, 437, 495, 592

Healing earth, see Clay

Health, looking after, 92–96
  hazards, 563
  basic rules for, 635–637

Hearing, hard of, 74, 399

Heart, 55, 116, 141–144, 147, 154, 365, 383–384, 400
  attacks (infarction), 117–118, 148–150, 646

Heart, damage, 177
  dilation of the, 116, 146, 152, 384
  disturbance, 27, 152, 411
  function, 142
  hormones, 143, 151
  loss of tone, 152
  muscles (cardiac muscles), 56, 150, 365, 383, 585
  pain in the, 153
  palpitations, 144, 156, 367, 391, 400
  poisons, 145–148
  rhythm, 142, 143
  spasms of the, 142, 153–154
  tonic, see also Cardiaforce and Crataegisan, 56, 214
  trouble, 5, 645
  weak, 152, 365, 452, 491

Heartburn, 5–6, 448, 526

Heartsease, see Wild pansy (Viola tricolor)

Heat, danger of, 575–576

Hedera helix, see Ivy

Heels, high, 331

Helianthus tub. (Jerusalem artichoke), 162, 201, 205

Hellebore, European (Veratrum album) poison, 152

Hemp nettle (Galeopsis ochroleuca), 29, 69, 79, 95, 152, 172, 326, 337, 363

Hepar sulph., 73, 176, 325

Herbaforce, 94, 270, 410, 478, 489, 549, 552, 557

Herbal baths, infusions, 4, 10, 25, 522

Herbal packs, poultices, 9, 48, 170, 182, 252, 255, 336, 441–444

Herbal seasoning salts, see Herbamare and Trocomare

Herbal soups (for sluggish bowels), 7, 224–225

Herbamare, 9, 118, 127, 157, 159, 416, 479, 492, 549, 557, 647

Hereditary disposition, factors, 193–195

Hernias, 337, 398

Herpes zoster, see Shingles

Herter's disease, see Coeliac disease

Hippophae rhamnoides, see Sea buckthorn

Hoarseness, 3, 375

Hodgkin's disease, see Lymphoadenoma

Honey, 79, 94, 260, 270, 454–5, 510, 561

Hookworm, 234

Hops, tea, 16, 188

Hormone
  glands, 60, 312
  fresh, 260–261
  product ACTH, 268
  treatment, 33–34

Horse chestnut (Aesculus hippocastanum), 27, 34, 120, 135

Horseradish, 92, 110, 116, 125, 177, 204, 326, 413–414, 478, 650
  poultice, 9, 51, 62, 78, 414
  syrup, 414
  tincture (how to make), 414

Horsetail, tea, 13, 20, 24, 29, 36, 38, 47, 52, 69, 78, 175, 249, 252, 337, 362–363

Hot flushes, 163, 390

Hot water treatments, 433

House building (construction), 590–593

Houseleek (Sempervivum tectorum), 358

Housing problems, 589

Humulus lupus, see Hops

Hutchinsia, alpine cress (Hutchinsia alpina), 412

Hydrochloric acid, 206, 208

Hydrotherapy, 433

Hypericum perforatum, see St. John's wort

Hyperisan, 120

Hyperthyroidism, 144, 155, 156, 157, 158, 167, 366, 424

Hypophysis, see pituitary gland

Hypothermia (body temperature below normal), 19

Hypothyroidism, 158, 161–162, 194

Hyssop (Hyssopus off.), 130, 407

Iceland moss (lichen), 8

Ignatia, 163
Immunity, building up resistance, 86, 88, 93
Immunity laws, 86–88
Imperarthritica, 263, 270
Imperatoria ostruthium, see Imperial
masterwort
Imperial masterwort (Imperatoria ostruthium),
77, 78, 263, 394
Impetigo, 324
Indurations, 275
Infant care, 35–39
Infantile eczema, 44–46
Infant nutrition, 39, 41, 101–102
Infectious diseases, 30, 47, 51, 54–57, 85,
88, 89, 92, 100, 175, 216, 236, 258,
324, 365, 390, 392, 464, 488, 502, 504
Infertility, 521
Inflammations, 261, 408
Influaforce, 56, 57
Influenza, 54–57, 74, 75, 365
Injections, homoeopathic, 367
Injuries, 27
Insect bites, stings, 14–15, 407
Insect pests, 90
Insomnia, 187–189, 611
Insulin, 61, 254, 267
Intestines, bowels, 24–25, 85, 89, 213–215,
217, 228, 240, 399, 408, 422, 465,
481, 547, 581, 641
care of, 12, 119, 642
cleansing, 252, 441, 641–643
Intestinal bacteria (flora), 89, 91, 219,
225–226, 254, 472, 479, 505, 541,
542, 551, 642
Intestinal catarrh (enteritis), 368, 542
disorders, 8, 62, 399, 406, 547
gases, fermentation, 408, 541, 551
mucous membranes (inflammation), 10,
372, 441, 505, 541, 642
parasites, 12, 226–233, 372, 399, 410,
446, 489, 495, 501
poisoning, 212–215
putrefaction, 541
ulcer (duodenal), 497
worms, 12
Iodine, iodised salt, 42, 130, 155, 158–162,
203, 412, 468, 554–557
deficiency, 157, 161
Ipecac, Ipecacuanha (Cephaelis ipecacuanha)
poison, 29, 51, 214

Iron, 397, 487, 496
Islets of Langerhans, 254, 368, 551
Itching of the skin, 12, 241
Ivy (Heder helix), ivy tincture, 14

Jam-making, 506
Jaundice (hepatitis), 11, 106, 228, 252–253,
483
Joint(s)
diseases of, see Arthritis
inflammation of (arthritis), 397
painful, 357, 367, 394
Juice(s), 495–499
day, 8, 226, 641
diets, 471, 641
fasting, 119, 183, 226, 645, 649
Juniper (Juniperus communis)
berries (Fructus juniperi), 11, 384
needles, leaves, 20, 25, 56, 81, 263, 328
432, 441
Juniperosan, 81, 328, 329, 331
Juniperus communis, see Juniper

Kale, see savoy cabbage
Kali chloricum (potassium chlorate), 399
Kali iodatum (potassium iodide), 72, 79, 98,
394
Kali phosphoricum (potassium phosphate),
49, 131, 185, 487
Kamala powder (Glandulae Rottlerae), 232
Kelp (seaweed), 9, 124, 130, 145, 155, 157,
161, 192, 205, 394, 424, 449, 459,
557
Kelpamare/Swiss Alpamare, 116, 549, 557
Kelpasan, 116, 118, 130, 161, 205, 270,
325, 374, 424, 451, 522
Kidneys, 12, 20, 24, 38, 51, 54, 55, 81, 85,
113, 124, 164–169, 179, 363, 385,
393, 405, 410, 420, 442, 472, 479, 509
care of, 12
elimination of toxins, 54, 56, 420, 645
inflammation (nephritis), 385
stones, 104, 488, 509
(stone) colic, 167–168
tea, 55, 78, 81, 172, 178, 252
Kneipp, treatments advocated by, 3, 47, 85,
152, 190
Kohlrabi (turnip cabbage), 84, 157, 178
Kuhne, treatment according to, 16, 33, 98,
163, 190, 436–438, 522

Lachesis, 48, 57, 78, 135, 137, 139, 213, 249, 271, 295, 394, 450
Lacrimal fluid, 68
  glands, 68
Lactic acid, bacteria, 80, 89, 255, 293, 324, 448, 450, 540, 541, 546
  fermentation, 342, 541
Lactose, 13
Lacto-vegetarian, 256
Lady's mantle (Alchemilla vulgaris) tea, decoction, 36, 163, 364
Lanolin cream, 33, 37, 45, 72, 79, 136, 176, 178, 312, 313, 319, 325, 329, 439
Larch (tree), 2
  moss (Usnea barbata), 84, 90, 99, 538,
Laryngitis, 448
Laxatives (herbal), 20, 24, 42, 51, 55, 85, 140, 152, 216, 251, 641–642, 650
Leanness, underweight, 201–203, 452
Leeks, 8, 52, 116, 408
Legs, tired, 4
  broken, 355
  ulcers, 27, 137, 356, 402, 418
Lemon (Citrus limonia), 4, 13, 78, 99
Lemon juice, 2, 16, 55, 78, 418, 498
Lemon balm, 36, 73, 153, 184, 188, 407, 431, 435, 441
Lettuce, 522
Leucocytes, 75, 80
Leucorrhoea, 25, 79
Leukemia, 649
Libido, excessive, 16
Lice, 569
Liquorice, 211
Ligaments, strained, 335
Lily of the valley (Convallaria majalis), 98, 144, 365
Lime fertiliser (calcium manure), 440
Limewood charcoal, 5, 10–11, 15
Linoforce, 95, 140, 216, 642, 650
Linseed (Semen lini), 7, 13, 41, 85, 95, 152, 221, 251, 440, 476, 497, 520, 533
Liquid soap, 13
Liver, 56, 113, 164, 179, 208, 221, 243–248, 290, 422, 452, 468, 471, 476, 479, 483, 494, 495, 497, 504, 536, 636
  diet, 12, 243, 247, 489
  disease (infections), 249

function of the, 208, 221, 239–243, 487
  inflammation of the (hepatitis), 106
  patients, 452, 471
  trouble, 11, 12, 24, 69, 88, 208, 241, 400, 482, 533
Loranthus europaeus, see Oak mistletoe
Lovage (Levisticum off.), 33, 318, 408
Lowland plants, 344–347
Lung(s), 56, 70, 351, 414, 455
  abscess on, 395
Lycopodium clavatum, see Club moss
Lycopus europaeus, see Bugleweed
Lymph, system, 107–111
Lymphatic glands, 30, 409, 435, 503–514, 562
  disorders, 369, 648
Lymph nodes, 107, 108
Lymphocytes, 75, 80, 107
Lymphoadenoma (Hodgkin's disease), 111

Madder (Rubia tinctorum), 164, 169
Magnesium phos., 167, 385, 487–488
Maize porridge, 11
Malaceous fruit (e.g. apples), 94
Malaria, 235, 238, 401, 570
Mallow (Malva silvestris), leaves, tea, 33, 216, 329, 642
Manna stick (Cassia fistula), 224
Manure, manuring liquid (cesspool), 230, 240, 470
Marigold (Calendula off.), 36, 50, 73, 137, 171, 184
Marjoram (Origanum majorana), 94, 127, 405
Massage, 95, 168
Mastitis, 32–33
Matricaria chamomila, see Camomile
Meadow saffron (Colchicum autumnale) poison, 263
Measles, 48, 74, 86, 165, 392, 395
Medicago sativa, see Alfalfa
Medicinal plants in the lowlands, 344–347
Medicine chest (cabinet), 353, 392
Melissa off., see Lemon balm
Memory, weak, poor, 361, 396, 452
Meningitis, 59, 73, 392
Menopause, 163, 201, 390, 491
Menstrual cramps, pains, disorders, 25, 162, 186, 352, 353, 399, 407, 451
Mentha piperita, see Peppermint

INDEX

Mercurius solubilis (mercury chloride), 50,
72, 74
Metabolic toxins, 51, 119, 306
cure, treatment, 422, 449
disturbances, 36, 38, 68, 121, 166, 274,
400, 435, 459, 471, 475, 483, 536
wastes, elimination, 55, 662, 605
Metabolism, 59, 114, 161, 175, 306, 326,
422, 449, 451, 521
Metallic salts, 562
Metastases, 279, 283, 292, 354
Mezereum, see Daphne
Midday meal (lunch), 126, 256–257, **476**,
498, 634, 652
Middle ear, inflammation of (otitis media),
73, 74, 76, 487
Migraine headaches, 6, 62, 186, 352, 399,
457, 592
Milk
cold compresses, 216, 448
milk and diary farming, 42, 102, 212,
244, **448**, 472, 536–540
milk fever, 33
Millefoil, see Yarrow
Millefolium, see Yarrow
Millet, gruel, 11, 208, 492
Mineral metabolism, 123, 191, 218, 262,
274, 497, 351
Minerals, deficiency of, 100, 124, 289, 398,
424, 449, 459, 463, 512, 519
Miscarriage, 522
Mistletoe (Viscum album), 95, 122, 129,
138, 271, 292, 349, 366, 467, 650
Molkosan, 1, 12, 22, 38, 44, 49, 50, 56, 77,
80, 84, 175, 176, 178, 208, 219,
226, 249, 255, 257, 293, 311, 319,
321, 324, 329, **448–450**, 476, 498,
570, 576, 647
Monkshood (Aconitum napellus)
poison, 47, 49, 163, 250, 364, 390
Mother of thyme, see Wild thyme
Mother's milk, 39, 42
Mothers, expectant, **26–29**
Mountain ash, 3
Mouth, suppuration in the, **69–70**
Mucous membranes, mucosa, 79, 82, 395,
416, 418
inflammation of (catarrh), 80
Muesli, 125, 222, 467, 476
Mugwort (Artemisia vulgaris), **367**

Multiple sclerosis, 87, 258–262, 436, 439,
463
Multi-vitamin capsules, 29
Mumps, 50, 85, 175
Muscles, spasms, cramps, 185
Music, healing power of, **619**
Mustard poultice, 51, 75, 98
Mustard seeds, 11, 103
Myocarditis, 85
Myxoedema, 161, 195, 555

Nail mycosis (mould), 450, 455
diseases of the nails, **325–326**, 396,
401
Naja, 152
Nasal discharge, 395
Nasturtium (Tropaeolum majus), 90, **412**
Nasturtium off., see Watercress
Natrum muriaticum (sodium chloride,
common salt), **399**
Natrum sulphuricum (sodium sulphate;
Glauber's salt), **400**
Nature protection, **593**
Nephrosolid, 38, 47, 57, 78, 81, 124, 165,
169, 171, 176, 178, 252, 270, 318,
397
Nerve
cells, 53, 451
flu (head flu), 56
Nerves, 81, 198, 371, 411, 489, 491, 521,
551
natural food for the, 371, **484–486**
weak, 407–457
Nervous asthma, **96**
Nervousness, irritability, 144, 156, 592
Nettles (Urtica urens/dioica), 6, 13, 29, 38,
101, 103, 123, 141, 177, 271,
368–370, 419, 420, 477, **487**
Nettle calcium, see Urticalcin
Nettle Hair Tonic, 311
Nettle rash (urticaria), 12, **181**
Neuralgic pain, spasms, 9, 391, 392
Neuritis, 182, 302, 357, 440
Neurodystonia, autonomic nervous disorder,
155–156
Neuroforce, 81, 156, 185
Nicotine, dangers of poisoning, 31, 42, 112,
116, 147, 153, 279, 584
Nitroglycerine, 153
Nose, 70–73, 75, 416

Nose bleeding, 5, 27, 48
  breathing (through the), 578
Nursing mothers, **26–29**
Nutmeg (Myristica off.), 94, 474
Nutrients, 58, 449, 463
Nutrition, natural diet, 21, 31, 45, 55, 87,
  94, 99, 135, 138, 139, 247, 269–270,
  289, **463**, 519
Nutritional therapy, 99, 197, 269–270
Nutritive salts, 22, 40, 58, 128, 449, 519
Nux vomica, see Poison nut

Oak bark (infusion), 337, 441
Oak mistletoe, yellow-berried mistletoe
  (Loranthus europaeus), 192
Oat flakes (porridge), 5, 7, 95, 209, 218
Oats (Avenaforce), 41, 56, 69, 81, 111, 116,
  144, 162, 188, 370– 372
Obesity, 162, 201–203, 400, **452, 648**
Occupational therapy, 199, 200
Oedemas, 416
Oil, 3, 118, **527–532**
  Body oil massage/Toxeucal, 9, 10, 37,
  271, 321–322, 436
Oil cure for gallstones, **250–252**
Oil fruits and seeds, oil-producing, 532–534
Old age, signs of, **123–129**, 467, 756
Olive oil, 4, 7, 95, 250, 528
Onion (Allium cepa), 2, 20, 72, 257, 313,
  411
Onion Hair Tonic, 311, 313
Onion poultice, 2, 6, 9, 62
Oral hygiene, 48–49, 56, 77
Orange juice, 39, 55, 99, 204
Orchitis (inflammation of the testicles),
  174–175
Ornithogalum caudatum, see False sea onion
Orthodox medicine, 266
Ovaries, 130, 163, 197, 201, 312, 368, 430,
  475, 504, 522
Ovarium, 130, 163, 197, 390
Overacidity, 5, 10, 509
Oversensitive (hypersensitive)
  babies, 41
  to influences, 468
Overtiredness, 60, 69, 604
Overweight, 157, 203
Overwork, 62, 69, 323
Oxygen, 31, 83, 114, 116, 118, 123, 135,
  583, 636

  lack of, 274, 290
Oyster shells (powder), 103

Pain, 10, **23–25**, 27, 50, 73, 141, **352**, 356,
  392–393
Pancreas, 6, 61, 85, 211, 222, 223, 224,
  241, 253, 267, 368, **374**, 477, 503,
  505, 551
Pancreatic disturbance, 241, 413, 440, 494
Papain, **445–448**
Papaya (Carica papaya), 228, 255, 298,
  372–374, **445–448**
Papayasan (Papayaforce), 228, 229, 232,
  447, 502
Paraffin, 4
Paralysis, 53
Parasites (see also Intestinal parasites), 233,
  236, 237–238, 240, 374, 446, 569
Paratyphoid fever, 19, 235
Parsley (Petrosselinum crispum), 7, 20, 24,
  85, 126, 487
Pasqueflower (Pulsatilla vulgaris), 27, 74,
  120
Passiflora incarnata, see Passion flower
Passion flower (Passiflora incarnata), 188
Pathogenic agents, 88
Peace and quiet, **621–623**
Pepper, 94, 474
Peppermint (Mentha piperita), 232, 318,
  435
Pepsin, 206
Periodontal disease, **308**
Periostitis, **334**, 356
Peritonitis, 211, 217, 228
Perspiration, profuse, 555
Pesticides, insecticides, 558
  poisoning, **564**
Petadolor, 9, 62, 98, 156, 185, 352
Petaforce, 98, 283, 353, 354, 404
Petasites off., see Butterbur
Pharyngitis, 394
Phenol, 284
Phlebitis, 26, 137, 358, 399
Phosphates, 202, 521
Phosphorus, 386, 487
Piles, see Haemorrhoids
Pimpernel root (Pimpinella saxifraga), 3, 77,
  374–375
Pimpinella saxifraga, see Pimpernel
Pines, pinaceous trees, 2

Pine buds, shoots, 2, 85, 335
Pine bud syrup, see Santasapina
Pine kernels, 84
Pituitary gland, 60–62, 261, 268, 388, 504
Plantaforce, 94, 549, 552
Plantain, greater or common (Plantago major), 343
Plantago major, see Plantain
Pneumonia, 22, 82, 365, 487
Podophyllum, 56, 69, 221, 250, 252, 292
Po-Ho-Oil, 436
Poison(s), toxins, 22, 557–562, 636
Poisoning, 13, 245, 508
Poison ivy (Rhus toxicodendron), 12, 176, 184, 213, 271
Poison nut (Strychnos nux vomica), 29, 54, 98, 187, 214, 216
Poliomyelitis, 53–54
Pollen, 97
Pollen, bee pollen, pollinosan, 79, 184 (warning for patients with high blood pressure), 131, 204, 458–460
Pollinosan, 79, 184
Polyp, adenoids, 72, 581
Poppy seed, oil, 251, 258
Populus (Balm of Gilead), 174
Potassium permanganate, 237
Potato (Solanum tuberosum), 5, 12, 13, 444, 477, 486, 492, 525–526
  in their jackets (boiled), 52, 486
  juice (raw), 5, 11, 208, 211, 263, 445, 471, 496, 497, 526
  starch, 223
  water (from boiling), 4
Potentilla anserina, see Silverweed
Potentilla tormentilla, see Tormentil
Poultice, packs, compresses, 11, 21, 24, 47, 48, 51, 53, 55, 62, 68, 73, 74, 76, 85, 137, 158, 168, 172, 185, 252, 255, 410, 429, 440
Pregnancy, 26, 29, 30–32, 61, 133, 488
  morning sickness due to, 29
Premature birth, 522
Priessnitz, 47
Prostasan, 174, 452
Prostate, hypertrophy, 164, 430
  trouble, 173–174, 452
Protein, 22, 43, 45, 57, 116, 118, 177, 202, 244, 269, 274, 374, 446, 475, 477, 521, 535, 616, 635

deficiency, 492–493
Provitamin A, 69, 388, 488, 495
Prunes, 85, 222, 251
Psoriasis, 175, 179–181
Psychological balance, 7
Psychosomatic illnesses, 195–200
Psyllium (Plantago psyllium), 7, 42, 85, 138, 152, 221, 251, 497, 642, 650
Pulmonary abscesses, 395
Pulmonary diseases, 99–100, 394, 401, 462, 487
  bronchial infection, catarrh, 394
Pulsatilla vulgaris, see Pasqueflower
Pulse, irregular, 400
Pulses (beans, peas, lentils), 475
Purging cassia (Cassia fistula), 224
Purple coneflower (Echinacea purpurea), 44, 84, 137, 213, 293, 295, 299, 343, 376–380

Quark, see Cheese

Radiation, 31, 290, 443
  damage, 31
Radioactivity, 290
Radish, black (Raphanus sativus)
  juice, 24, 253, 409, 415, 421
  syrup, 415
Raisins, 7, 84, 94, 260
Rasayana Treatment, 140, 216, 221, 232, 423, 642
Raspberry, juice and shrub (Rubus idaeus), 249, 420, 422, 502
Rauwolfia (Rauwolfia serpentina), 116, 130, 152
Rauwolfavena, 116, 152, 200, 367
Raw food, 55, 92, 111, 180, 191, 295, 298, 496–502
Raw juices, 496–499
Relaxation, relaxing, 7, 60, 334, 588, 599–601, 636
Remedies, herbal (how developed), 338–341
  (how used), 341–344
Rennin, 206, 253, 448, 541
Resistance, 84, 88
Respiratory organs (and diseases), 70, 92–96, 100, 351, 363, 415
Restharrow (Ononis spinosa), 263
Revulsion therapy (drawing away from focus), 75, 438–439

INDEX

Rh factor, 105

Rheumatism, articular, 9, 11, 15, 105, 385, 391, 404, 433, 441, 445, 496, 505, 568, 651–653
rheumatic fever, 22, 46, 76, 306, 554

Rheumatism Cure (A. Vogel's), 651

Rheumatoid arthritis, 265–272, 306

Rhus toxicodendron, see Poison ivy

Rhythm of life, 603–605

Ribwort, lance-leaf plantain (Plantago lanceolata), 37, 73, 422, 468

Rice, 41, 52, 117, 124–125
brown, whole, natural, 41, 52, 94, 101, 111, 116, 118, 122, 124, 128–129, 199, 208, 222, 223, 239, 459, 464–466, 467, 477, 498, 524
diet, 128–129

Rickets, 39, 315, 369

Ricinus communis (seeds are deadly poisonous), 375

Risopan, 518, 636, 648

Rosa canina, see Rose hips

Rose hip conserve (how to make), 387, 418

Rose hips, 20, 38, 184, 252, 385–387, 418, 485, 502

Rose hip tea, 387, 636

Rosemary (Rosmarinus off.), 405

Rosemary Toothpaste, 306

Roundworms (ascarid), 227, 240, 447–448

Rowanberries (Fructus sorbi), 3, 387

Rowan tree (European mountain ash), 3

Royal jelly (Gelée Royale), 294–295, 456–458

Rubiaforce, 169

Rubia tinctorum, see Madder

Rules, basic, for healthy and sick people, 635–637

Runny-nose (during a cold), 72, 412

Ruptures, see Hernias

Rye, 41, 94, 208, 518, 520

Sabal serrulata (Florida palm, saw palmetto), 171, 174, 452

Sage (Salvia off.), 8, 163, 319

Salivary glands (in mouth, liver, abdomen, stomach), 217, 300

Salsify, 8

Salt, common, cooking, table (Sodium chloride), 4, 94, 399, 550

Salt, as medicine, 157, 165, 169, 176, 415
packs, 4

water, 2, 14, 77–78

Salvia off., see Sage

Sanguinaria (Canadian bloodroot), 62

Sanicle (Sanicula europaea), 33, 216, 329, 358, 432

Santasapina Cough Syrup, 51, 78, 84, 375, 394, 418, 455

Sauerkraut, 29, 102–103, 157, 178, 418, 450, 471, 485, 545–547
how to make your own, 546

Sauna, 53, 119, 191, 316, 318, 420

Savory (Satureja hortensis), 94, 406

Savoy cabbage (kale), 1, 487

Scarlet fever, 74, 75, 165, 395

Schlenz bath (immersion bath of increasing water temperature), 10, 53, 98, 196, 199, 433–436

Sciatica, 11, 410

Scilla maritima, see Sea onion/squill

Scrofula, 104, 315, 369, 401

Sea, bathing (therapeutic value), 427–428, 553

Sea buckthorn (Hippophae rhamnoides), 387, 419, 486, 502

Sea onion/squill (Scilla, Urginea maritima), 98, 144, 380

Sea salt, 4, 9, 72, 118, 159, 415–416, 479

Seasoning, 127, 426, 547–550

Seasonings, spices, herbs, 404–409, 474

Seasoning salts (herbal), see Herbamare, Trocomare

Seaweed, 554, 555, 556
calcified, fertiliser, 470

Sebaceous glands, 314, 322, 324

Senna leaves, pods, tea, 7, 224, 232

Sepia off. (cuttlefish), 81, 163, 396

Septicaemia, 395

Sesame seed (Semen sesami), 247–248, 258–259, 534
oil (Oleum sesami), 247–248, 258–259, 534

Sex glands (gonands), 60, 130, 162, 290, 311, 323, 452, 459

Sexual weakness, impotence, 161, 451, 459, 488

Shallot (Allium ascalonicum), 412

Shave grass, see Horsetail

Shepherd's purse (Capsella bursa pastoris), 141, 162

Shingles (Herpes zoster), 184–185, 395

INDEX

Showers, cold, 16
  warm, hot, 62, 186, 255
  of long duration, 6, 185
Sick without a sickness, 154
Silica (Terra silicea purificata), 401–402
Silicea, see Silica
Silica deficiency, 29, 39, 50, 74, 95, 363, 397
Silverweed (Potentilla anserina), 8
Silvery lady's mantle (Alchemilla alpina), 7, 364
Sinew sprain, strain, 335
Sinusitis, 9, 73, 75
Sitz baths, 25, 33, 50, 52, 81, 163, 168, 172, 197, 201, 222, 312, 430–433
  of long duration, 5
Skin, 20, 37, 95, 313–324, 357–358, 363, 401, 420, 435, 495
  cancer, 450
  disorders, 175–182, 219, 396, 400, 435, 503
  effects of the sun on, 315
  eruptions, 4, 12, 50, 175–182, 400, 435, 449–450
  fungal infections, 325
  redness (babies), 37
Sleep, 7, 60, 124, 163, 606–612
Sleeping pills, 42, 189–191
Sleeping sickness, 238
Sleeplessness, see Insomnia
Slimness, 8
Slimming, see also Obesity, 8, 203
Slimming diet, 8–9
Sloes, blackthorn, 508
Slug syrup, 461–462
Smallpox, 395
Smoker's cancer, 284, 587
Smoking, 146, 584–587
Snow blindness, 2
Soda, 16
Sojaforce, 118
Solidago virgaurea, see Goldenrod
Soreness (in babies, nappy rash), 37
Sore throats, 22, 30, 74, 76–78, 84–85, 395, 448, 450
Sorrows, anxieties, worries, 212, 276, 288
Sour milk, 256, 498
Soybeans, protein, 45, 177, 245–246, 492, 522, 634
Soya mixes, 634

Spasms, cramps, 104, 185–186, 225, 261, 288, 352, 568
Sphincter
  weakness of, 171
Spigelia (Worm grass), 144
Spilanthes, 325
Spinach, 123
Spirea (Spirea ulmaria), 263
Spleen, 109
Spots, 219
Spring cures (treatments), 419–424
Spring fever (fatigue), 424, 504
Spurge (Euphorbia lathyrus), 141
Staphisagria (Stavesacre, seeds of), 174
Staphylococcus, 170, 324
Starchy foods, 8, 223
Stavesacre (Delphinium staphisagria), 174
St. John's wort (Hypericum perforatum), 26. 38, 120, 135, 137, 141, 171, 319, 343, 358, 402, 442, 468
  oil, 1, 9, 27, 33, 37, 44, 50, 75, 95, 136, 175, 178, 182, 207, 315, 319, 322, 343, 436, 440, 445
Stream baths, 430
  herbal, 430
Stellaria media, see Chickweed
Stomach
  cramps, 206–212, 214, 349, 408, 438, 546
  disorders, 207–208
  poisoning, 212–215
  ulcers, 187, 207, 210–212, 445, 462, 471, 497, 526
Stone fruit, 94, 505–506
Stools, 22, 24, 52, 399
Strains and sprains, 335
Strawberries, 12, 94, 420, 422, 486
Streptococcus, 170, 324
Stress, 145, 150, 207, 428, 587–589
Stroke (apoplectic), 27, 58, 131, 392, 395, 528
Strophanthus (Strophanthine), 144, 382
Sugar
  natural, 202, 511
  white (refined), 178, 509
Sulphur, 49, 74, 176, 397
Sulphuric acid, crystals, 166
Sun bathing, 573, 576
Sunbeams, solar radiation, 572–574, 576
Sundew (Drosera rotundifolia), 51, 393

Sunflower seeds, 533
  oil, 251, 528, 533
Suppuration, 15, 401, 487
Suprarenal gland, 60
  adrenal cortex, 267
Sweat, 314, 316, 390, 394, 396, 555
  glands, 53, 55, 78, 85, 119, 420
Sweet clover (Melilotus off.), 27, 135
Swellings, lumps, 7, 13, 350, 434, 439, 441,
  443, 448
  on fingers, see Whitlows
Sympathetic nervous system, 140, 142, 186
Symphosan, 216, 263, 270, 319, 320, 323,
  357–359, 432, 455, 651
Symphytum off., see Comfrey
Syphilis, 59
Syringing ear, 73

Tabacum, 151
Tapeworms, 230
Tapeworm tea, 232
Tarentula cubensis, 396
Taraxacum off., see Dandelion
Taste, sense of, 63
TB, see Tuberculosis
Teeth, 29, 39, 100, 104, 306–309, 398, 512
  bad teeth (decay), 398, 512, 514, 518
  care of the, 303–308
Television, 596–598
Temperature below normal (hypothermia),
  19
Tenseness, 275, 288, 392–393, see Silica
Testicles, 201
  inflammation of the (orchitis), 174–175
Teucrium marum (cat thyme), 72
Threadworm, pinworm (Oxyuris
  vermicularis), 227, 234, 447, 448
Throat
  inflammation of the, 76–78, 88
  sore, 15, 72, 375, 395, 448, 468
Thrombosis, 26, 119, 134, 216
Thydroca, 49, 51, 393
Thyme, wild, Mother of thyme (Thymus
  vulgaris), 4, 56, 81, 94, 127, 163,
  319, 329, 405, 431, 441
Thymus gland, 61
Thymus serpyllum, see Thyme
Thyroid, 60, 142, 201, 412, 415, 428, 452,
  468, 503, 504, 555
Tincture (how made), 342

Tiredness, getting tired, 53, 459, 592,
  601–605
Tobacco, see Smoking
Tobacco tar, 586
Tomatoes, 264, 478
Tomato juice, 496
Tongue, 49, 56, 63–65
Tonics, 451, 456, 520
Tonsillitis, 74, 76–78, 85, 165, 365, 394,
  395, 450
Tonsils, 76, 108
Tooth
  decay, cavities, 398, 512, 514, 518
Toothache (headache), 410, 411
Tormentavena, 51, 95, 141, 162, 169, 218
Tormentil (Tormentilla erecta), 5, 7, 38, 95,
  141, 162, 218, 363, 400, 508
Tormentilla erecta, see Tormentil
Toxins, 22, 53, 107, 262, 265, 306, 557–562
Trace elements, 459, 463, 464, 496
Treatments, courses of cures, diets, 417–444
Trocomare, 91, 116, 158, 413, 416, 479,
  492, 549, 557, 647
Tropical diseases, 88, 232–239
Tropics, visits to the, dangers in the, 232–239
Tuberculosis, 19, 49, 86, 89, 92, 104, 110,
  171, 175, 293, 370, 550
Tumours, 276, 278, 442, 435, 450, 587
Turpentine, 12
Typhoid fever, 235, 293, 395, 502, 569

Ulcers
  chronic, 395, 462, 523
Uraemia, 164
Uric acid, 10, 113, 445, 475
  (combatting)
Urinary bladder, 170
Urine (urinalysis), 24, 104, 166, 170, 171,
  213, 405, 412
  retention of, 10, 430
Urticalcin, 2, 15, 29, 39, 41, 45, 53, 54, 69,
  72, 78, 80, 81, 83, 84, 95, 99, 101,
  105, 110, 120, 122, 135, 138, 139,
  144, 155, 157, 172, 175, 192, 198,
  261, 302, 326, 337, 370, 538, 648
Urtica urens/dioica, see Nettles
Usnea barbata, see Larch moss
Usneasan, 91, 95, 137, 171, 172, 261, 270

Vaccinium myrtillus, see Bilberries

INDEX

Valerian (Valeriana off.), 188, 232
Valeriana off., see Valerian
Varicose veins, 26, 119, **132–136**, 140, 216,
   399
Varicosis, 2/
Veal, **2**
Vegetable juices, 10, 41, 125, 127, **471**,
   499, 639, **643–645**
   mixed vegetable juices, 641, 644, 646,
   650, 653
Vegetables, 8, 99, **467–469**, 497, 547
   fresh, raw, 99, 105, 118, 123, 135, 199,
   471, 476, 494
Vegetable water, from boiling, **4**
Vegetable bouillon, 549
Vegetarians, 475, 492, 539
Veins, venous system, 26, 134, 137, 468
Venous problems, obstructions, 27
Veratrum alba, see White hellebore
Vespétro, see Angelica liqueur
Vinegar, 99
Vinegar, socks soaked in, 21
Violaforce, 43, 45, 176, 178, 182, 319, 321,
   323, 535
Viola tricolor, see Wild pansy
Virus influenza, 55
Viruses, 86, 55–57, **293–299**
Viscum album, see Mistletoe
Vitaforce, 30, 110, 192, 453
Vitality, 468, 491
Vital substances
   deficiency, 301
Vitamin deficiencies, 13, 47, **83**, **417**, 490,
   503, 512
Vitamins, 22, 39, 58, 92, 202, 463, 519
   A, 84, 169, 417, **486**, 503, 556
   B (Complex), 94, 248, 388, **489–490**, 501
   B12, 404, 490, 542, 648
   C, 29, 84, 293, 385, 411, 413, 418, 485,
   502–505, 546
   D, 30, 39, 103, 109, 193, 301, 340, 369
   E (tocopherol), 201, 248, 388, 451, 453,
   464, 488, 490, 521, 570
   F, 320
   K, 488
Vocal breathing exercises, 199
Vogel's Rheumatism Cure, 651
Vomiting, 53

Walking, hiking, 31, 163, 173, 420

barefoot in the snow, 3
   on dewy grass, 198, **334**
Wallwosan, see Symphosan
Walnut(s), 222, 535–536
   oil, 241
   tea made from woody partitions, 144,
   153–154
Wasp stings, 15, 407
Water, **424–427**
   dangers in the, 286
   pollution, 594–595
   treading, 3, 199
   treatments, 5, 10, 252, 577, 610
Watercress (Nasturtium off.), 90, 116, 157,
   162, 412, 419, 468, 522
Way of life, natural, 112
Wheat, 1, 7, 94, 208, **466**, 497, 519–521
   bran, 466, 523
   coarse ground flour, 7
   germ, 34, 43, 118, 201, **521–523**
   germ and bran, 466, 523
   germ oil capsules, 34, 118, 148, **451–453**,
   491, 521
Whey, 1, 4, 12, 15, 45, 84, 255, 326, 448
Whipworm (Trichocephalus dispar), 234,
   448
White flour/sugar, 94, 102, 165, 178, 259,
   262, 304, **509**, **518**
White hellebore (Veratrum album), see
   Hellebore
Whitlows (felons), 13, 396, 401, 455
Wholemeal (flour made from whole grain),
   94, 222, 516
Wholegrain products, dishes, 105, 138, 199
Wholefood, natural, 11, 60, 79, 111, 119,
   137, 138, 199, 222, 269, 304, 463,
   472, 636
Wholefood Muesli (Full Value Muesli), 633,
   636, 651
Whooping cough, 49, 50–51, 74, 177, 392,
   393, 415, 457
Wild fruits, 382–389
Wild Thyme (Thymus serpyllum), 4, 37, 48,
   328, 430, 441
Wild pansy, heartsease (Viola tricolor), 13,
   43, 176, 178, 320, 323, 329, 431
Windflower, see Pasqueflower
Windpipe (trachea), 70
Witch grass, see Couch grass (Agropyron
   repens)

INDEX

Witch hazel (Hamamelis virginiana), 27, 120, 135, 141, 169, 208, 211, 319, 358

Wood ash, 5, 208, 209

Worms, intestinal, 501, 570

Wormwood, tea, 16, 226, 410

Worry, anxiety, anger, 266, 275

Wrinkles, 322, 357

Yarrow (Achillea millefolium), 26, 38, 120, 135, 137, 141, 169, 171, 399, 408, 468

Yeast, 551–552

Yeast extract, 13, 94, 474, 478, 489, 552
  pure culture (see Herbaforce)

Yeast fermentation, 342

Yoghurt, 89, 244, 256, 476, 540–541

Zincum valer., 98

Dr. Alfred Vogel— "The Nature Doctor" in Person

For most of this century Dr. Alfred Vogel has been learning the secrets of natural healing and the curative powers of herbs, and for almost as long has shared that knowledge with patients at the clinic he ran for many years and with countless readers of his many books. Born in 1902 near Basel, Switzerland, he eagerly absorbed herbal lore from his grandparents and parents, eventually becoming familiar with the whole body of European empirical folk medicine. In later years he traveled to the remotest parts of the world, and absorbed the curative lore of tribal peoples in Africa, Asia, Australia and the Americas. His stay with the Sioux Indians in South Dakota was among the most informative and inspiring of his many tribal encounters, and gave him some literally lifesaving information as well as deepening his sense of union with nature.

At his clinic in Teufen, treatment was based on naturopathic principles, using medicinal plants gathered at the foot of the Alps, and his great interest in all methods of natural healing led him to the study and use of homeopathic treatments as well. In his worldwide lectures and the newsletter he has published for more than sixty years, Dr. Vogel has brought his experience and wisdom to many thousands, but it is his books, beginning as far back as 1925, that have carried that wisdom, and a legion of practical instructions for the full range of health problems, to countless readers in many countries. His most famous work is *Der kleine Doktor,* published in English as *The Nature Doctor,* and translated into eleven languages. It has now been completely revised and substantially enlarged for this edition.

Dr. Vogel's decades of research and discovery have brought him professional recognition in many countries as well as the gratitude of those he has helped: he was granted an honorary doctorate in medical botany by the University of California at Los Angeles in 1952, and in 1982 was awarded the coveted Priessnitz Medal at the annual Congress of German Nature Cure Practitioners.

Though nearly ninety, Dr. Vogel still puts in a five-hour work day and attends many professional meetings and conferences, often discovering that the latest research "discovers" what he has been practicing for seven decades—and what folk medicine has known for centuries. "Only nature can heal and cure," Dr. Vogel is fond of observing, adding the corollary that "we can help and support nature and its laws that make a cure possible." This has been the basis of his lifelong work.

In 1963, Dr. Vogel founded Bioforce, now one of the major manufacturers of herbal extracts, homeopathic medicines, specialty health foods and biological body care products. The enterprise was started in the small farming community of Roggwil, but now has extensive production facilities in Switzerland and distributors and offices in many parts of the world.